CV Review Book - Vol. 1:

Invasive Basics

_____

6th Edition

by

J. Wesley Todd, BS, RCIS, RCES
Director, Cardiac Self Assessment
Spokane, WA 99216

ISBN-978-1-7326393-0-0

Self Published by:
Cardiac Self Assessment
1605 South Clinton Rd.
Spokane, WA 99216-0420
phone (509) 926-0344
Email w.t@westodd.com
Web Site http://www.westodd.com

ABOUT THIS SERIES

This book represents only one volume of a much larger series of 5 books. This vol. 1 combines material from the basic sciences, cardiovascular anatomy, physiology, and pathology. This book has been revised each time the author has taken one of the exams.

This book will serve those studying for all the cardiovascular registry exams for staff working in the cath lab, electrophysiology lab, ultrasound and vascular labs. Everyone needs knowledge of A&P, pathology, patient care, asepsis, BLS, and invasive lab protocols. Thus, volume 1 can be used to prepare for any of the CCI exams cardiovascular specialty exams or the ARRT exams (CI and VI). Those preparing for these cardiovascular invasive registries (RCIS, CI or VI) will also need additional books: Vol. 2, 3, 4 and 5 shown below:

INVASIVE REGISTRY - STUDY MATERIAL

Vol. #	Ch #	Chapter Content	Published	ISBN
Vol. I		Invasive CV Basics (this book)	2018	978-1-7326393-0-0
		A. CV Science		
		B. CV Anatomy & Physiology		
		C. CV Pathology		
Vol. II		CV Diagnostic Techniques	2018	978-1-7326393-1-7
Vol. III		Hemodynamics	2018	978-1-7326393-2-4
Vol. IV		Interventions	2018	978-1-7326393-3-1
Vol V		Registry Practice Exams	2018	978-1-7326393-4-8

All 5 the above books and CD are available as a bundled set. See: www.westodd.com

DISCLAIMER

The author and the many reviewers have made every effort to insure the current accuracy of the material in this book. Where possible, recognized authorities are referenced and quoted. Due to the fast-moving nature of the cardiovascular field, and the changing nature of accepted practice, we cannot accept any responsibility for the errors or omissions or for the consequences from application of the information in this book. Although we have made every effort toward accuracy, you should always check with hospital standards and company literature such as drug package inserts, before applying the information in this book.

We have tried to include information that we believe will be on the national CV Invasive Registry examinations. But, since the examination agencies frequently update and change their test questions and formats, the questions included here will be similar but not identical to the ones you find on your national exam.

PREFACE to 6th Edition:

This edition of Todd's CV Review Books has been revised to include the new question formats given by CCI. CCI calls these new types of questions "innovative items." The exams are no longer just four item multiple choice questions, as in the past. New formats include matching, drag and drop, multiple response (checkbox) and hot spot questions. Although we have always used these formats in our Todd CV Review CDs & USBs we have modified many questions in this new edition to match these "innovative" formats.

Hundreds of new questions have been added. This 6th edition now includes new structural heart information and new devices like TAVR, Impella, and Endovascular Aortic Repair (EVAR). Our new interactive CD & USB program should be available in 2019 to match the questions in this book and the current registry exams.

In 2019 CCI modified and clarified the RCIS exam content. It clarified that the large 80% procedure categories by dividing these into Diagnostic Procedure 42% and Interventional Procedures 33% of the exam. They also added a new category termed Responding to Emergencies 6%. These new categories match nicely with our books, where the Vol. 2 book is on Diagnostics and the Vol. 4 is on Interventions. Emergency procedures are in Vol. 4.

Wesley Todd, BS, RCIS, RCES 2018
Director, Cardiac Self Assessment

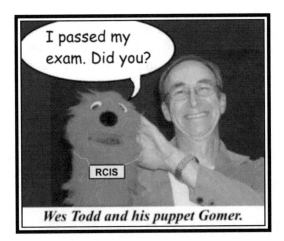

Wes Todd and his puppet Gomer.

INTRODUCTION

Volume I contains the background essential to all the CV registry exams taken by allied health and nursing staff. It is specifically designed for the Cardiovascular Invasive Exams (RCIS & CI).

I have organized this book around current exam content/matrix for the national CV exams, and designed it to be similar to the exam you will take. The content of each exam is detailed in this "Introduction to CV Exams." To prepare you for your exam, this book includes thousands of questions, answers, explanations, and references. It is up to you to match appropriate material from these volumes with the content of your exam. For example, RCIS and vascular candidates do not need the in depth EGM and action potential knowledge that EP candidates do.

GOALS OF THIS BOOK

Studying this book will improve your chances of passing the exam, but cannot replace formal education or clinical experience. This is not a "crash course." Neither can we cover all items that will appear on the exam. CCI's test bank includes more than 4000 test items, many more than in this book. If you have no formal training in your specialty, you will need extensive textbook study, tutoring, and clinical experience to gain the theoretical base necessary. These exams are difficult. Approximately 60-75% of the candidates pass these exams the first time. My experience shows that using this book to prepare for the exam can raise your exam score by as much as 20%.

This book will help you achieve your goal of passing the CV exams by helping you:
- evaluate your current Cardiovascular knowledge
- gain insight into your strengths and weaknesses
- form a directed plan of study to prepare for your exam
- gain confidence and reduce anxiety at test taking
- gain familiarity with the types of test items commonly used on these exams
- strengthen your test taking skills
- strengthen your problem-solving skills.
- Direct your study into recognized Cardiovascular references and textbooks. References for each question are included.

WHY SHOULD I BECOME CREDENTIALED?

Everyone working in a cardiovascular lab can attempt one of these examinations and become credentialed, both nurse and technician. Passing demonstrates competency to your co-workers, the physicians, and your patients. The medical professions have always relied heavily on credentials and titles. Consider a how an MD's walls are filled with diplomas and board certification credentials. JCAHO accreditation guidelines also heavily rely on credentials.

Passing one of these CV exams can be a source of great pride to you. Imagine how you will feel wearing the initials RCIS or CIT after your name. Imagine receiving the message that says "YOU PASSED, and will receive your credential in the mail?"

Becoming credentialed also has certain tangible benefits to improve your professional advancement.

● It may raise your salary by qualifying you for advanced skill categories. For example in Spokane Washington only registered and state licensed practitioners (Health Care Assistants) can make arterial punctures and place arterial sheaths. This also increases their salary.

● It may qualify you for advancement into administrative, research, or sales jobs.

● It may qualify you for state licensure. When your state develops laws for licensure of Invasive specialists, (as many now are). You will have to pass a recognized exam to prove your competency. Do it now while your training is still fresh in your mind. These exams only get harder, longer and more expensive with time.

● Many hospitals realize the educational benefits to employees who study for and pass these exams. They often pay for textbooks, study guides, and exam costs. It never hurts to ask.

● You will model personal incentive, intelligence, and courage to your peers.

● In this rapidly changing field, continuing education is your professional responsibility. All our professional organizations now require at least 12 annual hours of continuing education to maintain an invasive credential.

TESTING ORGANIZATIONS

Two organizations write these exams and register cardiovascular invasive professionals: Cardiac Credentialing International (CCI) and the American Registry of Radiologic Technologists (ARRT). Each provides specialty registry exams and credentials based on the needs of the cardiovascular invasive field. CCI members are mainly nurses and CVTs working in cardiovascular medicine. ARRT members are mainly X-ray technologists working in all aspects of radiology and ultasound. Each organization has specialty exams dealing with cardiac and vascular interventions, and each grants registry credentials. www.cci-online.org

EXAM APPLICATION

All the invasive exams consist of around 150 multiple choice questions. It will also include about 20 new questions that are not scored. They are just trying-out new questions that may be used on future exams.

After you have applied through CCI or ARRT to take one of the invasive exams, they will mail you about whether or not you are eligible. If you are eligible you will get an"Authorization to Test" letter. This will direct you to contact the "NCS Pearson Testing" organization, to set up a time and location for them to administer your computer based test. http://pearsontesting.com/cci/

The different exams for which these volumes were written are detailed below:

1.   **CCI - RCIS   (Registered Cardiac Invasive Specialist)**
2.   **CCI - RCES (Registered Cardiac Electrophysiology Specialist)**
3.   **ARRT - CI (Cardiac Interventional Technologist)**
4.   **ARRT - VI (Vascular Interventional Technologist)**

PASSING SCORES

CCI (RCIS & RCES Exams):

The final passing score is established by CCI or ARRT using a criterion-referenced passing score process. So, instead of an overall % score on your exam, you get an overall "scaled score." I will try to explain this process as I understand it.

There are several forms for each CCI exam. Form 1 might be 150 questions drawn randomly from the exam blueprint (E.g., 10% Pre-Procedural activities, 40% Procedural activities, 40 % Intra-Procedural activities, 10% Post-Procedural activities, etc.). Each form of the exam will have the same proportion of pre-, intra-, and post- procedural questions. You might take the Form 1 test. Another person might take Form 2. The questions will be different, but the proportion of each category of questions is the same (10 pre-, 40%intra-, 40% procedural, and 10% post- etc.). In addition they will throw in about 20 questions that are not scored, but are being evaluated for future exams. The results of these unscored questions will determine if they are used in future exams but do not effect your score. So, if you find a few questions that are "off-the-wall" or new to you, they might be one of those unscored questions that the testing organization is evaluating.

Statistically, each form of the exam will result in slight variations in overall difficulty based on the particular combination of test questions. The "scaled score" adjusts for variations in this overall exam difficulty. Harder tests will be assigned lower passing scores - perhaps 70%. Easier exams may require a 72% score to pass. They never tell you the overall % score you earned. You only see the scaled score, because you might feel it unfair if you were required to pass with over 72%, but someone else passed with 70%. To avid this confusion and to adjust for the difficulty of each exam, they use "scaled scores". Scaled scores range from 0 to 900. On CCI exams, everyone must earn a scaled score of 650 to pass. (Note that 650/900 = 72%) Thus, it does not matter which exam form you take. To make it fair, each passing score will reflect the overall difficulty of that exam.

At the end of the exam, you don't get your overall % score, only your "scaled score" and whether you passed or not. Above 650 is passing. But, they do give you the percentage of questions answered correctly for each section of the examination (E.g., Intra-Procedural, etc.). This information is provided to assist failing candidates target areas for further study.

ARRT (CI & VI Exams):

The final passing score is established by ARRT using a criterion-referenced passing score process. Their scaled scores range from 1 to 99.

ARRT says, "ARRT uses "scaled scores" to report examination results. Scaled scores are more meaningful than raw scores (i.e., number or percentage correct) because they take into account the difficulty of a particular test compared to other forms of the same test. Therefore, a scaled score of 75 represents the same level of test performance, regardless of what examination form was administered."

    "Total scores are reported on a scale that ranges from 1 to 99. The total scaled score does not equal the number or percentage of questions answered correctly. A total scaled score of 75 is required to pass the exam. The number of correct answers required to achieve a score of 75 was determined through a standard-setting (or passing score) study. ARRT and panels of consultants periodically review the passing score to assure its validity."

INVASIVE BASICS - Vol. 1

    This Volume I Review Book will help those studying for any of the Cardiovascular Exams. It is designed specifically for the invasive CV field, both cath lab and Interventional Radiology. We have written 2 other books for the electrophysiology exam, sold separately.

    This book has three major divisions. The A Chapters contain basic concepts including patient care. The B Chapters are on anatomy and physiology. The C Chapters cover pathology. All of these chapters are written from the invasive lab point of view and form a basis for the invasive CV registry exams - RCIS, CI, and VI. The list of duties that is expected of each invasive specialist forms the exam content. The following tables detail these duties and resulting exam contents for each of the four invasive exams. Additional details of each exam are on their respective web sites.

1. RCIS EXAM - Cath Lab - CCI

    This credential is for nurses and techs working in cardiac cath labs. Procedures done in the cath lab include heart catheterization, Coronary Arteriography, and Cardiac Interventions. A heart cath team usually consists of CVTs (Cath Techs), RN's (Nurses), and RT's (X-ray Techs). They assist cardiologists with invasive procedures.

    All school educated team members currently working in Cardiac invasive labs are eligible to take CCI's Invasive Registry Exams. In 2013 CCI eliminated the on-the-job (OJT) track for CVTs. Both school education and specific lengths of cath lab experience are now required. Workers with one year of health care college need 1 year experience. Bachelor degree health workers need 6 months experience to qualify for the RCIS exam. CVT graduates from CAAHEP approved schools can take the registry exams immediately upon graduation. Exceptions and other educational/experience qualifications exist. Check the latest candidate's handbook online at www.CCI-online.org or call the CCI national offices at 1-(800)-326-0268.

RCIS exam content (2019 blueprint)

RCIS CONTENT CATEGORY	Proportion of RCIS EXAM
A. Conducting Pre-Procedural Activities	10%
B. Conducting Diagnostic-Procedures	42%

C. Conducting Interventional Procedures	33%
D. Responding to Emergency Procedures and Protocols	6%
E. Conducting Post-Procedural Activities	9%
Total	100%

As you see, most of the RCIS exam is on diagnostic and interventional procedures. This covers duties common to all types of invasive procedures, such as monitoring, administering medications, and working with all types of intravascular catheters and devices.

CCI changed the content of this examination in 2019 to include emergency procedures. You can see the updated exam matrix outline and overview on the CCI website. The list of tested duties and supporting knowledge is lengthy and listed in the appendix.

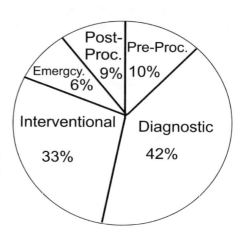

2. CI EXAM - Cath Lab - ARRT

Th Cardiac Interventional Technology (CI) exam is only for registered RTs (X-ray techs) who work in cath labs. If you are a CVT and nurse you are ineligible. ARRT says: "The purpose of the ARRT Examination in Cardiac-Interventional Technology is to assess the knowledge and cognitive skills underlying the intelligent performance of the tasks typically required of technologists employed in this specialized area. These content specifications are based on a comprehensive, nationwide job analysis of cardiac-interventional technologists."

"The table below presents the three major content categories and five procedural subcategories covered on the examination, and indicates the number of test questions in each category. The remaining pages list the specific topics addressed within each category, with the approximate number of test questions allocated to each topic appearing in parentheses."

CI EXAM Content - Cardiac Interventional -ARRT

CI Exam Specifications	Proportion of CI EXAM
A. Image Acquisition & Equipment	30 (20%)
B. Patient Care	35 (24%)
C. Cardiac-Interventional Procedures	80

1. Diagnostic Cardiac & Conduction Procedures	36 (25%)
2. Hemodynamics & Percutaneous Interventions	44 (30%)
Total (* There may be additional pilot questions.)	145 questions

As you see, the exam is very similar to CCI's RCIS content matrix, with increased emphasis on Patient Care and equipment. Some small categories are added such as "EP" and "Other." You can receive a free updated exam matrix outline and overview from ARRT on request for from their web site. RTs usually take this exam instead of the RCIS because they receive ARRT continuing education credits. Updates available on ARRT web site.

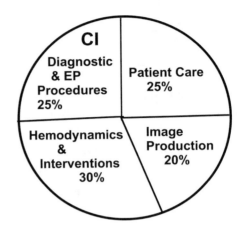

4. **VI Exam Content - Special Procedures -ARRT**

This Vascular Interventional Technolgist exam is for registered RTs (X-ray techs) who work in Vascular/Special Procedure labs. ARRT says: "The purpose of the ARRT Examination in Vascular-lnterventional Technology is to assess the knowledge and cognitive skills underlying the intelligent performance of the tasks typically required of technologists employed in this specialized area. These content specifications are based on a comprehensive, nationwide job analysis of vascular-interventional technologists employed in various f health-care settings."

"The table below presents the three major content categories and five procedural subcategories covered on the examination, and indicates the number of test questions in each category. The remaining pages list the specific topics addressed within each category, with the approximate number of test questions allocated to each topic appearing in parentheses. "

ARRT occasionally changes the content of these examinations. You may receive a free updated exam matrix outline and overview from ARRT on request. The 2002 exam content outline as stated by ARRT follows:

VI EXAM Content

VI Content Specifications	Number of questions and % of Vascular exam	
A. Equipment and Instrumentation	23	(14%)
B. Patient Care	37	(23%)
C. Procedures:	100	

1. Neurologic	15	(9%)
2. Genitourinary	19	(12%)
3. Gastrointestinal	26	(16%)
4. Peripheral	28	(18%)
5. Thoracic	12	(8%)
Total (160 questions) (* There may be additional pilot questions.)	160	(100%)

As you see, the Vascular Interventional Technology exam contains the same patient care and equipment categories as the other invasive exams, but it does not include cardiac procedures. It focuses on special procedures often performed by a radiologist on other organ systems. You can receive a free updated exam matrix outline and overview from ARRT on request for from their web site.

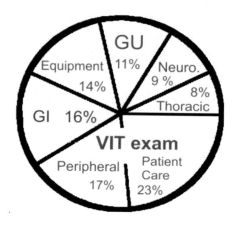

How to PREPARE for EXAMs

INTRODUCTION

This section will help you evaluate your "current skill level" and then tailor a plan of study to bring you to a "passing level." It will also make you "test smart," through explanations of the types of questions used on the cardiovascular examination.

STUDY SMARTER NOT HARDER

Don't just jump into a crash study program. Smart exam applicants best manage their own learning by selecting learning strategies that best suit their learning style, and they budget their study time appropriately. This book suggests specific strategies for different types of exam content. You can make this study memorable by becoming an "active learner" through self motivation and using memorable learning strategies.

1. **ESTABLISH YOUR MOTIVATION TO LEARN BY ASKING YOURSELF:**
   - Why is this material worth studying?
   - Is this concept likely to be on the exam?
   - Is there a practical use for this knowledge in the lab?

Throughout this book the detailed rationales show how and why each question is an important Cardio-Vascular concept.

2. **LEARNING STRATEGY:**

What learning strategy is most efficient and memorable for you? We all use different methods to learn. I tend to be a visual learner and have included hundreds of diagrams to explain the questions and answers.

- Analogies and memory crutches
- Repetition, Flash-cards
- Computer interaction - use associated Todd CD
- Comparing and contrasting with what you already know
- Verbal Paraphrasing, discussion, and teaching others
- Homework problems
- Reviewing commonly used graphics
- Practice innovative question formats (drag & drop, matching...)
    This is best done using my interactive program.
- Practice taking mock registry exams, as in our Vol #5.
    Your results on mock exams will point out your weak areas to study.

EXAM DIFFICULTY

How easy or difficult are these test questions? Exam questions are written at different "Performance Levels" to assure that the exam ranges from simple memorization to complex problem solving. Your exam will require you to think in many levels of difficulty.

RELEVANCY

Good exam writers test only relevant information. They stress facts that a competent cardiovascular professional should know. For example:

1. **In blood lab electrolyte tests, which number below is a normal serum Potassium (K+) level?**

          a. 1 mEq/L
    →   b. 4 mEq/L
          c. 10 mEq/L
          d. 20 mEq/L

Serum Potassium is an important number. When the K+ electrolyte blood level is reduced, CV patients are arrhythmia prone and are candidates for KCl infusion. Normal adult K+ levels are between 3.5 and 5.0 mEq/L. Irrelevant facts make poor questions and are seldom used on registry tests. You must know **why** this material is **clinically important**. It motivates you to store this into "**long term memory**."

Most anatomy questions employ simple memory recall. For example:

2. **What structure is anatomically cephalad from the Aortic Valve?**

          a. Pulmonary Valve
          b. Left Ventricle
          c. Pulmonary Artery
    →   d. Aortic Arch

Most CV Professionals know where the AO is located in relation to the aortic valve. But they may not know that "cephalad" means toward the head. Recall questions may ask you to identify anatomic structures or commonly used terms. For example:

3. **Which of the following forms the patient's right cardiac border marked #1 on this posterior-anterior (PA) chest film?**
→   a. RA
       b. RV
       c. PA
       d. LV

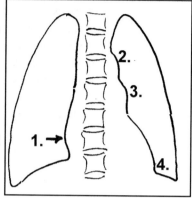

PA Chest film

There is always only one correct best answer. But, you should be able to identify all the other anatomic structures seen as well. Can you identify the structures labeled #2, #3, and #4? (See test section A1.)

Other types of recall questions might be:
      In electro-physiology what is an "Ectopic Focus":
      What is the normal arterial PO2 at sea level?
      Which artery bifurcates to form the Superficial Femoral and the Profunda arteries?

CRAMMING

Although, many students cram the night before an exam, they forget most of this information quickly. It pushes other useful information out of short term memory. You might remember the normal KCl level, but forget what time the test is to be given tomorrow. There is no doubt you can "cram" a lot of information into short term memory. Just be selective about what you memorize. Organize it, understand it's clinical use. And DON'T cram too much the night before. Only memorize useful information, things that may be needed to solve application questions like:

4. **What drug should be administered if a heart cath patient's serum Potassium level is 1.9 mEq/L?**
      a. PO_4
→   b. KCl
      c. HCl
      d. K_2SO_4

CRUTCHES

"Crutches" help you organize and remember important facts. Develop <u>acronyms</u> that organize groups of data. They will help you recall not just one, but several related facts or sequences. Examples of this are:
     • NAVL (Nerve, Artery, Vein, Ligament)
     • ABCs of CPR (Airway, breathing, Circulation)
     • The three I's of ECG (Injury, Ischemia, and Infarction)

● The five cyanotic congenital lesions "The 5 Terrible T's"
      (TET., Transposition, Tric. Atresia, Truncus, TAPVAR).

Other helpful "crutches" are catchy words or images that encapsulate difficult ideas. Develop your own humorous and catchy "crutches." Here is an example of a catchy "Myosin" concept.

5. **What is the central anatomic structure of the sarcomere with globular heads that facilitate cross-bridge linking and systole?**
        a. Actin or thick filament
        b. Actin or thin filament
→   **c. Myosin or thick filament**
        d. Myosin or thin filament

During systolic contraction the actin and myosin fibers are pulled together.

Remember, myosin as the thicker "workhorse" fiber. "Myo" means muscle, and these thicker muscled fibers have the heads (oars) on them. They pull the myosin fibers into the actin fibers and result in systolic contraction.

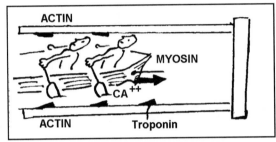

SARCOMERE

Other examples are:
      ● "Widow-maker" (A main-stem coronary lesion)
      ● "Shaker Can" (motion sensitive piezoelectric sensors in rate responsive pacemakers)
      ● "Strep. And Stretch" (Combination of Thrombolytic agent
          followed by Angioplasty).

TYPES OF MULTIPLE CHOICE QUESTIONS

All multiple choice items begin with a written question called the **"stem"**. The answers follow with one correct answer and several incorrect responses called **"distractors."** The following are examples.

COMPLETE QUESTION IN STEM:

6. **The prefix "centi-" corresponds to:**
        a. 1/10
→   b. 1/100
        c. 1/1000
        d. 1/1,000,000

FILL IN TYPE STEM:

7.   Normally_____ Pulmonary veins enter the _____.
     a. 2, RA
     b. 2, LA
     c. 4, RA
→   d. 4, LA

Watch out for negatively phrased questions including NOT or EXCEPT. For example:

8.   All of the following are names for normal arterial branches off the Aortic Arch EXCEPT:
→   a. Rt. Common Carotid Artery
     b. Left Common Carotid Artery
     c. Innominate Artery
     d. Brachycephalic Artery

Exams try to avoid "EXCEPT" type question. They can usually be converted to a multiple checkbox type of questions.

INCOMPLETE SENTENCE IN STEM:

9.   The most common vector for spread of infection in the hospital environment is:
     a. Airborne dust
     b. Airborne moisture droplets
     c. Soiled instruments
→   d. Human hands

MATCHING QUESTION:

10. The normal resting cardiac output varies with age, position, and BSA. Estimate the normal resting cardiac index (CI) for the patient #3 (reclining 70 year old adult) in the box.
     a.   2.0 L/min/M^2
→   b.   2.5 L/min/M^2
     c.   3.5 L/min/M^2
     d.   4.5 L/min/M^2

Patient # 10
1. Reclining 7 year old child
2. Standing 7 year old child
*3. **Reclining 70 year old adult**
4. Standing 70 year old adult

ANSWER b. 2.5 L/min/M^2. Grossman says, "the normal cardiac output appears to vary with age, steadily decreasing from approximately 4.5 L/min/M^2 at age 7 to approximately 2.5 L/min/M^2 at age 70... In addition to age, cardiac output is affected by posture, decreasing approximately 10% when rising from a lying to a sitting position and approximately 20% when rising (or after being tilted) from a lying to a standing position. Also, body temperature, anxiety, environmental heat and humidity, and a host of other factors influence the normal resting cardiac output." CORRECTLY MATCHED ANSWERS ARE:

    1. Reclining 7 year old child   = 4.5 L/min/M^2 (children have high metabolic rate)

    2. Standing 7 year old child   = 3.5 L/min/M^2 (reduced 20% from reclining CI)

    3. Reclining 70 year old adult= 2.5 L/min/M^2

    4. Standing 70 year old adult = 2.0 L/min/M^2 (reduced 20% from reclining CI)

This is a simple multiple choice question which asks about the "**reclining 70 year old adult**" cardiac index. It could be rewritten as 4 different multiple choice questions with each patient age and position in the stem. But, it could also be a matching question, where you match each number to an answer. When you see a question like this, for your own education match them all, not just the single multiple choice.

MULTIPLE ANSWER QUESTIONS

    With multiple answer questions you select several correct answers (numbered) then decide which combination of answers is correct. ARRT uses this type of question, but CCI does not. Multiple answer questions are included here for completeness. For example:

11. **Which of the following are associated with the Austin Flint cardiac murmur?**

    1. AS
    2. AI
    3. Increase with inspiration
    4. Increase with exercise
    5. Diastolic flutter of a mitral valve
    6. Systolic flutter of an aortic valve

        a . 1, 3, 5
        b. 1, 3, 6
→   **c. 2, 4, 5**
        d. 2, 4, 6

    Letter c. above is correct, indicating answers 2, 4, and 5 are the correct combination. ARRT uses this type of question, CCI does not. It can be rewritten into a multiple answer type of question such as the question below.

12. **Check the 3 correct answers below that are associated with the Austin Flint cardiac murmur?**

    1. ~~AS~~
→   **2. AI**
    3. ~~Increase with inspiration~~
→   **4. Increase with exercise**
→   **5. Diastolic flutter of a mitral valve**
    6. ~~Systolic flutter of an aortic valve~~

    Perhaps the best way to answer the above question is, circle the answers you KNOW to be correct and CROSS OUT those you <u>know</u> are incorrect. Circle answers (3, 4, & 5 as the final best choice.

You alone are responsible for your learning. So once you identify your weak areas, concentrate your study on these. You may need extra study time, discussion groups, additional clinical experience or to get help from local experts.

This book will help you prepare in your weak areas. By concentrating your study in your weakest areas you can best increase your overall exam performance. Each chapter in this book has an index at the front with comments as to their frequency on the RCIS exam. Study hardest on sections marked as **"know"**. It is less important to study sections marked as **"refresh only."**

Sample Drag and drop question:
Arrange these thoracic arteries in the order of blood flow, starting with the aortic arch.

Axillary
Brachial
Innominate
Subclavian

Ao Arch

Sample Checkbox question:
Check the 3 boxes below that are positive atrial pressure waves.

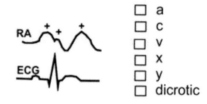

☐ a
☐ c
☐ v
☐ x
☐ y
☐ dicrotic

Sample Hot spot question:
On the Atrial pressure wave above click on the "c" wave. (2nd + sign)

Sample innovative questions like the "drag-and-drop" shown here require you to move your mouse:

YOUR EXAM PREPARATION PLAN

Sign up to take one of the national exams described. After filling out the application and paying for the exam you will receive a letter describing the exam and study directions from the national office. Application deadlines are usually two months in advance of the test date. You need all this time for concentrated preparation. For further information on the exam call or write the national offices of CCI or ARRT.

After assessing your basic knowledge, design a program of study adequate to the task. Most find that this exam requires a commitment of at least three months preparation - three months of persistent <u>daily</u> study. If the pre-test exams indicate severe weakness, you may have to prepare longer. I believe that ANY PRACTICING CV INVASIVE TEAM MEMBER (RN, RTR, or Technologist) CAN PASS THESE EXAMS with proper study and tutoring.

Each day set aside a time and place to study. Many exam candidates find that getting away to a hospital or public library provides the quiet time needed. Or If several people from your hospital or area are taking the exam together, you have an ideal study group. Group discussion is a great way to share experiences, especially the higher level application and problem solving skills. One group member will have experience that you don't - "I remember a patient like that . . . " Divide the topics among the group. Try tutoring others in an area in which you are strong. Teachers always learn more than their students. Teaching builds skill, confidence, and knowledge.

Question "why?" - and anticipate questions. You're smart enough! You've worked in the lab long enough to <u>prove that</u>. Set up a schedule of topics with deadlines. Ask your Cardiologists and Radiologists for help. They are usually flattered when asked for help with specific questions or with lectures. Additionally this will increase their respect for you. Select and purchase recognized textbooks, especially those recommended here and in your exam study guide.

EXAM TIPS <u>A multiple choice test is a "game"</u> and there are tricks to winning. Most of these can be learned by practicing and analyzing the questions in this book and interactive CD or USB.

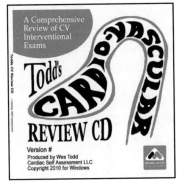

Todd's CV Review CD

Multiple choice questions are composed of a stem (question) one correct answer and 3-4 distractors (wrong answers). Read the stem carefully, with an open mind, yet reading nothing into it that is not there. Highlight key words in the stem. Eliminate obviously wrong answers, to narrow down the possible answers. Read all the possible answers before selecting one. Two answers may be close together.

Select the one **BEST** answer. When unsure of the correct answer to a question, mark it for review and come back to it later. Other questions may provide clues or jog your memory. So come back to it. Studies do NOT bear out the saying "Never change an answer." If upon review, you decide your first guess is incorrect - CHANGE IT! Always double check calculations a second time to double check your math!

You need to cover the entire exam with time to spare. Half way through the exam, check the time. If you are going fast - slow down - relax. Use a watch or wall clock to pace yourself. No rush. There is plenty of time.

There is no need to reread questions you have already answered. Only go back to those you were unsure and marked for review. Complete the exam. Double check to be sure you answered EVERY question. If you don't know - guess! You have one in four chances of getting it correct. No one is penalized for guessing.

CONCLUSION

If you systematically and thoroughly prepare for your exam, **you will pass**. Use this book to assess your knowledge through the associated mock exams. Evaluate your strong and weak areas. Concentrate your study on these weak areas, but do not neglect the basics. Formulate a study plan and study SMART by using the memory tools and study techniques discussed here.

The Exams include questions of different levels of difficulty - all the way from simple recall to problem solving. Establish an efficient learning method. Start early! Review and prepare thoroughly.

Become test smart by practicing the various forms of multiple choice questions enclosed. Keep practicing and studying until **you know** you are prepared for the exam. Build up your positive attitude about the exam and you will **be prepared** on exam day.

What additional help is available? Todd's review materials will help you prepare for the examination, including Todd's CD and online class. The testing agency (CCI) offers an exam handbook that itemizes its exam content. You can also get take review classes offered by professional organizations, hospitals, and medical product companies. Call the professional organizations ASCP (540)891-0079, or SICP (800)766-6014, or ARRT .

REVIEWERS AND CONTRIBUTORS INCLUDE:

Al Bennett, RCIS
Director Invasive Cardiology School
Carnegie Institute
550 Stephenson Hwy, Suite 100
Troy, Mi 48083

Todd Ginapp, RN, MSN, RN-BC, RCIS
West Houston Medical Center
Director of Cardiovascular Services
Houston, TX 77082

Jay Andrews, Technical Services

Prior edition contributors:
Connie Marshall, RT(R), RCIS, M.A.
Anthony Williams, MSM, RN, RCIS
Sabrina Black, BS, RDCS, FASE
Patrick Hoier, BS, RCSA, RCIS, FSICP
Polly Keller MBA, RRT, RCIS
Kristy Schultz, M.Ed., RTRM, RCIS

Dan Sullivan, BSN, RN
Al Bennett, RCIS
Allan Mirehouse, RCIS
Christie Hodge, RCIS
Robert Howard, RCIS
Syed Mustafa Khundmiri, BS, RCIS
Esma Campbell RT
Scott (William) Corson, RCIS
Lois Schaffer, MEd, RT®, RCIS
Marsha Holton, CCRN, RCIS, FSICP
Stephanie Ranck, BA, RCIS
Jeff Davis, RRT, RCIS, BS
Vicki Lemaster, BS, TR(R)(CV)
Chuck Williams, BS, RCSA, RPA/RA, RCIS, RT(R)(CV)(CI), CPFT, CCT,
Erwin Wuehr, BS, CP
Richard Merschen, MS, RT(R)(CV)

These knowledgeable reviewers have encouraged me and made suggestions throughout the years of book development. Although they have all proofed, critiqued, and edited my work I have not always taken their suggestions. And, they are not responsible for errors in the text. Full responsibility for the contents and accuracy of the book rests with the author.

Special thanks to all the others who have received advanced copies and made suggestions, whose names I have forgotten.

CONTENTS
Vol. I, Invasive Basics 6th Edition 2018

Chapters in 5 Volumes of Todd CV Review Books

General Concepts - Math & Units

INDEX: A1 - General Principles - Mathematics

1. General Units - On Exam

1. What does the MKS system use as the basic unit of distance?

   a.   Micron

   b.   Inch

   c.   Meter

   d.   Mole

ANSWER c.   MKS = Meter Kg Sec. other systems include: CGS (cm, gm. sec) and English (ft, lb, sec) **See:** math text **Keywords:** weight conversion

2. Which of the following are measurements of VOLUME? (Select 3.)

   a. ___ L

   b. ___ cc

   c. ___ mL

   d. ___ mm

ANSWERS: a, b, & c.

a. L - YES

b. cc - YES

c. mL - YES

d. mm - NO

L (liter), cc (cubic centimeter) and mL (milli-liter) are all measurements of volume. MM (millimeter) is length - 1/10 of a cm, or 1/1000 of a meter.

See: math text   **Keywords:** measures of volume

3. The prefix "centi" corresponds to:
- a. **1/10**
- b. **1/100**
- c. **1/1000**
- d. **1/1,000,000**

ANSWER b.   1/100 = "centi"   In the table below note how to move the decimal.

mega-			kilo-	hecto-	deka-	ONE	deci-	centi-	milli-			micro-
million			thousand	hundred	ten	1	tenth	hundredth	thousandth			millionth
10^6			10^3	10^2	10^1	10^0	10^{-1}	10^{-2}	10^{-3}			10^{-6}
1000000.			1000	100	10	1	0.1	0.01	.001			.000001

See: math text   **Keywords:** prefix centi-

4. Which prefixes listed below are correctly arranged from smallest to largest?
- a. **Milli, deci, centi, nano**
- b. **Nano, micro, milli, centi**
- c. **Nano, centi, micro, milli, deci**
- d. **Micro, nano, deci, centi, milli**

ANSWER b. Nano, micro, milli, centi. nano = 10^{-9}, micro =10^{-6}, milli = 10^{-3}, centi = 10^{-2}. These prefixes are used in measurements of ultrasound waves and microscopic measurements.
See: Reynolds, chapter on "Elementary Principles." centi

5. Which prefixes below are correctly arranged from largest to smallest?
- a. **Kilo, mega, giga**
- b. **Mega, giga, kilo**
- c. **Giga, kilo, mega**
- d. **Giga, mega, kilo**

ANSWER d. Giga, mega, kilo. Giga = 10^9= billion; Mega = 10^6 = million; Kilo = 10^3 = 1000. These prefixes are used in measurements of computer memory and astronomical measurements. **See:** Reynolds, chapter on "Elementary Principles."

2. Measures and Unit Conversion - On Exam

LENGTH

6. **How long is one micron?**

   a.   **10 meters**

   b.   **1 meter**

   c. 10^{-3} **meters**

   d. 10^{-6} **meters**

ANSWER d. 10^{-6} meters = one micro-meter **See:** math text **Keywords:** length conversion

7. **Convert 20 feet into meters.**

   a.   **3.1 M**

   b.   **4.1 M**

   c.   **5.1 M**

   d.   **6.1 M**

ANSWER d. 6.1 M. $20 \text{ ft} \left(\dfrac{12 \text{ in}}{\text{ft}}\right)\left(\dfrac{2.54 \text{ cm}}{\text{in}}\right)\left(\dfrac{M}{100 \text{ cm}}\right) = 6.1 \text{ M}$

(Memorize the length conversion factor 2.54 cm/in)

See: math text **Keywords:** length conversion

MASS & WEIGHT

8. **Convert 30 Kg into pounds.**

   a.   **44 lbs**

   b.   **55 lbs**

   c.   **66 lbs**

   d.   **77 lbs**

ANSWER c. 66 lbs.   30 Kg (2.2 lb/Kg) = 66 Kg.

See: math text **Keywords:** convert Kg to Lbs.

9. **One gram contains how many milligrams?**

   a.   **10**

   b.   **100**

   c.   **1000**

   d.   **10000**

ANSWER c. 1000,   1/1000 = milli;   so 1000 mg = 1 gm
See: math text   **Keywords:** weight conversion

10.   **One kilogram equals how many pounds?**
  a.   **1.0 lb.**
  b.   **2.2 lb.**
  c.   **2.54 lb.**
  d.   **3.2 lb.**

ANSWER b.   2.2 lb = 1 kg (Memorize this conversion factor.)
See: math text   **Keywords:** weight conversion

11.   **A patient's weight drops 2.0 Kg. How much fluid loss would cause this?**
  a.   **1.5 liters**
  b.   **2.0 liters**
  c.   **1.5 lb.**
  d.   **2.0 lb.**

ANSWER b. 2.0 liters. One liter of water weights 1 Kg. So by proportion 2 liters equals 2
Kg. **See:** math text   **Keywords:** weight of water.

12.   **One cubic centimeter (cc) equals:**
  a.   **0.01 M^2**
  b.   **1.0 ml**
  c.   **10 ml^3**
  d.   **1 deciliter**

ANSWER b.   1 ml is 1/1000 L or 1 cubic centimeter **See:** math text

13.   **1000 ml is approximately equal to:**
  a.   **1 gallon**
  b.   **1 pint**
  c.   **1 quart**
  d.   **1 ounce**

ANSWER c. 1 quart, 1000 ml = 1 L = 1.056 Qt. (pretty close) See: math text

AREA & VOLUME

14. **A planimeter measures an area of 2.1 square inches. Convert this area into square centimeters.**
    a.   **5.30 cm^2**
    b.   **9.6 cm^2**
    c.   **13.5 cm^2**
    d.   **28.4 cm^2**

ANSWER c. 13.5 cm^2

$$2.1 \text{ in}^2 \times \left(\frac{2.54 \text{ cm}}{\text{in}}\right)\left(\frac{2.54 \text{ cm}}{\text{in}}\right) = 2.1 \text{ in}^2 \times 6.45 \text{ cm}^2/\text{in}^2 = 13.5 \text{ cm}^2$$

Unless you know the number of square cm per square inch, and few do, you need to use the linear conversion (2.54 cm/in) times itself or squared. Note that the number and the units become squared. Thus, (2.54 cm/in)^2 = 6.45 cm^2/in^2. If you have trouble with this math, continue on to the math concepts at the end of this chapter. **See:** math text

TIME

15. **A PR interval measures 4 mm long on an ECG strip which was run at paper speed 25 mm/sec. How long is the PR interval?**
    a.   **160 msec**
    b.   **200 msec**
    c.   **250 msec**
    d.   **400 msec**

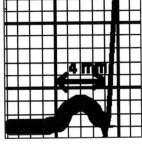

ECG grid

ANSWER a. 160 msec.
$$4 \text{ mm} \left(\frac{1 \text{ sec}}{25\text{mm}}\right)\left(\frac{1000\text{ms}}{\text{sec}}\right) = 160 \text{ msec.}$$

Notice how the units all cancel to result in milliseconds.
See: math text **Keywords:** time conversion

TEMPERATURE

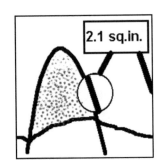

2.1 sq.in.

16. **100 degrees Fahrenheit equals ____ degrees Celsius.**
    a.   **51 ◦C.**
    b.   **46 ◦C.**
    c.   **40 ◦C.**
    d.   **38 ◦C.**

ANSWER d. 38∘C = $\dfrac{5}{9}$ (∘F - 32) = $\dfrac{5}{9}$ (68) = 38∘C

Here you must first solve the given equation for degrees C then plug in the number 100. Memorize one of the Fahrenheit, Celsius conversion formulas. You need to memorize one of the formulas, either F=(9/5) C + 32 or C =(5/9) (F - 32). If you have trouble with this math, continue on to the math concepts at the end of this chapter. **See**: math text

17.   **Convert 25 degrees Celsius into degrees Fahrenheit.**

    a.   **13 ° F**

    b.   **46 ° F**

    c.   **77 ° F**

    d.   **98 ° F**

ANSWER c. 77 ° F. Substitute 25 ° C into the formula and solve for degrees F. Of course you know human temperature of 98.6 ° F= 37 ° C. So you know 25 ° C is lower than 98.6 ° F. You can estimate it as around 70 or 80 degrees ° F. Using the formula: F= (9/5) C + 32 = (1.8 x 25) + 32 = 45 + 32 = 77° F. You need to memorize one of the formulas, either F=(9/5) C + 32 or   C =(5/9) (F - 32). You can always derive the second formula from the first algebraically.

| °F=(9/5) C + 32 |
| °C =(5/9) (F - 32) |

Temp. conversion formulas

See: math text **Keywords**: Celsius, Fahrenheit, temperature

18.   **A patient's temperature is 5° F. warmer than normal. What is his temperature in °C?**

    a.   **40 ∘C.**

    b.   **43 ∘C.**

    c.   **45 ∘C.**

    d.   **52 ∘C.**

ANSWER a. 40 ∘C.

Convert 5 degrees F to degrees C with the formula ∘C = (5/9) (∘F) to calculate what this is in degrees C. Remember 37 ∘C = 98.6 ° F and 0 ∘C = 32 ° F.

∘C = $\dfrac{5}{9}$ (5) = $\dfrac{25}{9}$ =   2.78 ∘C

So add this 2.78 ∘C to normal of 37 yields 39.78 or approximately 40 ∘C

See: math text **Keywords**: temp. conversion

OTHER

19.   **One microvolt equals:**

    a.   **0.000001 v**

    b.   **0.0001 v**

    c.   **0.001 v**

d.   0.01 v

ANSWER a. 0.000001 v   Micro = 10^{-6}. So 1×10^{-6} is a 1 with the decimal point moved six places to the left. 1/ (1 million).
See: math text   **Keywords:** scientific notation

20.   **In physics, the amount of energy it takes to heat one ml. of water one degree C. is termed one:**
   a.   **Joule**
   b.   **Newton**
   c.   **Calorie**
   d.   **Kilo-Pascal**

ANSWER c. Calorie = 1∘C change in 1 ml H_2O. This principle is used to develop the equations used to calculate thermodilution CO. Note that in metabolic calculations and dieting a Kilo-Calorie is 1000 small calories. This K-Calorie unit is used more in medicine than this small calorie.
See: math text   **Keywords:** energy conversion

21.   **Your new computer has 4 gigabytes of memory (RAM). How many bytes is this?**
   a.   **400,000**
   b.   **4,000,000**
   c.   **40,000,000**
   d.   **400,000,000**
   e.   **4,000,000,000**

ANSWER e. 4,000,000,000. Giga is a billion. 4 gigs is 4 billion, or 4 with 9 zeroes after it. See chart of decimals in 3rd question in this chapter.

22.   **If a person's liver weighs 3.5 times more than his heart, what percentage is this? His liver weight is _____ % of his heart's weight.**
   a.   **0.35 % larger**
   b.   **3.5% larger**
   c.   **35% larger**
   d.   **350% larger**

ANSWER d. 350% larger. The ratio here is 3.5 to 1. To change to percentage multiply by 100%, which is unity. This makes 350%. This is equivalent to moving the decimal point 2 places to the right. This means if his heart weighs 100 grams, the liver weighs 3.5 times that or 350 grams. Note that "of" is always associated with multiplication. If you have trouble with this math, continue on to the math concepts at the end of this chapter. **See:** math text

23.   **What are the appropriate units used to measure aortic valve area?**
   a.   mm diameter
   b. cm^2
   c. cm^3
   d.   inch circumference

ANSWER b. cm^2. Valve area is measured in square cm units. Each square cm is about the size of one finger. Surgeons customarily measure in finger sizes.
See: Reynolds, chapter on "Elementary Principles" **Keywords:** area measure, aortic area

24.   **The continuity equation states that area times velocity equals flow or $A_1 V_1 = A_2 V_2$. The area of the LV outflow track is 4 cm^2 and the velocity there is 40 cm/sec. What is the area of the aortic valve if the aortic valve velocity is 100 cm/sec?**
   a.   0.63 cm^2
   b.   1.6 cm^2
   c.   2.4 cm^2
   d.   3.2 cm^2

ANSWER b. 1.6 cm^2. $A_1 V_1 = A_2 V_2$; Rearrange to solve for A_2; $A_2 = (A_1 V_1) / V_2$ Plugging in numbers: $A_2 = (4 \times 40) / 100 = 1.6 \, cm^2$. This the way echocardiography finds the aortic valve area using Doppler - a simple ratio. See: math text

3. Fractions, Ratios, & Percent - Not on Exam (Refresher Only)

25.   **Divide 4.5 by 1.125.**
   a.   1/4
   b.   4
   c.   8/9
   d.   9/8

ANSWER b. 4
4.5/1.125 = 4

26.   **Divide 1/5 by 1.50.**
   a.   1.33
   b.   0.33
   c.   1/10
   d.   2/15

ANSWER d. 2/15 or 0.133.

Dividing 1/5 by 1.5 is dividing 0.2 by 1.5 = 0.133. However, this answer is not available above. Doing it in fractions - 1/5 divided by 3/2 - we need to invert the denominator and multiply. So: 1/5 x 2/3 = 2/15 See: Math Text.

27. **The ratio 1:3 equals:**

   a.   **0.1333**

   b.   **0.333**

   c.   **1.333**

   d.   **3.0**

ANSWER b. 0.333 A ratio is a fraction. So 1:3 = 1/3 = 0.333333...
See: math text **Keywords**: ratios, fractions

28. **A CV Tech uses ½ his vacation time fishing, 1/5 his vacation time visiting relatives and 1/4 of it camping. What part of his vacation time was left to relax at home?**

   a.   **1/5**

   b.   **1/20**

   c.   **1/3**

   d.   **3/20**

ANSWER b. 1/20 $\frac{1}{2} + \frac{1}{5} + \frac{1}{4} = \frac{10}{20} + \frac{4}{20} + \frac{5}{20} = \frac{19}{20}$ only 1/20 remains to use.

See: math text **Keywords**: fraction problem

29. **A doctor's Mercedes-Benz car has a gasoline tank which holds 20 gallons. When this gauge reads 1/4 full, how many gallons are needed to fill the tank?**

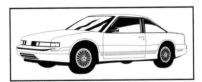

Drs. car 1/4 full

   a.   **5**

   b.   **10**

   c.   **12**

   d.   **15**

ANSWER d. 15 gal.

$\left(\frac{1}{4}\right)$ 20 = 5 in tank, 20 - 5 = 15 gal. to add

See: math text **Keywords**: algebraic solution

30.   **Write 4.5 % as a fraction.**

    a.   **9/2**

    b.   **9/20**

    c.   **9/200**

    d.   **9/2000**

ANSWER c. 9/200.   4.5% = 4.5/100 = 9/200

See: math text   **Keywords:** fraction

31.   **What is 62.5 % of 80?**

    a.   **.5**

    b.   **5**

    c.   **50**

    d.   **500**

ANSWER c. 50.   62.5% of 80 = .625 x 80 = 50. Whenever you see "of" multiply.

See: math text   **Keywords:** percentage

32.   **80 is 40% of what number?**

    a.   **20**

    b.   **32**

    c.   **200**

    d.   **320**

ANSWER c. 200.   80 = 40% x;   80 = .4x,   x = 80/0.4 = 200

See: math text   **Keywords:** percentage

33.   **Divide ½ by 1/50.**

    a.   **5**

    b.   **12.5**

    c.   **25**

    d.   **100**

ANSWER c. 25. To divide fractions, invert the denominator and multiply. So ½ divided by 1/50 is ½ x 50 = 25. Or you can reduce the fractions to decimals and divide: .50 / .02 = 25.

See: math text   **Keywords:** percentage

34. **Solve: ½ + 3/4 - 5/6 = ?**
   a.   **5/12**
   b.   **7/24**
   c.   **1/3**
   d.   **5/6**

   ANSWER a. 5/12 $\frac{1}{2} + \frac{3}{4} - \frac{5}{6} =$ $\frac{6}{12} + \frac{9}{12} - \frac{10}{12} = \frac{5}{12}$

   See: math text   **Keywords:** fractions

35. **In the proportion 5/10 = X/6, solve for the unknown X.**
   a.   **3**
   b.   **9**
   c.   **12**
   d.   **18**

   ANSWER a. 3 $\frac{5}{10} = \frac{x}{6}$ $x = 6\left(\frac{5}{10}\right)$ $= 6(.5) = 3$

   See: math text   **Keywords:** proportion

36. **Subtract 3/4 from 9/10.**
   a.   **3/20**
   b.   **1.40**
   c.   **3/5**
   d.   **3/40**

   ANSWER a. 3/20. $\frac{9}{10} - \frac{3}{4} =$ $\frac{18}{20} - \frac{15}{20} =$ $\frac{3}{20}$

   Find lowest common denominator (20) and subtract numerators.

   See: math text   **Keywords:** fractions

37. **The product of (-3)(+4)(- ½)(- 1/3) is:**
   a.   **-1**
   b.   **-2**
   c.   **+2**
   d.   **- 6**

   ANSWER b. -2 $(-3)(4)\left(\frac{-1}{2}\right)\left(\frac{-1}{3}\right) = \left(\frac{-3}{1}\right)\left(\frac{4}{1}\right)\left(\frac{-1}{2}\right)\left(\frac{-1}{3}\right) = \frac{-12}{6} = -2$

   See: math text   **Keywords:** fractions

4. Exponents and Powers - On Exam

38. **Multiply:** $10^2 \times 10^3 \times 10^{-1} = ?$
   a.   **10**
   b.   **100**
   c.   **1000**
   d.   **10000**

ANSWER d. 10,000 $10^2 \times 10^3 \times 10^{-1} = 10^{2+3-1} = 10^4 = 10,000$
Multiply all numerators together. Multiply all denominators together. Reduce fraction. **See:** math text   **Keywords:** scientific notation

39. **Find the value of** $(5/4)^3$**.**
   a.   **1.25**
   b.   **1.95**
   c.   **2.65**
   d.   **3.35**

ANSWER b. 1.95 can be done by 1.25^3 or

$$\frac{5}{4} \times \frac{5}{4} \times \frac{5}{4} = \frac{25 \times 5}{16 \times 4} = \frac{125}{64} = 1.95$$

See: math text **Keywords:** cube a fraction

40. **Using powers of ten,** 1.0×10^6 **equals:**
   a.   **1000**
   b.   **10,000**
   c.   **100,000**
   d.   **1,000,000**

ANSWER d. 1,000,000. Mega = 10^6. So 1×10^6 is a 1 with the decimal point moved six places to the right (1 million). Common computer prefix where memory is commonly expressed in mega-bytes. **See:** math text **Keywords:** scientific notation

41. **Using the powers of ten,** 1.0×10^{-3} **equals:**
   a.   **0.01 or centi-**
   b.   **0.001 or milli-**
   c.   **0.0001 or micro-**
   d.   **0.00001 or hecta-**

ANSWER b. 0.001 or milli. The decimal is moved 3 places to the left. So the power of ten is -3. This is the commonly used milli-gram or milli-meter prefix.

See: math text **Keywords:** scientific notation

42. **Using the powers of ten, 0.000000133 equals:**
   a. $1.33 \times 10^{(-4)}$
   b. $1.33 \times 10^{(-5)}$
   c. $1.33 \times 10^{(-6)}$
   d. $1.33 \times 10^{(-7)}$

ANSWER d. $1.33 \times 10^{(-7)}$. The decimal is moved 7 places to the right. So the power of ten is -7. Remember, to make the whole number on the left, larger; you must make the exponent on the right smaller. So making 0.000,000,133 more usable and larger, the decimal must be moved to the right 7 places. To balance this the exponent must be made equally smaller -7 powers of ten. This could also be written as $0.133 \times 10^{(-6)}$, 0.133 Micro-units, or 0.133 μ units. **See:** math text **Keywords:** scientific notation

43. **Expressed in exponential scientific notation, 1540 equals:**
   a. $1.54 \times 10^{(2)}$
   b. $1.54 \times 10^{(3)}$
   c. $1.54 \times 10^{(4)}$
   d. $1.54 \times 10^{(5)}$

ANSWER b. $1.54 \times 10^{(3)}$. To express as a single digit to the left of the decimal the decimal must be moved 3 places to the left. So the power of ten is 3. See: math text

44. **Take three to the third power and that answer to the third power as expressed in the box.**
   a.   9
   b.   27
   c.   729
   d.   19,683

$$\left(3^3\right)^3$$

ANSWER d. 19,683

   Starting inside the brackets: $3^3 = 3 \times 3 \times 3 = 27$
   Then: $27^3 = 27 \times 27 \times 27 = 19,683$

See: math text **Keywords:** powers

45. **The number of capillaries in the body is approximately $3.0 \times 10^{+9}$. This is:**
   a.   3 hundred thousand
   b.   3 million
   c.   3 hundred million
   d.   3 billion

ANSWER d. $3.0 \times 10^{+9}$ is a 3 with 9 zeroes behind it, or 3,000,000,000. This is 3 billion.

See: Berne & Levy, chapter on "The Circuit" **Keywords:** scientific notation

46. **Express 30,800,000 in the scientific exponential notation system.**
   a. $3.08 \times 10^{+4}$
   b. $3.08 \times 10^{+5}$
   c. $3.08 \times 10^{+6}$
   d. $3.08 \times 10^{+7}$

ANSWER d. $3.08 \times 10^{+7}$ 30,800,000 moved 7 places = 3.08×10^{7} See: math text

47. **Multiply these terms expressed in exponential notation: $3.2 \times 10^{1} \times 4.4 \times 10^{1}$ =**
   a. 1.408×10^{1}
   b. 1.408×10^{2}
   c. 1.408×10^{3}
   d. 1.408×10^{4}

ANSWER c. 1.408×10^{3}
        $3.2 \times 10 \times 4.4 \times 10 = 14.08 \times 100 = 1408 = 1.4 \times 10^{3}$ **See:** math text

48. **State the numerical value of absolute zero in degrees Celsius, where the Kelvin temperature = 0. Use the formula: K = C+ 273**
   a.   0 degrees C.
   b.   -100 degrees C.
   c.   +273 degrees C.
   d.   -273 degrees C.

ANSWER d.   -273.∘ C = Absolute zero

C = K - 273 = 0 - 273 = - 273 degrees Celsius (That's AS COLD AS IT GETS!)

All the gas laws require that gas temperature be expressed in absolute temperature.

About the only time you might use this is in converting gas volumes from ATPS (ambient temp. & pressure saturated) to STPD (standard & pressure dry).

See: math text   **Keywords:** absolute temp

Statistics section removed from book 2018.
No statistics on RCIS Exam.

Patient Care

INDEX: A2 - Patient Care

1. Medical Terminology

49. Medical terms are commonly built by adding a prefix in front of a root word. Match the prefix with its meaning.

1. PERI-_____
2. ENDO- _____
3. RETRO-_____
4. HYPER- _____
5. HYPO- _____
6. TRANS-_____

     a. Behind
     b. Deficient
     c. Excessive
     d. Within
     e. Surrounding
     f. Across

ANSWER
1. PERI-   e. Surrounding or around (E.g., Pericardium)
2. ENDO- d. Within or inward (E.g., Endocardium)
3. RETRO- a. Behind or backward (E.g., Retroperitoneal)
4. HYPER- c. Excessive, above, beyond, or more than normal (E.g., Hyperkalemia)
5. HYPO-   b. Deficient, beneath, under, or below normal (E.g., Hypothermia)
6. TRANS- f. Across or beyond (E.g., Trans-thoracic)
Be able to match all prefixes above. **See:** Medical Dictionary   **Keywords: prefix**

50. **Medical terms are commonly built by adding a prefix in front of a root word. Match the prefix with its meaning. Note a (o) indicates an o may be added to the combining form.**

1. Vaso _____
2. Phlebo _____
3. Arterio _____
4. Ather(o) _____
5. Cholangi(o) _____

    a.   **Vessel**
    b.   **Systemic vessel containing deoxygenated blood**
    c.   **Fatty degradation**
    d.   **Systemic vessel containing oxygenated blood**
    e.   **Bile duct**

ANSWERS
1. Vas(o) -   a. Vessel or canal for carrying a fluid (E.g., vasoconstriction)
2. Phlebo-   b. Vein or venous or Systemic vessel containing deoxygenated blood (E.g., phlebitis)
3. Arteri(o)-   d. Systemic vessel containing oxygenated blood (E.g., arteriosclerosis)
4. Ather(o) -   c. Fatty degradation (E.g., atheromatous plaque)
5. Cholangi-   e. Bile duct (E.g., cholangiogram)
Be able to match all prefixes above. **See:** Medical Dictionary **Keywords:** prefix

51. **Medical terms are commonly built by adding a suffix to the end of a root word. Match each suffix with its meaning.**

1. Blood condition _____
2. Formation _____
3. Enlargement _____
4. Disease condition _____
5. Deficiency _____
6. Inflamation _____

    a. - poiesis
    b. - pathy
    c. - emia
    d. - penia
    e. - megaly
    f. -itis

ANSWERS
1. Blood condition   c. - emia (E.g., anemia)
2. Formation   a. - poiesis (E.g., erhythropoiesis)
3. Enlargement   e. - megaly (E.g., cardiomegaly)
4. Disease condition   b. - pathy (E.g., myocardopathy)
5. Deficiency   d. - penia (E.g., thrombocytopenia)
6. Inflamation   f. -itis (E.g., phlebitis)

52. Surgical terms are commonly built by adding a suffix to the end of a root word. Match each suffix with its meaning.
1. Surgical repair _____
2. Surgical removal or incision _____
3. Surgical tap _____
4. Surgical opening between organs _____
       a. -centesis (E.g., thoracentesis
       b. -ostomy (E.g., colostomy)
       c. - plasty (E.g., angioplasty)
       d. -ectomy (E.g., Pericardiectomy)

ANSWER
1. Surgical repair   c. - plasty (E.g., angioplasty)
2. Surgical removal/incision   d. -ectomy (E.g., pericardiectomy)
3. Surgical tap   a. -centesis (E.g., thoracentesis
4. Surgical opening between organs   b. -ostomy (E.g., colostomy, pericardiostomy or pericardial window into pleural cavity)

Be able to match all suffixes above. **See:** Medical Dictionary **Keywords:** suffix

53. A patient with oliguria may be treated with a:
a.   **Foley catheter**
c.   **Fogarty catheter**
d.   **Urethroscope**
e.   **Kidney catheter**

ANSWER: a. Foley catheter is a dual lumen rubber catheter which is positioned in the bladder to drain it when patients are unable to void adequately. This condition of decreased urine output in relation to the intake is termed oliguria, hypouresis or oligouresis. Olig- means "deficient." **See:** Mosby's Comprehensive Review of Nursing for NCLEX-RN, Chapter on "Urinary systems" **Keywords:** Oliguria, Foley cath

54. Infiltration of fluids or blood around an arterial or IV access site is termed:
a.   **Extravasation**
b.   **Extravenous irrigation**
c.   **Extramural tamponade**
d.   **Extra-parenteral discharge**

ANSWER: a. Extravasation or infiltration is the accidental administration fluids or blood into the surrounding tissue, either by leakage or direct infusion from a needle that has come out of the vein. Extravasation implies a more serious infiltration by a caustic agent and occurs more often with geriatric patients whose vessels are hardened by atherosclerosis. **See articles:** https://www.ncbi.nlm.nih.gov/pmc/articles/PMC3664495/ and https://academic.oup.com/annonc/article-lookup/doi/10.1093/annonc/mds294 Keywords: Extravasation or infiltration

55. **The opening in a single use sterile femoral drape sheet is called a:**
    a.   **Lumen**
    b.   **Window**
    c.   **Foramen**
    d.   **Access site**
    e.   **Fenestration**

ANSWER: e. A fenestrated drape has a round or slit-like opening in the center. "Single use/disposable drapes are composed of nonwoven natural and synthetic materials ... These fabrics include a fluid-proof polyethylene film laminated between the fabric layers at strategic locations of the drape, usually around the drape fenestration..." From: Essential of Perioperative Nursing", chapter on Aseptic Practices, by Cynthia Spry, Jonas and Bartlett Publishers **Keywords:** fenestrated drape

56. **Match each medical directional term with its anatomic meaning.**
    1. Ventral _____
    2. Dorsal _____
    3. Cranial _____
    4. Caudal _____
        a. Anterior
        b. Posterior
        c. Superior
        d. Inferior

ANSWER
1. Ventral = a. Anterior, The face is anterior
2. Dorsal = b. Posterior, The butt is posterior
3. Cranial = c. Superior, The head or higher
4. Caudal = d. Inferior, Toward feet or lower
Be able to match all terms above. **See:** Spence, chapter "Introduction to A & P"

2. Positioning & IVs

57. **When caring for a patient with an IV drip infusion of a 1 liter bag of saline, the container/bag should be _____ to maintain flow.**
    a.   **Kept below the level of the infusion site**
    b.   **Kept above the level of the infusion site**
    c.   **Turned wide-open position**
    d.   **Turned off, then turned back on at completion of exam**

ANSWER b. Kept above the level of the infusion site. IVs run by gravity and must be kept above the infusion site to continue dripping. If the IV bag goes below the infusion site, backflow may occur, which may lead to coagulation and contamination. Carefully support the arm so as not to dislodge the IV in the vein or cause clotting of the access site. Also, use

caution to avoid trapping or kinking the IV line.
See: Nursing Text **Keywords**: IV bag above

58. **An ambulatory patient is:**
   a.   **Able to walk**
   b.   **Unable to walk**
   c.   **Breathing adequately**
   d.   **Not breathing adequately**

ANSWER a. Patients are able to walk, means the patient is "ambulatory" or able to "ambulate." An ambulatory lab, is one where patients are able to get up and walk soon after their heart cath - on the same day.
See: Medical dictionary **Keywords:** ambulatory

59. **Match the medical directional terms with their anatomic meaning.**
   1. **Toward the midline** _____
   2. **Away from the midline** _____
   3. **Closer to a point of reference** _____
   4. **Farther from a point of reference** _____
      a. **Distal**
      b. **Proximal**
      c. **Medial**
      d. **Lateral**

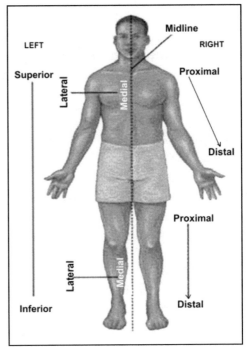

ANSWER
1. Toward the midline = c. Medial (E.g., Heart is medial to the lungs)
2. Away from the midline = d. Lateral (E.g., Lungs are lateral to the heart)
3. Closer to a point of reference = b. Proximal (E.g., Arm is proximal to the hand)
4. Farther from a point of reference = a. Distal (E.g., Hand is distal to the arm)
Be able to match all terms above. **See:** Spence, chapter "Introduction to A & P"

60. **A patient in acute pulmonary edema should be positioned in a:**
   a.   **Prone position**
   b.   **Sitting up Fowler's position**
   c.   **Trendelenburg position**
   d.   **Right or left lateral position**

ANSWER b. Sitting up Fowler's position to facilitate breathing and decrease venous return. A patient with dyspnea is usually uncomfortable in a lying supine position (orthopnea). This is because reclining increases venous fluid pooling (preload) in the lungs which increases edema in CHF patients. They breath easier sitting up, in either a semi-sitting (mid- Fowler's) position 30°, sitting (high- Fowler's) position 45°, or reverse Trendelenburg position (body tilted head up). **See:** Medical Dictionary **Keywords:** orthopnea - sit up

61. **A major safety guideline to a person transferring a premedicated patient from a bed onto a gurney is:**
a.   **Transfer patients slowly**
b.   **Wear protective gloves and mask**
c.   **Get adequate assistance**
d.   **Use a heavy sheet to pull him over**

ANSWER c. Get adequate assistance. Torres says:"A patient must never be moved without adequate help; to do so may cause injury to the patient or the RT [Health Care Provider]." Don't try to do it alone unless the patient is conscious and can move himself over. If the patient has been premedicated generally 4 assistants will be needed, 2 on each side to assist in pulling the patient with the supporting sheet.
See: Torres, chapter on "Basic Patient Care in Diagnostic Imaging" **Keywords:** move patient with assistance only

62. **In general, when selecting an IV site in the arm at the beginning of a case start with the:**
a.   **Largest vein available**
b.   **Vein closest to the heart**
c.   **Most medial site**
d.   **Most peripheral (distal) site**

ANSWER d. Most peripheral (distal) site. Intermed says, "Generally IV's are started at the most peripheral site that is available and appropriate for the situation. This allows cannulation of a more proximal site if your initial attempt fails. If you puncture a proximal vein first, and then try to start an IV distal to that site, the fluid may leak from the injured proximal vessel. The preferred site in the emergency department is the veins of the forearm, followed by the median cubital vein that crosses the antecubital fossa.... In circumstances in which no peripheral IV access is possible a central IV can be started. [subclavian, IJ...]"
See: http://med.uottawa.ca/procedures/iv/

63. **Where should you start the IV when a radial artery catheterization is scheduled?**
a.   **Ipsilateral arm**
b.   **Contralateral arm**
c.   **A vein distal to the radial access**
d.   **A vein medial to the radial access**

ANSWER b. Contralateral arm. Use the alternate arm so you can access the IV site during the case. Normally the right arm will be used for the arterial access and will be covered with sterile drapes and inaccessible to the nurse. Thus, the IV is placed in the patients left (contralateral) arm. See: personal experience

64. **For a cardiac cath, usually the first vascular access is the _____ because _____.**
    a.   **Femoral artery, it is the largest artery**
    b.   **Brachial artery, it is the safest artery**
    c.   **IV, it provides a drug lifeline**
    d.   **IV, it provides needed electrolytes & ACT draws**

ANSWER: c. IV, it provides a drug lifeline. Kern says, "the second lifeline is the IV access. (His first lifeline is the ECG.) Emergency drugs to counteract vagal or allergic reaction or other problems are best administered by the IV route...additional analgesia. The IV line is also important for hydration after cardiac catheterization." See: Kern, chapter on "The Catheterization Lab"

3. Documentation

65. **When charting in the medical record you should:**
    a.   **Avoid generalizations like "appears, inadvertently, seems to..."**
    b.   **Avoid writing with fountain pens with liquid ink**
    c.   **Avoid documenting routine safety measures**
    d.   **Chart care as you are planning it, not after it is given**

ANSWER a. Avoid generalizations like "appears, inadvertently, seems to..." Kern says: "Information in the medical record should reflect only accurate facts regarding the particular patient. Avoid generalizations and speculating by charting only what you see, hear, feel, and smell. Do not use words such as inadvertently, unfortunately, appears, resembles, and the like.... Chart after the delivery of care, not before. Never make an entry in anticipation of something to be done...The chart note should identify precautionary or protective measures that have been taken for the safety of the patient, including the use of side rails and restraints." Charting should always be done with a permanent ink pen, although especially runny ink may smear.
See: Kern, chapter on "Documentation in the Cardiac Catheterization Laboratory"
Keywords: Charting, no generalizations

66. **Prior to any cardiac invasive procedure the ultimate responsibility for obtaining informed consent lies with the:**
    a.   **Assigned risk manager**
    b.   **The operating physician (cardiologist)**
    c   **Circulating nurse assigned to the case**
    d.   **Patient's primary care referring physician (GP)**

ANSWER b. The operating physician (cardiologist). The ultimate responsibility for obtaining permission is the operating physician's, usually the operating cardiologist. The cath lab staff are responsible for checking that the consent is on the chart, properly signed, and that the information on the form is correct.

Kern says, "The cardiologist has the nondelegable duty to provide the patient or responsible party with adequate information about the planned procedure(s). "Some PAs & CRNPs also gain consent depending on state laws.... Failure to properly obtain informed consent is assault and battery." **See:** Allmers, Review for Surgical Tech. Exam, chapter on "Fundamentals"

67. **Your alert patient states that he is having a defibrillator implant, but the consent form is for a bi-ventricular pacemaker. What should you do?**
    a.   **Contact the implanting MD**
    b.   **Check the chart for diagnosis**
    c.   **Set up for what the patient says**
    d.   **Set up for what the consent form says**

ANSWER: a. Contact the implanting MD. Only he knows what procedure he scheduled for this patient. It is possible this patient is scheduled for CRT-D, which is a biventricular pacemaker with an ICD combination. – as opposed to a CRT-P, which is pacing only. **Reference:** Ellenbogen, chapter on "Cardiac Resynchronization Therapy" **Keywords:** Consent unclear, call physician

68. **To be legally valid, what is the LATEST that the patient should sign the informed consent form?**
    a.   **Before administration of preoperative antiplatelet agents (such as Plavix)**
    b.   **Before administration of conscious sedation (such as Versed)**
    c   **Before any invasive incisions or percutaneous punctures are made**
    d.   **Before any interventions are made (PTCA, Stent...)**

ANSWER b. Before administration of conscious sedation (such as Versed). Consent forms must be signed before the administration of sedative medications. This is to ensure that the patient fully understands and is informed about the procedure and the risks involved. If the patient's is mind is clouded by preoperative medications such as Demerol or sedatives such as Versed the consent is not legally valid. **See:** Allmers, Review for Surgical Tech. Exam, chapter on "Fundamentals" **Keywords:** Get consent before premeds

69. **The intent of informed consent for cardiac procedures is to:**
    a.   **Authorize all routine hospital procedures**
    b.   **Protect patient from high risk procedures**
    c   **Protect the operating physician and the hospital from claims of an unauthorized operation**
    d.   **Authorize the physician to withhold lifesaving measures as he deems appropriate**

ANSWER c. Protects the operating physician and the hospital from claims of an unauthorized operation. An informed consent (operative permit) protects the operating physician and the hospital from claims of an unauthorized operation. A general consent authorizes the physician and staff to render treatment and perform procedures which are routine duties normally carried out at the hospital. It also protects the patient from procedures they have not been informed about. The physician cannot perform different procedures or withhold lifesaving measures unless it has been approved by the patient. **See:** Allmers, Review for Surgical Tech. Exam, chapter on "Fundamentals"   **Keywords:** Consent protects MD & hospital

70. **Which of the statements below are true regarding informed consent for cardiac catheterization? (Select 3.)**
   a. **Discussion should cover alternative treatments**
   b. **Only considered legal for 2-3 days from date of signature**
   c. **Consent must be obtained before patient receives sedation**
   d. **If not obtained, the patient has the right to sue for malpractice**

   ANSWERS: a, c, & d.

   a. Discussion should cover alternative treatments - YES.
   b. Only considered legal for 2-3 days from date of signature - NO.
   c. Consent must be obtained before patient receives sedation - YES.
   d. If not obtained, the patient has the right to sue for malpractice - YES.

   According to the University of Virginia: *"Legally, informed consent is valid for a reasonable period of time. Per Joint Commission, this reasonable period of time consists of 30 days. In cases where treatments are planned in advance, such as chemotherapy, consent may be obtained for the treatments to be provided up to 6 months in advance. If informed consent is not obtained, the patient has the right to sue for medical malpractice....The legal requirement to obtain informed consent rests with the <u>attending (or operating) physician</u>.... Informed consent should include discussion of the following:*
       1. Diagnosis
       2. Purpose of proposed treatment / procedure
       3. Possible risks and benefits of proposed treatment / procedure
       4. Possible alternatives to proposed treatment / procedure
       5. Possible risks of not receiving treatment / procedure
   Consent may not be required for treatment in the case of emergency." **See:** http://www.med-ed.virginia.edu/courses/rad/consent/   **Keywords:** Consent legal 30 days

71. **The cardiologist gives the nurse a verbal telephone order to administer a medication to her patient stat. She should:**
   a. **Immediately give the medication.**
   b. **Tell him telephone orders cannot be accepted.**
   c. **Write the order down, then read it back to the physician for approval.**
   d. **Restate the order in your own words to the physician, then write it down.**

   ANSWER: c. Write the order down, then read it back to the physician for approval
       Univ. Texas policy is "Verbal and telephone orders may only be given by a provider.

• When verbal and telephone orders are issued, they must be written and read back to the physician. The physician then becomes responsible for the order that is to be treated as any other physician order and carried out by the appropriate hospital personnel.

• The health care worker receiving the verbal order shall transcribe the order onto the medical record and Physician Order Sheet , identifying the order as a verbal order and the name of the provider who issued it. The health care worker will then sign the Physician Order Sheet." **See:**

https://www.utmb.edu/policies_and_procedures/IHOP/Clinical/Personnel_Issues/IHOP%20-%2009.11.05%20-%20Physician%20Orders.pdf

Kern says, "When taking telephone orders, drug names should be confirmed by spelling them back to the physician." **See:** Kern, chapter on Risk Management

72. **Besides asking a patient his name, an adequate identifier is:**
   a. **Birthday on bracelet**
   b. **Room number on bracelet**
   c. **Name of operating physician**
   d. **Asking the type of case he is expecting**
   e. **Asking the patient what limb he expects will be accessed**

ANSWER: a. Birthday on bracelet. The Joint Commission says: "The intent of using two patient identifiers is two-fold: first, to reliably identify the individual as the person for whom the service or treatment is intended; second, to match the service or treatment to that individual. Therefore, the two patient-specific identifiers must be directly associated with the individual and the same two identifiers must be directly associated with the medications, ...or procedures.

   For those patients with armbands, patient name and ID number compared to the order/MAR could be the two identifiers. The two identifiers may be in the same location, such as a wristband. It is the person-specific information that is the "identifier," not the medium on which that information resides. Acceptable identifiers may be the individual's name, an assigned identification number, telephone number, or other person-specific identifier. Electronic identification technology coding, such as bar coding or RFID, that includes two or more person-specific identifiers (not room number) will comply with this requirement."

73. **The Joint Commission evaluates & protects:**
   a. **Safety & quality of patient care**
   b. **Confidentiality of patient information**
   c. **Physician and staff competence**
   d. **Equipment and facility adequacy**

ANSWER: a. Safety & quality of patient care. The Joint Commission (JCAHO) Mission Statement is: "To transform health care into a high-reliability industry by developing highly effective, durable solutions to health care's most critical safety and quality problems in collaboration with health care organizations..."

   HIPPA is more concerned with the confidentiality of patient information, health insurance coverage, and electronic billing.

74. **Signed informed consent documents will <u>not</u> be valid if:**
  a.   **Patient is under age 18 even though guardian is present**
  b.   **Patient does not speak English even though translator is present**
  c.   **Patient has received antiarrhythmic drugs**
  d.   **Patient has mental retardation, or other lack of capacity to understand**
  e.   **Patient's condition has changed to increased risk and was not discussed.**

ANSWER: Patient's condition changes to increased risk and was not discussed. Some other examples of lack of informed consent are:
1. "Where a new procedure is offered, the patient must be informed about whether it was FDA approved, has been tested, and the <u>short and long-term risks</u>."
2. "The patient was talked into the procedure with subtle coercion as the health provider had a financial interest in performing the procedure, prescribing the medication, or using a particular implant device."
3. "The patient was not given enough information that a reasonably prudent physician or health provider would have disclosed."
4. "Safer alternatives were not disclosed along with the advantage and disadvantages of using them."
See: http://www.sswpa.com/informed-consent.asp

4. Transport

75. **To avoid injury to yourself use your strongest muscles while lifting and positioning pati.ents. A cardiovascular specialist should use the strongest muscles in his/her body, which are in the:**
  a.   **Upper extremities**
  b.   **Lower extremities**
  c.   **Core lumbar spinal areas**
  d.   **Core thoracic spinal areas**

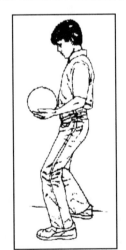

Lifting after Torres

ANSWER b. Lower extremities. The strongest muscles are in the legs or lower extremities. The smaller back muscles frequently are injured because excess strain is placed on them. Besides the legs, your bicep arm muscles are also strong. Both should be used in conjunction with good posture when lifting. Flexing the legs slightly makes the legs a shock absorber and increases balance.
See: Torres, chapter on Basic Patient Care in Diagnostic Imaging." **Keywords:** Body mechanics, use legs

76. How should wheelchair footrests be positioned when moving the patient to or from the wheelchair?
    a.   Moved aside
    b.   Parallel to the floor
    c.   Beneath the patient's feet
    d.   Above the patient's feet

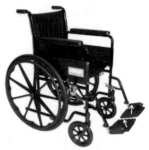

ANSWER a. Moved aside or removed so the patient won't trip over them. In addition when moving a patient into or out of a wheelchair the big wheels must be locked to prevent its rolling.
See: Torres, chapter on "Basic Patient Care in Diagnostic Imaging"
Keywords: Wheelchair

77. What is the best method to move an ambulatory patient from a wheelchair onto a bed or gurney? After lifting the wheelchair foot rests you should assist the patient by standing:
    a.   With 3 other assistants alongside the wheelchair to lift him onto the table with a draw sheet
    b.   Between the patient and the cath. table, one arm on the table and one to help the patient
    c.   With your foot between the patient's feet, and the other close to the cath. table, knees bent
    d.   With both your feet between the patient's feet, knees locked

ANSWER c. With your foot between the patient's feet, and the other close to the cath. table, knees bent. This is a body mechanics question, to make sure the patient is well supported and that you don't hurt your back as you assist him. Of course, you never want to lock your knees. Remain bent to absorb the patient's weight should he fall. One foot should be between the patient's feet to provide direct lifting support from that leg.
See: Torres, chapter on "Basic Patient Care in Diagnostic Imaging" **Keywords:** moving from wheelchair

78. Which of the following are important when moving a patient from the bed to a wheelchair? (Select 4.)
    a.   Get adequate assistance
    b.   Elevate the head of the bed first
    c.   Lower the bed to the level of the wheelchair
    d.   Have the patient swing his legs over the side of the bed
    e.   As you support the patient, twist at your waist while moving him onto the wheelchair

ANSWERS: a, b, c, & d.
a. Get adequate assistance - YES.
b. Elevate the head of the bed first - YES

c. Lower the bed to the level of the wheelchair - YES
d. Have the patient swing his legs over the side of the bed - YES
e. As you support the patient, twist at the waist moving him onto the wheelchair - NO.

MDA says, "To get started lower the patient's bed as far as it will go and raise the head. Support the patient's head and knees. Lift and rotate the patient to a sitting position with their legs hanging over the edge of the bed. At this point some patients will be able to stand and get to the wheelchair on their own.

To prevent back injury to you (the caregiver), bend at the knees, not at the waist, as you prepare to lift someone; then straighten at the hips and knees as you lift.

Keep a wide base of support by spreading your feet apart. If you're transferring someone from one place to another, stagger your feet in a walking position, and shift your weight from front to back as you lift, while keeping the person as close to you as possible.

To avoid back injury: When turning, pivot on your feet or move them. Don't twist at the waist. **See:**
www.mda.org/sites/default/files/publications/Everyday_Life_with_ALS_P-532.pdf

5. Patient Safety & Risk Management

79. **What does this symbol with 3 broken semicircles stand for?**
  a.   **Poison**
  b.   **Fire danger**
  c.   **Biohazard**
  d.   **Radiation hazard**

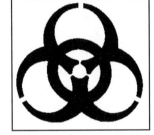

What is this symbol?

ANSWER c. Biohazard. OSHA says: "Labeling: The standard requires that fluorescent orange or orange-red warning labels be attached to containers of regulated waste, to refrigerators and freezers containing blood and other potentially infectious materials, and to other containers used to store, transport, or ship blood or other potentially infectious materials" Used on "sharps" containers and "biohazard bags".
See: OSHA Regulations on Bloodborne Pathogens **Keywords:** Biohazard symbol

80. **Your patient has a latex allergy. What should be avoided because it typically contains rubber?**
  a.   **R2 pads**
  b.   **Endotracheal tubes**
  c.   **Swan-Ganz catheter**
  d.   **Silastic pacemaker leads**

ANSWER: c. Swan-Ganz catheter balloon contains latex. Non-rubber based balloon catheters are available. Myers article states, "almost all Swan-Ganz catheters contain at least a latex balloon...If a hypersensitivity reaction occurs, without a history of prior allergic reaction, consider latex as a potential allergen and remove all latex products from patient contact...A completely latex-free environment should be provided for such [hypersensitive] patients..." "Arrow" makes a latex free Swan. **See:** Myers, "Latex Versus Iodinated Contrast Media Anapylaxis in the Cardiac Cath Lab" in Catheterization and Cardiovascular Diagnosis 35:228-231 (1995) **Keywords:** latex allergy

81.   **You inserted an IV catheter and started a dopamine drip on a patient 30 minutes ago. Now the patient is complaining of coldness and swelling at the IV site. What should you do FIRST?**
a.   **Stop the IV and attempt to aspirate**
b.   **Stop the IV and apply pressure to the swollen area**
c.   **Open up the IV to see if it flows freely**
d.   **Lower the IV bag below the level of the heart to see if you get blood or fluid coming back**

ANSWER: a. Stop the IV and attempt to aspirate. Hadaway says, "Extravasation occurs when a peripheral catheter erodes through the vessel wall at a second point, when increased venous pressure causes leakage around the original venipuncture site, or when a needle pulls out of the vein. Signs and symptoms of extravasation include edema and changes in the site's appearance and temperature, such as swelling, blanching, and coolness. The patient may complain of pain or a feeling of tightness around the site.... antibiotics, electrolytes or vasopressors cause severe tissue injury or destruction when they extravasate....If extravasation occurs... Immediately stop the infusion and disconnect the tubing as close to the catheter hub as possible. Attach a syringe to the hub and attempt to aspirate the remaining drug from the catheter....If aspiration was unsuccessful, remove the catheter without placing pressure on the site. Elevate the affected arm. ...For most extravasations, you'll apply ice for 20 minutes at least four times a day for 24 to 48 hours." Consider injecting an antidote to the infused drug if necessary. **See:** online: "Preventing and managing peripheral extravasation" Nursing, May 2004 by Hadaway, Lynn C **Keywords:** Extravasation - Stop the IV and attempt to aspirate

82.   **You are alone in the cath lab. Your patient arrives early on a stretcher outside the cath lab entrance. The orderly says he has to leave, but the side rails are up and safety strap is in place. You note that she is sleeping and secure, so you go next door to get some last minute supplies. While you are gone she somehow climbs off the stretcher, falls and breaks her hip.**
a.   **You can be charged with assault**
b.   **You can be charged with abandonment**
c.   **The orderly can be charged with malpractice**
d.   **You cannot be charged because all safety devices were in place**

ANSWER b. You can be charged with abandonment in court, because standard procedures say that a patient should never be left alone at any time while in the care of cath lab personnel. You cannot be charged with assault because you did not even touch the patient. Your job should have been to inform the orderly that he cannot leave because you have not set up the room yet. **See:** Allmers, Review for Surgical Tech. Exam, chapter on "Fundamentals" **Keywords:** Leaving patient alone = abandonment

6. Communication and Instruction

83.   You have just completed an echocardiogram. Your patient asks you to interpret the results of his diagnostic examination. Your response as a healthcare professional should be to:
    a.   Say you don't know how to interpret results
    b.   Explain that the physician will interpret it and report the results
    c.   Explain that the final results are inconclusive
    d.   Honestly interpret it to the best of your ability

ANSWER b. Explain that the physician will interpret it and report the results. One of the 10 principles of professional conduct adopted by the ARRT is "Radiologic Technologists shall not diagnose, but in recognition of their responsibility to the patient, they shall provide the physician with all information they have relative to radiologic diagnosis for patient management." We do not possess all the information or training necessary to diagnose the patient. Diagnosis, pathology and treatment are the physician's final responsibility. We can often reinforce his comments, clarify things and respond to our patient's questions, but always with the qualification that the physician has the final say.
See: Torres, chapter on "The Radiologic Technologist and professionalism" **Keywords:** Professionalism, when patient wants diagnosis

84.   Your patient is noncompliant in taking his medications for systemic hypertension. He should be taught that a common complication of uncontrolled hypertension is:
    a.   Arterial calcification
    b.   Cerebral hemorrhage
    c.   Congestive heart failure
    d.   Pulmonary fibrosis with pulmonary hypertension

ANSWER b. Cerebral hemorrhage leading to stroke. Hemorrhaging and occlusion of blood vessels in the body are common complications of uncontrolled hypertension. This complication can occur in the brain (stroke), the eyes, the heart (myocardial infarction) and the kidneys. It is our professional duty to educate such patients and alert them to the risks of not taking their medication. **See:** Lippincott's State Board Review for NCLEX-PN.
Keywords: Untreated Hypertension = stroke

85.   Your patient is told that he has a poor prognosis, but says he believes there is some mistake. According to Dr. Elisabeth Kubler- Ross, this patient is most probably in what grief stage?
    a.   Anger
    b.   Denial
    c.   Bargaining
    d.   Depression

ANSWER b. Denial. "When a terminally ill person states that there must be a mistake or that he is being confused with someone else, he is most probably denying his impending death. These 5 stages of grief are described by Dr. Elisabeth Kubler- Ross:

1. **Denial & disbelief**   "What! There must be some mistake "
2. **Anger**   "Why me?"
3. **Bargaining**   "If I'm healed, I promise to..."
4. **Depression**   "Oh God! Wherefore art thou?"
5. **Acceptance**   "OK. Thy will be done."

See: Lippincott's State Board Review for NCLEX-PN. **Keywords:** Stages Grief

---

86.   **A lack of demonstrated care or skill, which is unreasonable or imprudent from a medical professional, is termed:**

a.   **Assault**
b.   **Abandonment**
c.   **Negligence**
d.   **Battery**

ANSWER c. Negligence is legally defined as the omission to do something which a reasonable and prudent person would do, or doing something which a reasonable and prudent person would not do. For example a circulating nurse who fails to establish a patient's identity prior to an invasive procedure is negligent.
See: Medical Dictionary

---

87.   **The legal rule that holds each individual responsible for his or her own actions is termed:**

a.   **Legal duty**
b.   **Liability**
c.   **Contract law**
d.   **Malpractice**

ANSWER b. Liability holds each individual responsible for his or her own acts. If our actions cause injury, loss, or damage to a patient, we are liable. Liability means we are legally bound, answerable, and responsible to our patients. Patients or family members may institute civil actions against any person who does not fully meet their obligations to protect the patient from injury and provide the best care possible.
See: Medical Dictionary **Keywords:** Liability

---

88.   **Criteria that identifies, measures, monitors, and evaluates patient care come from:**

a.   **OSHA regulations**
b.   **Medicare guidelines**
c.   **Automated information systems**
d.   **Quality assurance programs**

ANSWER d. Quality assurance programs establish criteria, identify, measure, monitor, and evaluate patient care. Such programs are often mandated by Joint commission (JCAHO). This agency sets the standards for optimal care, patient safety and continuity of patient care in medical facilities. Occupational Safety and Health Administration (OSHA) is a US

federal agency that regulates workplace safety and health.
See: Allmers, chapter on "Fundamentals" **Keywords:** Quality assurance programs

89. **What worldwide registry collects clinical data for hospital quality improvement? Their quarterly reports compare your hospital to others in relevant cardiac areas like: Door to Balloon time, STEMI Mortality, and other outcome metrics.?**
   a. **The Joint Commision(TJC)**
   b. **World Health Organization (WHO)**
   c. **Occupational Safety and Health Administration (OSHA)**
   d. **ACC's National Cardiovascular DataBase Registry (NCDR)**

ANSWER: d. ACC's National Cardiovascular DataBase Registry (NCDR) promotes quality improvement through the collection and use of clinical data for benchmarking, as well as linked quality tools and quality initiatives, education, and outcomes research. Over 2,400 hospitals participate in NCDR programs. A sample of their quarterly report comparing your hospital to others is shown below. Note that your #18 STEMI mortality rate is below average.

   ACC says, "ACC, Quality Improvement for Institutions, A Comprehensive Suite of Registries: Currently, the NCDR suite of cardiovascular data registries like...

ACC NCDR Registry for quality improvement		PCI Process Metrics
2 Proportion of elective PCIs with prior positive stress or imaging study		
My Hospital	US Hospitals 50th Pctl	US Hospitals 90th Pctl
74.5 %	67.51%	90.02%
Proportion of elective PCI procedures (excluding patients with ACS) with an antecedent stress or imaging study with a positive result (suggestive of ischemia) or with a fractional flow reserve value of <=0.8 during the PCI procedure [Detail Line:1513]		
19 PCI in-hospital risk adjusted mortality (STEMI patients excluded)		
My Hospital	US Hospitals 50th Pctl	US Hospitals 90th Pctl
59%	0.87	0.41
Your hospital's PCI in-hospital risk adjusted mortality rate for patients with other diagnoses (not STEMI) using the NCDR® risk adjustment model. [Detail Line:2054]		
18 PCI in-hospital risk adjusted mortality (patients with STEMI)		
My Hospital	US Hospitals 50th Pctl	US Hospitals 90th Pctl
7.7	6.50	3.44
Your hospital's PCI in-hospital risk adjusted mortality rate for patients with STEMI adjusted using the NCDR® risk adjustment model. [Detail Line:2045]		

Acute myocardial infarction treatment and Diagnostic cardiac catheterization and PCI....Door to Balloon (D2B), Hospital to Home (H2H), Surviving MI, and other campaigns.... seeks to use data to increase the adoption of evidence-based strategies associated with lower 30-day risk standardized mortality rates (RSMR) for patients hospitalized with acute myocardial infarction (AMI).... Quarterly risk-adjusted benchmark reports with performance measures and quality metrics to compare an institution's performance with that of peer groups and the national experience." See, https://cvquality.acc.org/NCDR-Home/reports

90. **Most invasive malpractice claims could be avoided by:**
   a. **Thinking before you act**
   b. **Obtaining properly informed consent**
   c. **Clearer handwriting in the medical record**
   d. **Better communication with the patient**

ANSWER d. Better communication with the patient. Kern says: "Medical malpractice actions are frequently initiated as a result of unresolved anger and frustration of the part of the patient.... The best advice in this area is to try always to keep lines of communication

open between the provider (Dr., nurse, technologist) and the patient. Remember to take the time to let your patient know that he or she is important to you."
See: Kern, chapter on "Documentation in the Cardiac Catheterization Laboratory"
Keywords: malpractice = frustrated patient, communicate

91. **Which of the following are included in the "Patient's Bill of Rights"? (Select 3.)**
   a. **Refusal of treatment**
   b. **Continuity of care**
   c. **Possession of their medical images**
   d. **Confidentiality of their medical records**

ANSWERS: a, b, & d.
a. Refusal of treatment - YES.
b. Continuity of care - YES.
c. Possession of their medical images - NO.
d. Confidentiality of their medical records - YES.

The American Hospital Association identifies 12 important areas in their "Patient's Bill of Rights." These rights do not include the right to possess their original medical images. Although, most physicians will freely give image copies to patients, they are not qualified to interpret them. And the originals remain in the medical record as property of the hospital or laboratory. **See:** Appleton & Lange's Review for the Radiographic Examination, chapter on "Patient Care" **Keywords:** Patient's Bill of rights

92. **When teaching a patient to care for his femoral artery puncture site following angiography, which instruction below is correct?**
   a. **"Try to cough up any fluid in your lungs"**
   b. **"Keep you hand on the bandage to feel for wetness or bleeding."**
   c. **"Don't sit up by yourself. But, the nurse may elevate your bed to a slight sit up position."**
   d. **"Occasionally raise your head to look down at your groin to see if it's bleeding. If it is, call the nurse."**

ANSWER: c. "Don't sit up by yourself. But, the nurse may elevate your bed to a slight sit up position." Kern says, "The patient should be given the following instructions:
   1. Keep your head down
   2. Hold the groin site when coughing
   3. Keep punctured leg straight
   4. Stay in bed
   5. Drink fluids
   6. Call a nurse for assistance if there is bleeding, leg numbness or pain, or chest pain."
See: Kern, chapter on "Arterial and Venous Access" **Keywords:** Hemostasis teaching

93. Your patient had a diagnostic left heart cath with 6F catheters. When giving instructions after holding manual pressure post-cath, which of the following are correct? (Select 4.)
  a. "Drink lots of fluids."
  b. "Don't lift your head off the pillow."
  c. "Keep your leg straight. Don't bend it."
  d. "If after 2 hours you still can't urinate, sit up and try harder."
  e. "Don't cough. If you must cough, hold pressure on the puncture site."
  f. "Don't laugh. If you must laugh, hold your hand over your mouth."

ANSWERS: a, b, c, & e.

  a. "Drink lots of fluids." - YES
  b. "Don't lift your head off the pillow." - YES
  c. "Keep your leg straight. Don't bend it." - YES
  d. "If after 2 hours you still can't urinate, sit up and try harder." - NO
  e. "Don't cough. If you must cough, hold pressure on the puncture site." - YES

Two things are WRONG: don't sit up and don't force urination. Kern says, "Depending on the catheter and sheath size, the patient is kept at bed rest for 2 to 6 hours after femoral artery puncture. With small diameter catheters (i.e. ≤5F) shorter times (<2 hrs) can be used. The patient should be given the following instructions:
  1. Keep your head down
  2. Hold the groin site when coughing
  3. Keep punctured leg straight
  4. Stay in bed
  5. Drink fluids
  6. Call a nurse for assistance if there is bleeding, leg numbness or pain, or chest pain."
See: Kern, chapter on "Arterial and Venous Access" **Keywords:** Hemostasis teaching

7. History, Physical Exam & Patient Assessment

94. If the following items appear in your patient's health history, which one is most significant in terms of predisposing her to hypertension?
  a. Having had 3 children in less than 4 years
  b. Having had childhood German measles (rubella)
  c. Having two grandparents who died of the disorder
  d. Having been underweight all of her life, including during pregnancies

ANSWER c. Having two grandparents who died of the disorder. The exact cause of primary hypertension is unknown. However, heredity appears to play an important role, because strong familial tendencies are often noted. Other factors that appear to bring on hypertension include obesity, emotional stress, smoking, and high blood sodium and cholesterol levels.
See: Lippincott's State Board Review for NCLEX-PN. **Keywords:** hereditary hypertension

95. Identify 3 predisposing factors for acute myocardial infarction (MI).
   a.   Hyperglycemia
   b.   Hypertension
   c.   Hyperlipidemia
   d.   Hyperestrogenism
   e.   Elevated high-density lipoprotein cholesterol (HDL-C)

ANSWERS: a, b, & c.
a. Hyperglycemia - YES
b. Hypertension - YES
c. Hyperlipidemia - YES
d. Hyperestrogenism (high estrogen levels) - NO
e. Elevated high-density lipoprotein cholesterol (HDL-C)
Estrogen, is in a group of hormones found in women, that protect women from heart disease. After menopause, when estrogen levels fall in women, they begin to develop coronary disease akin to men. Hyperglycemia, hypertension, and hyperlipidemia (high cholesterol) are all risk factors for atherosclerosis. When both men and women pass middle age their sex hormones decline and they develop increasing risk for CAD. Metabolic syndrome develops. HDL-C is protective against heart disease. LDL is bad.
See: Braunwald, chapter on "Coronary Risk Factors" **Keywords:** Estrogen protective MI

HEART SOUNDS

96. If you suspect that your patient has an organic heart murmur, the cause of such a murmur would probably be a defect in the:
   a.   Conduction system
   b.   Coronary arteries
   c.   Mixing of blood
   d.   Action of the heart valves

ANSWER d. Action of the heart valves. An organic heart murmur is caused by a defect in the action of heart valves such as stenosis or leakage (regurgitation or shunt). A functional heart disorder, in contrast to an organic heart disease, is a disturbance in function only with no organic cause. A functional heart murmur is often caused by anxiety or exercise.
Heart murmurs are unrelated to oxygenation of blood, the heart's ability to pump, or the capacity of coronary arteries.
See: Lippincott's State Board Review for NCLEX-PN. **Keywords:** organic heart murmur

97. Your patient reports having had an illness which predisposed her to having a heart murmur. What childhood disease was this?
   a.   Measles
   b.   Mononucleosis
   c.   Rheumatic fever
   d.   Whooping cough

ANSWER c. Rheumatic fever. Patients who have had rheumatic fever often have heart valve problems, such as mitral stenosis, later in life. Although mostly eliminated in the USA due to the advent of antibiotics, it is common in tropical countries. **See:** Lippincott's State Board Review for NCLEX-PN. **Keywords:** Rheumatic fever =heart valve stenosis

98. **Where is the point of maximum intensity (PMI) normally seen and felt on the chest?**
   a.   **LV apex**
   b.   **Right precordium**
   c.   **V6 lead position**
   d.   **V2 lead position**

ANSWER a. LV apex hits the chest wall during systole making a palpable thump. This location is normally felt around th V4 ECG position beneath the left nipple. However, it can shift leftward in LV hypertrophy. PMI means "Point Maximum Intensity" on the chest. **See:** Braunwald, chapter on "Physical Exam" **Keywords:** PMI = LV apex = V4

99.   **Moist or crackling auscultatory sounds heard at the base of the lung are termed:**
   a.   **Bruits**
   b.   **Murmurs**
   c.   **Rales**
   d.   **Wheezes**

ANSWER c. Rales are crackling sounds heard best at the base of the lung, like crinkling cellophane or pop fizzing. They indicate fluid in bronchi & alveoli. Moist rales are the bubbling or gurgling lung sounds due to transudation of fluid into the alveoli. This fluid then moves into the airways and gurgles on inspiration. These sounds are often accompanied by expectoration of frothy, blood-tinged sputum.

Pulmonary RALES

OTHER ABNORMAL SOUNDS LISTED ARE:
1. **BRUITS:** Blowing sound heard over an aneurysm or
      stenosis
2. **MURMURS:** Heart sound
3. **RALES** (moist): Abnormal respiratory sound due to fluid in the air passage
4. **WHEEZES:** whistling or high pitched buzzing breath sound.
See: Braunwald, chapter on "Clinical Aspect of Heart Failure" also, see Todd's, Vol. I, chapter on "Heart Failure and Shock." **Keywords:** CHF, inadequate emptying LA

100. **Murmurs on the _____ side of the heart are affected the most by _____.**
   a.   **Right heart, respirations**
   b.   **Right heart, stress/exercise**
   c.   **Left heart,   respirations**
   d.   **Left heart,   stress/exercise**

ANSWER a. Right heart, respirations. The right side of the heart supplies the lungs. And, intrapleural pressure effect the right side more than the left because of the lower pressures generated there. For example, the negative pleural pressure associated with inspiration pulls in more venous blood to the RA, forcing the RV to increase its stroke volume and delay pulmonary valve closure. Respiration has a dramatic effect on right sided heart murmurs. **See:** Braunwald, chapter on "Physical Examination" **Keywords:** Right side murmurs affected by respiration

101. **The term "thrill" is used to describe which of the following?**
   a.   **Soft murmurs**
   b.   **Loud murmurs**
   c.   **A palpable heart sound or murmur**
   d.   **A palpable venous pulse**

ANSWER c. A palpable heart sound or murmur. When the examiner uses his hands to palpate a patient he may feel a low frequency vibration over the area of a heart murmur. If it is palpable it is probably a severe murmur.
See: Braunwald, chapter on "The Physical Examination." **Keywords:** thrill

102. **A bruit is a:**
   a.   **Type of hematoma**
   b.   **Lung sound, caused by fluid accumulation in the alveoli**
   c.   **Red spot on the skin caused by a small arterial embolus**
   d.   **Sound heard over a blood vessel**

ANSWER d. Sound heard over a blood vessel. These are like murmurs, but heard with a stethoscope over an artery that is stenosed, especially the carotid and femoral arteries. A bruit is usually a soft blowing sound heard loudest in systole.
See: Braunwald, chapter on "Physical Exam." **Keywords:** Bruit

103. **When a systolic murmur suddenly develops in a patient 12 hours after an MI you should suspect:**
   a.   **Aortic insufficiency**
   b.   **Papillary muscle dysfunction**
   c.   **Ventricular aneurysm**
   d.   **Early pericarditis**

ANSWER b. Papillary muscle dysfunction or rupture leads to severe mitral regurgitation and associated systolic murmur. This may occur when a papillary muscle becomes necrotic following an MI. The mitral valve leaflet is then not supported during systole. It prolapses and leaks. See: Braunwald, chapter on "Valvular Heart Disease." **Keywords:** Papillary muscle dysfunction post MI

104. Loud 3rd or 4th heart sounds are termed:
   a.   Gallops
   b.   Murmurs
   c.   Palpitations
   d.   Click or snaps

ANSWER: a. Diastolic gallop sounds. The first two heart sounds separate systole and diastole. The last sounds S3 & S4 are the diastolic filling sounds. S3 is due to rapid ventricular filling and S4 is due to atrial contraction. The normal heart rhythm contains two audible heart sounds called S1 and S2 that give the well-known "lub-dub" rhythm caused by the closing of heart valves. A gallop rhythm contains additional 3rd or 4th heart sounds. It can also contain both of these sounds forming a quadruple gallop, and in situations of very fast heart rate can produce a summation gallop where S3 and S4 occur so close as to be indistinguishable.

FOLEY CATHETERIZATION (Removed from RCIS exam 2013)

105. A Foley retention catheter is positioned in the _____ and the balloon is inflated with _____.
   a.   Intestine, air
   b.   Intestine, saline
   c.   Bladder, air
   d.   Bladder, saline

ANSWER: d. Urinary bladder, saline or other fluid. A Foley retention catheter drains urine from the bladder into a collection bag. It is retained in place with a rubber balloon at the tip which is inflated with fluid.
See: Mosby's Comprehensive Review of Nursing for NCLEX-RN, Chapter on "Urinary systems" **Keywords:** Foley in bladder filled with saline

106. When a Foley retention catheter is placed it should be inserted in the urethra until:
   a.   Urine flows
   b.   The balloon opens
   c.   Resistance is felt
   d.   A decrease in resistance is felt

ANSWER a. Urine flows when the catheter enters the bladder. As a urinary catheter passes the urethral sphincter and enters the bladder, urine will begin to flow through the catheter into the drainage bag. Then it should be inserted several cm. more to enter the urinary bladder. The catheter tip should be lubricated and passed easily without undue resistance. Only after the catheter tip is properly positioned should the retention balloon be inflated.
See: Mosby's Comprehensive Review of Nursing for NCLEX-RN, Chapter on "Urinary systems" **Keywords:** Insert Foley until urine flows

107. When a patient arrives in your vascular lab with a Foley catheter bag, it is important to:
   a.   Place the drainage bag above the level of the bladder
   b.   Place the drainage bag below the level of the bladder
   c.   Clamp the Foley catheter for the time of the study
   d.   Not touch the tubing or bag

ANSWER b. Place the Foley drainage bag below the level of the bladder so it can properly drain by gravity. **See:** Appleton & Lange's Review for the Radiographic Examination, chapter on "Patient Care" Never place the bag on the patient during transport. It could lead to urinary track infection. **Keywords:** Foley lower than bed

108. During cardiac catheterization, a patient with congestive heart failure in the cath lab becomes extremely short of breath. The physician orders furosemide (Lasix) 40 mg given IV. The physician will probably follow up this order by ordering a/an:
   a.   Foley catheter
   b.   Fogarty catheter
   c.   Multipurpose catheter
   d.   Additional IV line for the furosemide infusion

ANSWER a. Foley catheter. The usual initial dose of furosemide is 20 mg to 40 mg given as a single dose, injected intramuscularly or intravenously. The intravenous dose should be given slowly (1 to 2 minutes). Ordinarily a prompt diuresis ensues. A Foley catheter will prevent you having to give the patient a urinal or a bedpan every few minutes. The urine volume is measured to evaluate patient fluid output. E.g., One sign of shock is low urine output. See: Mosby's Comprehensive Review of Nursing for NCLEX-RN, Chapter on "Urinary systems"

8. Patient Assessment - Signs and Symptoms

109. Which factors below may precipitate angina pectoris? (Select 3.)
   a.   Alcohol consumption
   b.   Eating a large meal
   c.   Smoking
   d.   Emotional stress
   e.   Straining (ValSalva)

ANSWERS: b, c, & d. (Eating a large meal, smoking, and emotional stress.)
Alcohol consumption in moderation does not precipitate angina. Recent studies suggest that one alcoholic drink daily may be beneficial for atherosclerosis especially red wine. Stable angina comes on with exertion, smoking, or cold temperatures, eating large meals, and is relieved by rest or nitroglycerine.
See: Braunwald, chapter on "Chronic Coronary Artery Disease." **Keywords:** Alcohol OK

110. **Signs and symptoms of a distal aortic dissecting aneurysm include:**
- a.　**Hypotension, tachycardia, radiating back pain**
- b.　**Hypotension, bradycardia, EKG changes**
- c.　**Anterior chest pain, radiating to the left arm, dyspnea, syncope**
- d.　**Hypertension, vomiting, EKG changes**

ANSWER a. Hypotension, tachycardia, radiating back pain. The pain associated with aortic dissection is described as: ripping, tearing, or stabbing. This pain is often "cataclysmic" in onset. It may be all but unbearable, and patients may writhe in agony. It is unlike angina pain in that it is usually as severe as it is going to get during the initial dissection, whereas angina usually increases as time goes on. Neither does this pain migrate down the arm as angina does. The location of the pain is usually in the anterior chest for proximal dissections, in the neck or jaw for arch dissections, or in the back for distal dissections. **See:** Braunwald, chapter on "Diseases of the Aorta." **Keywords:** AO dissection = PAIN

111. **Retrosternal chest pain that is associated with sweating, nausea or vomiting, and not relieved by rest and nitroglycerine is most likely due to:**
- a.　**Pericarditis**
- b.　**Crescendo angina**
- c.　**Aortic dissection**
- d.　**Myocardial infarction**

ANSWER d. Myocardial infarction. Braunwald says about MI: "The pain of AMI is variable in intensity; in most patients it is severe...prolonged. described as constricting, crushing, oppressing,... The pain is usually retrosternal in location, spreading frequently to both sides of the anterior chest, with predilection for the left side. Often the pain radiates....Nausea and vomiting occur in more than 50 percent of patients with transmural MI and severe chest pain,...." **See:** Braunwald, chapter on "Acute Myocardial Infarction" **Keywords:** Symptoms MI

112. **What signs and/or symptoms are associated with dependent edema?**
- a.　**Swollen legs**
- b.　**Swollen sore joints**
- c.　**Pulmonitis and coughing**
- d.　**Pulmonary congestion**

ANSWER a. Swollen & puffy legs. Being dependent (meaning the part of the body nearest the ground) fluid may accumulate in the lowest parts of the body, usually the legs. This is often associated with heart failure, where the right heart cannot pump out adequate venous return. Fluid and electrolyte balance is important in regulating all forms of edema. **See:** Medical Dictionary **Keywords:** dependent edema

113. **A patient tells you that he has "awful palpitations" meaning he:**
   a.   Feels a sensation of heat and flushing
   b.   Feels that his heart rate is rapid or irregular
   c.   Feels that he cannot get his breath
   d.   Feels a sense of impending doom

ANSWER b. Feels that his heart rate is rapid or irregular. Palpitations are a patient's subjective awareness that his heart rate is unduly rapid, irregular or fluttering. This is usually an arrhythmia or series of PVCs.
See: Medical Dictionary   **Keywords:** Palpitations

114. **Your patient is in atrial fibrillation. For the most accurate HR:**
   a.   Count pulses for 1 min
   b.   Measure HR in morning before eating
   c.   Measure on ECG as 1 RR interval, divided into 60
   d.   Average half-way between the fastest rate and the slowest rates

ANSWER: a. Count pulses for 1 min. to get the most accurate average heart rate .The problem with atrial fibrillation is the complete irregularity of the heart rate. Often every beat has a different RR interval. So, measuring one beat will not give an accurate average heart rate. The longer you can measure the pulse, the more accurate the average.
Reference: Personal experience   **Keywords:** AF count HR

115. **The admitting nurse reports that your patient has tachypnea. This means that your patient has:**
   a.   Rapid heart rate
   b.   High blood pressure
   c.   Rapid respiratory rate
   d.   Labored breathing

ANSWER c. Rapid respiratory rate. Tachy means fast, as in tachycardia. Tachypnea means rapid respirations. Dyspnea is a term to describe labored or difficult respirations. Noisy respirations are referred to as stertorous breathing. Moist respirations are often associated with pulmonary edema, and may be termed rales or ronchi. There is no term for describing shallow respirations. **See:** Medical Dictionary **Keywords:** tachypnea

116. **You observe your African-American patient for cyanosis. The area of the patient's body where cyanosis is most likely to be apparent in dark skinned individuals is:**
   a.   Scalp
   b.   Ear lobes
   c.   White of the eyes
   d.   Oral mucosa

ANSWER d. Oral mucosa. Cyanotic blue discoloration due to oxygen desaturation is usually easiest to detect first where the body's vessels are near the surface. These areas are the nail-beds, the lips, the earlobes, and the oral mucous membranes. In the person with dark skin, cyanosis usually is observed best in the oral mucosa.
See: Lippincott's State Board Review for NCLEX-PN. **Keywords:** Cyanotic blue lips

117. One indicator of cardiogenic shock is:
a.   **Bradycardia**
b.   **Hypertension**
c.   **Pyrexia**
d.   **Oliguria**

ANSWER d. Oliguria is decreased urine production. It is one of the signs of cardiogenic shock. Other signs are hypotension, tachycardia, cold clammy skin, and cyanosis. These signs can also be caused by hypovolemia. Braunwald states that "Shock encompasses the syndromes associated with an acute reduction in effective blood flow with failure to maintain the transfer and delivery of essential substrates to sustain the function of vital organ systems." In shock, blood is shunted to vital organs (such as the brain), and away from less essential tissues (skin). **See:** Braunwald, chapter on "Acute Circulatory Failure (Shock)." **Keywords:** Shock Signs

118. Amaurosis fugax is a symptom that involves the patient's:
a.   **Sight**
b.   **Hearing**
c.   **Equilibrium**
d.   **Sensation of pain**

ANSWER a. Sight. Amaurosis fugax is a temporary episode of blindness in one eye, or partial blindness. It is often a sign of TIA or cerebral ischemia suggesting carotid stenosis. **See:** Medical dictionary **Keywords:** Amaurosis fugax = blindness in one eye

119. Identify 4 signs of acute stroke. (Select 4 below.)
a.   **Weakness or numbness on one side of the body/face**
b.   **Trouble speaking or understanding**
c.   **Trouble seeing in one or both eyes**
d.   **Loss of coordination**
e.   **Severe chest or left arm pain**

ANSWERS: a, b, c, & d.
a. Weakness or numbness on one side of the body/face - YES.
b. Trouble speaking or understanding - YES.
c. Trouble seeing in one or both eyes - YES.
d. Loss of coordination - YES.
e. Severe chest or left arm pain - NO.

Current guidelines say, "The signs and symptoms of stroke include sudden weakness or numbness on one side of the body; sudden confusion; trouble speaking; trouble seeing in one or both eyes; trouble walking, dizziness, loss of coordination; or sudden severe headache." Severe chest or arm pain is associated with heart attack, not brain attack. **See:** http://circ.ahajournals.org/content/122/18_suppl_3/S818.full

120. **What is the scoring system used to assess the effects of conscious sedation on patients in 5 different areas?**
a.   **Aldrete**
b.   **Apgar**
c.   **Ramsay**
d.   **Mallampati**

ANSWER: a. Aldrete.
The Aldrete scoring system evaluates patients in 5 areas to assess the effects of sedation on the patient's major body systems. Most labs use the "Modified Aldrete" with a maximum score is 10. A score of 0, 1, or 2 is given for the level of respiratory ability, O2 saturation, level of consciousness, circulation (blood pressure), and activity (movement). (See chart 1 - "The Modified Aldrete scale." in the next question.) Before a patient is discharged to the floor, after careful monitoring, the Aldrete score should have returned to baseline, usually 8 or greater. Another scoring system is the Mallampati score that determine the patient's ease of intubation. **See:** Ginapp, Cath Lab Digest, 7/12

121. **A patient post anesthesia is fully alert & has recovered his normal motor functions and BP. However, he still is dyspneic and requires O2 to maintain his O2 sat >90%. What would the modified Aldrete score be?**
a.   **2**
b.   **4**
c.   **6**
d   **8**
e.   **12**

Chart 1. The 'modified' Aldrete Scale

	2	1	0
RESPIRATION	Able to take deep breath and cough	Dyspnea/Shallow Breathing	Apnea
O2 SATURATION	Maintains > 92% on room air	Needs O2 inhalation to maintain O2 saturation > 90%	Saturation < 90% even with supplemental O2
CONSCIOUSNESS	Fully awake	Arousable on calling	Not responding
CIRCULATION	BP ± 20mmHg pre op	BP ± 20-50mmHg pre op	BP ± 50mmHg pre op
ACTIVITY	Able to move 4 extremities voluntarily or on command	Able to move 2 extremities voluntarily or on command	Able to move 0 extremities voluntarily or on command

From: Ginapp, "Ask the Instructor." Cath Lab Digest, July 2012

ANSWER: d. 8 on the Modified Aldrete score, because 2 of the evaluations on the chart are down from 2 to 1.
Dyspnea takes one point off the Respiration index and requiring O2 takes one point off the O2 Sat. index. Maximum Aldrete score is 10. So, 2 points have been deducted, giving a total of 8. He should probably be monitored further until the Aldrete score raises to at least 9. This assumes he is not normally short of breath or on oxygen. See Chart 1 above.
See: Ginapp, Cath Lab Digest, 7/12

122. An ex-smoker comes to the cath lab with a BP of 155 systolic and an O2 sat of 92% on low flow nasal oxygen. He received conscious sedation during his PCI. After successful hemostasis he is moved to the Post-Anesthesia Care Unit (PACU) and monitored for 2 hours. His reflexes are now normal and he is alert. When should the patient be discharged back to the floor?

a. If fully conscious he is able to be moved now

b. Only when the O2 sat on oxygen exceeds 95%

c. When his Aldrete score has returned to baseline

d. Only when all monitored parameters are within normal limits

ANSWER: d. When his Aldrete score has returned to baseline the patient may be discharged. This patient comes to the lab with a lowered Aldrete score due to low O2 sat and elevated BP. His score is probably 8 pre-cath. That is his normal. He should not be moved until he has returned back to his normal level. He may never reach the full 9 or 10 score expected of normal individuals. See: Cath Lab Digest 2012

Ginapp says, "One of the requirements of patient assessment and care after sedation is to evaluate the patient's recovery as the sedation wears off... The staff will utilize this scale to decide when the patient is "recovered" enough to move through the phases of PACU, and ultimately to go home or back to their room. To apply this scale, it is very important to know the patient "pre-anesthesia" score. Some patients may have "normal" abnormalities that change the score. To know, and have documented, what the pre-sedation assessment was is very important in order to determine the post-sedation assessment as the patient returns to their "normal" status."

Kerns says, "Patients who receive conscious sedation should be monitored for 1 to 2 hours before discharge. During this time the patient should be assessed and monitored with the same parameters used in the preprocedural assessment. When the patient returns to baseline, discharge is appropriate." See: Kern, chapter on "The Catheterization Laboratory"

123. An apparently normal female patient received conscious sedation during a coronary intervention. After being monitored for 2 hours post-cath in the PACU her Aldrete score is 7. Based on this score, she will generally be:

a. Returned to the OR or cath lab

b. Transferred out of the PACU into the ICU

c. Discharged to her hospital bed and room

d. Retained in the PACU until condition improves

ANSWER d. Retained in the PACU until condition improves

Kern says: " The following discharge criteria should be met before the patient is sent back to the floor or home:

1. The Aldrete score has returned to baseline (summed Aldrete scores of 9 or 10).

2. At least 2 hours have elapsed since the last dose of sedative agents.

3. Vital signs have returned to baseline.

4. Ventilation (respiratory rate and oxygen saturation) has returned to baseline.

5. The patient is mentally alert, and all protective reflexes are intact."

See: Kern, chapter on "The Catheterization Laboratory"

BLOOD PRESSURE

124. Before placing the bell of your stethoscope over your patient's brachial artery to obtain the blood pressure, you should first:
a.   Feel for the patient's pulse at the radial artery
b.   Pump up the pressure cuff on the patient's arm
c.   Feel for the patient's pulse at the brachial artery
d.   Raise the patient's arm above his/her head momentarily

ANSWER c. Feel for the patient's pulse at the brachial artery. When obtaining the blood pressure, before adjusting the bell of the stethoscope, you should feel for the patient's pulse at the brachial artery. This technique allows you to place the stethoscope bell directly over the artery where she will listen for characteristic sounds when obtaining blood pressure. **See:** Lippincott's State Board Review for NCLEX-PN. **Keywords:** BP - Feel for the pulse

125. To take an accurate auscultatory blood pressure:
a.   Talk frequently to the patient to relax him
b.   Read pressures to nearest 2 mmHg.
c.   After pumping up the cuff, deflate the cuff 5-10 mmHg/sec
d   Be sure the inflatable bladder in the cuff encircles 100% of the arm circumference
e.   Prior to placing the stethoscope on the arm, pump up the pressure cuff to around 300 mmHg

ANSWER: b. Read pressures to nearest 2 mmHg. is correct. Trying to read to the nearest mmHg is difficult or impossible.   Most analog BP devices are graduated in 2 mm intervals.
The mercury column should be deflated at 2 to 3 mm/s, and the first and last audible sounds should be taken as systolic and diastolic pressure. When the auscultatory BP is taken, the cuff should be inflated to a pressure approximately 30 mmHg greater than systolic, as estimated from the disappearance of the pulse in the brachial (or radial) artery by palpation. Initial estimation of the systolic pressure by palpation avoids potential problems with an auscultatory gap and locates the best spot to place the stethoscope.
The patient should be seated comfortably with the back supported and the upper arm bared without constrictive clothing. The legs should not be crossed. The arm should be supported at heart level, and the bladder of the cuff should encircle at least 80% of the arm circumference. Neither the patient nor the observer should talk during the measurement.
 See: http://medind.nic.in/maa/t03/i1/maat03i1p51.pdf **Keywords:** BP, Read to nearest 2 mmHg

126. When obtaining a patient's blood pressure, the first clear tapping sound you hear is called the:
a.   Venous pressure
b.   Systolic pressure
c.   Diastolic pressure
d.   V wave pressure

ANSWER b. Systolic pressure. As you drop the cuff pressure, the first appearance of faint but clear tapping sounds that slowly increase in intensity is called the systolic pressure. You should read the level of mercury in the manometer carefully when you first hear a tapping sound and record this as systolic pressure.
See: Lippincott's State Board Review for NCLEX-PN. **Keywords**: BP Systolic pressure

127. **Of the following factors, the one that has the LEAST effect on most adult patient's resting blood pressure is:**
    a.   **Their age**
    b.   **Hardening of the arteries**
    c.   **Being angry or fearful when obtaining the blood pressure**
    d.   **Sitting or lying down when obtaining the blood pressure**

ANSWER d. Sitting or lying down when obtaining the blood pressure has the least affect the blood pressure. The difference when the person is sitting or lying down is very small and usually is considered clinically insignificant. The person's age, sex, and emotional status affect blood pressure. Some diabetics have arteries so hard, that you cannot compress them with a BP cuff, and thus cannot get a BP from that artery. Just be sure the limb where you measure your BP is at the same level as the heart. E.g. If the arm were up in the air the measured BP would be too low, similar to a transducer being set above the patients mid-chest level. **See:** Lippincott's State Board Review for NCLEX-PN.

128. **What are the sounds heard through the stethoscope when a blood pressure is taken?**
    a.   **Murmurs**
    b.   **Purkinje sounds**
    c.   **Rales and Ronchi**
    d.   **Korotkoff sounds**

ANSWER d. Korotkoff sounds. These are the tapping and swishing sounds you hear when taking a BP. They occur when the blood pressure overcomes the cuff pressure and squirts into the column of arterial blood distal to the cuff forming turbulence.
See: Lippincott's State Board Review for NCLEX-PN. **Keywords**: Korotkoff sounds

129. **Evaluate a patient's blood pressure of 80/45 and heart rate of 56.**
    a.   **Hypertensive with tachycardia**
    b.   **Hypertensive with bradycardia**
    c.   **Hypotensive with tachycardia**
    d.   **Hypotensive with bradycardia**

ANSWER d. Hypotensive with bradycardia. Normal blood pressure is 120/80. Below 100 is hypotensive. Normal HR is 60-100. Bradycardia is below a heart rate of 60 bpm. However, in resting athletic young people the rate may normally go as low as 50 bpm. **See:** Lippincott's State Board Review NCLEX-PN. **Keywords**: Hypotensive, bradycardia

130. Aneroid manometers used to measure BP utilize a:
   a.   Digital readout
   b.   Mercury column
   c.   Pressure transducer
   d.   Mechanical gauge

ANSWER d. Mechanical gauge BP manometers utilize a metal gauge and numeric dial. This is opposed to the digital manometers using a strain gauge or mercury manometers where mercury is pumped into a glass tube marked in cm. Aneroid manometers should be calibrated annually against the more accurate mercury manometers.
See: Braunwald, chapter on "Physical Examination" **Keywords:** Aneroid manometers

131. If you use your thumb to obtain a patient's pulse rate, you are likely to:
   a.   Feel your own pulse
   b.   Cut off circulation in the patient's blood vessel.
   c.   Obtain a pulse rate that is too rapid
   d.   Obtain a pulse rate that is too slow

ANSWER a. Feel your own pulse. The only danger of using the thumb to obtain a patient's pulse rate is that you may feel your own pulse in your thumb rather than that of the patient. To take a pulse you should place your index finger and middle finger over the patient's radial artery.
See: Lippincott's State Board Review for NCLEX-PN. **Keywords:** No pulse with thumb

TEMPERATURE

132. The normal adult body temperature is:
   a.   98.6 °F, or 32 °C
   b.   98.6 °F, or 37 °C
   c.   100 °F, or 32 °C
   d.   100 °F or 37 °C

ANSWER b. 98.6 °F, or 37 °C are the normothermic temperatures of people.
See: Lippincott's State Board Review for NCLEX-PN. **Keywords:** Normal temp °F & °C

133. Your patient does not want to gain weight. She asks you, "What is a calorie?" You should respond that a calorie is best defined as the amount of heat necessary to raise the temperature of 1 kilogram of water by:
   a.   1 ° F
   b.   10 ° F
   c.   1 ° C
   d.   10 ° C.

ANSWER c. 1 ° C. A calorie is a measure of heat that derives from the food we eat. It is defined as the amount of heat necessary to raise the temperature of one kilogram of water 1 °c. Nutritionists also refer to a calorie as a kilocalorie, or the so- called big calorie. It may be abbreviated Kcal. The "small" calorie, which is 1/1,000 of a large calorie, is used in chemistry and physics. In thermodilution CO each ml of cool injectate contains 1 calorie of heat energy for each degree C below body temperature. This heat is transferred to the blood. **See:** Lippincott's State Board Review for NCLEX-PN. **Keywords**: Calorie

9. Standards & Regulations

134. According to the Joint Commission what is the minimum number of patient identifiers that should be checked before you proceed with a case? (e.g., Name band, birthday, SS#, ask patient his name, hospital room number?, etc.)

a. 2
b. 3
c. 4
d. 5

ANSWER: a. 2 patient identifiers are required before proceeding with an invasive procedure.

Joint Commission says: "Acceptable identifiers may be the individual's name, an assigned identification number, telephone number, or other person-specific identifier. Electronic identification technology coding, such as bar coding or RFID, that includes two or more person-specific identifiers (not room number) will comply with this requirement....The two identifiers may be in the same location, such as a wristband....the two patient/client/resident-specific identifiers must be directly associated with the individual and the same two identifiers must be directly associated with the medications, blood products, specimen containers (such as on an attached label), other treatments or procedures." **See:** https://www.jointcommission.org/search/?Keywords=npsg.01.01.01&f=sitename&sitename=Joint+Commission&sort=Date **Keywords**: 2 acceptable patient identifiers

135. Which federal agency creates regulations to protect *"patient's rights"*?

a. HIPAA
b. FDA
c. OSHA
d. Joint Commission

ANSWER: a. HIPAA. The "Health Insurance Portability and Accountability Act" (HIPAA) of 1996.... address the security and privacy of health data. The standards are meant to improve the efficiency and effectiveness of the nation's health care system by encouraging the widespread use of electronic data interchange in the U.S. health care system....and the security and privacy of health data"

136. Which of the following are part of a pre-cath "time-out", as according to the Joint Commission? (Select 4.)
    a.   Confirm correct patient identity
    b.   Confirm availability of special equipment
    c.   Agreement on the procedure to be done
    d.   Include only the major team members in the case
    e.   Identify the intended side and site of incision or insertion
    f.   Confirm type and route of anesthesia

ANSWERS: a, b, c, & e.
a. Confirm correct patient identify - YES.
b. Confirm availability of special equipment - YES.
c. Agreement on the procedure to be done - YES.
d. Include only the major team members in the case - NO. Not just the "major", but ALL
e. Identify the intended side and site of incision of insertion - YES.

It must involve **THE ENTIRE CATH TEAM** present on the case, not just the "major" members. Time-out is: "active communication among <u>all</u> members of the surgical/procedure team, consistently initiated by a designated member of the team, conducted in a "fail-safe" mode, i.e., the   procedure is not started until any questions or concerns are resolved." "Time out? the surgical pause that counts", AORN Journal, Dec, 2004 by Nancy Charlton
        NPSG.01.02.01 Chapter: National Patient Safety Goals: "The final verification process involves the entire team, uses active communication, and includes the following:
        - Correct patient identity
        - Correct side and site
        - Agreement on the procedure to be done
        - Correct patient position
        - Availability of appropriate documents, correct implants, and any special equipment
        - Involves the <u>entire</u> operative team in the time out using active communication.
See: http://www.jointcommission.org/assets/1/18/UP_Poster.pdf

137. The risk of contracting a disease by performing mouth to mouth resuscitation is quite small. Patients with which disease would be most contagious to health care-givers giving mouth-to-mouth ventilation?
    a.   Hepatitis B virus
    b.   Hepatitis C virus
    c.   AIDs virus
    d.   Tuberculosis

ANSWER d. Tuberculosis and other airborne diseases may be transmitted during mouth to mouth ventilation. ACLS guidelines say: "The actual risk of disease transmission during mouth-to-mouth ventilation is quite small; only 15 reports of CPR related infection were published between 1960 and 1998, and no reports have been published in scientific journals from 1998 through 2000.... At last report (1998), the cases of disease transmission during CPR include *helicobacter pylori, Mycobacterium tuberculosis, meningococcus, herpes simplex, Shigella, Streptococcus, Salmonella, and Neisseeia gonorrhoeae.* **No reports on transmission of HIV, HBV, hepatitis C virus, or cytomegalovirus were found.**... The theoretical risk of infection is greater for salivary or aerosol transmission of herpes simplex, *Neisseria meningitidis,* and airborne diseases such as tuberculosis and other respiratory infections.... The emergence of multidrug-resistant tuberculosis and the risk of tuberculosis to emergency workers is a cause for concern. Rescuers with impaired immune systems may be particularly at risk."

See: AHA Guidelines 2000 for CPR, Chapter on "Adult BLS"   **Keywords:** TB airborne

138. **Which body fluid is LEAST likely to transmit HIV to a health care worker?**
    a.   **Semen**
    b.   **Blood**
    c.   **Pericardial fluid**
    d.   **Saliva**

ANSWER d. Saliva. The CDC says: "HIV has been isolated from blood, semen, saliva, tears, urine, vaginal secretions, cerebro-spinal fluid, breast milk, and amniotic fluid, but only blood and blood products, semen, vaginal secretions, and possibly breast milk, have been directly linked to transmission of HIV. Contact with fluids such as saliva and tears has not been shown to result in infection. Although other fluids have not been shown to transmit infection, all body fluids and tissues should be regarded as potentially contaminated by HBV or HIV, and treated as though they were infectious...." HIV may also be transmitted by sexual contact, including semen.

See: Dept Labor/Dept Health & Humans Services, Joint advisory Notice, "Protection against occupational exposure to HBV and HIV"   **Keywords:** HIV in body fluids

139. **Which body fluid is MOST likely to transmit the Hepatitis B virus to a health care worker?**
    a.   **Urine**
    b.   **Blood**
    c.   **Pericardial fluid**
    d.   **Vomitus**

ANSWER b. Blood. The CDC says: "Blood contains the highest HBV titers of all body fluids and is the most important vehicle of transmission in the health- care setting. HBsAg is also found in several other body fluids, including breast milk, bile, cerebrospinal fluid, feces, nasopharyngeal washings, saliva, semen, sweat, and synovial fluid. However, the concentration of HBsAg in body fluids can be 100- 1000- fold higher than the concentration of infectious HBV particles. Therefore, most body fluids are not efficient vehicles of transmission because they contain low quantities of infectious HBV....Feces, nasal secretions, saliva, sputum, sweat, tears, urine and vomitus are not considered potentially infectious unless they contain blood. The risk for transmission of HBV, HCV, or HIV infection from these fluids and materials is extremely low."

See: Dept Labor/Dept Health & Humans Services, Joint advisory Notice, "Protection against occupational exposure to HBV and HIV"   **Keywords:** Blood = highest HBV

140. **Which of the following poses the greatest risk for bloodborne pathogen infection?**
  a. **A nurse sustains a needle-stick while drawing up insulin to administer to a patient with diabetes**
  b. **A lab worker is splashed in the eye with urine from a patient with HIV**
  c. **A scrub tech who gets blood on his chapped hands while assisting in a surgery on a patient with hepatitis B infection**
  d. **While cleaning the bathroom, a housekeeper's intact skin has contact with feces**

ANSWER c. A scrub tech who gets blood on his chapped hands while assisting in a surgery on a patient with hepatitis B infection. Blood is the most infectious body fluid, especially when it gets into an open wound as may be found on chapped hands. The nurse's needle-stick appears to be from a clean needle. CDC says: "Feces, nasal secretions, saliva, sputum, sweat, tears, urine and vomitus are not considered potentially infectious unless they contain blood." **See:** Dept Labor/Dept Health & Humans Services, Joint advisory Notice, "Protection against occupational exposure to HBV and HIV" **Keywords:** BB pathogens

141. **Which virus is commonly transmitted by food workers who fail to wash their hands?**
  a. **Hepatitis A**
  b. **Hepatitis B**
  c. **AIDS**
  d. **HIV**

ANSWER a. Hepatitis A is a food borne virus. HAV is found in the feces of HAV-infected persons. It is commonly spread by food workers who don't wash their hands after using the toilet. HIV, Hepatitis B and Hepatitis C viruses are found in the body fluids of infected individuals; and can be transmitted to health workers during invasive procedures via needle sticks, skin lesions, or splashing body fluids onto mucous membranes. HIV virus leads to the AIDS syndrome, which occurs in the final stages of the HIV infection. See: http://www.immunize.org/catg.d/p4075.pdf **Keywords:** Hepatitis A, B, & C

142. **Many health care workers who develop hepatitis B viral infections have not been exposed to HBV infected patients. How were these workers probably infected?**
  a. **Tattooing or ear piercing**
  b. **Inhalation of aerosolized nasal secretions**
  c. **Ingestion of contaminated food or drinking water**
  d. **Direct contact with dried blood on environmental surfaces**

ANSWER d. Contact with dried blood on environmental surfaces. Such secondary infection is the main reason all blood spills and spatters must be cleaned up and disinfected and why it is so important to wash your hands frequently. The CDC says: "Although percutaneous injuries are among the most efficient modes of HBV transmission, these exposures probably account for only a minority of HBV infections among health care professionals (HCP). In several investigations of nosocomial hepatitis B outbreaks, most infected health care professionals could not recall an overt percutaneous injury, although in some studies, up to one third of infected HCP recalled caring for a patient who was HBsAg- positive. In addition, <u>HBV has been demonstrated to survive in dried blood at room temperature on environmental surfaces for at least 1 week.</u> Thus, HBV infections that occur in health care professionals with no history of nonoccupational exposure or occupational percutaneous injury might have resulted from direct or indirect blood or body fluid exposures that inoculated HBV into cutaneous scratches, abrasions, burns, other lesions, or on mucosal surfaces..., There is no evidence that HBV or HIV can be transmitted via food, drinking water, or airborne aerosols." There is lots of evidence that HBV can also be transmitted by unprotected sex. **See:** Dept Labor/Dept Health & Humans Services, Joint advisory Notice, "Protection against occupational exposure to HBV and HIV" **Keywords:** dried BB pathogens

143. **For which viruses currently are there NO immunizing vaccines?**
a. **HIV and HBV**
b. **HIV and HCV**
c. **HAV and HBV**
d. **HAV and HCV**

ANSWER b. HIV and HCV have NO immunizing vaccines as of year 2018. These are the Human Immunodeficiency Virus and the Hepatitis C Virus. Unfortunately both of these virus can be spread by blood or body fluids from infected individuals. **See:** http://www.immunize.org/catg.d/p4075.pdf **Keywords:** NO vaccines for HIV and HCV

144. **After an accidental needle-stick from the needle used on an infected patient, which bloodborne pathogen poses the greatest risk of infection to health care workers?**
a. **Hepatitis A**
b. **Hepatitis B**
c. **Hepatitis C**
d. **HIV**

ANSWER b. Hepatitis B is most contagious. The Dept. of Labor says: "Despite the similarities in the modes of transmission, the risk of HBV infection in health-care settings far exceeds that for HIV infection. For example, it has been estimated that the risk of acquiring HBV infection following puncture with a needle contaminated by an HBV carrier ranges from 6% to 30% - far in excess of the risk of HIV infection under similar circumstances, which the CDC estimates to be less than 1%." HCV is not transmitted efficiently through occupational exposure to blood. And, HAV is transmitted via food.
See: Dept Labor/Dept Health & Humans Services, Joint advisory Notice, "Protection against occupational exposure to HBV and HIV" **Keywords:** Hep. B most contagious

145. Your ICU patient needs arterial line monitoring. He develops sepsis and tenderness at the insertion site. Besides systemic antibiotics therapy you should:
a.   Apply povidone-iodine related ointment at puncture site
b.   Change the continuous flush, transducer, and pressure tubing
c.   Remove the catheter and replace it with a new one at a different access site
d.   Exchange the arterial line and catheter with the Seldinger technique

ANSWER c. Remove the catheter and replace it with a new one at a different access site. CDC Guidelines say: "Do not use guide wire assisted catheter exchange whenever catheter-related infection is documented. If the patient requires continued vascular access, remove the implicated catheter, and replace it with another catheter at a different insertion site."

"If catheter-related infection is suspected, but there is no evidence of local catheter-related infection (e.g., purulent drainage, erythema, tenderness), remove the existing catheter and insert a new catheter over a guide wire. Send the removed catheter for ... culture. Leave the newly inserted catheter in place if the catheter culture result is negative. If the catheter culture indicates colonization or infection, remove the newly inserted catheter, and insert a new catheter at a different site."
See: CCD, Guideline For Prevention of Intravascular Device-Related Infections" **Keywords:** Art Line sepsis - remove

146. The primary purpose for placing immune-suppressed patients in reverse (protective) isolation is to help prevent microorganisms from reaching:
a.   Visitors
b.   Health workers
c.   Housekeeping personnel
d.   The immune-suppressed patient

ANSWER d. The immune-suppressed patient. Lewis says: "Using reverse (protective) isolation primarily helps to prevent organisms from reaching the patient. In other types of isolation, the purpose is to help to prevent organisms from the patient from spreading to others." **See:** Lippincott's State Board Review for NCLEX-PN. **Keywords:** Reverse isolation

147. Which of the following areas of a patient's body is the LEAST likely place for bloodborne pathogens to enter?
a.   The nose
b.   The intact skin
c.   The genital tract
d.   The urinary tract

ANSWER b. The intact skin. The CDC says: "Both HBV and HIV appear to be incapable of penetrating intact skin, but infection may result from infections fluids coming into contact with mucous membranes or open wounds (including unapparent lesions) on the skin. If a procedure involves the potential for skin contact with blood or mucous membranes, the appropriate barriers to skin contact should be worn. e.g., gloves." Organisms enter the nose, the genital tract, and the urinary tract with greater ease than intact skin. Since we commonly touch or eyes, nose and mouth good hand washing is critical. **See:** Dept Labor/Dept Health & Humans Services, Joint advisory Notice, "Protection against occupational exposure to HBV and HIV" **Keywords:** skin protects against BB pathogens

148. **If a patient acquires an infection in the hospital where he is a patient, it is called:**
   a.   **A local infection**
   b.   **An enteric infection**
   c.   **A primary infection**
   d.   **A nosocomial infection**

ANSWER d. A nosocomial infection. Any infection acquired in a health agency is called a nosocomial infection. This is one of the main reasons to get patients out of the hospital as early as possible. An enteric infection is spread by feces containing the causative organism. A local infection, such as an abscess, is limited to the body's tissues and remains there. A primary infection is one that occurs before a subsequent infection develops. **See:** Lippincott's State Board Review for NCLEX-PN. **Keywords:** nosocomial infection

149. **Eye-wear, goggles, and/or face-shields need to be worn only:**
   a.   **On invasive procedures (where blood may spatter)**
   b.   **On interventional procedures (not diagnostic cases)**
   c.   **On cases who are in isolation (with bloodborne pathogens)**
   d.   **On positive HIV or HBV cases (with end stage disease)**

ANSWER a. On invasive procedures of vascular access. Health care workers need to wear protective barriers on all cases where blood or body fluids may splash. Basically that includes all invasive procedures. You can best protect yourself by shielding your eyes, nose, and mouth mucus membranes from blood spatter; and by wearing gloves whenever touching any patient's body fluids. OSHA says: "Masks in combination with eye protection devices, such as goggles or glasses with solid side shields, or chin-length face shields, shall be worn whenever splashes, spray, spatter, or droplets of blood or other potentially infectious materials may be generated and eye, nose, or mouth contamination can be reasonably anticipated."
See: OSHA Regulations on Bloodborne Pathogens **Keywords:** Goggles =blood splash

150. **You are working around a patient with an IV. You are wearing gloves but accidentally get some patient blood on your forearm where you have a small cut. The CDC recommends that your first action should be to:**
   a.   **Rinse it off with warm water**
   b.   **Wash forearm and the cut with soap and water**
   c.   **Wash forearm and rinse your cut with a mild bleach solution**
   d.   **Wash your forearm and cut with antiseptic and squeeze to make it bleed**

ANSWER b. Wash it with soap and water. The CDC says: "Wounds and skin sites that have been in contact with blood or body fluids should be washed with soap and water. Mucous membranes should be flushed with water. No evidence exists that using antiseptics for wound care or expressing fluid by squeezing the wound further reduces the risk of bloodborne pathogen transmission; however, the use of antiseptics is not contraindicated. The application of caustic agents (e.g. bleach) or the injection of antiseptics or disinfectants into the wound is not recommended." This same procedure should be used for blood contaminated needle-sticks. **See:** CDC, Guidelines for Occupational Exposures to HBV, HCV, and HIV **Keywords:** Blood on your wound = wash with soap and water

151. **While working to place an IV you accidentally spatter patient blood in your mouth and eye. The CDC recommends that your first action should be to:**
a.   Flush your mouth and eye with water
b.   Flush your mouth and eye with soap and water
c.   Flush your mouth and eye with a mild bleach solution
d.   Flush your mouth and eye with antiseptic

ANSWER a. Flush your mouth and eye with water. The CDC says: "mucous membranes should be flushed for several minutes with copious amounts of water. No evidence exists that using antiseptics for wound care or expressing fluid by squeezing the wound further reduces the risk of bloodborne pathogen transmission; however, the use of antiseptics in not contraindicated. The application of caustic agents (e.g. bleach) or the injection of antiseptics or disinfectants into the wound is not recommended." Many labs contain eye-wash sinks or eye-cups for irrigation. **See:** CDC, Guidelines for Occupational Exposures to HBV, HCV, and HIV **Keywords:** Blood splash = Flush your mouth and eye with water

152. **What is a hospital's responsibility to provide hepatitis B vaccination to employees who are exposed to patient body fluids?**
a.   None, totally up to the employee
b.   Must be made available
c.   Must be made available and free of charge
d.   Required for all such employees and free of charge

ANSWER c. Must be made available and free of charge. OSHA requirement is: "The employer shall make available the hepatitis B vaccine and vaccination series to all employees who have occupational exposure,...at no cost to the employee" The vaccine and follow-ups are not required of the employee. However, if an employee refuses these free services, they cannot be forced and must sign a release form. **See:** CDC, Guidelines for Occupational Exposures to HBV, HCV, and HIV **Keywords:** OSHA hepatitis B vaccination

153. **You are accidentally exposed to a patient's blood. What is a hospital's responsibility to provide post-exposure follow-up and blood testing to employees after an exposure incident?**
a.   None, totally up to the employee
b.   Must be made available
c.   Must be made available and free of charge
d.   Must be made available and free of charge only if the patient is a known carrier of bloodborne pathogens or the employee is not immunized
e.   Required for all exposed employees and free of charge

ANSWER c. Must be made available and free of charge. OSHA requirement is: "The employer shall make available the hepatitis B vaccine and vaccination series to all employees who have occupational exposure, and post-exposure evaluation and follow-up to all employees who have had an exposure incident...at no cost to the employee...all laboratory tests are conducted by an accredited laboratory at no cost to the employee." However, you cannot force an exposed employee to take these follow-ups services. If they refuse these free services they must sign a release form. **See:** CDC, Guidelines for Occupational Exposures to HBV, HCV, and HIV **Keywords:** HIV post-exposure follow-up

154. **After a blood spill it is best to disinfect the area of the spill with:**
    a. **Soap and water**
    b. **Betadine 5%**
    c. **One part bleach to 10 parts water**
    d. **One part alcohol to 10 parts water**

    ANSWER: c. One part bleach to 10 parts water is an excellent disinfectant. If alcohol were used it should be much stronger than 1:10 concentration. Betadine is an antiseptic for skin use, not as a disinfectant. Gloves should be worn, the area mopped up and then disinfected with diluted beach. It will kill all pathogens. See: Saia, Radiography Exam, chapter on "Patient Care" **Keywords:** bleach disinfectant 1:10

155. **What should be done with needles used for patient injection or IV infusion?**
    a. **Bent and then placed in the sharps disposal container**
    b. **Cut in half and then placed in the sharps disposal container**
    c. **Removed from the syringe and then placed in the sharps disposal container**
    d. **Recapped on the syringe and placed in the sharps disposal container**
    e. **Both needle and syringe should be placed together in the sharps disposal container**

    ANSWER e. Both needle and syringe should be placed together in the sharps disposal container without bending, shearing, or recapping. OSHA says that: "Contaminated needles and other contaminated sharps shall not be bent, recapped or removed [from the syringe] unless the employer can demonstrate that no alternative is feasible or that such action is required by a specific medical or dental procedure." **See:** CDC, Guidelines for Occupational Exposures to HBV, HCV, and HIV **Keywords:** sharps disposal

156. **How should laundry contaminated by patient body fluids, such as bloody patient drapes, be handled?**
    a. **Sort it, bag it in heavy cloth, and remove it at the end of the day**
    b. **Wear gloves, sort it, bag it in heavy cloth, & remove it at the end of the day**
    c. **Bag it in plastic, and remove it at the end of each case**
    d. **Wear gloves, bag it in plastic, and remove it at the end of each case**

    ANSWER d. Wear gloves, bag it in plastic, and remove it at end of each case. OSHA says: "Contaminated laundry shall be placed and transported in bags or containers labeled or color-coded....Whenever contaminated laundry is wet and presents a reasonable likelihood of soak-through of or leakage from the bag or container, the laundry shall be placed and transported in bags or containers which prevent soak-through and-or leakage of fluids to the exterior. The employer shall ensure that employees who have contact with contaminated laundry wear protective gloves and other appropriate personal equipment." **See:** CDC, Guidelines for Occupational Exposures to HBV, HCV, and HIV **Keywords:** Bagging contaminated laundry

157. **According to "universal or standard precautions", in emergency situations which body fluids are to be considered infectious?**
   a.   **Blood and certain body fluids of infected patients**
   b.   **All body fluids of infected patients**
   c.   **Blood and certain body fluids of all patients**
   d.   **All body fluids of all patients**

ANSWER d. All body fluids of all patients are considered infectious because in an emergency it is difficult to distinguish one body fluid from another and blood may be mixed within any of them. According to OSHA: "Universal [Standard] precautions must be observed. This method of infection control requires the employer and employee to assume that all human blood and specified human blood fluids are infectious for HIV, HBV, and other bloodborne pathogens. Where differentiating of types of body fluids is difficult or impossible [as in emergency trauma] , all types of body fluids are considered to be potentially infectious." CDC says that feces, nasal secretions, saliva, sputum, sweat, tears, urine and vomitus are probably not potentially infectious unless they contain blood. And the risk for transmission of HBV, HCV, or HIV infection from these fluids and materials is extremely low. But, who wants to take the chance? For this reason, hospital workers consider ALL body fluids as potentially infectious. **See:** OSHA Regulations on Bloodborne Pathogens **Keywords:** Universal [Standard] precautions for ALL

References

Allmers, Nancy M., and Verderame, Joan, *Appleton & Lange's Review for Surgical Technology Examination,* Fourth Edition, Appleton & Lange, 1996
Aston & Brown, *Medical Instrumentation for Nurses and Allied Health-Care Professionals,* Jones and Bartlett Publishers, 1994
Braunwald, Eugene, Ed., *HEART DISEASE A Textbook of Cardiovascular Medicine,* 8th Ed., W. B. Saunders Co., 2008
2000 CDC, *MMWR Weekly Report,* Updated U.S. Public CCD, Guideline For Prevention of Intravascular Device-Related Infections" 1995
          www.cdc.gov/ncidod/hip/Iv.htm
Ellenbogen & Wood, Cardiac Pacing and ICDs, 5th edition, Blackwell Publishing, 2008
Guidelines 2005 for Cardiopulmonary Resuscitation and Emergency Cardiovascular Care, International Consensus on Science, and Supplement to Circulation
Health Service Guidelines for the Management of Occupational Exposures to HBV, HCV, and HIV and Recommendations for Postexposure Prophylaxis.
Kern, M. J., Ed., *The Cardiac Catheterization Handbook,* 2nd Ed., Mosby-Year Books, 1995
Lewis, LuVerne Wolff, RN, *Lippincott's State Board Review for NCLEX-PN,* 3rd Ed., J.B. Lippincott, 1990

OSHA, US Dept. *Labor Regulations (Standards - 29 CFR) Bloodborne pathogens* -1910.1030

Saia, D.A., Appleton & Lange's Review for the Radiographic Examination, 1991

Spence, Alexander P., and Mason, Elliot B., *Human Anatomy and Physiology*, 3rd Ed.,
    Benjamin/Cummings Publishing Co., 1987

Saxon, Dolores F., *Mosby's Comprehensive Review of Nursing for NCLEX-RN*, 16th Ed., 1999

Tilkian, A. G., and Daily, E, J, *Cardiovascular Procedures, Diagnostic Techniques and
    Therapeutic Procedures*, C. V. Mosby Company, 1986

Torres, L. S., *Basic Medical Techniques and Patient Care for Radiologic Technologists*,
    3rd Ed., J. B. Lippincott Co., 1989

Underhill, S. L., Ed., *CARDIAC NURSING*, 2nd Ed., J. B. Lippincott Co., 1989

OUTLINE: A2 - Patient Care

1. PREFIX
   a. Peri- Surrounding or Around (E.g., Pericardium)
   b. Endo-. Within or Inward (E.g., Endocardium)
   c. Retro. Behind or Backward (E.g., Retroperitoneal)
   d. Hyper-. Excessive, Above, or More than Normal (E.g., Hyperkalemia)
   e. Hypo- Deficient, beneath, under, or below normal (E.g., Hypothermia)
   f. Trans- Across or beyond (E.g., Trans-thoracic)
   g. Vas(o)- Vessel or canal for carrying a fluid (E.g., vasoconstriction)
   h. Phlebo- Vein or venous (E.g., phlebitis)
   i. Arteri(o)- Vessel containing oxygenated blood (E.g., arteriosclerosis)
   j. Ather(o-) Fatty degradation (E.g., atheromatous plaque)
   k. Cholangi(o)- Bile duct (E.g., cholangiogram)
2. SUFFIX
   a. -emia =Blood condition - (E.g., anemia)
   b. -poiesis =Formation - (E.g., erhythropoiesis)
   c. -megaly =Enlargement - (E.g., cardiomegaly)
   d. -pathy =Disease condition - (E.g., myocardopathy)
   e. -penia =Deficiency - (E.g., thrombocytopenia)
   f. -itis =Inflamation (E.g., phlebitis)
   g. - plasty =Surgical repair   (E.g., angioplasty)
   h. -ectomy =Surgical removal/incision (E.g., Pericardiectomy)
   i. -centesis =Surgical tap (E.g., thoracentesis
   j. -ostomy =Surgical opening between organs

   k. -fenestrated, hole in drape
   l. -ambulatory = able to walk
   m. -oliguria, use Foley catheter
      i. Foley catheterization
         (1) Urinary bladder, saline or other fluid
         (2) Urine flows when the catheter enters the bladder
         (3) Place the drainage bag below the level of the bladder
3. Positional terms
   a. Ventral = Anterior, The face is anterior
   b. Dorsal = Posterior, The butt is posterior
   c. Cranial = Superior, The head or higher
   d. Caudal = Inferior, Toward feet or lower
   e. Media = Toward the midline
   f. Lateral= Away from the midline
   g. Proximal = Closer to
   h. Distal = Farther away from
   i. Sitting up position for acute pulmonary edema
4. Documentation
   a. Charting in medical record
      i. Avoid generalizations
      ii. Only accurate facts
      iii. Only what you see
      iv. Chart only after the delivery of care
      v. Note protective measures
      vi. Pen only
5. Lifting or moving patients
   a. use lower extremities
   b. good posture
   c. get adequate assistance
   d. Wheelchair
      i. Footrests, Moved aside or removed
      ii. Position your foot between the patient's feet
      iii. Elevate the head of the bed 1st
      iv. Lower the bed to the level of the wheelchair
      v. Swing patients legs over the side of

the bed
6. Patient Safety
   a. Biohazards
      i. Latex allergy - non-latex Swan
   b. IVs
      i. Extravasation or IV infiltration
         (1) -Stop the IV and attempt to aspirate
      ii. Infusion bag kept above the level of the infusion
7. Communications & patient teaching
   a. Patient asks you to interpret/diagnose - don't
   b. Medication compliance
      i. teach importance
      ii. teach complications
      iii. hypertensive meds-
         (1) Cerebral hemorrhage, stoke
      iv. Post stent
         (1) Plavix, aspirin
   c. vein stripping - blood rerouted
   d. Stages of grief: -Kubler- Ross
      i. Denial & disbelief
      ii. Anger
      iii. Bargaining
      iv. Depression
      v. Acceptance
8. Legal issues
   a. Negligence =omission to do something reasonable and prudent
   b. Liability =individual responsible for his or her own acts
   c. Quality assurance programs (JCAHO)
      i. optimal pt. care
      ii. patient safety
      iii. continuity of care
   d. Malpractice - claims:
      i. Avoided by better communication
      ii. Angry frustration patients cause
      iii. Patient is most important

   e. Patient's rights include:
      i. Refusing treatment
      ii. Continuity of care
      iii. Not Possessing their medical images
      iv. Confidentiality of medical records
      v. Knowing who is treating & their relationships
      vi. HIPAAs mission = protect patient's rights
   f. Informed consent
      i. Protects operating physician and hospital
      ii. Physician responsible for obtaining
      iii. Discuss diagnosis & alternative treatments
      iv. Only considered legal for 30 days from date of signature
      v. Must be obtained before patient receives sedation
      vi. If not obtained, the patient has the right to sue for malpractice
   g. Patient teaching - care of puncture site:
      i. Keep your head on pillow

      ii. Hold groin site when coughing
      iii. Keep punctured leg immobile & straight
      iv. Stay in bed
      v. Don't sit up
      vi. Don't force urination or BP
      vii. Drink lots of fluids
      viii. Call a nurse if bleeding, numbness or pain
   h. "Time-out" - purpose:
      i. Confirm correct patient identity
      ii. Confirm availability of special equipment
      iii. Agree on the procedure to be done
      iv. Include ALL team members in the case
      v. Identify the intended access sites
      vi. Check 2 patient identifiers
9. Pt. Assessment
   a. Predisposing factors for MI
      i. Hyperglycemia
      ii. Hypertension
      iii. Hyperlipidemia
      iv. Estrogen protective
   b. Organic heart murmur
      i. Defect in heart valves (stenosis, regurg.)
      ii. Functional heart murmur - innocent
      iii. Rheumatic fever (MS...)
   c. PMI = LV apex = V4
10. Auscultation
   a. BRUITS: Blowing sound heard over a vessel
   b. MURMURS: abnormal valve sound
   c. RALES (moist): respiratory sound due to fluid in lungs
   d. WHEEZES: whistling or high pitched breath sound.
   e. THRILL: A palpable heart sound or murmur
   f. Korotkoff sounds during taking of BP
   g. Diastolic gallop sounds - S3 - S4
   h. Right heart murmurs effected by respiration
11. Signs and Symptoms
   a. Things that precipitate angina pectoris
      i. Smoking
      ii. Emotional stress
      iii. Cold temperatures
      iv. Eating a large meal
   b. Aortic dissecting aneurysm symptoms
      i. Hypotension BP<90
      ii. Tachycardia HR >100
      iii. Radiating back pain
   c. Dependent edema =Swollen legs
   d. Palpitations
      i. Sensation of rapid or irregular heart rate
      ii. atrial fibrillation HR- count pulses for 1 min
   e. Tachypnea =Rapid respiratory rate
   f. Cyanosis = blue coloration
      i. in African Americans -check Oral mucosa

g. Signs of cardiogenic shock
    i. oliguria
    ii. hypotension
    iii. tachycardia
    iv. cold clammy skin
    v. cyanosis
h. Amaurosis Fugax
    i. temporary blindness in one eye
i. Normal temp = 98.6 °F, or 37 °C
    i. Calorie - heats 1 ml H20 1 degree C. Aneroid, mercury manometers

12. Auscultatory blood pressure:
  a. Read pressures to nearest 2 mmHg.
  b. After pumping up the cuff, deflate the cuff 2-3 mmHg/sec
  c. Be sure the bladder in the cuff encircles 80% of the arm circumference
  d. Pump up the pressure cuff to 30 mmHg over expected systolic
  e. 1st sound to disappear = systolic
  f. Auscultatory BP effected by:
    i. Patient age
    ii. Hardening of the arteries
    iii. Being angry or fearful when obtaining the blood pressure
    iv. *Sitting or lying down - no effect*
  g. Take pulse - with your index and middle fingers
  h. Hypotensive = <90 mmHg
  i. Bradycardia HR<60

13. Pathogens
  a. Isolation
    i. - protects staff from patient organisms
  b. Reverse (protective) isolation
    i. - prevents organisms from reaching the patient
    ii. Immuno-suppressed patient
  c. Nosocomial infection = hospital acquired infection
  d. Sepsis in patients invasive art. Line
    i. Remove and replace - use different access site
  e. Mouth to mouth ventilation can transmit:
    i. TB & other airborne diseases
    ii. Herpes
    iii. Strep & Salmonella
    iv. Gonorrhea
    v. *Not: HIV, HBV, hepatitis C virus*
  f. Transmit Hepatitis B virus:
    i. transmitted mainly via - blood or dried blood
      (1) also, breast milk, bile, cerebrospinal fluid, feces, saliva, semen, sweat, pericardial fluid, and synovial fluid
    ii. Open wound (E.g., cuts, chapped hands)
    iii. Hepatitis A - food workers
    iv. Hepatitis B is most contagious
      (1) Needle sticks contagious
    v. Intact skin = best barrier
    vi. No immunizing vaccines for:
      (1) HIV or HCV
  g. Universal or Standard precautions
    i. Protection against blood borne pathogens
    ii. Use around ALL body fluids & ALL patients
    iii. Eye-wear, goggles, Gown, & gloves
      (1) Worn on all invasive procedures
    iv. Blood to skin contact - Wash area with soap and water
    v. Blood contact on mucous membranes - flush with large amounts of water
    vi. Hospital must:
      (1) provide hepatitis B vaccination to employees
      (2) made available free of charge
      (3) provide post-exposure follow-up
      (4) made available free of charge
    vii. Blood spill
      (1) - clean with 1:10 bleach/water solution
    viii. Sharps disposal container
      (1) Discard both needle and syringe together
    ix. Handling contaminated laundry
      (1) Wear gloves, bag it in plastic, & remove it at end of each case

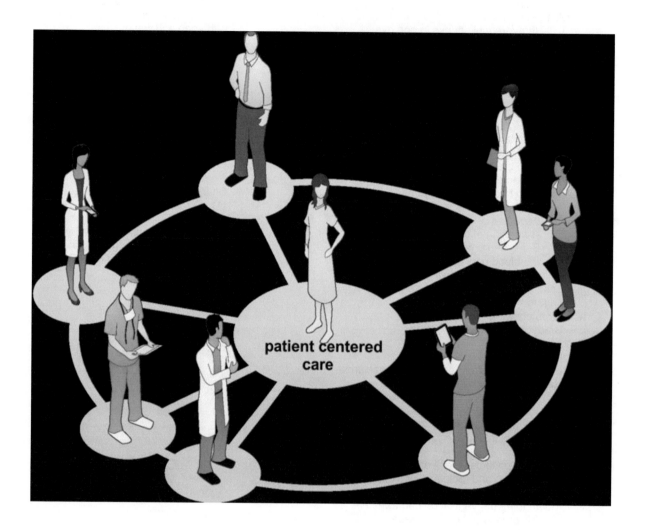

Instrumentation

INDEX: A3 - Instrumentation

1. Electricity and Magnetism

BASIC DEFINITIONS

158. Match the physical quantity labeled #1 in the box (frequency) with its Standard International (SI) unit of measure below.

- **a. Watt**
- **b. Newton**
- **c. Joule (or erg)**
- **d. Hertz**

#1. Frequency
2. Force
3. Energy
4. Power

Physical quantities

ANSWER d. Hertz measures the frequency of a repetitive wave in cycles / sec. Other commonly used physics units are:

1. Frequency	= Hertz	= cycles / sec
2. Force	= Newton	= m kg/sec^2 (also weight in grams - CGS)
3. Energy or work	= Joule	= m^2 kg/sec^2 (also Ergs or Watt Sec)
4. Power	= Watt	= m^2 kg/sec^3 (also rate of doing work)

See: Curry, chapter on "Radiation" **Keywords:** SI Physical Units

159. Match the electric quantity labeled #1 in the box (Charge) with its Standard International (SI) unit of measurement below.

a.   Tesla (Gauss)
b.   Weber
c.   Volt
d.   Farad
e.   Coulomb

| #1. Charge |
| 2. Potential |
| 3. Capacitance |
| 4. Magnetic flux |
| 5. Mag. induction (flux density) |

Electric quantities

ANSWER d. Coulomb is a quantity of negatively charged electrons. An ampere of flow occurs when this quantity of electrons flow past a point in the circuit each second. One amp = one coulomb/sec.

1. Charge	= Coulomb	= Amp sec = quantity of electron charges
2. Potential	= Volt	= driving force or pressure
3. Capacitance	= Farad	= short term charge storage
4. Magnetic flux	= Weber	= quantity of magnetic flux
5. Mag. induction	= Tesla (Gauss)	= density of magnetic lines (flux density)

See: Curry, chapter on "Radiation"   Keywords: SI Physical Units

160. The flow of electric current is measured in:

a.   Ohms
b.   Volts
c.   Watts
d.   Amperes

ANSWER d. Amps = 1 coulomb/sec. Electric current flow is similar to fluid flow through tubes. Current (I) is analogous to fluid flow, except the units change. Hemodynamic flow is expressed in L/min. Electric current flow is in coulombs/sec.
See: Electronic text   Keywords: electric current = amps

161. What is the term used to denote the total opposition to flow of alternating current in a circuit?

a.   Reactance
b.   Impedance
c.   Inductance
d.   Capacitance

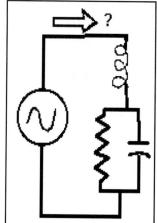

ANSWER b. Impedance or resistance (ohms). Resistance is the term used to denote opposition to DC current flow. Impedance is the complex resistance to alternating or pulsating flow. Impedance changes with the frequency, amount of capacitance, resistance, and inductance - as shown in the diagram. The same is true in fluid systems composed of pulsatile flow, compliant vessels, and dynamic inertial forces.
See: Aston, Chapter #1 on "Definitions, components..."

Opposition to AC flow

162. **The device by which alternating current is changed to direct current is known as a/an:**
   a.   Inverter
   b.   Rectifier
   c.   Amplifier
   d.   Collector

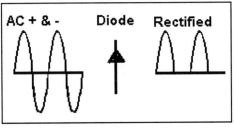
AC to DC Rectifier

ANSWER b. Rectifiers (diodes) are one way valves for electricity, converting AC to DC. That is how battery chargers work. First they have to convert the 120 volt AC current into DC. This is done with diodes.
See: Aston, chapter on "Definitions, components..." **Keywords:** rectifier

163. **What is the most common DC electric power source?**
   a.   60 cycle wall outlet
   b.   A charged capacitor
   c.   Transformer
   d.   Battery

ANSWER d. Battery. Batteries are an electrochemical source of direct current. DC current only travels in one direction. Defibrillators use batteries to charge a capacitor.
See: Physics text **Keywords**: battery, DC power

164. **Electric battery current has a frequency of:**
   a.   0 Hz
   b.   60 Hz
   c.   120 Hz
   d.   1000 Hz

ANSWER a. 0 Hz. DC current flows steadily from - to +. It does not alternate back and forth like AC current does. **See:** Aston, chapter on "Definitions, components..." **Keywords:** rectifier

165. **In the USA, most electrical wall outlets provide:**
   a.   DC current at 60 volts
   b.   DC current at 120 volts
   c.   60 cycle AC current at 60 volts peak to peak
   d.   60 cycle AC current at 120 volts RMS

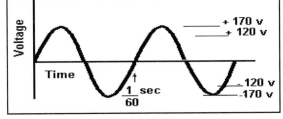
AC Voltage

ANSWER d. 60 cycle AC is 120 volts root

mean squared (RMS). The RMS voltage is the "effective" voltage of 120 volts. The actual peak voltages reach ± 170 volts, as shown. In a 60 cycle AC circuit, electrons vibrate back and forth at a rate of 60 cycles each second.
See: Aston, chapter on "Definitions, components..." **Keywords:** 60 cycle AC electric current

166. **The force which initiates the flow of electric current is termed:**

a.   **Amperage**
b.   **Wattage**
c.   **Resistance**
d.   **Voltage**

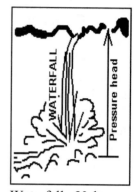

Waterfall - Voltage

ANSWER d. Voltage is electricity's driving force. Just as in hemodynamic systems the pressure head imparts energy to the fluid, voltage is force driving current through a conductor. In the waterfall shown we see the potential "pressure head" energy being dissipated into kinetic energy as if falls. In the case of electricity potential voltage energy is dissipated in heat as current flows.
See: Aston, chapter #1 on "Definitions, components..."

167. **The ability of a system to clearly distinguish between closely spaced targets is termed that system's:**

a.   **Resolution**
b.   **Clarity**
c.   **Specificity**
d.   **Sensitivity**

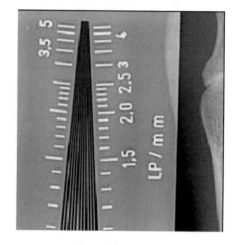

ANSWER a. Resolution. Tiny wires may be placed side by side and imaged. The more line pairs/mm clearly seen, the smaller the object that can be imaged and the better the resolution. Echocardiography distinguishes between axial and lateral resolution, depending on whether the line pairs are along the ultrasound beam axis or transverse to it. The higher the resolution the more clarity and detail seen. **See:** Reynolds, chapter on "Doppler" **Keywords:** resolution

ELECTRICAL SAFETY

168. **Match the number on the 3 prong standard AC outlet shown to its electrical use in the USA.**

a.   **Hot 60 cycle wire (120 volt)**
b.   **Chassis ground (0 volts)**
c.   **Return wire (0 volts)**

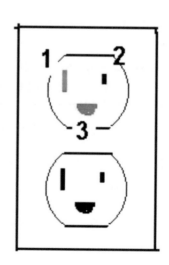

Correctly matched answers are:
1. c.   Return wire (red) (0 volts)
2. a.   Hot 60 cycle wire (black)(120 volts)
3. b.   Chassis ground (green) (0 volts)

The smallest black flat outlet is the dangerous hot wire that will conduct 60 cycle current to any ground. It is the smallest plug for safety reasons. The wire inside is black because it appears burnt.

The large flat red outlet normally conducts all the current from #2 back to ground. Sometimes this case ground outlet is T shaped.

The crescent shaped outlet is another ground that is connected to the chassis of the machine. It is only used to drain off dangerous current when there is an electrical short to the chassis. The wire inside is green to represent ground.

All electrical outlets in cath labs are checked regularly by biomed. Hospital outlets also have ground fault detectors or other safety features.

169. **With temporary pacing wires, it is important to avoid microshock. Which of the statements below are electrical safety rules when using temporary pacing wires? (Select 3.)**
  a. **Wear rubber gloves when handling pacer wires attached to the patient**
  b. **Do not touch electrical equipment and the pacing wires simultaneously**
  c. **Discharge any static electricity onto a grounded metal surface prior to touching the patient**
  d. **Cover exposed electrode connections with sterile saline soaked 4 x 4s**

ANSWERS: a, b, & c.
  a   Wear rubber gloves when handling pacer wires - YES.
  b   Do not touch electrical equipment and the pacing wires simultaneously - YES.
  c   Discharge any static electricity onto a grounded metal surface prior to touching the patient. - YES.
  d   Cover exposed electrode connections with sterile saline soaked 4 x 4s - NO.
       Covering exposed electrode connections with 4 x 4s soaked in saline would "short out" the pacer and prevent pacing. Watson says: " Electrical safety is a major concern for this patient population, as the pacing lead provides a direct route for current flow to the heart tissue. Pacing leads must always be protected from any potential source of electrical current whether environmental or equipment related. Nurses caring for patients should ensure proper maintenance and grounding of equipment. In addition they should discharge any potential static electricity on a metal surface prior to contact with patients. Rubber gloves should be worn when handling pacing leads (wires) and exposed pacing wires should also be protected with insulating material (i.e., a rubber glove). Contact between two pacing wires should be avoided. Nurses should not simultaneously touch electrical equipment and pacing wires. A recent study suggests that policies for electrical safety may not be adequate in many facilities." **See:** Watson, chapter on "Cardiac Pacing"

170. **The greatest danger of accidental electric micro-shock to patients in the cath lab is:**
  a. **Ablation of conduction pathways, resulting in heart block**
  b. **Ablation of myocardium resulting in pericardial tamponade**
  c. **Stimulating ventricular tachycardia**
  d. **Stimulating ventricular fibrillation**

ANSWER d. Ventricular fibrillation resulting in cardiac arrest. Minute currents when applied directly to the heart may induce cardiac arrest, especially when a pacing wire is in the heart. Aston defines micro-shock as "A physiological response to a current applied to the surface or in the close vicinity of the heart that produces an unwanted stimulation, muscle contraction or tissue injury." The most serious result is ventricular fibrillation and cardiac arrest. **See:** Underhill, chapter on "Electrical Hazards in the Cardiac Care Unit."

171. **Which patient has the greatest risk of receiving electric micro-shock?**
   a.   **CCU patient on counterpulsation therapy**
   b.   **ICU patient intubated and ventilated**
   c.   **Cath lab patient with central venous line**
   d.   **CCU patient with temporary dual chamber pacemaker**

ANSWER d. CCU patient with temporary dual chamber pacemaker.

The temporary pacemaker leads are passed through venous sheaths either the external jugular veins, common femoral veins or subclavian veins. The external connections can inadvertently conduct small currents by touching another electrical device, such as an electric bed that is improperly grounded to "mother earth." in Aston says "Micro-shock is most often caused when currents on excess of 10 microamps flow through an insulated catheter (electrode) to the heart . . . This accounts for the 1000:1 ratio of macro-shock to micro-shock current levels." E.g., It takes 10 milli-amps to contract the muscles through the skin (let-go current), but only 10 µamps to fibrillate the heart when in direct contact with it.

The electrical resistance of fluid-filled catheters is much greater than that found in a pacemaker electrode. This makes fluid-filled-catheter induced micro-shock somewhat less hazardous, although still possible. Underhill says, "Fluid-filled central venous and pulmonary artery catheters (without pacing electrodes) appear to pose much less of a hazard than do cardiac pacing wires." **See:** Aston, Chapter on "Electrical Shock."

172. **Which frequency of electric current is the most lethal at inducing ventricular fibrillation?**
   a.   **Direct current**
   b.   **60 Hz**
   c.   **1000 Hz**
   d.   **1 megahertz**

ANSWER b. 60 Hz

It is a dangerous coincidence that AC wall current happens to be the most lethal at inducing fibrillation. For this reason it is especially important to follow all electrical safety precautions when operating 60 cycle AC electrical equipment around patients. Higher frequencies used during electrocautery and radio-frequency ablation equipment may cauterize or burn but do not cause fibrillation. Sixty-cycle current is actually used to fibrillate patients during open heart surgery. A quivering heart is easier to operate on than a beating heart. **See:** Aston, Chapter on "Electrical Shock." **Keywords:** Most dangerous frequency = 60 Hz

173. **Hospital codes for electrical safety require electrical power cords to be:**
   a.   **3-wire conductor, with 3-prong plug**
   b.   **Shielded coaxial 1-wire conductor, with 2-prong plug**
   c.   **Shielded coaxial 2-wire conductor, with 3-prong plug**
   d.   **Shielded coaxial 3-wire conductor, with 3-prong plug**

ANSWER a. 3 wire insulated conductor, with 3 prong plug
        In the cardiac laboratory all receptacles and plugs must be the 3-pin grounded type. This requires that 3 wires be used in all power cables and lab wiring. The green ground wire must be larger than normal, to drain off small currents and voltages from the equipment chassis. Only ECG and some low voltage video cables are routinely shielded. **See:** Tilkian, Chapter on "Electrical Hazards" **Keywords:** 3 prong plug, electrical safety

174. **In electrical injury, the pathway of current most likely to be fatal is:**
   a.   **Hand-to-hand**
   b.   **Hand-to-foot**
   c.   **Foot-to-foot**
   d.   **Foot-to-ground**

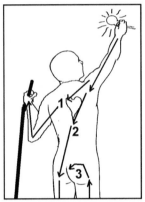

ANSWER a. Hand-to-hand. Most of the current passes though the chest and heart using much the same path as defibrillation. It is the path most likely to cause ventricular fibrillation. Hand-to-foot current path is more associated with cardiac muscle damage. To prevent shock, electricians avoid the practice of working with both hands on live circuits.
        Lightning strikes on an individual are DC current that is less hazardous than 60 cycle AC current. Also, protective in lightning strikes is a "flash over" phenomenon, where the current travels along the outer surface of the body. DC shock is more associated with asystole. **See:** ACLS manual, Chapter on "Special Resuscitation Situations."

Electric shock body-paths

175. **For maximum electrical safety, ECG monitored patient's should be _____ , and the monitor chassis should be _____ or nonconductive.**
   a.   **Grounded, Grounded**
   b.   **Grounded, Ungrounded**
   c.   **Ungrounded, Ungrounded**
   d.   **Ungrounded, Grounded**

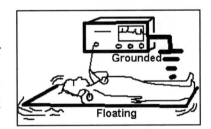

ANSWER d. Ungrounded, Grounded. Patients should never be connected directly to ground. This is analogous to standing in a pool of conductive water. A grounded patient becomes a "lightning rod" available to conduct any potential leakage currents. Whereas, if the patient is ungrounded, or floating, he does not provide himself a ready conductor to ground.

Safe isolation/grounding

Most medical instruments at a patient's beside are encased in a metal box (chassis). For safety these should always be grounded through the 3rd prong of the plug (green wire). Properly grounded medical equipment safely conducts stray leakage currents away from the patient to ground. Some new devices are encased in a plastic non-conductive case which makes leakage current flows negligible. Plastic cases need not be grounded because they are insulators and cannot conduct leakage currents. **See:** Aston, Chapter on "Electrical Shock." **Keywords:** patient ungrounded, chassis grounded

176. In the ICU when recording an intracardiac ECG from a pacing electrode or pericardiocentesis needle it is safest to:
   a.   Ground the ECG monitor to a water pipe
   b.   Ground the patient to a water pipe
   c.   Use a battery powered monitor
   d.   Use low resistance defibrillation pads as the limb electrodes

ANSWER c. Use a battery powered monitor to reduce microshock hazard.
Underhill says. "to record the electrocardiogram from a pacing wire, or to help guide a pericardiocentesis needle, it is safest to operate the monitor on battery power, if possible. Otherwise, only use an instrument known to have a leakage current of less than 10 µA..." Because batteries are not referenced to ground, battery power provides a safe method of preventing leakage current. **See:** Underhill, chapter on "Electrical Hazards in the CCU."

177. When you plug in an electric instrument, you are alarmed when sparks fly from the wall outlet as shown. The most likely electrical safety problem is a:
   a.   Outlet miswired
   b.   Broken insulation on the power cord
   c.   Machine off-on switch was left turned-on
   d.   Machine fuse shorted out

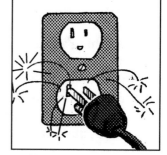

Pulling hot plug

ANSWER c. Machine **off-on switch** was never turned-off. Electrical equipment should not be turned off (or on) by pulling the plug from (or plugging it into) an electric outlet. Switches are designed to safely do this. Pulling the plug of a piece of equipment while it is operating can also damage the equipment, melt the plug, and present a fire hazard. Consider how computers can be damaged if turned off incorrectly. **See:** Aston, Chapter on "Electrical Shock."

FILTERS

178. The elimination of vibrations at certain frequencies is accomplished through the use of electronic devices known as:
   a.   Diodes
   b.   Grids
   c.   Filters
   d.   Rectifiers

ANSWER c. Filters. Most amplifiers have high and low limits beyond which they do no amplify. ECG amplifiers typically incorporate a "band Pass filter" that cuts off low frequencies < 0.1 Hz and high frequencies >100 Hz. Pressure amps are a low pass filter, because they pass all low frequencies - down to 0 Hz or DC. The upper limit may be changed to increase fidelity and/or reduce motion artifacts. **See:** Aston, chapter on "Definitions, components..."

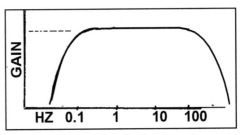

100 Frequency Response curve - Bandpass filter

179. **When filtering a physiologic signal, a high pass filter setting of 30 means:**
   a.   **Signals over 30 mV will be amplified**
   b.   **Signals under 30 mV will be amplified**
   c.   **Frequencies <30 Hz will be eliminated**
   d.   **Frequencies >30 Hz will be eliminated**

ANSWER: c. Frequencies <30 Hz will be eliminated. Such settings would be used in electrophysiology to record intracardiac electrograms.

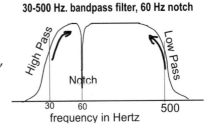

30-500 Hz. bandpass filter, 60 Hz notch

High Pass — Low Pass — Notch — 30 — 60 — 500 — frequency in Hertz

Issa says, "Defining a band of frequencies to record, such as setting the high-pass filter to 30 Hz and the low-pass filter to 500Hz, defines a band of frequencies from 30 to 500 Hz that are not attenuated (i.e., band pass filtering). A notch filter is a special case of band pass filtering, with specific attenuation of frequencies at 50 or 60 Hz to reduce electrical noise introduced by the frequency of common AC current."

Note in the diagram how the high pass filter is really on the low end, and the low pass end of the filter is really on the high end. Every frequency between the high and low pass filter ends passes; everything else is eliminated. The high pass filter passes frequencies over 30 Hz. The low pass filter only passes frequencies lower than 500 Hz. **See:** Issa, chapter on "EP Testing"

180. **For best fidelity, surface ECG leads should be filtered to allow frequencies between:**
   a.   **0.1 to 100 Hz**
   b.   **1 to 100 Hz**
   c.   **30 to 300 Hz**
   d.   **50 to 500 Hz**

ANSWER: a. 0.1 to 100 Hz. Some ECGs are filtered at an even a wider bandwidth of 0.05 to 300 Hz.

Reducing the high-pass filter to less than 0.1 Hz means T waves and ST changes will be accurately measured. One problem with such a low setting is baseline drift.

Issa says, "The surface ECG is usually filtered at 0.1 to 100.0 Hz. The bulk of the energy is in the 0.1- to 20.0-Hz range. But, because of interference from alternating current (AC), muscle twitches, and similar relatively high-frequency interference, it is sometimes necessary to record the surface ECG over a lower frequency range (reduce the low pass filter) or to use notch filters (which filter out 60 Hz noise)." **See:** Issa, chapter on "EP Testing"

2. Implantable Devices

DEFIBRILLATORS

181. When a DC defibrillator "charges" it stores electrical energy in its:
a. Batteries
b. Capacitors
c. Transformers
d. Photovoltaic cells

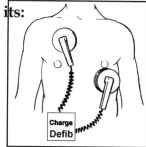
Defibrillator charging

ANSWER b. Large capacitors store the charge. When you charge a defibrillator, large capacitors become polarized and charged up to several thousand volts. This allows for a large amount of electricity to be temporarily stored. When the "fire" button is depressed, this charged capacitor is suddenly discharged into the patient (defib. pulse).

Pacers and defibrillators both charge a capacitor slowly from a battery or transformer, then discharge the capacitor's stored current rapidly into the patient. The unit of capacitance is the Farad. A large capacitor of 1000 microfarads may charge to 500 V and store 125 Joules of energy. Pacemakers require much less energy, and thus use smaller capacitors. **See:** Aston, Chapter #1 on "Definitions, components..."

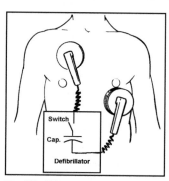
Defibrillator circuit

182. During daily testing of your cath lab defibrillator:
a. Fire it with paddles in their wells
b. Do not touch the paddles
c. Biomed. should calibrate its output
d. Fire it with paddles pressed together

ANSWER: a. Fire it in its holder. Most defibrillators are made to be tested in their holder. Firing with the paddles touching will cause a spark and pit the electrodes. Of course do not touch the electrodes, but touching the paddle handles is expected. Some daily automated defibrillator test are at low voltage (30 joules) to save battery power and electronic circuits.

183. Synchronized cardioversion (countershock):
a. Is the primary treatment for all forms of cardiac arrest
b. Is used only for rhythms with ventricular responses of < 60/min.
c. Is triggered from the patient's P wave
d. Delivers a shock a few milliseconds after the peak R wave.

ANSWER: d. Delivers a shock a few milliseconds after the peak R wave - within the QRS. Some machines show you exactly where in the QRS the pulse will fire. You don't want to fire during the vulnerable relative refractory period, on the downslope of the T wave. Emergent high energy defibrillation is used in VF and pulseless VT cardiac arrest. We cardiovert arrhythmias with reentry loops (like AF) which only need to be interrupted. This can be done with low energy pulses. But in the automatic ventricular rhythms (like VF) the defibrillation pulses must be large enough to depolarize the entire ventricle - RV & LV. **See:** AHA, ACLS Provider Manual, chapter on "Advanced Skills" **Keywords:** Cardioversion synchronized to R wave

184. **Most defibrillators are constructed such that you CANNOT cardiovert when monitoring the patient's ECG through the:**
    a.   **Limb leads (4 wire)**
    b.   **Monitor leads (3 wire)**
    c.   **Quick look paddles**
    d.   **Disposable defibrillation pads**

ANSWER: c. Quick look paddles. ACLS guidelines say: "cardioverters synchronize only to the signal from the monitor electrodes and never through the hand-held quick-look paddles. An unwary practitioner may try to synchronize - unsuccessfully in that the machine will not discharge - and may not recognize the problem." Quick look paddles are for emergency use only. **See:** AHA, ACLS Provider Manual, chapter on "Stable Tachycardias"

185. **Your physician decides to cardiovert a patient with SVT. After placing the cardioverter/defibrillator in synchronization mode and administering a sedative and analgesic to the patient, the patient suddenly becomes unresponsive and pulseless. The ECG rhythm is** as shown. **The Dr. says "SHOCK HER NOW!" But, when you hold down the discharge buttons on the defibrillator - nothing happens. Why?**

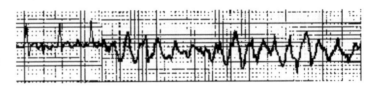

    a.   **The defibrillator battery is low**
    b.   **The SYNC switch is not functioning properly**
    c.   **Fibrillation waves won't trigger the synchronizer**
    d.   **Low energy shocks are inadequate to convert VF**

ANSWER: c. Fibrillation waves won't trigger the synchronizer circuit. In VF the fibrillation waves are usually rounded and low in amplitude. A synchronized defibrillator waits until it senses an adequate R wave, then fires. The R waves must be high enough in voltage and have steep enough slope to trigger the monitors threshold. Many defibrillators automatically start in "defib." mode to prevent this problem.

        There is no evidence that the battery or SYNC switch have failed. It is true that cardioversions normally start at lower energy (50-100J) because, cardioversion is designed to break up a small reentry loop in the atrium with a low energy pulse. In VF the defibrillation pulses must be large enough to depolarize the entire ventricle, both RV & LV. **See:** AHA, ACLS Provider Manual, chapter on "Unstable Tachycardia"

ICDs

186. **When placing an ICD, where is the initial shock level usually set for effective defibrillation of a patient's VF?**
a.　　At defibrillation threshold
b.　　Twice the defibrillation threshold
c.　　10 J below maximum ICD output
d.　　10-15 Joules

ANSWER: c.10 J below maximum ICD output
　　　Kanjwal, et. al, say: "Early studies in defibrillation revealed that a tested and confirmed safety margin at implantation of >10 J (i.e. 10 J below the maximum output of the device) was adequate to ensure success in the event of a "real-life" arrhythmic episode . . . Presently it is . . . common to ensure a repeated successful defibrillation 10 J or more below the maximum output of the device or at least once 15–20 J or more below the maximum output of the device. This testing protocol does not determine the actual defibrillation threshold but does establish defibrillation efficacy . . . "
　　　"Ideally the defibrillation threshold would exist as a fixed point above which it would always be successful and below which it would likely fail, similar to the threshold for pacing. Unfortunately, defibrillation is inherently a probabilistic phenomenon meaning that the same energy cannot be counted on to always defibrillate the patient. A variety of factors including ischemia, metabolic or electrolyte derangements, autonomic tone, and medications can affect the success of defibrillation. The mechanisms by which these factors affect defibrillation are not well understood, but likely they have an impact on the number and size of the eddy currents existing during fibrillation and the voltage gradient necessary to terminate them. The defibrillation threshold has been loosely defined as the shock amplitude at which there is roughly a 50% success rate in terminating ventricular fibrillation. The hope is that an ICD at implant will have enough of a safety margin between the defibrillation threshold and its maximum output so as to expect that it will reliably defibrillate the patient when clinically necessary . . . " **See:** Khalil Kanjwal, et al. "Defibrillation Threshold Testing: A Primer" in Journal of Innovations in Cardiac Rhythm Management 2012

187. **When a modern ICD detects a tachyarrhythmia it will initially attempt antitachycardia pacing, then cardioversion and finally defibrillation at higher and higher output levels until the arrhythmia terminates. This is termed:**
a.　　Arrhythmia Triage
b.　　Progressive AED
c.　　Titrating response
d.　　Tiered response

ANSWER: d. Tiered response. Watson says: "Tachycardia is based on rate and duration of rate as programmed by the practitioner. Most devices allow for the definition of two or three different tachycardia zones, based on rate. A maximal duration for the heart rate to be in that zone may also be programmed. If rate and duration criteria are met, therapy is initiated. For example, a ventricular tachycardia may be defined as a heart rate between 150 and 180 bpm for 16 consecutive beats to meet detection criteria. [Then antitachy pacing maneuvers start] Ventricular fibrillation may be defined as a heart rate above 180 bpm. However, the criteria for the duration of ventricular fibrillation are typically less stringent. Instead of requiring 16 beats in a row, any 12 of 16 beats may need to be classified as VF to meet detection." Once VF rate is detected the tiered response automatically goes to defibrillation. **See:** Watson, chapter on "Implantable Cardioverter Defibrillator"

188. **Current ICDs use high efficiency cardioversion and defibrillation. The most efficient shock waveforms are:**
   a.   Monophasic
   b.   Biphasic
   c.   Sinusoidal
   d.   Square waves

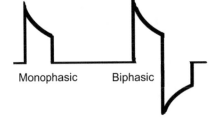
Monophasic   Biphasic

ANSWER b. Biphasic waveforms convert patients with less energy then the traditional monophasic waveform. In the biphasic defibrillation current goes from cathode to anode then reverses and returns in a push-pull manner. Watson says: "Much investigation has gone into developing the optimal shock waveform. As a result, the shape of the defibrillation waveform has changed and become more efficient. The biphasic or bidirectional waveform has proven to be more efficient than the unidirectional or monophasic waveform, thus providing lower defibrillation thresholds." See: Watson, Chapter on "Implantable Cardioverter Defibrillator"

Recent atrial fibrillation (AF) studies indicate that 200 J biphasic energies are as effective as 360 J monophasic shocks, suggesting that biphasic shocks are almost twice as effective as monophasic shocks.

189. **The energy unit of defibrillation is joules. "1 joule" is the same as:**
   a.   1 Gray
   b.   1 Watt Second
   c.   1000 Volt Amps
   d.   10,000 Milliwatts

> 1 Joule = 1 Watt sec

ANSWER b. 1 Watt Second. Defibrillator output energy is rated in joules or watt seconds. Since the joule is also a watt-second and the common unit for electricity sales to homes is the kW·h (kilowatt-hour), a kW·h is thus 1000 (kilo) watt × 3600 seconds = 3.6 MJ (megajoules). Prior to standardization of SI units, defibrillators were rated in watt seconds.

190. **With ICDs the lowest energy that consistently achieves successful defibrillation is termed:**
   a.   Minimum Defibrillation Level (MDL)
   b.   Pre-Defibrillation Force (PDF)
   c.   Cardioversion Threshold (C-T)
   d.   Defibrillation Threshold (DFT)

ANSWER d. Defibrillation threshold testing (DFT) is performed to assure adequate detection of ventricular fibrillation and efficacy of device therapy. The defibrillation threshold can be defined as the lowest energy at which successful defibrillation occurs at least two times. Other authors suggest the DFT is the lowest level at which defibrillation is achieved 50% of the time.
See: Watson, chapter on "Implantable Cardioverter Defibrillator"

191. **The energy ranges available for ICD shocks range from:**
  a.   **0.01 to 2 joules**
  b.   **0.1 to 40 joules**
  c.   **5 to 100 joules**
  d.   **20 to 360 joules**

ANSWER: b. 0.1 to 40 joules. High efficiency ICD devices may need as little as 0.1 joules to cardiovert VT, but may need to go as high as 40 joules in refractory VF.
See: Watson, chapter on "Implantable Cardioverter Defibrillator"

PACEMAKERS

192. **In the pacemaker circuit shown what happens when switch S1 is closed?**
  a.   **Capacitor charges**
  b.   **Pacemaker discharges into patient**
  c.   **Battery charges**
  d.   **Diode changes AC to DC**

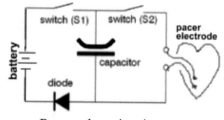
Pacemaker circuit

ANSWER: a. Capacitor charges. First you have to charge the capacitor by connecting it to the battery or power source. Then S1 opens and S2 closes to discharge the capacitor to the patient's pacer electrodes or through the defibrillator paddles. The diode rectifies the current flow to force it to go one direction. This happens with every discharge and is done automatically. Both pacemaker and defibrillator circuits are similar, except in a pacemaker an internal Lithium battery source is used instead of a transformer. Since the battery is DC, the diode shown is unnecessary.

193. **During a pacemaker implant when connecting a pacing lead, the negative terminal of the pacer should be connected to the:**
  a.   **Proximal electrode**
  b.   **Distal electrode**
  c.   **Pacer can**
  d.   **Subcutaneous tissue via a metal clip**

ANSWER: b. Distal electrode. Slightly lower thresholds result when the distal electrode is the negative pole. Moses says: "The distal electrode is usually attached to the negative terminal (cathode) because the heart is generally more easily stimulated if electrons travel from the distal electrode, which usually has the best myocardial contact . . . " Exceptions exist. **See:** Moses, chapter on "Pacemaker Technology"

194. An MI patient has an intrinsic rate of 60-80 bpm with a stimulation threshold of 2 mA. With the external pacemaker shown, when the switch is turned to "on" with the settings shown, what will occur?

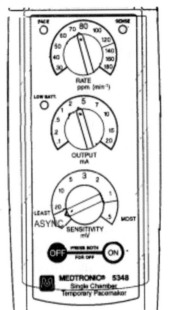

a. No pacing will occur
b. Demand pacing (fires if HR falls below 75)
c. Demand pacing (fires if HR exceeds 75)
d. Fixed rate pacing at 75 bpm with competition

ANSWER d. Fixed rate pacing at 75 bpm with competition. This is termed "asynchronous pacing."

Since the pacer output exceeds the stimulation threshold it will capture the ventricle at a rate of 75. Since it is set to asynchronous mode, it will fire at a fixed rate. If the patient's intrinsic SA rate exceeds 75 the two pacers will compete to capture the ventricle. This is dangerous, since the pacer spike may fire into the T wave and cause cardiac arrest. The sensitivity switch should be turned up until it is sensitive enough to detect the patient's QRS. This will cause the pacer to inhibit (stop pacing) when the patient's intrinsic

Temporary Pacer

rate exceeds 75 bpm. Unlike the pacer shown here, most modern pacemakers are digital. **See:** Moses, chapter on "Types of Pacemakers and Hemodynamics of Pacing"

195. Which of the following pacemaker electrodes use PASSIVE FIXATION?

a. Ring electrode
b. Helical screw-in
c. Tined tip
d. Epicardial sutured electrode

ANSWER: c. Tined tip. Passive leads usually have fins or tines to anchor them into the trabeculations. Active fixation uses wires imbedded into the myocardial surface. One type of active lead is a tiny metal helix that screws into the muscle. If the screw is on the end of a lead it is an active transvenous lead. Some are retractable to allow safe passage through the vein. If the screw goes on the outside of the heart it is termed an epicardial active lead, that may be placed during cardiac surgery. **See:** Moses, chapter on "Pacemaker Technology"

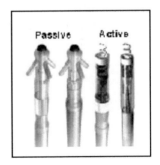

196. **Compared to the permanent pacemaker, the temporary pacer output uses:**
- a.   Constant voltage and generates up to 20 volts
- b.   Constant voltage and generates up to 5 volts
- c.   Constant current and generates up to 20 volts
- d.   Constant current and generates up to 5 volts

ANSWER: c. Constant current and generates up to 20 volts. Temporary pacers use a 9.5 v alkaline battery whose voltage can be doubled to almost 20 volts. That's a big pacer spike. Temporary pacers use a method to generate their pacer spikes different from permanent pacers. They generate a constant current spike, whereas permanent pacers use a constant voltage spike.
See: Moses, chapter on "Electrophysiology of Pacing"

197. **Before using a temporary pacer put in a new:**
- a.   2.8 volt alkaline battery
- b.   2.8 volt lithium battery
- c.   9 volt alkaline battery
- d.   9 volt lithium battery

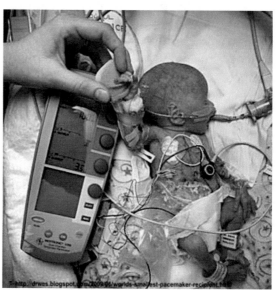

ANSWER: c. 9 volt alkaline battery. Watson says, "Batteries that are used to power pacemakers must be reliable and long lasting. Temporary pacers are typically powered by 9 V batteries. [The rectangular type used in home smoke detectors.] In temporary generators, batteries are usually changed before instituting pacing and at regularly scheduled intervals.... Permanent pulse generators are typically powered by a 2.8 V lithium iodine battery."
See: Watson, chapter on "Cardiac Pacing"

Neonate needs temp. pacer

198. **From this recording of a pacemaker threshold measurement determine the stimulation threshold.**
- a.   2 v
- b.   2.5 v
- c.   3 v
- d.   3.5 v

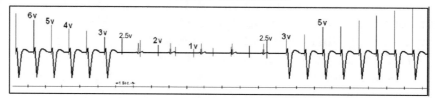

ANSWER: c. 3 v is the threshold. As you turn down the pacer amplitude below 3 volts, you lose pacing and the patient returns to his intrinsic rhythm - sinus bradycardia. Then as you increase the pacer output it captures the rhythm again at 3. volts. In this example to capture the patient's rhythm consistently you must program the pacemaker voltage over 3 volts, preferably double that, around 6 volts.

This tracings shows the same voltage threshold when lowering the voltage as when increasing it. However, it may vary slightly, depending on whether you are increasing or decreasing the voltage. Normally the threshold is slightly lower (0.1-0.2 V) when increasing from sub-threshold. So, the right side of the tracing should start capturing around 2.8 V instead of 3.0 Volts. However, this slight difference **termed the Wedensky effect**, is usually clinically insignificant. **See:** Moses, chapter on "Electrophysiology of pacing"

199. **When defibrillating a patient in VF, what is your LAST step just before you discharge the defibrillator?**
   a.   **Recheck pulse and ECG rhythm**
   b.   **Ensure that no one is in contact with the patient or stretcher ("clear the victim")**
   c.   **Press with 25 lb. of pressure and press the discharge button on the apex paddle**
   d.   **Be sure the defibrillator is fully charged to the appropriate energy level**

ANSWER: b. Ensure that no one is in contact with the patient or stretcher ("clear the victim"). Although all the listed answers are important, it is most important to not create a second victim by shocking someone on your own team. ACLS current guidelines say: "The person who presses the SHOCK button is responsible for ensuring that no one is touching the victim when a defibrillatory shock is provided . . . state in forceful voice before each shock, for example, 'I'm going to shock on three. One, I am clear . . . Two, you are clear . . . Three, everybody is clear.'" You must press BOTH buttons, one on each paddle.
See: AHA, ACLS Provider Manual, chapter on "VF treated with CPR and AED"

CRTs - BIVENTRICULAR PACERS

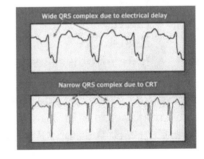

200. **What is the purpose of CRT devices?**
   a.   **Synchronize right and left ventricular contractions**
   b.   **Synchronize atrial and ventricular contractions**
   c.   **Defibrillate lethal arrhythmias**
   d.   **Antitachycardia pacing**

ANSWER: a. Synchronize right and left ventricular contractions especially in heart failure patients with bundle branch block where one ventricle contracts late. A lead placed in the left coronary vein usually paces the LV 1st then the RV pacer fires in the RV so both ventricles contract together in synchrony. CRT - Cardiac Resynchronization Therapy. Note how with CRT the QRS is much narrower as the 2 ventricles contract together.
        There are two types of CRT Devices. Depending on the patients heart failure condition, a Cardiac Resynchronization Therapy Pacemaker (CRT-P) or a Cardiac Resynchronization Therapy Defibrillator (CRT-D) may be indicated. **See:** http://www.webmd.com/heart-disease/heart-failure/cardiac-resynchronization#1

201. **What the type of pacemaker is shown in this X-ray?**
   a.   (S-ICD) Subcutaneous - ICD
   b.   (DP) Dual chamber pacing
   c.   (MLP) Multi-lead transvenous pacing
   d.   (CRT) Cardiac resynchronization therapy

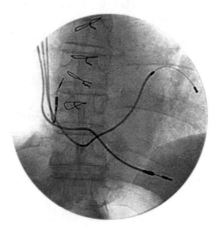

ANSWER: d. (CRT) Cardiac Resynchronization Therapy is also termed biventricular pacing, or just BiV.

   A biventricular pacemaker, also known as CRT (cardiac resynchronization therapy) is a type of pacemaker that can pace both RV and LV to coordinate ventricular contraction. LV pacing comes through a lead in the coronary sinus and posterolateral coronary vein. Poor asynchronous ventricular contraction occurs when one ventricular chamber beats before the other resulting in inefficient ejection of blood. This is usually due to bundle branch block. If the side that is blocked receives a pacemaker stimulus timed appropriately early, it may resynchronize contraction of the two ventricles so they beat at the same time. This helps remodel the dilated heart in CHF patients. In the X-ray image, note the 3 leads: RA, RV and LV (Cor. vein in upper right paces LV).

OHM'S LAW

202. **The Watt Second (or Joule) is a unit of:**
   a.   Current
   b.   Energy
   c.   Resistance
   d.   Rate of power usage

ANSWER: b. Energy - defibrillators are charged from 50-360 Joules. Watt second units are similar to the units on your home electricity/energy bill in Kilowatt hours.
See: Curry, chapter on "Radiation"

203. **What is the current drawn by a resistor of 100 ohms if a 10 volt battery is applied across it? V = I x R**
   a.   0.1 amp
   b.   10 amp
   c.   100 amp
   d.   1000 amp

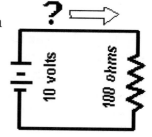

ANSWER a. 0.1 amp. I = V/R = 10v/100Ω = 0.1 amp or 100 milliamps. Ohm's law relates current, voltage and resistance just the way cardiac output relates to driving pressure and resistance. If you can't remember Ohm's law use this triangle. Cover up the letter you want to solve for. E.g., Cover up the V on top, to get the formula I x R on the bottom of the triangle. **See:** Aston, Chapter #1 on "Definitions, components..."

Ohm's Law

204. Use Ohm's law to calculate the flow when an average pressure of 100 mmHg is applied across 33 HRUs. (Same as current through a 33 ohm resistor with 100 volts applied as shown.)

    a.   ⅓ L/min

    b.   1 L/min

    c.   3 L/min

    d.   33 L/min

> **Ohm's Law:** $I = V/R$, or
> Flow = (Δ pressure)/ Resistance

ANSWER c. 3 L/min. Rearrange the Ohm's law resistance formula from R = pressure gradient/flow, to flow or CO = pressure gradient/R = 100 mmHg/33 mmHg/L/min = 3. L/min. Fluid flow problems are analogous to simple electric circuits, where current flow equals fluid flow. In fact, I use Ohm's law to remember the resistance equation. Use the Ohm's law triangle described earlier. **See:** Baim, chapter on "Clinical Measurement of Vascular Resistance **Keywords:** Ohm's law for fluids

3. Transducers

205. What instrument converts one form of energy into another?

    a.   Transformer

    b.   Transistor

    c.   Transducer

    d.   Rectifier

ANSWER c. Transducer. Medical pressure transducers convert blood pressure energy into electrical energy. Thermistors transducer temperature into electrical energy. Piezoelectric transducers (crystals) convert electrical waves into ultrasound waves. Then they record the reflected pressure waves and convert them back into electrical energy so we can view the echogram. **See:** Medical dictionary text **Keywords:** transducer, piezoelectric

206. What type of sensor is used in a thermodilution catheter to detect temperature changes?

    a.   Diode

    b.   Thermocouple

    c.   Thermometer

    d.   Thermistor

ANSWER. d. Thermistor. This is a semiconductor element whose resistance varies dramatically with temperature. Placed near the end of each thermistor catheter, it detects and measures the temperature change in blood caused by cool saline injected upstream. **See:** Aston, chapter on "Transducers & Amplifiers"

207. The hydrostatic pressure due to water at the bottom of a tank filled with water to a depth of 1 meter is:
a. $1\ gm/cm^2$
b. $10\ gm/cm^2$
c. $100\ gm/cm^2$
d. $1000\ gm/cm^2$

ANSWER c. $100\ gm/cm^2$. Facts: density of water is $1\ gm/cm^3$ and $1\ M = 100\ cm$. Use the formula, Pressure = Density x ht. = $(1\ gm/cm^3)\ (100\ cm) = 100\ gm/cm^2$. In the same way a column of mercury is used to measure pressure. The density of mercury is 13.6 times that of water. **See:** basic physics text   **Keywords:** pressure, Pressure = Density x Ht.

208. What new unit of pressure equals 1/760th of the barometric pressure at sea level?
a.   1 Bar
b.   1 Torr
c.   1 Joule
d.   1 cmHg

ANSWER b. 1 Torr. This is the new unit of pressure. One Torr = 1 mmHg or 1/760 th of the barometric pressure at sea level. Torr is named after the physicist Torrichelli who carried a mercury barometer to the top of a mountain and observed the pressure drop. At sea level the barometric pressure will push a column of mercury up 760 mm. Thus, one atmosphere at sea level exerts a pressure of 760 mmHg, 760 Torr, or 1 Bar. Some blood gas labs are now reporting ABGs, not in mmHg, but in Torr. **See:** Medical Dictionary

ULTRASOUND

209. Ultrasound transducers are usually composed of a:
a.   Bonded Strain gauge
b.   Electromagnetic induction coil
c.   Capacitance array
d.   Piezoelectric crystal

ANSWER d. Piezoelectric crystal. Transducers convert one form of energy into another. Ultrasonic transducers convert electric signals into ultrasonic energy. This is transmitted into the tissues, and some of it bounces back. The reflected ultrasonic waves are then converted by the same crystal into electric energy. The time for a signal to be reflected back is a measure of the depth of the structure off which it was reflected.

The thickness of the ultrasound crystal transducer determines its resonant frequency. The crystal is "struck" with a sharp voltage spike, and just like a pipe in a pipe organ, it resonates at one natural frequency. Typically a 1 mm thick crystal resonates at 2 MHZ. **See:** Curry, chapter on "Ultrasound.

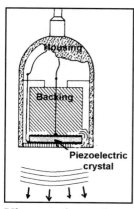

Ultrasound transducer

210. A change in electrical charge on a crystal following mechanical stress is termed the:
   a.   Crystalloid ionization
   b.   Crystallization
   c.   Photoelectric effect
   d.   Piezoelectric effect

ANSWER d. Piezoelectric effect. Ultrasound waves hitting a crystal deform it, causing it to generate an electric charge on its surface. This charge is measured by an amplifier and is displayed as a tissue interface on the echogram. Crystals can transform energy in both directions, from mechanical to electrical and from electrical to mechanical. Ultrasonic transducers typically first generate ultrasound vibrations that are transmitted into the tissues. Some of these vibrations bounce back. These echos are then converted by the same crystal into electric energy that reads out on the echocardiogram machine.
See: Reynolds, chapter on "Elementary Principles" **Keywords:** photoelectric effect

211. The period of the wave emitted from a 5 megahertz continuous wave ultrasound transducer is:
   a.   0.2 milliseconds
   b.   0.2 microseconds
   c.   5.0 milliseconds
   d.   5.0 microseconds

ANSWER b. 0.2 microseconds. Period (T) is the time per cycle. Since wavelength or period is 1/frequency, wavelength = $1/(5 \times 10^6) = 0.2 \times 10^{-6} = 0.2$ micro seconds. Know the formula $f = 1/period$ or $f = 1/T$ **See:** Reynolds, chapter on "Elementary Principles"

212. The period of an ultrasound wave is determined by the:
   a.   Source (transducer)
   b.   Medium (tissue)
   c.   Source and medium
   d.   Sonographer (machine controls)

ANSWER a. Source (crystal). The frequency of the ultrasound transducer is the only factor determining the frequency or period (wavelength) of the ultrasound wave. To increase frequency for a child's echo, you must change to a higher frequency transducer.
See: Reynolds, chapter on "Elementary Principles" **Keywords:** period, source (transducer)

213. The speed of an ultrasound wave varies. Which tissues below would conduct sound with an increasing propagation speed?
   a.   Air, bone. soft tissue
   b.   Air, soft tissue, bone
   c.   Bone, air, soft tissue
   d.   Bone, soft tissue, air

ANSWER b. Air, soft tissue, bone. The denser the tissue the faster the sound moves. For example you can hear a train coming through the steel railroad tracks long before you hear its whistle. **See:** Reynolds, chapter on "Elementary Principles" **Keywords:** ultrasound speed

214. **Which of the following are considered to be improvements from increasing the frequency of ultrasound? (Select 3.)**
   a. **Axial resolution (better detects closely spaced objects along direction of the sound beam)**
   b. **Lateral resolution (better detects closely spaced objects perpendicular to direction of the sound beam)**
   c. **Depth of penetration (penetrates deeper tissues)**
   d. **Beam diameter (extends near zone length)**

ANSWERS: a, b, & d.
a. Axial resolution (better detects closely spaced objects along direction of the sound beam) - YES.
b. Lateral resolution (better detects closely spaced objects perpendicular to direction of the sound beam) - YES.
c. Depth of penetration (penetrates deeper tissues) - NO.
d. Beam diameter (extends near zone length) - YES.

Reynolds says, "Increasing the frequency improves axial resolution because it decreases the wavelength, spatial pulse length, period, and pulse duration. Increasing the frequency also improves lateral resolution because it extends near zone length thus decreasing overall beam diameter and beam divergence...Also, increasing the frequency reduces depth of penetration." **See:** Reynolds, chapter on "Propagation of Ultrasound Through Tissue."

215. **As the frequency of ultrasound increases its:**
   a. **Resolution increases**
   b. **Velocity increases**
   c. **Beam penetration increases**
   d. **Pulse repetition rate increases**

ANSWER a. Resolution increases. Smaller structures can be better visualized with shorter wavelength sound waves (higher in frequency). That is why transducers as fast as 3.5 MHZ are use in infant echocardiography. The resolution of a particular frequency ultrasound beam is only 1.5 x the wavelength of the ultrasound wave. At higher frequencies, as the resolution increases, the penetration decreases. **See:** Curry, chapter on "Ultrasound." **Keywords:** increased ultrasound frequency increases resolution

216. **Calculate the wavelength of a 1.5 megahertz ultrasound wave.**
   a. **.1 Meter**
   b. **.001 Meter**
   c. **.000001 Meter**
   d. **.00000001 Meter**

ANSWER b. .001 M or 1 mm. Remember the speed of sound in soft tissue is 1540 m/sec and from the formula above: Wavelength = Velocity/Frequency.

$$\left(1.54 \times 10^3 \; \frac{M}{sec}\right) \Big/ \left(1.5 \times 10^6 \; \frac{cy}{sec}\right) \approx 10^{-3} \; \frac{M}{cy} \approx 1 \; mm$$

Memorize the formula: Velocity = Frequency x Wavelength
See: Curry, chapter on "Ultrasound." **Keywords:** wavelength

217. **Calculate the frequency of transducer that produces a wavelength of 0.5 mm.**
  a. **2.5 MHZ**
  b. **3.1 MHZ**
  c. **4.8 MHZ**
  d. **12.4 MHZ**

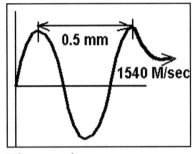
Ultrasound wave

ANSWER b. 3.1 MHZ. Remember the speed of sound in soft tissue is 1540 m/sec and from the formula above: Frequency = Velocity/Wavelength.
 0.5 mm = 0.5 mm/(1000 mm/M) = 0.0005 M

$$\left(1.54 \times 10^8 \; \frac{M}{sec}\right) \Big/ \left(0.5 \times 10^{-3} \; M\right) \approx 3.10 \times 10^6 \; \frac{cy}{sec} = 3.1 \; MHZ$$

Memorize the formula: Wavelength = Velocity/Frequency.
See: Curry, Chapter on "Ultrasound." **Keywords:** wavelength

218. **The active element in ultrasound transducers is a/an:**
  a. **Bonded strain gauge**
  b. **Electromagnetic induction coil**
  c. **Capacitance array**
  d. **Piezoelectric crystal**

ANSWER: d. Piezoelectric crystal. Transducers convert one form of energy into another. Ultrasonic transducers convert electric signals into ultrasonic energy. This is transmitted into the tissues, and some of it bounces back. The reflected ultrasonic waves are then converted by the same crystal into electric energy. The time for a signal to be reflected back is a measure of the depth of the structure off which it was reflected.

The thickness of the ultrasound crystal transducer determines it resonant frequency. The crystal is "struck" with a sharp voltage spike, and just like a pipe in a pipe organ, it resonates at one natural frequency. Typically a 1 mm thick crystal resonates at 2 MHZ. **See:** Curry, chapter on "Ultrasound."

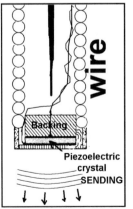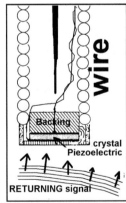
Doppler Flo-wire

219. **A change in electrical charge on a crystal following mechanical stress is termed/the:**

a.   Crystalloid ionization
b.   Crystallization
c.   Photoelectric effect
d.   Piezoelectric effect

ANSWER: d. Piezoelectric effect. Ultrasound waves hitting a crystal deform it, causing it to generate an electric charge on its surface. This charge is measured by an amplifier and is displayed as a tissue interface on the echogram. Crystals can transform energy in both directions, from mechanical to electrical and from electrical to mechanical. Ultrasonic transducers typically first generate ultrasound vibrations that are transmitted into the tissues. Some of these vibrations bounce back. These echos are then converted by the same crystal into electric energy that reads out on the echocardiogram machine. **See:** Reynolds, chapter on "Elementary Principles" **Keywords:** photoelectric effect

220. **The speed of ultrasound in soft tissue (water) is:**

a.   875 m/sec
b.   1200 m/sec
c.   1540 m/sec
d.   5280 m/sec

ANSWER: c. 1540 m/sec. Although the speed of sound is faster in denser tissues, medical ultrasound assumes a velocity of 1540 m/sec in all soft tissues.

Helguera says: "Wavelength depends on the frequency and propagation speed: Wavelength (mm) = Propagation Speed (mm/microsecond) / Frequency(MHZ) Propagation speed depends on the medium. In soft tissue it averages 1540 m/s, or 1.54 mm/μs." With a frequency of 10 MHZ, or 10,000,000 Hz used in ICE, this ratio gives a wavelength of 0.15 mm; which results in very fine resolution. Using this math you can see that IVUS at 30 MHZ is even better at about 0.05 mm resolution. **See:** https://www.cis.rit.edu/research/ultrasound/ultrasoundintro/ultraintro.html

IVUS

221. **One difference between mechanical IVUS and solid state (phased array) IVUS is:**

a.   Mechanical IVUS has a guide wire artifact
b.   Mechanical IVUS displays a pie shaped image
c.   Mechanical IVUS has a lower frequency with less resolution
d.   Mechanical IVUS cannot do pull backs

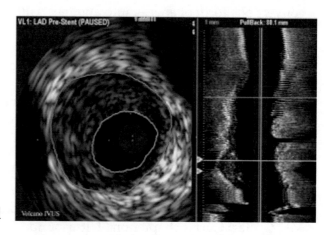

ANSWER: a. Mechanical IVUS has a guide wire artifact - true. Since the rotating crystal occupies the entire IVUS catheter tip, the tracking guide wire is usually seen as a reflecting echo in the vessel alongside the IVUS catheter. It is not seen in this phased array image. It actually has a higher frequency than the phased array, and can also be pulled back. It is the phased array ICE catheter that displays as a pie shaped sector scan.

DOPPLER

222. **Whose law is this? "The relative frequency of a reflected wave increases as the relative motion of the reflector approaches the observer."**
   a. **Hertz**
   b. **Doppler**
   c. **Bernoulli**
   d. **Laplace**

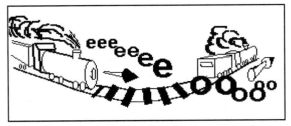

ANSWER b. Doppler. Doppler measures velocity of any reflectant object/fluid by evaluating the change if frequency of the reflected ultrasound. You have heard a Doppler frequency shift. When a whistling train approaches, you hear the "eeee" sound. As soon as it passes, the frequency of the whistle suddenly drops to a "oooo."

Doppler principle - train whistle example

This change to a lower pitch is an indication that approaching objects compress the sound waves to make them sound higher pitch. Objects moving away rarefy the sound waves coming from them and sound lower in pitch. Objects perpendicular to the beam do not shift the Doppler frequency. Ideally the ultrasound beam should be pointed into the vector direction of oncoming blood cells. See question below. **See:** Curry, chapter on "Ultrasound." **Keywords:** Doppler principle

223. **In Doppler echocardiography what is the usual target from which the ultrasound is reflected?**
   a. **Plasma eddies**
   b. **Red blood cells**
   c. **Cardiac valves**
   d. **Endocardium and/or pericardium**

ANSWER b. Red blood cells. Doppler is used to measure blood flow or velocity. The RBCs carried within the blood reflect the sound waves. RBCs moving towards the transducer increase the reflected velocity and the pitch of the Doppler sound heard. Micro-bubbles are also easily recorded within the blood, making limited contrast flow studies possible. **See:** Braunwald, chapter on "Echocardiography." **Keywords:** echo Doppler

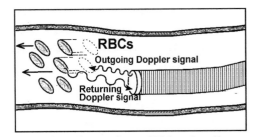

Doppler - bouncing off blood cells

target - RBCs

224. **When a Doppler device measures flow away from the transducer, the returning ultrasound wave has a:**
   a.   **Higher relative frequency**
   b.   **Lower relative frequency**
   c.   **Higher relative amplitude**
   d.   **Lower relative amplitude**

ANSWER: b. Lower relative frequency. Doppler measures velocity of any reflecting object/fluid by evaluating the frequency change of the reflected ultrasound. You have heard a Doppler frequency shift with cars and trains. When a whistling train approaches, you hear the "epee" sound. As soon as it passes, the frequency of the whistle suddenly drops to an "oooo." This change in pitch indicates that approaching objects compress the sound waves to make them sound higher pitch. Objects moving away, slow the sound waves bouncing from them. They thus sound lower in pitch. The more parallel the moving object is the ultrasound beam the greater the change in pitch; thus the cosine in the formula below. Objects moving perpendicular to the beam do not shift the frequency. Doppler's law says that the relative frequency of a reflected wave increases as the relative motion of the reflector approaches the observer. The Doppler equation uses the variables shown (no need to memorize this):

V = velocity of blood flow
F_1 = returning frequency
F_0 = transmitting frequency
C = Constant speed of sound in blood
φ = angle of incidence.

$$V = \frac{(F_1 - F_0)}{2F_0} \; \frac{C}{\cos \varphi}$$

See: Curry, Chapter on "Ultrasound." **Keywords:** Doppler principle

225. **Which below best describes turbulent blood flow?**
   a.   **Laminar and parallel blood streaming**
   b.   **Complex non-laminar fluid motion with vortex-like eddies.**
   c.   **Back and forth particle motion parallel to the direction of travel**
   d.   **Organized flow distribution where blood cells move with a uniform direction and velocity**

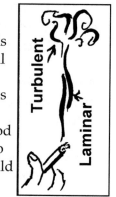

Turbulent
Laminar

Reynold's #

ANSWER b. Complex non-laminar fluid motion with vortex-like eddies. This chaotic blood flow pattern is important because it is found in areas of arterial and valvular stenosis. Here the kinetic energy of flow creates vortex-like eddies or vortices at the base of a waterfall. The overall fluid motion becomes complex. Heart murmurs are associated with turbulence. Even though the driving pressure increases across a stenotic valve, there is no increase in blood flow volume. Turbulence is generally bad in blood. It makes it more prone to clot, waste energy, and develop stenosis. The only place turbulent flow should normally occur is in the RV.

A simple example is seen in rising cigarette smoke. Smoke initially rises straight up in laminar flow. But it eventually rises so fast that it begins curling around in a turbulent pattern. **See:** Reynolds, chapter on "Doppler" **Keywords:**

turbulent flow

226. **What type of Doppler modality is shown in the lower half of the image as a time based graph with ECG?**

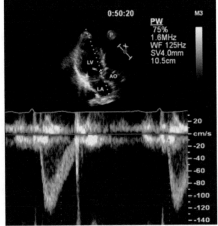

    a.   **Color Flow Doppler**
    b.   **Single Crystal Doppler**
    c.   **M-mode Doppler**
    d.   **Spectral Doppler**

ANSWER: d. Spectral Doppler. There is a tight band of flow away from the transducer at the lower edge of the display. This suggests normal aortic flow with no turbulence or spectral broadening. Flow occurs only during systole immediately following the QRS. The spikes in flow after the T wave are the aortic valve closing. This pulsed wave spectral Doppler uses the sample volume shown on the 2D echo in the upper half of the image positioned at the aortic valve.

PRESSURE TRANSDUCERS

227. **When a pressure transducer is balanced, it should be set to the patient's mid-chest level. What is the name of this zero pressure point?**

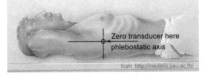

    a.   **Mid-axillary line**
    b.   **Zero reference**
    c.   **Phlebostatic axis**
    d.   **Hydrostatic CVP point**

ANSWER: c. Phlebostatic axis is the reference point for all cardiac pressures. With the patient reclining, it is a level mid-chest plane that passes approximately through the patient's RA. All pressure transducers must be set at this level for accurate readings prior to recording. When the zeroing transducer stopcock is open to air, adjust it to the patient's mid-chest level. This is most accurately set by measuring the patient's chest thickness, dividing this in two and then moving the transducer to that level using a ruler and level.

    "With the head of bed at 60 degrees or less, the phlebostatic axis is located at the fourth intercostal space at the mid-anterior-posterior diameter of the chest wall. This is the location of the right atrium, where the tip of a CVP catheter would lay. Maintaining the device stopcock at the phlebostatic axis will help ensure a proper reading. If the stopcock is positioned below the phlebostatic axis, the readings will be erroneously high; if above the phlebostatic axis, the readings will be erroneously low" from, Nursing Made Incredibly Easy, Understanding the phlebostatic axis, LWW Journal, 2011

228. **The patient is sitting up in bed. A pressure transducer accidentally set below the patient's phlebo-static axis (LA) position will result in a measured pressure that is:**
   a.   Too high
   b.   Too low
   c.   Overdamped
   d.   Underdamped

ANSWER: a. Too high. The real pressure gains energy as it drops down to the transducer. There is a head of pressure above the transducer pressing on it. All measured pressures will be too high by a fixed mmHg. Every inch too low will result in a pressure that is 2 mmHg high since mercury is 13 times heavier than water. Conversely, a transducer placed above the true zero position will furnish a measure pressure lower than the actual pressure. These small pressure changes caused by improper zeroing may lead to significant errors in diagnosis and perhaps, inappropriate therapy. See: Ragosta, chapter on Normal Waveforms.

229. **The diamond shaped arrangement of resistors in a pressure transducer or strain gauge is termed a:**
   a.   Carrier amplifier
   b.   Zeroing circuit
   c.   Modulator - circuit
   d.   Wheatstone Bridge

ANSWER: d. Wheatstone Bridge or strain gauge is an electrical circuit used to measure movement or pressure. This circuit contains four resistors which are balanced to give zero output. When one of these resistors is stretched (strained) by applied pressure the voltage across the bridge increases and is proportional to the pressure applied. See: Todd, Chapter E3 "Pressure Recording Systems"

4. Computers

230. **On a computer the LCD display is called a:**
   a.   CPU
   b.   Printer
   c.   Monitor
   d.   Scanner

ANSWER c. Monitor. Monitor is another word for display screen, however, the term usually refers to the entire device. Display screen can mean just the screen.

If you get up close to an LCD monitor, you'll see that the picture is made up of millions of tiny blocks or picture elements. Each element is effectively a separate red, green, or blue light that can be turned on or off very quickly using liquid crystals to rotate the polarized light thus making a moving color picture.

Before LCDs, cathode-ray tubes (CRT) were used in TVs and monitors. Within each tube were 3 electron guns - red, green, and blue - that would quickly and precisely "paint" a moving image on the back of the screen that you could see.
See: http://www.webopedia.com/TERM/M/monitor.html

231. Which item below is an input device?
   a.   **Monitor**
   b.   **Printer**
   c.   **Scanner**
   d.   **Speakers**

ANSWER: c. Scanner. A computer scanner is one of the many ways to input data into a computer. A keyboard, scanner or mouse are all examples of input devices. In computing, an image scanner—often abbreviated to just scanner— is a device that optically scans images, printed text, handwriting, or an object, and converts it to a digital image. See: http://www.webopedia.com/TERM/I/input_device.html

232. Which of the following is an example of a binary code?
   a.   **1238**
   b.   **1011**
   c.   **http://**
   d.   **1b5a4c**

ANSWER: b. 1011. A binary numbering system uses a system of numbers with two as its base, employing the digits 0 and 1. For example the binary numbers for 0, 1, 2, & 3 are written as 00, 01, 10, 11. The binary number shown 1011, is converted to decimal by remembering that each place from the right is a power of 2. E.g., 2^3, 2^2, 2^1, 2^0; 2^3 is 8; 2^2 is 4; 2^1 is 2; 2^0 is 1. Thus the number in this question, "1011" binary = 8 + 0 + 2 + 1 or "11" decimal. Four memory bits like this can store a binary number from 0 to 15. The binary system is used internally by all modern computers. See: http://www.webopedia.com/TERM/B/binary.html

233. An example of an output device is a:
   a.   **Mouse**
   b.   **Printer**
   c.   **Scanner**
   d.   **Keyboard**

ANSWER: b. Printer. An output device is any piece of computer hardware equipment used to communicate the results of data processing carried out by a computer to the outside world. Examples of output devices are: Speakers, Headphones, Screens (Monitor), and Printers. See: http://www.webopedia.com/TERM/O/output_device.html

234. The programed instructions that tell a computer what to do, that usually comes on a CD are termed:
 a. Software
 b. Hardware
 c. Processor
 d. Operating system

ANSWER: a. Software. Computer software, or just software, is the collection of computer programs and related data that provide the instructions telling a computer what to do. The term was coined to contrast with the term hardware (meaning physical devices). In contrast to hardware, software is intangible, meaning it "cannot be touched." See: http://www.webopedia.com/TERM/S/software.html

235. The main processing chip in a computer that tells it what to do is the:
 a. CPU
 b. Ram
 c. Rom
 d. Core

ANSWER: a. CPU is the brain and the single most important chip in the computer that tells it what to do. The central processing unit (CPU) or the "processor" carries out the instructions of a computer program. The "microprocessor" (E.g., Intel Pentium) incorporates a computer's central processing unit (CPU) on a single integrated circuit. See: http://www.webopedia.com/TERM/C/CPU.html

236. One kilobyte is
 a. 1,000 bytes or 2,000 bits
 b. 1,000 bytes or 8,000 bits
 c. 1,000,000 bytes or 2,000,000 bits
 d. 1,000,000 bytes or 8,000,000 bits

ANSWER: b. 1,000 bytes or 8,000 bits. Kilo mean one thousand, a byte is 8 bits. 1,000 x 8 = 8,000 bits. See: http://www.webopedia.com/TERM/S/software.html

237. A type of memory that <u>cannot</u> have information written to it, is termed:
 a. DRAM
 b. RAM
 c. ROM
 d. SRAM

ANSWER: c. ROM is Read Only Memory. This contains the basic startup instructions, which are set by the computer manufacturer. In its strictest sense, ROM refers only to mask ROM (the oldest type of solid state ROM), which is fabricated with data permanently stored in it, and thus can never be modified. However, more modern types such as EPROM and flash EEPROM can be erased and re-programmed multiple times; they are still

described as "read-only memory"(ROM). The other kind of memory to which you can both write and read is termed "Random Access Memory" (RAM). See:
http://www.webopedia.com/TERM/R/ROM.html

238. **The smallest spot on a digital image is termed a:**

a.   **Pixel**
b.   **Raster**
c.   **Bit**
d.   **Byte**

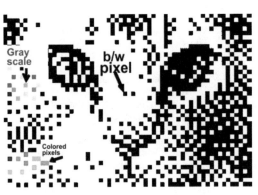

ANSWER: a. Pixel. Each small dots in the image is a pixel. "Short for **Pic**ture **El**ement, a pixel is a single point in a graphic image. Graphics monitors display pictures by dividing the display screen into thousands (or millions) of pixels, arranged in rows and columns. The pixels are so close together that they appear connected."

"The number of bits used to represent each pixel determines how many colors or shades of gray can be displayed. For example, in 8-bit color mode, the color monitor uses 8 bits for each pixel, making it possible to display 2 to the 8th power (256) different colors or shades of gray. On color monitors, each pixel is actually composed of three dots -- a red, a blue, and a green one. Ideally, the three dots should all converge at the same point." See:
http://www.webopedia.com/TERM/P/pixel.html

References

Aston & Brown, Medical Instrumentation for Nurses and Allied Health-Care
        Professionals, 1994, Johns and Bartlett Publishers
Baim, D. S. and Grossman W., *Cardiac Catheterization, Angiography, and Intervention*,
        6th Ed., Lea and Febiger, 2006
Braunwald, Eugene, et.al. Ed., *HEART DISEASE A Textbook of Cardiovascular Medicine*, 8th Ed., W. B. Saunders
        Co., 2012
Curry, Dowdey, and Murry, Christensen's Introduction to the Physics of Diagnostic   Radiology,
3rd Ed., Lea & Febiger Publisher
Khalil Kanjwal, et al. "Defibrillation Threshold Testing: A Primer" in Journal
        of Innovations in Cardiac Rhythm Management 2012 Medtronic.com
Moses, K. Weston, et al., *A Practical Guide to Cardiac Pacing*, 4th Ed., Little and
        Brown Co., 1995
Nave and Nave, Physics for the Health Sciences, W. B Saunders Co.
Reynolds, Terry, RDCS, BS, ULTRASOUND PHYSICS, Registry Exam Preparation
        Guide, Arizona Heart Institute Foundation, Phoenix, AZ 1996
Todd, J.W., Cardiovascular Invasive Review Book, Vol. IV, Hemodynamics, 2012
Watson, Sandy, Ed., *Invasive Cardiology, A manual for Cath Lab Personnel*, 2nd Ed., Physicians Press, 2005

OUTLINE: A3 - Instrumentation

1.   Electricity and Magnetism - Definitions
     a.   Frequency   = Hertz
     b.   Force= Newton
     c.   Energy or work = Joule
     d.   Power=Watt
     e.   Charge=Coulomb= Amp sec = quantity of electron charges
     f.   Potential=Volt=driving force or pressure

g. Capacitance=Farad= short term charge storage
h. Magnetic flux =Weber=quantity of magnetic flux
i. Mag. induction =Tesla (Gauss)
j. Energy = WattSec = joules
k. Impedance = resistance (ohms)
l. Components: Capacitor, resistor, etc.
2. Electrical Concepts
   a. Rectifiers (diodes) are one way valves
   b. Rectifiers (diodes) are one way valves = battery = 0 Hz.
   c. Elimination of certain frequencies =filter
      i. ECG filtering: 0.1 - 100 Hz
      ii. High pass, Low Pass filters
      iii. Notch filter
   d. Capacitors store charge for defibrillators
   e. Voltage is electricity's driving force
   f. Ohm's Law, I = V/R
      i. Series, parallel resistors
      ii. Pacer lead: Broken wire or insulation
   g. Thermistor resistance varies with temp. for TDCO
   h. Transducer converts one form of energy into another
3. Defibrillator Concepts
   a. Function of battery, capacitor, diode
   b. Daily Testing - test fire in unit, document
   c. Synchronized Cardioversion - on R wave
   d. Quick Look paddles - not in sync mode
   e. ICD concepts
      i. Coil electrodes
      ii. DFT
      iii. 1- 40 joules
      iv. Joules = watt sec
      v. Cardioversion, defibrillation
4. Pacemaker Concepts
   a. Leads
      i. Unipolar, bipolar
      ii. Fixation: active (tined), passive
      iii. Distal tip electrode - polarity
      iv. Ring or can electrode + polarity
   b. Threshold measurement
      i. 1 volt RV minimum
      ii. Acute /chronic threshold
   c. Chamber paced
      i. RA, RV, BiV, dual chamber
      ii. CRT / BiV pacer = CS / LV lead
         (1) Resynchronization in CHF
   d. Types:
      i. Permanent: constant voltage
      ii. Temporary: constant current (mA)
   e. Sensing & inhibition
      i. Asynchronous pacing
      ii. Demand pacing
      iii. Inappropriate pacing (on T wave)
5. Electrical Safety Concepts
   a. Macroshock
      i. Hand to hand most lethal
      ii. 60 cycle most lethal frequency
   b. Skin Resistance/ intracardiac resistance through pacing lead
   c. Microshock
      i. 10 microAmps safe limit
      ii. Discharge static electricity
   d. Biomed. check all equipment
   e. Grounding

   i. 3 prong plug
   ii. Hot, return, ground wires
   f. Use battery powered equipment
   g. no earth ground
   h. Plastic nonconductive chassis
   i. Turn Machines off when not in use
   j. Don't pull or insert plug when equipment turned on
   k. Don't pull power cord, pull plug
   l. Sparks = danger
6. Ultrasound Concepts
   a. Ultrasound transducers = Piezoelectric crystal
   b. Piezoelectric effect
   c. Period (T) is the time per cycle
   d. f = 1/period or f = 1
   e. US Frequencies used:
      i. Adult TTE = 2.5 – 3 MHz
      ii. Infant TTE = 5 – 7.5 MHz
      iii. ICE = 5- 10 MHz
      iv. IVUS = 20 – 40 MHz
   f. Speed of an ultrasound wave varies in Air, soft tissue, bone
      i. 1540 M/sec in soft tissue
   g. Higher frequency of ultrasound
      i. reduces depth of Penetration
      ii. improves lateral resolution
   h. Frequency = Vel./Wavelength
7. ICE - Intracardiac Echo
   a. Phased array: pie shaped display
   b. Mechanical / rotating (Boston Sci.)
      i. 360 degree display
8. TEE = Transesophageal Echo
   a. Evaluate clots in LAA
9. IVUS - Intravascular Ultrasound
   a. Phased Array: multiple crystals
   b. Mechanical / rotating (Boston Sci.)
   c. Pullback recording = 0.5 - 1 mm/sec
10. Doppler Concepts
   a. Measures frequency shift
      ii. Evaluate blood Velocity
      iii. Laminar / turbulent flow
      iv. Target = RBC
11. Transducers
   a. Converts one form of energy to another
   b. Thermistor
   c. Pulse oximeter
   d. Xray detector
   e. Piezoelectric, echo transducer
   f. Pressure transducer
      i. Wheatstone bridge modulation / demodulation
      iv. Phlebostatic axis = mid chest
      v. 13 mm H20 = 1 mmHg
      vi. 1 mmHg = 1 Torr
12. Pressure Concepts
   a. H2O hydrostatic pressure 1 meter =100 gm/cm2
   b. One Torr = 1 mmHg or 1/760 th BP
13. Computer Concepts
   a. Input / output devices
   b. Memory: Ram, ROM, hard drive...
   c. CPU
   d. Pixel
   e. Binary / analog

Sterilization & Asepsis

INDEX: A4 - Sterilization and Asepsis

1. General Asepsis

239. Identify the meaning of the term labeled #1 in the box.

a. Destroys all microorganisms
b. Inhibits or stops growth of bacteria
c. Kills bacteria
d. Destroys most pathogens on living tissues
e. Destroys most pathogens on instruments, unsafe for living tissues
f. Destroys all pathogens

TERMS
1. Disinfect
2. Bacteriostatic
3. Bactericidal
4. Antiseptic
5. Sterilize
6. Aseptic

ANSWER e. Destroys most pathogens on instruments, unsafe for living tissues. Know all the terms and their meanings. **BE ABLE TO MATCH ALL ANSWERS.**

TERM	MEANING
1. Disinfect	Destroys most pathogens on instruments. Unsafe for living tissues.
2. Bacteriostatic	Inhibits or stops growth of bacteria (-static = hold steady).
3. Bactericidal	Kills bacteria (-cidal = kill).
4. Antiseptic	Destroys most pathogens on living tissue, safe to use on skin.
5. Sterilize	Destroys all microorganisms.
6. Aseptic	Destroys all pathogens (-sepsis = infection).

See: Burton, chapter on "Control of Microbial Growth."   **Keywords:** Disinfect

239. Identify an agent that performs the aseptic function labeled #1 (disinfect) in the box.

a. Penicillin, Amoxicillin
b. Clorox, Glutaraldehyde (Cidex)
c. Hexachloraphene, Benzalkonium Chloride (Zephiran)
d. Alcohol (70%), Povidone-iodine
e. Autoclave, ETO gas

TERMS
1. Disinfect
2. Bacteriostatic
3. Bactericidal
4. Antiseptic
5. Sterilize

ANSWER b. Clorox, Glutaraldehyde. Know all the agents, classes and functions listed below. **BE ABLE TO MATCH ALL ANSWERS.**

AGENTS	CLASS	FUNCTION
1. Clorox, Glutaraldehyde (Cidex)	Disinfect	Destroys most pathogens on instruments, unsafe for living tissues
2. Hexachlorophene, Benzalkonium chloride (Zephiran)	Bacteriostatic	Inhibits or stops growth of bacteria. Often put in soap to inhibit growth of skin flora for several hours.
3. Penicillin, and other antibiotics	Bacteriocidal	Kills bacteria but not virus in vivo
4. Alcohol (70%), Povidone-iodine	Antiseptic	Destroy most pathogens on living tissue, safe to use on skin
5. Autoclave, ETO Gas	Sterilize	Destroys **ALL** microorganisms if certain precautions are taken (time, temp, packing, circulation...)

See: Burton, chapter on "Control of Microbial Growth." **Keywords:** Disinfectants = Clorox, Glutaraldehyde

240. Medical ASEPTIC SKIN PREP is directed at cleanliness and:
   a.   Killing all microbial agents
   b.   Inhibiting the growth of all microbial agents
   c.   Reducing the numbers of all infectious agents (pathogens)
   d.   Elimination of all infectious agents (pathogens)

ANSWER d. Elimination of all infectious agents (pathogens). Asepsis means the **absence of infectious agents.** The problem is that **skin cannot be sterilized.** Even after the best scrubbing and antiseptic application, there always exist resident microorganism deep in the crevices and folds of the skin. Since resident skin flora live with us constantly, they are considered not pathogenic and their minimal presence must be tolerated in medical asepsis. **See:** Gruendemann & Meeker, chapter on "Principles and Procedures of Asepsis." **Keywords:** Asepsis

241. Cardiovascular personnel should use strict infection control and universal/standard precautions when dealing with:
   a.   Any patient with recent history of infection
   b.   Any patient with a known communicable disease
   c.   Any patient suspected of having a communicable disease
   d.   All patients

ANSWER d. All patients. You cannot tell which patients have an infectious disease (such as hepatitis or are HIV+) because laws protect patients from public disclosure. "UNIVERSAL PRECAUTIONS or STANDARD PRECAUTIONS" means that everyone should be treated as if they are potential pathogen carriers. Universal precautions require you to treat **all body fluids from anyone** as potentially infectious.
See: Torres, chapter on "Infection Control."   **Keywords:** universal precautions

242. **The chief purpose of hospital "infection control" is to prevent:**
   a. **Nosocomial infections**
   b. **Opportunistic infections**
   c. **Airborne infections**
   d. **Vector infections**

ANSWER a. Nosocomial infections. These are infections originating in the hospital, that were not present prior to admission. Infections developing within 3 days after admission are suspected to be "nosocomial" in origin. Hospital-acquired infections most frequently arise from poor aseptic technique within the hospital.
See: Burton, chapter on "Control of Microbial Growth."   **Keywords:** nosocomial infections

243. **In the cath lab, which patient would be most susceptible to infection?**
   a. **Neonates**
   b. **Cancer patients**
   c. **Heart transplant patients**
   d. **Open heart surgery patients**

ANSWER c. Heart transplant patients are susceptible to infection because they are taking immuno-suppression drugs. Immuno-suppressants reduce the chance of tissue rejection to heart transplant patients. That's why they often wear a mask. Other patients susceptible to infection include those with diseases that suppress the autoimmune system, such as AIDS or chemotherapy patients.
See: Gruendemann & Meeker, chapter on "Principles and Procedures of Asepsis."
Keywords: infections most susceptible in immune suppressed patients

244. **Bacteria that CANNOT live in the presence of AIR are known as:**
   a. **Aerobes**
   b. **Anaerobes**
   c. **Mesophiles**
   d. **Bacteriophiles**

ANSWER b. Anaerobes can live only in the absence of air because oxygen is poisonous to these germs. Pathogens such as tetanus and botulism are anaerobic bacteria. The opposite type of germs are "aerobes" such as TB, cholera, and diphtheria that require oxygen and thrive in the lungs.
See: Gruendemann & Meeker, chapter on "Principles and Procedures of Asepsis."
Keywords: anaerobic organisms

2. Sterilization Technique

245. The most complete, practical, efficient, and inexpensive method to sterilize metal instruments involves:
   a.   Chemicals
   b.   Dry heat
   c.   Steam heat
   d.   Ethylene oxide gas

ANSWER c. Steam heat. Burton says, "Heat is the most practical, efficient, and inexpensive method of disinfection and sterilization of objects that can withstand high temperatures. Because of these advantages, it is the means most frequently employed." ETO gas sterilization is effective but it is more expensive and takes a long time. Gruendemann says, "Any item that can be steam sterilized should never be gas sterilized."

In a rush, metal instruments may be "flash" sterilized with dry heat. Burton says, "Heat applied in the presence of moisture, such as boiling, or steaming, is more effective than dry heat because moist heat causes the proteins to coagulate... Moist heat is faster than dry heat, and can be done at lower temperatures..." The effectiveness of dry heat depends on how deeply the heat penetrates. So, the items to be "baked" must be arranged so the hot air circulates freely among them.
See: Burton, chapter on "Control of Microbial Growth."   **Keywords:** heat sterilization

246. Effective sterilization by autoclave depends on adequate:
   a.   Temperature and pressure
   b.   Temperature and time
   c.   Time and pressure
   d.   Time and concentration

ANSWER b. Temperature and time. Adequate autoclave sterilization requires a minimum of 120 degrees C for 20 minutes. An autoclave is a pressure cooker with pressures of 15 psi. The circulating pressurized steam increases the temperature above regular boiling point. The autoclave time and temperature cycles are recorded on a graph to document the adequacy of the cycle.

Resistant microorganisms such as spores and viruses may survive autoclaving if they are hidden inside blood or tissue due to the insulation provided by the surrounding material. Thus, pay careful attention to packaging and quality control.
See: Burton, chapter on "Control of Microbial Growth." **Keywords:** autoclave sterilization requires: time & temp.

247. Sterilization of most plastic materials is best achieved with:
   a.   Benzalkonium chloride (Zephiran)
   b.   Ethylene oxide (gas)
   c.   Povidone-iodine
   d.   Steam autoclaving

ANSWER b. Ethylene oxide (gas). Gruendemann says, "As a sterilizing agent, ethylene

oxide has the advantage that it is easily available, is effective against all types of microorganisms, easily penetrates through masses of dry material, does not require high temperatures, humidity, or pressure, and is noncorrosive and non-damaging to items....In general ethylene oxide sterilization should be used only if the materials are heat sensitive and will not withstand sterilization by saturated steam under pressure. Any item that can be steam sterilized should never be gas sterilized." There is a long aeration period, and it is more expensive than steam.
See: Gruendemann & Meeker, chapter on "Principles and Procedures of Asepsis."
Keywords: ethylene oxide gas

248. **Why would you elect to sterilize certain items with gas sterilization instead of steam?**
   a.   **It is less expensive**
   b.   **It is less damaging to items**
   c.   **It is more effective**
   d.   **It is faster**

ANSWER b. It is less damaging to items. EO gas is an effective substitute for most items that cannot be sterilized by heat and pressure, or that would be damaged by repeated exposure to heat. Can you imagine steam sterilizing a pacemaker, with all its electronic components? No. EO gas is noncorrosive and does not damage items. It completely penetrates porous and most plastic packaging.
See: Allmers, Review for Surgical Tech. Exam, chapter on "Fundamentals" **Keywords:** gas sterilization less damaging

249. **What is the most common vector for spread of infection within the hospital?**
   a.   **Insects and parasites**
   b.   **Coughing (air borne)**
   c.   **Failure to wash hands**
   d.   **Soiled linen and instruments**

ANSWER c. Failure to wash hands.
Torres says, "Microbes are most commonly spread from one person to another by human hands. It follows that the best means of preventing the spread of microorganisms is hand-washing...even if gloves have been worn....Any exposed breaks in your skin must be covered by a waterproof protective covering." Hepatitis B virus can live for over a week in dried blood. It can easily be picked up by your hands and spread.
See: Torres, chapter on "Infection Control." **Keywords:** hand washing

250. "Shelf life" is the length of time a sterilized pack may be considered "sterile." What is the shelf life of items labeled #1 (single cloth wrap)?

a.   Not sterile
b.   21-30 days
c.   6 months - 1 year
d.   Indefinitely

SHELF LIFE
1. Single cloth wrapping
2. Double cloth wrapping
3. Heat-sealed plastic wrapping
4. Non-woven envelopes encased in sealed plastic wrapping

ANSWER a. Not sterile. **(Be able to match all 4 shelf-life items.)**
1. Single cloth wrapping = Not sterile. Can only be sterilized if double wrapped in appropriate cloth.
2. Double cloth wrapping = 21-30 days
3. Single-layer heat-sealed plastic wrapping = 6 months - 1 year
4. Sealed envelopes encased in sealed plastic wrapping are sterile indefinitely if not damaged, stored incorrectly, or handled roughly.
Shelf life is really more event dependent than time dependent. Things that must be considered in determining "shelf-life" are: type and number of layers of packaging, imperviousness of cover, package handling, and conditions of storage.
See: Gruendemann & Meeker, chapter on "Principles and Procedures of Asepsis."

251. The most positive assurance that the inside of a surgical pack is sterile is by checking its:

a.   Mechanical sterilization indicators
b.   Heat-sensitive tape
c.   Biological indicators
d.   Chemical indicators

ANSWER c. Biological indicators provide positive assurance that a pack is sterile. These consist of living spores. When properly sterilized, the biological indicator turns color indicating all organisms have been killed. Unlike heat-sensitive tape, biological indicators are placed inside packs to provide the final proof that even the most resistant of micro-organisms (spores) deep in the pack have been destroyed. The CDC recommends weekly use to assure steam sterilization kills everything deep within the pack. **See:** Allmers, Review for Surgical Tech. Exam, chapter on "Fundamentals"indicator

252. A packaged sterilize item that is accidentally dropped on the floor is considered sterile only if it has not been damaged and is:

a.   Used immediately
b.   Enclosed in impervious material (plastic)
c.   Wrapped in 3 or more layers of woven cloth
d.   In a surgically clean area

ANSWER b. Enclosed in impervious material (plastic). Such airtight packaging prevents entry of dust and moisture, but only if the integrity of the packaging is maintained. Dropped cloth-wrapped items should no longer be considered sterile.

See: Allmers, Review for Surgical Tech. Exam, chapter on "Fundamentals" **Keywords:** dropped item - only if plastic wrapped

253. **Identify 3 acceptable wrappers for gas sterilized items.**
   a.   **Nylon**
   b.   **Muslin**
   c.   **Paper**
   d.   **Plastic**
   e.   **Tinfoil or other metal**

ANSWERS: b, c, & d.
   a.   Nylon - NO
   b.   Muslin - YES
   c.   Paper - YES
   d.   Plastic - YES

Cloth, fabrics, paper, and most other plastic can be safely penetrated by the ethylene oxide gas. Nylon, because of inadequate permeability to the gas, is considered unacceptable. **See:** Allmers, Review for Surgical Tech. Exam, chapter on "Fundamentals"

254. **Which of the following is the ONLY acceptable plastic wrapper for steam sterilized items?**
   a.   **Polyethylene**
   b.   **Polyvinyl chloride (PVC)**
   c.   **Polyamide**
   d.   **Polypropylene**

ANSWER d. Polypropylene plastic film is the only plastic that is acceptable and will not melt under the extreme heat. Polypropylene pouches come pre-sealed on 3 sides. Items are placed in the pouch and the open side is then heat sealed.
See: Allmers, Review for Surgical Tech. Exam, chapter on "Fundamentals" **Keywords:** Polypropylene plastic only

255. **Which skin prep is the least harmful to skin and provides the longest lasting asepsis?**
   a.   **Alcohol rub**
   b.   **Povidone-iodine**
   c.   **Chlorhexidine (Hibiclens)**
   d.   **Parachlorometaxylenol (PCMX)**

ANSWER: c. Chlorhexidine (Hibiclens) or ChloraPrep, have excellent residual activity and are excellent against Gram-Positive bacteria. The others listed have poor to fair residual effect. **See:** Surgical Technology: Principles and Practice, by Fuller, 2013

256. **Which 3 of the following help reduce permanent pacemaker implant (PPI) infection? (Select 3.)**
   a.   **The best prep is povidone-iodine**
   b.   **The best wound dressings contain silver**
   c.   **Administer antibiotic one hour before procedure**
   d.   **Compulsive attention to sterile technique**
   e.   **Mesh jacket around pacemaker**

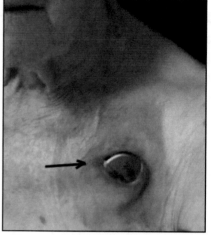

ANSWERS: b, c, & d.
   a.   The best prep is povidone-iodine - NO. It is chlorhexidine-alcohol.
   b.   The best wound dressings contain silver - YES
   c.   Administer antibiotic one hour before procedure - YES
   d.   Compulsive attention to sterile technique - YES

Pacer pocket infection

   e.   Jackets are placed to prevent movement in the pocket (E.g., twiddlers syndrome). Some may contain silver or other antibacterial compounds.

These are AHA, Recommendations for Antimicrobial Prophylaxis at the Time of CIED (Cardiovascular Implantable Electronic Devices) Placement 2010.

"Preoperative antiseptic preparation of the skin of the surgical site should be done....Preoperative skin cleansing with chlorhexidine-alcohol is superior to povidone-iodine, ... Intraprocedurally, compulsive attention to sterile technique is mandatory.... Prevention of CIED infection can be addressed before, during, and after device implantation. Before device implantation, it is important to ensure that patients do not have clinical signs of infection. A parenterally administered antibiotic is recommended one hour before the procedure. Data ... strongly support the administration of antibiotic prophylaxis for CIED implantation. Most experts continue to advocate a first-generation cephalosporin, such as cefazolin, for use as prophylaxis." (or Gentamicin)
http://circ.ahajournals.org/content/121/3/458.full

....."It has been known for many years that silver has antimicrobial properties. Arglaes (Medline Industries, Inc., Mundelein, IL) dressings use silver antimicrobial technology and are designed to prevent SSIs [Surgical Site Infections]. The dressings are transparent, designed for wound care and were the first antimicrobial, sustained-release dressings on the market. Arglaes provides a continuous and controlled release of silver ions, which act as an antibacterial agent. The ionic silver creates an environment that is hostile to bacteria and fungi, yet non-cytotoxic (e.g. will not harm healthy tissue), and the sustained-activity ionic silver maintains full efficacy for up to 7 days."
http://www.innovationsincrm.com/cardiac-rhythm-management/2010/october/25-prevention-of-bacterial-infections-cied

257. **Cleaning the room of dust and wiping it down is termed:**
   a.   **Asepsis**
   b.   **Case turnover**
   c.   **Case disinfection**
   d.   **Terminal decontamination**

ANSWER: d. Terminal decontamination follows every case. It follows removal of instruments and contaminated disposables. It focuses on areas soiled with blood, tissue or body fluids. A disinfectant is used to clean surfaces and fixtures. Decontamination of instruments, devices, table, floors, operating table & pad is critical to prevent transmission of infection. **See:** Surgical Technology: Principles and Practice, by Fuller, 2013

258. The opening in a single use sterile femoral drape sheet is called a:

a. Lumen
b. Window
c. Foramen
d. Access site
e. Fenestration

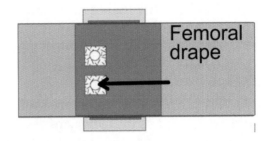

ANSWER: e. A fenestrated drape has a round or slit-like opening in the center. "Single use/disposable drapes are composed of nonwoven natural and synthetic materials ... These fabrics include a fluid-proof polyethylene film laminated between the fabric layers at strategic locations of the drape, usually around the drape fenestration..." **See:** Essential of Perioperative Nursing", chapter on "Aseptic Practices" by Cynthia Spry, Jonas and Bartlett Publishers

3. Sterile Principles and Techniques

259. How should a circulator open the first flap of cloth-wrapped sterile packs? First place the sterile pack on the back table, pull off the sterile indicator tape, then:

a. Move first flap towards you (over front of table)
b. Move first flap away from you (over the top of the pack)
c. Move the right flap over the right side of the table
d. Grasp both flaps and spread them right & left over both sides of the table

ANSWER b. Move first flap **AWAY** from you (over the top of the pack). This prevents you from touching the open sterile field, because it is away from you. Finally, the near flap is opened **TOWARDS** you as you back away, preventing contamination. This sequence is opposite to that used by a sterile person opening a pack as seen below. **See:** Burton, chapter on "Control of Microbial Growth." **Keywords:** circulator first opens pack away

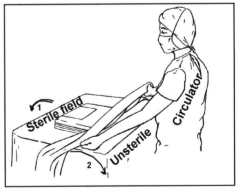

Unsterile person opens last flap towards

260. How should the skin be prepped with each chlorhexidine sponge prior to heart cath?
   a. Soaked overnight with a soaked sponge, then scrubbed briskly back and forth
   b. Shaved the day before, then scrubbed in the same direction as the hair grows
   c. Begin at the inside and scrub away from the puncture site in a spiraling manner
   d. Start at incision area with gentle back and forth motions, progressing out to periphery of the field.

ANSWER d. **Start at incision area with gentle back and forth motion of sponge, progressing out to periphery of the field.** ChloraPrep 10.5 ml applicator IFU says, "Pinch the wingts only once to activate the ampoule and release the antiseptic. Allow the solution to partially load in the sponge. Gently press the applicator against the treatment area to evenly distribute the solution throughout the sponge. Once the solution is visible on the skin, completely wet the treatment/incision area with the antiseptic, using gentle back-and-forth strokes for 30 seconds or two minutes, progressing from the incision site to the periphery of the surgical field."
See: Gruendemann & Meeker, chapter on "Principles and Procedures of Asepsis."

261. How should a sterile scrub assistant open a sterile pack? Open the first flap ___ you and the last flap ___ you.
   a. Towards, Away
   b. Towards, Towards
   c. Away, Towards
   d. Away, Away

ANSWER a. Towards, Away. This establishes a sterile field between you and the pack so you can protect the sterile pack and your gown from contamination. The final sterile flap is moved AWAY from you over the top of the pack as shown. Note that this is opposite to the circulator's sequence described above. **See:** Gruendemann & Meeker, chapter on "Principles and Procedures of Asepsis."

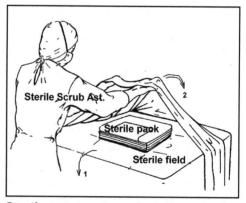

Sterile person opens last flap away

262. Which of the following statements about surgical asepsis are true? (Select 3.)
   a. When in doubt about the sterility of an item, consider it unsterile
   b. The front and back of a wrap-around gown are considered sterile
   c. The sides of sterile tables are considered unsterile
   d. Instruments used in contact with the skin such as sponge forceps are discarded and not reused
   e. Only steam sterilized items are considered sterile

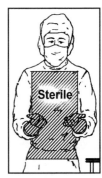

ANSWERS: a, c, & d.

a. When in doubt about the sterility of an item, consider it unsterile - YES. For the patient's safety, anyone who sees a break in aseptic technique should immediately mention it to the person in charge.

b. The front and back of a wrap-around gown is considered sterile - NO. For this reason, arms should not be crossed and tucked under the armpit. Because they cannot be carefully watched, the backs of gown are considered contaminated. They are only considered sterile in the front, from the waist (table) level, and only from 2 inches below the elbow down to the gloves.

c. The sides of sterile tables are considered unsterile - YES. Only the top surface of the table is sterile. A sterile person rolling a sterile table should hold it by the top surface only, not the sides.

Gown, Sterile areas

d. Instruments used in contact with the skin such as sponge forceps are discarded and not reused - YES. Sponge sticks should NOT be put back among the other sterile instruments. Remove them from your sterile field. They have touched the patient's skin.

e.   ETO gas sterilization is acceptable.

See: Gruendemann, chapter on "Principles... of Asepsis." **Keywords:** gown sterile area

263. **You are setting up the sterile table for a probable PCI. The patient is brought in and put on the angio table. The physician then calls and cancels the procedure. What should you do with the sterile table that is set up in the room?**
a.   **Leave it open and save it for the next case immediately to follow.**
b.   **Tear it down and discard all disposable items. Start a new table for next case.**
c.   **Cover it with a sterile cloth drape. It is considered sterile for only 6 hours**
d.   **Discard all solutions and cover it with a sterile plastic drape. It is considered sterile for 12 hours.**

ANSWER: b. Tear it down and start completely over for the next case. Surgery encyclopedia says, "The environment contains potential hazards that may spread pathogens through movement, touch, or proximity... restrict traffic in the operating room. Sterile packages or fields are opened or created as close as possible to time of actual use." The safety of the next patient to enter the room is the most important. If you can cover the dry table before the patient enters the room it may be saved and used on the next case.
See: http://www.surgeryencyclopedia.com/A-Ce/Aseptic-Technique.html

264. **Identify the gloving method labeled #1 (closed) in the box.**
a.   **Gown sleeves are used to handle gloves**
b.   **First glove is grasped by bare hand inside of cuff**
c.   **Glove is stretched open with both hands**

GLOVING METHODS
*1. Self-gowning closed
2. Self-gowning open
3. Another individual

ANSWER a. Gown sleeves are used to handle gloves

GLOVING METHODS (Be able to match all 3 above.)

1. SELF-GOWNING CLOSED METHOD: In this method your hands are surrounded "closed in" and protected by the gown sleeve that is used to handle the gloves. Left glove is placed palm down on your left sleeve as shown. Grasp the cuff of the glove through the gown with your left hand. With your right hand protected by the sleeve, grasp the top of the glove, and stretch it over your left hand. Insert your left hand into the glove through the gown sleeve.

2. SELF-GOWNING OPEN METHOD: In this method your hands are unprotected, and are "open" to the air. The first glove is grasped by your bare hand inside of the cuff. Grasp left glove cuff with right hand. Insert left hand into glove. Pick up right glove with cuff as shown. Insert right hand into glove. Roll back cuffs over sleeves.

3. GLOVING ANOTHER INDIVIDUAL: Glove is stretched open with both hands. After one individual has gowned and gloved herself, she grasps the preferred glove by the cuff, as shown. The second individual inserts his hand into opened glove. Be able to match all above answers. **See:** Gruendemann & Meeker, chapter on "Principles and Procedures of Asepsis."

265. **You are gowned and gloved. The operating physician has just scrubbed and enters the lab looking at you. Which of the statements below are true regarding gowning him? (Select 3.)**

a.   **Open the hand towel and lay it on the doctor's hand**
b.   **Place the folded gown into the hands of the doctor.**
c.   **Keep your hands on the outside of the gown under a protective cuff**
d.   **Open the gown and hold it so the doctor can insert his dry hands into the sleeves.**
e.   **Glove the Dr. Before he dons his gown**

ANSWERS: a, c, & d.
a. Open the hand towel and lay it on the doctor's hand - YES.
b. Place the folded gown into the dry hands of doctor - NO.
c. Keep your hands on the outside of the gown under a protective cuff - YES.
d. Open the gown and hold it so the doctor can insert his dry hands into the sleeves - YES.
e. The gown should be put on 1st, then the gloves - NO.
Before handling a gown, grasp it at the neckband, hold it up and let the lower parts unfold. While keeping your hands protected on the outside of the gown, open it and hold it by its outside shoulders so the doctor can insert his hands into the sleeves. Do all this while protecting yourself from contamination. The physician must dry his hands before donning his sterile gown. **See:** Allmers, Review for Surgical Tech. Exam, chapter on "Fundamentals"

266. You are scrubbed-in on a pacemaker implant procedure when you contaminate your right glove. The circulator should help you by:
   a.   Helping you re-gown and re-glove using the closed technique
   b.   Helping you re-gown and re-glove using the open technique
   c.   Pulling off your right glove and opening a new pair for you
   d.   Pulling off both your gloves and opening a new pair for you

ANSWER c. Have the circulator pull off your right glove, and open a new pair for you. You can use your sterile left hand to don the right glove using either the open or closed technique. You need not replace the left glove or re-gown unless they were contaminated.
See: Allmers, Review for Surgical Tech. Exam, chapter on "Fundamentals"

267. At the end of a case you remove your gown and gloves. Which of the statements below are true? (Select 3.)
   a.   Remove the gloves first before the gown
   b.   Remove your gloves inside out
   c.   Have the circulator untie your gown
   d.   Pull the gown off inside out

ANSWERS: b, c, & d.
a. Remove the gloves first before the gown - NO.
b. Remove your gloves inside out - YES.
c. Have the circulator untie your gown - YES.
d. Pull the gown off inside out - YES.

After the circulator unties it, your gown is always removed first. It is pulled downward from the shoulders, turning the sleeves inside out as it is pulled off the arms. Likewise, gloves are removed inside out, using the glove-to-glove then skin-to-skin technique.
See: Allmers, Review for Surgical Tech. Exam, chapter on "Fundamentals"

268. When doing a surgical scrub, how high should you scrub up your arm?
   a.   Scrub to the mid-forearm
   b.   Scrub to 2 inches below the elbow
   c.   Scrub to the elbow
   d.   Scrub to 2 inches above the elbow

ANSWER d. 2 inches above the elbow. The surgical scrub should include the hands, wrists, forearms, elbows, antecubital fossa up to 2 inches above the elbow.
See: Allmers, Review for Surgical Tech. Exam, chapter on "Fundamentals"

269. When pouring a sterile solution from a screw top bottle onto a sterile field:
   a.   Open, pour only once, then discard left-over solution.
   b.   Once opened, solutions may be poured again from same bottle, but only on the same case.
   c.   Use sterile procedure to pour again during same case, as long as sterile cap

is replaced between uses.

    d.   Use sterile procedure to pour as many times as you wish, as long as sterile cap is replaced between uses.

ANSWER a. Open, pour only once, then discard left-over solution. After a sterile bottle is opened, the contents must be used or discarded. The cap cannot be replaced without contamination of the pouring edges. The edges of anything that encloses sterile contents are considered unsterile. **See:** Allmers, Review for Surgical Tech. Exam, "Fundamentals"

270. Draped sterile tables are considered sterile on the top:
    a.   And sides as long as table is watched by scrub person
    b.   And sides, down to 1 inch from the bottom edge
    c.   And patient's side only
    d.   Top only - not any sides

ANSWER d. On the top surface only, not any sides. A sterile table is considered sterile only on the top. The edges and sides extending below the table level are not considered sterile. **See:** Allmers, Review for Surgical Tech. Exam, chapter on "Fundamentals" **Keywords:** Table top sterile only

271. Which of the statements below are true regarding sterility? (Select 3.)
    a.   Wrapper edges are unsterile
    b.   Instruments or sutures hanging over the table edge are discarded
    c.   Sterile persons pass each other back to back
    d.   A sterile person faces a nonsterile person when passing
    e.   Instruments exposed to the patient's blood are considered unsterile

ANSWERS: a, b, & c.
a. Wrapper edges are unsterile - YES.
b. Instruments or sutures hanging over the table edge are discarded - YES.
c. Sterile persons pass each other back to back - YES.
d. A sterile person faces a nonsterile person when passing - NO. A sterile person turns his back to a nonsterile person or area when passing. This is to protect the scrub assistant's sterile frontal area.
e. The patient's blood is considered sterile.
See: Allmers, Review for Surgical Tech. Exam, chapter on "Fundamentals" **Keywords:** Turn back to a nonsterile person when passing

272. Which of the statements below are true about wearing <u>shoe covers</u> in surgical environments? (Select 3.)
    a.   Are usually considered optional
    b.   Reduce the risk of surgical site infections
    c.   May NOT be worn outside the surgical suite
    d.   Wash your hands after removing shoe covers
    e.   Reduce spread of infections to staff around hospital

ANSWERS: a, c, & d.

a. Are usually considered optional - YES.

b. Reduce the risk of surgical site infections - NO.

c. May NOT be worn outside the surgical suite - YES.

d. Wash your hands after removing shoe covers - YES.

Spry says,"Shoe covers are usually optional and have not been shown to contribute to reducing surgical site infection rates. Shoe covers may be worn to protect personnel footwear from becoming soiled. [unless the cases involves gross contamination].... Shoe covers should be removed and deposited in a designated receptacle before leaving the operating room suite. [not worn outside the lab] Removal of shoe covers can permit transfer of microorganisms from the shoe covers to the hands. Hands should be washed after shoe cover removal." Some hospitals may require shoe covers, but they are not proven to reduce infection. Some surgeons wear their own special shoes or boots that they reserve for surgery, instead of using covers.

See: Essential of Perioperative Nursing", chapter on Aseptic Practices, by Cynthia Spry, Jonas and Bartlett Publishers   **Keywords:** Shoe covers optional

273. **Which of the statements below are true about surgical scrub and alcohol-based hand rubs prior to gowning and gloving for the first heart cath of the day? (Check all 4 that apply.)**

  a.   **Apply to both hands and forearms**

  b.   **Rub in the alcohol-based product until dry**

  c.   **Hands must be cleaned, washed and dried first**

  d.   **Alcohol rubs are less effective than traditional scrub-brush methods**

  e.   **Nails and subungual areas of both hands must be cleaned with a nail file first**

ANSWERS: a, b, c, & e.

a. Apply to both hands and forearms - YES.

b. Rub in the alcohol-based product until dry - YES.

c. Hands must be cleaned, washed, and dried first - YES.

d. Alcohol rubs are less effective than traditional scrub-brushed methods - NO.

e. Nails and subungual areas of both hands must be cleaned with a nail file first - YES.

Spry says, "Alcohol-based hand rub products....have been shown to save time and reduce costs, are more effective than products used in the traditional scrub method, and because of added emollients are gentle to the hands...The procedure should include the following:

  -Hands and forearms are washed with soap and running water.

  -The nails and subungual areas of both hands are cleaned with a nail file.

  -Hands and forearms are rinsed and thoroughly dried with a clean towel.

  -Hands and forearms are rubbed until dry.

  -An FDA approved antiseptic rub is used.

  -Manufacturer's instructions must be followed.

See: Essential of Perioperative Nursing", chapter on Aseptic Practices, by Cynthia Spry, Jonas and Bartlett Publishers

274. **What is the recommended patient skin preparation prior to central line or vascular catheter insertion?**
　　a.　2% chlorhexidine in alcohol (Chloraprep), air dry
　　b.　2% chlorhexidine in alcohol (Chloraprep), sterile towel dry
　　c.　Povidine iodine in saline, 1 minute air dry
　　d.　Povidine iodine in alcohol, sterile towel dry

ANSWER: a. 2% chlorhexidine (ChloraPrep), air dry
　　CDC recommendations say: "A 2% chlorhexidine based preparation (e.g., Chloraprep) for skin antisepsis is preferred during central line insertion, but tincture of iodine (an iodophor) or 70% alcohol may be substituted. Allow the antiseptic to remain on the insertion site (do not swab excess) and air dry before catheter insertion when possible. Povidine iodine is most effective when allowed to remain on the skin for at least 2 min or longer if it is not yet dry."
　　"For patient skin preparation in the operating room, iodophors, alcohol-containing products, and chlorhexidine gluconate (CHG) are most commonly used. CHG achieved both a greater reduction in skin microflora and had a greater residual activity after a single application when compared with povidine-iodine. Further, CHG is not inactivated by blood or serum protein, whereas iodophors my be. CHG is bacteriostatic and effective as long as it is present on the skin."
　　See: Catheterization and Cardiovascular Interventions, ACC/AHA/SCAI 2005 guideline update for percutaneous coronary intervention - summary article: Infection control guidelines for the cardiac catheterization laboratory: Society guidelines revisited, by Charles E. Chambers, at al., 2006
http://onlinelibrary.wiley.com/doi/10.1002/ccd.20589/full

275. **What is the recommended disinfectant to apply to your hands prior to donning pre-surgical sterile gloves, according to the World Health Organization?**
　　a.　Antimicrobial medicated soap scrub with water via brush
　　b.　Povidine iodine scrub with water via sponge
　　c.　Chlorhexidine based handrub
　　d.　Alcohol based handrub

ANSWER: d. Alcohol based handrub.
　　Alcohol based handrubs have been proven to be more effective than the traditional 5 minute scrub with povidine iodine and a scrub brush. These handrubs destroy bacteria faster, are cheaper, have greater residual activity and have fewer side-effects on the hands.
　　WHO says: "...the antibacterial efficacy of products containing high concentrations of alcohol by far surpasses that of any medicated soap presently available. In addition, the initial reduction of the resident skin flora is so rapid and effective that bacterial regrowth to baseline on the gloved hand takes more than six hours. This makes the demand for a sustained effect of a product superfluous. For this reason, preference should be given to alcohol-based products. Furthermore, several factors including rapid action, time savings,

less side-effects, and no risk of recontamination by rinsing hands with water, clearly favour the use of presurgical handrubbing." **See:** WHO Guidelines on Hand Hygiene in Health Care: First Global Patient Safety Challenge Clean Care Is Safer Care, https://www.ncbi.nlm.nih.gov/books/NBK144036/

276. What is the recommended first step in performing a pre-surgical hand rub?
- a. Dipping fingertips for 5 seconds into 5 ml of alcohol based hand rub solution
- b. Dipping fingertips for 10 seconds into 10 ml of alcohol based hand rub solution
- c. Rub 5 ml of alcohol based hand rub solution into both hands at the same time up to the wrists for 10-20 seconds
- d. Rub 10 ml of alcohol based hand rub solution into both hands at the same time up to the wrists for 20-30 seconds

ANSWER: a. Dipping fingertips for 5 seconds into 5 ml of alcohol based hand rub solution.

WHO surgical handrub technique poster recommends the following initial steps:
1. Put approximately 5 ml (3 doses) of alcohol based handrub in the palm of your left hand, using elbow of your other arm to operate the dispenser.

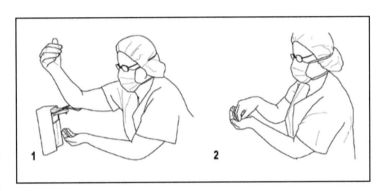

2. Dip the fingertips of your right hand in the handrub to decontaminate under the nails (5 seconds). Fingernails and all dirt should be cleaned before using hand-rubs.
See: www.who.int/infection-prevention/countries/surgical/NewSurgicalA3.pdf

277. Before an average sized person dons sterile gloves, how much total alcohol based hand rub solution should be used during surgical hand preparation, at a minimum, according to the World Heath Organization?
- a. 10 ml, 5 for the forearms and 5 for the hands
- b. 15 ml, 5 for each forearm and 5 for the hands
- c. 20 ml, 5 for each forearm and 5 for each hand
- d. 40 ml, 10 for each forearm and 10 for each hand

ANSWER: b. 15 ml, 5 for each forearm and 5 for the hands.

World Health Organization says: "The hands should be wet from the alcohol-based rub during the whole procedure, which requires approximately 15 ml depending on the size of the hands. One study demonstrated that keeping the hands wet with the rub is more important than the volume used. The size of the hands and forearms ultimately determines the volume required to keep the skin area wet during the entire time of the handrub....

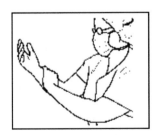

Institutions opting to use the WHO-recommended formulations for surgical hand preparation should ensure that a minimum of three applications are used, if not more, for a period of 3 to 5 minutes. For surgical procedures of more than a two hours' duration, ideally surgeons should practise a second handrub of approximately 1 minute, even though more research is needed on this aspect.... the time required for surgical alcohol-based handrubbing depends on the compound used. Most commercially available products recommend a 3-minute exposure, although the application time may be longer for some formulations, but can be shortened to 1.5 minutes for a few of them." **See:** WHO Guidelines on Hand Hygiene in Health Care: First Global Patient Safety Challenge Clean Care Is Safer Care, https://www.ncbi.nlm.nih.gov/books/NBK144036/

278. **When using an alcohol based hand rub solution for pre-surgical hand preparation, your hands must be: (Check 2 requirements below.)**
   a.   **Still damp with hand rub solution when donning sterile gloves**
   b.   **Dried of hand rub solution when donning sterile gloves**
   c.   **Washed clean and damp when first applying the hand rub**
   d.   **Clean and dry when first applying the hand rub**
   e.   **Scrubbed for 5 minutes with a medicated sponge when first applying the hand rub**

ANSWERS: b & d. Dried of hand rub solution when donning sterile gloves and clean and dry when first applying the hand rub.
   Prior to donning sterile gloves the handrubbing technique for surgical hand preparation must be performed on perfectly clean, dry hands. Gloves should not be put on until hands are completely dry. **See:** WHO Guidelines on Hand Hygiene in Health Care: First Global Patient Safety Challenge Clean Care Is Safer Care, https://www.ncbi.nlm.nih.gov/books/NBK144036/

279. **You are scrub assistant on several surgical cases today. What hand preparation is recommended between consecutive cases prior to donning sterile gloves?**
   a.   **Perform a 1 minute simple hand washing, then use the handrub solution**
   b.   **Perform a 5 minute scrub with a medicated sponge, then use the handrub solution**
   c.   **Perform a 5 minute scrub with a medicated sponge only**
   d.   **Wash your hands with medicated soap, then use the handrub solution**
   e.   **Use the handrub solution only**

ANSWER: e. Use the handrub solution only.
   WHO recommends washing of hands at the beginning of the day, when first entering the operating room or whenever your hands become contaminated with blood or soiled, but not between cases. Hand scrubbing is good for basic hand cleanliness, but can irritate the skin. In addition, the water you wash with may not be free of bacteria.
   World Health Organization says: "It is not necessary to wash hands before handrub unless hands are visibly soiled or dirty. The hands of the surgical team should be clean upon entering the operating theatre by washing with a non-medicated soap. While this handwash may eliminate any risk of contamination with bacterial spores, experimental

and epidemiological data failed to demonstrate an additional effect of washing hands before applying handrub in the overall reduction of the resident skin flora. The activity of the handrub formulation may even be impaired if hands are not completely dried before applying the handrub or by the washing phase itself. A simple handwash with soap and water before entering the operating theatre area is highly recommended to eliminate any risk of colonization with bacterial spores. Non-medicated soaps are sufficient, and the procedure is necessary only upon entering the operating theatre: repeating handrubbing without prior handwash or scrub is recommended before switching to the next procedure. **See:** WHO Guidelines on Hand Hygiene in Health Care: First Global Patient Safety Challenge Clean Care Is Safer Care, https://www.ncbi.nlm.nih.gov/books/NBK144036/

280. **Your cardiologist requests preoperative hair removal prior to cath from both groins of your patient. To minimize surgical site infections remove the patient's groin hair with a/an:**
 a. **Disposable razor**
 b. **Straight razor**
 c. **Electric clipper**
 d. **Depilatory cream**

ANSWER: c. Electric clipper reduces the chance of infection and is recommended by CDC infection control guidelines. Dross says, "..shaving damages the skin and increases the risk of infection. The source pathogens for most nosocomial infections are skin-dwelling microorganisms. Razor shaving increases the risk of infection by creating microabrasions in the skin that allow skin-dwelling microorganisms to collect and multiply. These organisms may then migrate into the incision site and may also collect on catheters or sheaths that must remain in place for a period of time following the procedure. The longer a catheter or sheath is in place, the higher the risk for catheter-associated infection."

"In contrast to shaving, clipping hair using a rechargeable electric trimmer with a disposable head does not damage the skin and is associated with lower infection rates. In a prospective study that compared infection rates among 1,980 surgical patients whose hair was either shaved or clipped pre-operatively, patients who were clipped had a statistically significantly lower infection rate than patients who were shaved (p = 0.024)."

"Hair should be removed as close to the time of surgery as possible and in an area away from the sterile field (in the pre-catheterization holding area, for example) to prevent loose hair clippings from dispersing onto sterile surfaces and causing contamination. A rechargeable electric clipper with a disposable head or one that can be removed and disinfected should be used."

Depilatory cream use is safer than shaving with a razor, but it has separate problems of causing allergy and skin irritation. Cutdown procedures also have a higher incidence of local infections than percutaneous. **See:** http://www.cathlabdigest.com/articles/Clipping-versus-Shaving-Who-Wins-End-Infection-Risk-and-Hair-Removal-Guidelines, Dave Droll, RT(R)(T)(CV), RCIS

References:
Allmers, Nancy M., and Verderame, Joan A., *Appleton and Lange's Review for Surgical Tech. Exam*, Appleton and Lange, Fourth Edition, 1996
Gruendemann and Meeker, *Alexander's Care of the Patient in Surgery*, CV Mosby Co., 1987

Torres, *Basic Medical Techniques and Patient Care for Radiologic Technologists*,
    J.B. Lippincott Co., 1989
Burton, R.W., *Microbiology for the Health Sciences*, J.B. Lippincott Co., 1988
Dave Droll, Cath Lab Digest, Clipping versus Shaving: Who Wins in the End?
    Infection Risk and Hair Removal Guidelines, Sept 2005

OUTLINE: A4 - Sterilization & Asepsis

1. **General Asepsis**
   a. **Disinfect** = Destroy most pathogens on instruments. Unsafe for living tissues
      i. Clorox, Glutaraldehyde (Cidex)
      ii. destroy most pathogens on instruments
      iii. unsafe for living tissues
   b. **Bacteriostatic**= Inhibits or stops growth of bacteria (-static = hold steady)
      i. E.g., Hexachlorophene, Benzalkonium chloride (Zephiran)
      ii. inhibits or stops growth of bacteria.
   c. **Bactericidal**= Kills bacteria (-cidal = kill)
      i. E.g., Penicillin, and other antibiotics
      ii. kills bacteria- but not virus in vivo.
   d. **Antiseptic**= Destroys most pathogens on living tissue, safe to use on skin
      i. E.g., Alcohol (70%), Povidone-iodine
   e. **Sterilize**= Destroys all microorganisms
      i. E.g., Autoclave
      ii. ETO Gas
   f. **Aseptic**= Destroys all pathogens (-sepsis = infection)
   g. **Aseptic Skin Prep** =Elimination of all pathogens
2. **Sterile Principles and Techniques**
   a. When in doubt about the sterility, consider it unsterile
   b. Patient should never be left alone at any time
   c. Spread of infection = poor hand washing
   d. Use standard precautions on All patients
   e. Nosocomial infections =originate in the hospital
      i. Heart transplant patients susceptible to infection
   f. Anaerobic bacteria = live only in the absence of air
   g. Aerobic bacteria = live only in the presence of air
3. **Sterilization Technique**
   a. Steam heat =autoclave
      i. Requires temperature and time
      ii. Biological indicators
      iii. Ethylene oxide (gas) = less damaging
         (1) Wrap in Polypropylene plastic film Not nylon
4. **Shelf Life - packaging**
   a. Single Cloth wrapping = Not sterile
   b. Double cloth wrapping = 21-30 days
   c. Single-layer plastic wrapping = 6 months - 1 year

    d. Sealed envelopes + plastic = sterile indefinitely
5. **Scrub**
   a. Scrub 2 inches above the elbow
   b. Alcohol hand rubs:
      i. Clean nails and subungual areas first
      ii. Hands must be cleaned, washed and dried first
      iii. Rub in until dry
      iv. Are as effective as scrub-brush methods
      v. Skin prep = wipe spiral out motion
6. **Gloving**
   a. Self-gowning closed method
   b. Self-gowning open method
   c. Gloving another individual
   d. Contaminated glove, circulator pulls it off
   e. Remove your gloves inside out
7. **Gowning**
   a. Open the hand towel and lay it on the Drs. hand
   b. Keep your hands on the outside of the gown under a protective cuff
   c. Open the gown and hold it so the Dr. can insert his dry hands into the sleeves
   d. Have the circulator untie your gown
   e. Pull the gown off inside out
   f. Sterile persons pass each other back to back
8. **Shoe covers**
   a. Are usually considered optional
   b. May NOT be worn outside the surgical suite
   c. Wash hands after removing shoe covers

Open sterile packs
   d. Circulator open the first flap away
   e. Sterile scrub assistant open first flap towards
9. **Sterile table**
   a. Pour solutions only once, then discard left-over solution
   b. Draped sterile tables, sterile on the top surface only
   c. Wrapper edges are unsterile
   d. Instruments or sutures hanging over the table edge are discarded
   e. If patient in room & physician cancels case= Tear table down
10. **Hair removal - shave groin**
   a. Electric clipper= less chance of infection

Fetal Circulation

INDEX: B1 -Fetal Circulation

1. Fetal Circulation and Normal Shunts

281. Which normal cardiovascular fetal shunt normally closes off immediately after the infant's first breath?

- a.   Patent foramen ovale
- b.   Sinus venosus
- c.   Ductus venosus
- d.   Patent ductus arteriosus

ANSWER a. The patent foramen ovale normally closes at the first breath. When the lungs inflate and decrease the PVR and PA pressures, then the RA-LA pressure gradient reverses. Since the LA pressure exceeds RA pressure the LA flap (septum primum) closes and covers the foramen ovale. It normally seals itself to the atrial septum and eventually grows into it.

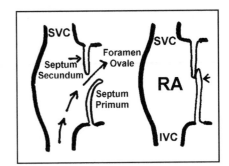
Patent foramen closing

       The umbilical arteries and veins close when the umbilical cord is tied. The ductus venosus remains as a potential channel to shunt blood, but eventually closes. The patent ductus arteriosus is dependent on O2, PH and vasoconstrictor levels. It may not close for weeks after birth. Sinus venous is a type of ASD.
See: Braunwald, chapter on "Congenital Heart Disease."

282. After the newborn takes its first breath and the umbilical cord is tied the right sided pressures will drop. This drop in pressure change normally causes immediate closure of the:

- a.   VSD
- b.   PDA
- c.   Ostium primum
- d.   Ostium secundum

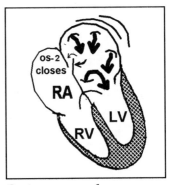
Ostium secundum

ANSWER d. Ostium secundum. The ASD (Atrial Septal Defect) is also called the "secundum defect" or the foramen ovale. It closes immediately after the first breath when the RA-LA pressures reverse. The flap of tissue (septum secundum) normally held open by the R-L shunt is closed like a trap door. This channels all right heart blood into the

PA and lungs.**See:** Rushmer, chapter on "Congenital Malformations of Heart."

283. Which shunt normally closes off several days after a full term birth?
   a.   VSD with right to left shunt
   b.   VSD with left to right shunt
   c.   Patent ductus arteriosus
   d.   Patent foramen ovale

ANSWER c. Patent ductus arteriosus. Normally the arterial PO2 increases with the first breath. This along with local vasoconstrictor secretion begins the process of shrinking the PDA into the vestigial "ligamentum arteriosus," but it takes time to totally close off. After increase in the PA O2 sat. vasoconstricts the PDA (1-3 days) the PDA fibroses, develops intimal hyperplasia and should be completely closed by 1-2 weeks after birth.
See: Braunwald, chapter on "Congenital Heart Disease." **Keywords:** PDA closes at 1 week

284. A patient with normal "situs" will have a PA chest radiograph showing abdominal contents with:
   a.   Left sided stomach bubble & left hepatic shadow
   b.   Left sided stomach bubble & right hepatic shadow
   c.   Right sided stomach bubble & right hepatic shadow
   d.   Right sided stomach bubble & left hepatic shadow

ANSWER b. Left sided stomach bubble & right hepatic shadow. "Situs Inversus" is bilateral switching of body parts (as in dextrocardia). The stomach bubble and liver are easily seen markers for situs. Normally the stomach bubble is on the patient's left with the liver on his right.
See: Braunwald, chapter on "Congenital Heart Disease."

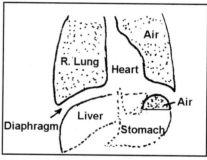

Normal situs - liver & stomach

285. In the normal fetal circulation, what percentage of the cardiac output goes through the lungs?
   a.   0-6%
   b.   10-12%
   c.   30-40%
   d.   50-60%

ANSWER b. 10-12%. Since the fetal blood is oxygenated by the placenta, significant pulmonary blood flow is not needed. Since about ½ of the RA blood goes through the foramen ovale (ASD) and 1/3 of it goes through the PDA (PA-AO), this leaves only 10-12% to go to the lungs. (Braunwald says 10%.)
See: Berne and Levy's chapter on "Special Circulations."

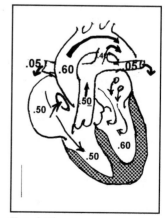

Fetal Flow

286. The normal fetal shunt between the AO and PA is termed the _____ and it shunts blood in a _____ direction before birth.
   a. PDA, R-L
   b. PDA, L-R
   c. Foramen Ovale, R-L
   d. Foramen Ovale, L-R

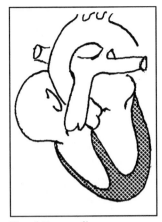
Fetal Lung flow

ANSWER a. PDA, R-L. Both normal fetal shunts (PDA & ASD) redirect arterialized blood from right to left. This oxygenated blood is shunted into the systemic circulation for the brain and other developing tissues.
See: Berne & Levy, chapter on "Special Circulations." **Keywords:** Shunts, PDA

287. Which normal fetal shunt carries the most oxygen rich blood? (i.e., Which has the highest O2 saturation)?
   a. Ostium secundum
   b. PDA
   c. VSD
   d. Ductus venosus

ANSWER d. Ductus venosus. This major blood channel develops in the embryonic liver from the left umbilical vein (80% O2 sat) to the inferior vena cava. The foramen ovale shunts most of this red blood to the LA, LV, and AO where it supplies the fetal brain with O2 and nutrition. Structures numbered in the diagram are:

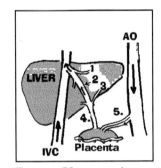
Ductus Venosus in fetus

   1. Hepatic veins
   2. Ductus venosus
   3. Portal vein
   4. Umbilical vein
   5. Umbilical arteries
See: Berne & Levy, chapter on "Special Circulations." **Keywords:** Shunts, Ductus Venosus

288. What is the normal anatomic position of the aorta and IVC in relation to the backbone? Normally the aorta descends to the _____ of the vertebral column and IVC comes up the _____ side of the vertebral column.
   a. Right, Right
   b. Right, Left
   c. Left, Right
   d. Left, Left

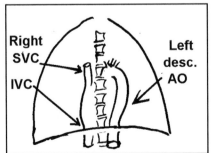
IVC - vertebra - AO

ANSWER c. Left, Right. Normally the aorta descends to the left of the patient's backbone. IVC venous return comes up to the right of the patient's backbone and empties into the RA, as shown. This is "Normal Situs."

Embryologically there are both right and left IVCs. The left side becomes the normal left sided AO and right side becomes the IVC.
See: Braunwald, chapter on "Congenital Heart Disease."

289.   In prenatal life the fetal lung alveoli are:
a.   **Filled with blood**
b.   **Filled with amniotic fluid**
c.   **Filled with inert gases**
d.   **Collapsed**

ANSWER d. Collapsed. The fetal alveoli are collapsed. The surfactant that is produced by the lung just before birth, allow the alveoli to expand and fill with air immediately after birth. Preterm infants often have inadequate surfactant, and the work of inflating the lungs and breathing is increased. That's why most preemies are on ventilators.
See: Underhill, chapter on "Development of CV System."

290.   When the umbilicus is clamped at birth what happens to the aortic and pulmonary blood pressures? The AO pressure _____ and the PA pressure _____.
a.   **Increases, increases**
b.   **Increases, decreases**
c.   **Decreases, increases**
d.   **Decreases, decreases**

ANSWER b. Increases, decreases. As the first breath opens the alveoli, the pulmonary capillaries also open. This drops the resistance to blood flow through the lungs, and the PA pressure drops from around 60 to 35 mmHg.

Tying of the umbilical cord removes the low resistance through the ductus venosus and increases systemic arterial resistance. This causes the aortic pressure to rise immediately after birth and to continue to rise from 60 to more normal levels of 120 mmHg. Thus after birth the arterial system continues to handle more pressure than the pulmonary system. And the pressure diverge.
See: Rushmer, chapter on "Congenital Malformations of the Heart."

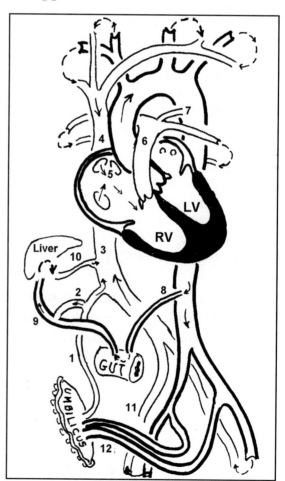

Prenatal Circulation

BOTH QUESTIONS BELOW REFER TO THIS DIAGRAM.

291. This is a diagram of the normal prenatal circulation. Identify the structure seen at # 1 (exiting the umbilicus).
a.   Portal Vein
b.   Hepatic Vein
c.   Iliac Artery
d.   Umbilical Vein
e.   Ductus Venosus

292. Which prenatal vessel in this diagram has the highest O2 saturation?
a.   Aorta
b.   Pulmonary Vein
c.   Umbilical Artery
d.   Umbilical Vein

ANSWERS TO BOTH QUESTIONS BELOW.

291. ANSWER d. The umbilical vein brings O2 rich blood from the placenta to the IVC. This is the fetus' only source of oxygen.   **CORRECTLY MATCHED**
ANSWERS ARE: 1. Umbilical Vein

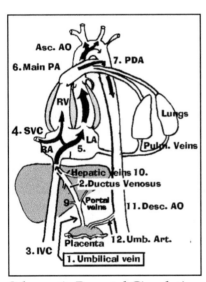

Schematic Prenatal Circulation

2. Ductus Venosus
3. IVC
4. SVC
5. Patent Foramen Ovale
6. PA
7. PDA
8. Mesenteric Artery - not shown
9. Portal Vein
10. Hepatic Vein
11. Descending AO.
12. Umbilical Artery
The chief structures of interest are:
    #2. Ductus Venosus, an extension of the umbilical veins which supplies the liver and IVC with the only source of oxygenated blood - the placenta.
    #5. Patent Foramen Ovale (Ostium Secundum) between the RA and LA. It is a normal R-L shunt carrying the oxygenated blood (approx. 62% sat.) into the LV, ascending AO and brain (which badly needs it).
    #7. PDA which carries the PA blood (52% O2 sat.) into the descending AO and lower trunk and extremities. Note how all 3 of these normal shunts bridge other structures to get the most O2 rich blood to the tissues that need it most - the liver and the brain.
See: Braunwald, chapter on "Congenital Heart Disease." **Keywords:** ID structures in prenatal circulation

292. ANSWER d. Umbilical Vein. Placenta is the only source of O2 for fetal life. Oxygen

and CO_2 are exchanged across the placenta. The umbilical arteries bring the dark venous blood and the umbilical vein carries blood averaging only 80% O2 saturation. That's as good as it gets for the fetus. It survives and grows with less oxygen than we "air breathers" are used to.

Some of this oxygenated blood passes through the liver. The brain gets the next highest concentration of O2 and that only averages 62% O2 sat. The blackest blood comes back from the SVC (approx. 25% sat.) because the brain extracts so much O2.

The blood going into the lungs is only 52% O2 sat. and the pulmonary veins lower yet at 42%. **See:** Braunwald, chapter on "Congenital Heart Disease."

293. **In the normal fetal circulation, oxygenated blood from the placenta preferentially goes through the _____ and the blue blood from the SVC preferentially goes through the _____ .**
   a.   **Ductus venosus; umbilical artery**
   b.   **Umbilical artery, Umbilical vein**
   c.   **Ductus arteriosus; foramen ovale**
   d.   **Foramen ovale; ductus arteriosus**

ANSWER d. Foramen ovale; ductus arteriosus. Oxygenated umbilical vein blood passes through the ductus venosus, into the IVC, RA and through the patent foramen ovale into the LA, LV, and ascending AO. The dark SVC blood (25% O2 sat.) is preferentially directed down into the RV, PA, PDA and descending AO. These normal shunts get the O2 rich blood to the tissues that need it most - the brain and coronary arteries.
See: Braunwald, chapter on "Congenital Heart Disease." **Keywords:** Normal fetal flow

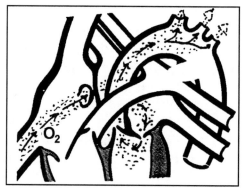
Oxygenated blood path

2. Fetal / Congenital Defects - Know Basic Defects Only

294. **What abnormality of development is shown? The central portion of the heart failed to develop, omitting the medial AV valve cusps.**
   a.   **Ostium secundum with VSD**
   b.   **Truncus arteriosus**
   c.   **Tricuspid atresia**
   d.   **AV canal**

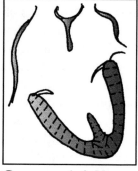
Common A & V

ANSWER d. The AV canal or endocardial cushion forms the central crux of the heart including: Upper ventricular septum, lower atrial septum, and the septal cusps of the AV valves. When it fails to develop (endocardial cushion defect) shunts can develop between any of the four chambers. If the endocardial cushions do not fuse, the AV valves fail to develop medial leaflets, also the upper part of the IVS and lower IAS will not meet. This results in a shunt in the center of the heart that may shunt in any direction. Depending on the severity of the endocardial cushion defect a partial or complete AV canal may be formed. Partial AV canal results in a primum ASD and a cleft mitral valve with mitral regurgitation.

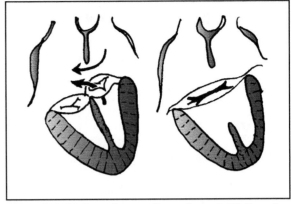

Partial A V Canal   -   Complete A V Canal

Complete AV canal usually results in a common AV valve overriding the ventricular septum. **See:** Rushmer, chapter on "Congenital Malformations of the Heart." **Keywords:** Defects, Endo. Cushion

295. **Between the 24th and 28th day of gestation the truncus arteriosus must divide and spiral. What congenital defect develops if the truncus fails to spiral as it divides?**

    a.   **Dextrocardia**
    b.   **Tetralogy of Fallot**
    c.   **Total anomalous venous return**
    d.   **Transposition of the great vessels**

ANSWER d. Transposition of the great vessels. This embryological spiral is why the PA and AO cross over each other. In embryology the large single great vessel (truncus arteriosus) out of the ventricles normally divides to form the PA and AO. If it just divides without spiraling, a cyanotic heart defect develops termed "Transposition of the Great Vessels." If TGV develops, the RV dumps into the AO, and the LV pumps into the PA. Transposition is fatal unless shunts are present. It may be fatal because the systemic circulation may not pick up oxygen from the pulmonary circulation. **See:** Rushmer, chapter on "Congenital Malformations of Heart."

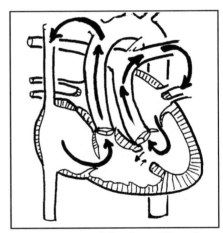

Transposition of the Great Vessels

BOTH QUESTIONS BELOW REFER TO THIS DIAGRAM.

296. **Identify the congenital shunt labeled #1 on the diagram.**
- a. PDA
- b. VSD
- c. ASD
- d. Truncus Arteriosus
- e. Total Anomalous Venous Return
- f. Transposition Great Vessels

297. **The congenital defect labeled at #4 would normally cause:**
- a. Cyanosis
- b. Acyanosis
- c. Anemia
- d. Polycythemia

BOTH ANSWERS LISTED TOGETHER BELOW.

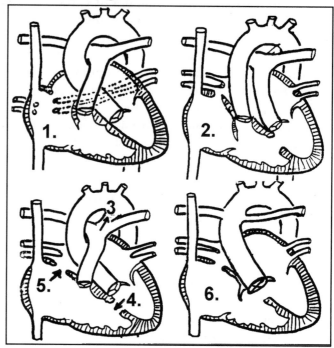

Congenital Shunt Defects

296. ANSWER e. Total Anomalous Venous Return. In this defect the pulmonary veins all drain into the right atrium. Other shunts (ASD - not shown) must exist for arteriolized blood to get into the systemic circulation. **CORRECTLY MATCHED ANSWERS ARE:**
  1. Total Anomalous Venous Return
  2. Transposition Great Vessels
  3. PDA
  4. VSD
  5. ASD
  6. Truncus Arteriosus
See: Rushmer, chapter on "Congenital Malformation of Heart."

297. ANSWER b. Acyanosis. #4 is a L-R VSD. These simple lesions shown at #3, 4, & 5 are considered the acyanotic lesions. Unless pulmonary hypertension develops these defects normally shunt from left to right. Here the left heart's red blood dumps into the right heart's blue blood. This blood goes to the lungs where it is further oxygenated. These are NOT the *blue baby* defects which have incompletely oxygenated (blue) systemic blood. **See:** Braunwald, chapter on "Congenital Heart Disease." **Keywords:** acyanotic defects

298. A congenital narrowing (stenosis) shown at #1 on the diagram is termed:
  a.   Subvalvular Obstruction
  b.   Valvular Aortic Stenosis
  c.   Supravalvular Obstruction
  d.   Preductal Coarctation
  e.   Postductal Coarctation

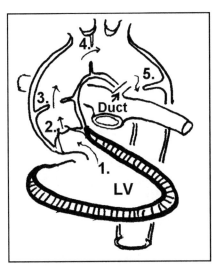
Aortic Obstructions

ANSWER a. Subvalvular Obstruction
CORRECTLY MATCHED ANSWERS ARE:
1. **Subvalvular Obstruction:** also termed HOCM or IHSS.
2. **Valvular Aortic Stenosis**: Note doming of valve - shaped like a dome.
3. **Supravalvular Obstruction**
4. **Preductal Coarctation**
5. **Postductal Coarctation:** It is believed that some of the aortic tissue near the ductus arteriosus may be composed of "ductal type tissue" which constricts, just as the PDA constricts after birth. This can result in a coarctation either above (Pre-ductal) or below (post-ductal) coarctation.
See: Braunwald, chapter on "Congenital Heart

299. Inversion of the atria (RA on left side) is usually associated with _____ and a _____ sided IVC.
  a.   Situs solitis, left
  b.   Situs solitis, right
  c.   Situs inversus, left
  d.   Situs inversus, right

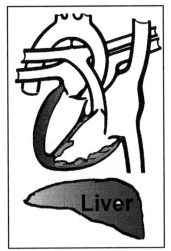
Total Inversion

ANSWER c. Situs inversus, left sided IVC. "Situs" refers to the Rt-Lt. sidedness of the viscera and atria. When "inverted" the situs inversus creates a left sided liver, IVC, IVC, and RA. This diagram shows complete inversion at all three levels of the heart: Atria, ventricles, and great vessels. Here everything is reversed: Situs inversus (viscera and atrial reversed), ventricular inversion (dextrocardia), and right-sided descending AO (dextroposition). The ventricle is identified by the trabeculations. The most heavily trabeculated chamber is the RV. The LV has a smooth walled endocardium. **See:** Braunwald, chapter on "Congenital Heart Disease."

REFERENCES:

Rushmer, R. F.,*CARDIOVASCULAR DYNAMICS*, W. B. Saunders Co., 1976

Braunwald, Eugene, Ed., *HEART DISEASE A Textbook of Cardiovascular Medicine*, 5th
       Ed., W. B. Saunders Co., 1997

Underhill, S. L., Ed., *CARDIAC NURSING*, 2nd Ed., J. B. Lippincott Co., 1989

Hurst, J. W., and Logue, R. B., et. al., *THE HEART Arteries and Veins*, 3rd Ed., McGraw-
       Hill Book Co., 1974

pappano and Wier, *Cardiovascular Physiology*, 10th Ed., Mosby Year Book, 2013

Netter, *CIBA Collection of Medical Illustrations*, *"The Heart"*, CIBA Pharmaceuticals

OUTLINE: B1 - Embryology and Fetal Circulation

1. FETAL CIRCULATION
    a.   ID and trace Blood flow
       •. Foramen Ovale
       i.Ductus Arteriosus
       •. Ductus venosus
       ii.Placenta
       •. umbilical artery
       iii.umbilical vein
       •. IVC
       iv.SVC
       •. PA
       v.PDA
       •. Mesenteric Artery
       vi.Portal Vein
       •. Hepatic Vein
       vii.Hepatic Vein
       •. Iliac Artery
    b.   % blood flow through
       i.lungs
       ii.Ductus
       iii.RV/LV
       iv.O2 Saturation
       v.AO, Ductus, LV, RV, RA,
       i.Umbilical vein, IVC, SVC
    c.Birth and the First Breath
       i.Lung Inflation
       ii.Closure Foramen Ovale
       iii.Ductus Venosus cut/tied

       iv.Change in PVR
       v.Change in flow patterns

2.CONGENITAL HEART DEFECTS
    a.Pulmonary Hypertension
    b.Obstructive
       i.Subvalvular Obstruction
       ii.HOCM, Infundibular Stenosis
       iii.Valvular Aortic Stenosis
       iv.Pulmonic Stenosis
       v. Supravalvular Obstruction
       vi.Coarctation
       vii.Preductal coarctation
       viii.Postductal coarctation
    c.Shunts: Cyanotic = Rt.-Lt. shunts
       i.Truncus Arteriosus
       ii.Total Anomalous Venous Return
       iii.Transposition great vessels
       iv.Tetralogy Fallot
       v.Tricuspid Atresia
    c.   Shunts: Acyanotic = Lt.-Rt. shunts
       i. VSD
       ii.PDA
       iii.ASD: Ostium primum
       iv.ASD: Ostium Secundum
       v.ASD: Sinus Venosus

Blood

INDEX: B2 - Blood

1. Lipoproteins

300. **Which one of the following blood lipoproteins is the major carrier of cholesterol?**
   a.   **Triglycerides**
   b.   **Cholymicrons**
   c.   **LDLs**
   d.   **HDLs**

ANSWER c. LDLs = Low density lipo-proteins are the bad ones and are the major carrier of cholesterol (being low in density, they float like cream). High density lipo-proteins (HDL's) are beneficial by removing and excreting excess cholesterol from the body. Triglycerides are composed mainly of the very low density lipo-proteins (VLDL) which are of unknown importance in heart disease. The Framingham study has shown that the ratio of total cholesterol to HDL is one of the best predictors of CAD in asymptomatic persons.
See: Underhill, chapter on "Laboratory Tests using blood and Urine." **Keywords:** blood, cholesterol, LDL

301. **To reduce risk of heart attack, serum cholesterol should be kept below:**
   a.   **1.5 g/l**
   b.   **24 g/l**
   c.   **100 mg/dl**
   d.   **200 mg/dl**

ANSWER d. 200 mg/dl.   The Framingham study shows that men with elevated serum cholesterol levels have three times the incidence of CAD than those with cholesterol levels under 200. However, the average US male over 35 (and female over 45) years of age has a cholesterol over 200 mg/dl. Experts suggest that the ideal adult serum cholesterol should be around 180 mg/dl. or at least below 200 mg/dl. Cholesterol levels typically elevate with patient age. For CHD or diabetes patients who cannot bring down their cholesterol level with diet, the AMA recommends statin intervention to reduce the LDL level < 100 mg/dl and triglyceride level <150 mg/dl.
See: Braunwald chapter on "Prevention of CHD" **Keywords:** blood, cholesterol normal < 200 mg/dl

302. The worst dietary factors that increase serum cholesterol and its lipoprotein
fraction are increased:
   a.   Alcohol intake, soluble fiber, and simple sugars
   b.   Calories, saturated fats, and cholesterol
   c.   Alcohol intake, saturated fats, and fish high in oil
   d.   Salt intake, complex carbohydrates, and unsaturated fats

ANSWER b. Increased calories, saturated fats, and cholesterol. Animal fat and especially
cholesterol should be minimized in the diet. Increased risk of CAD is associated with a
high intake of dietary saturated fat and cholesterol, a low polyunsaturated fat intake and
low fiber intake. However bad fatty diets are, dietary carbohydrate can also be changed
into lipoprotein and cholesterol, as is evidenced by the many vegetarians who still have
elevated cholesterol blood levels. One alcoholic beverage per day may be beneficial.
See: Braunwald, chapter on "Risk Factors." **Keywords:** blood, diet, cholesterol

303. Which of the following blood lipoproteins is believed to have a PROTECTIVE or
preventative effect against the development of atherosclerotic heart disease?
   a.   Total cholesterol
   b.   Triglycerides
   c.   High density lipoproteins
   d.   Low density lipoproteins

ANSWER c. High density lipoproteins. One way to distinguish which is the good and
which is the bad cholesterol, remember that cream is bad for you. Because it is low in
density it <u>floats</u> on the top of milk, whereas the high density lipoproteins <u>sink</u>. Underhill
says, "Elevated serum total cholesterol and low-density lipoprotein (LDL) cholesterol are
associated strongly within increased risk of CHD. However, high concentrations of high-
density lipoprotein (HDL) cholesterol in the serum seem to have a protective effect against
the development of atherosclerosis." **See:** Underhill, chapter on Coronary Heard Disease
Risk Factors." **Keywords:** High Density Lipoproteins, Cholesterol

2. O2 and HGB

304. The actual amount of O2 carried in
blood (in vol.%) is defined as the
oxygen:
   a.   Content
   b.   Capacity
   c.   Saturation
   d.   Dissociation

ANSWER a. O2 content is the amount (cc.)
of O2 contained in 100 ml of blood. This O2

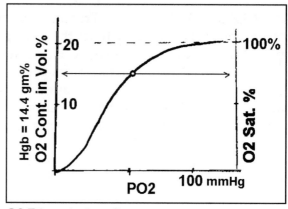

O2 Dissociation Curve

content and % O2 saturation varies non-linearly with the PO2 (see O2 dissociation curve). O2 content (CaO2) is calculated by 1.39 x O2 Sat. x Hgb.

CaO2 = 1.39 x O2 Sat x Hgb

The maximum amount which can be carried (at 100% saturation) is termed the "O2 capacity" in Volume % units. The top of the curve shown is the "O2 capacity." In a patient with Hgb of 14.4 gm% as shown 100% O2 saturation = 20 vol% (top of curve). Or it can be calculated by the formula O2 capacity (100% x 1.39 = 20 vol %). The formula for O2 capacity is: **O2 Cap = 100 %O2 sat x 1.39 x Hgb.**

The formula for O2 content is: **O2 Cont. = %O2 sat x 1.39 x Hgb.**

For O2 content of the 75% sample marked, use the calculation 75% x 1.39 x 14.4 = 15.0 vol %

Note that some labs use 1.34 or 1.36 instead of 1.39 vol%/gm% Hgb as their constant. These definitions are necessary to calculate Fick Cardiac Output.

See: Grossman, chapter on "Blood Flow and CO" **Keywords:** O2 content

305. **Which of the following will shift the oxyhemoglobin curve to the right and facilitate O2 unloading in the tissues?**
   a.   **Acidosis**
   b.   **Decreased PCO2**
   c.   **Decreased temperature**
   d.   **Decreased O2 content**

ANSWER a. Acidosis. The O2 dissociation curve is shifted to the right in venous blood and in disease. Although arterial O2 saturation will be decreased slightly (perhaps 1%), venous O2 sat will greatly decrease (perhaps 10%) for the same PO2 change. This makes for 9% more O2 delivered to tissues.

Things that shift the curve rightward often provide a beneficial effect. This is termed the "Bohr effect." They are the same compensatory changes associated with chronic lung disease:
- acidosis, decreased pH, increased H⁺ ions
- increased temperature
- increased 2,3 DPG
- increased PCO2

See: ACLS chapter on "Pharmacology I." **Keywords:** Shifts in O2 dissociation curve

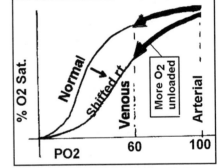

O2 Dissociation Curve - Shift

306. **How do elevated blood PCO2 and low pH levels effect tissue oxygenation?**
   a.   **Increased PaO2**
   b.   **Decreased PaO2**
   c.   **Increased oxygenation of tissues**
   d.   **Decreased oxygenation of tissues**

ANSWER c. Increased oxygenation of tissues results when the O2 dissociation curve shift to the right, as occurs with many disease states. Low arterial pH with high CO2 describes respiratory acidosis. This does not help O2 combine with hemoglobin. It helps O2 <u>release</u> at the tissues level, making it <u>easier to unload</u> oxygen from the hemoglobin molecule, where you really need it. This is termed the Bohr effect. This additional O2 unloading helps oxygenate the tissues and compensate for the acid base imbalance.

Elevated blood PCO2 and low pH levels also occur normally at the tissue level. As capillary blood picks up metabolically generated CO2 it becomes more acidic resulting in more O2 unloaded to the tissues - a good thing.

In PaO2, the "P" stands for partial pressure, as in a blood gas measurement; the "a" stands for arterial blood, not pulmonary artery (PA). The arterial partial pressure (PaO2) is mainly effected by alveolar PO2 in the lungs.
See: Guyton, chapter on "Transport of Oxygen and CO2" **Keywords:** Blood, Bohr effect

307. What is the normal adult male hemoglobin measurement?
 a. Hgb = 15 gm/deciliter
 b. Hgb = 23 gm/deciliter
 c. Hgb = 45 gm/deciliter
 d. Hgb = 75 gm/deciliter

ANSWER a. Hgb = 15 gm/deciliter is a normal adult male Hgb, comparable to a HCT of 45%. Women normally have a lower Hgb because of menses. The Hgb is a more accurate measure of hemoglobin in blood. Hgb is approximately 1/3 of the Hct level.
See: Underhill, chapter on "Acid Base Balance." Hemostasis." **Keywords:** Hct, Hgb.

308. Following angiography a patient's venous and arterial pressures have slowly fallen 20%. His hematocrit of 54% is consistent with a diagnosis of:
 a. Retroperitoneal bleed (hematoma)
 b. Hemolytic anemia (due to artificial valves)
 c. Excessive fluid intake and/or IV infusion
 d. Diuresis with insufficient hydration

ANSWER d. Diuresis with insufficient hydration. Normal hct is 45%. As patients become hypovolemic, the filling pressures fall due to lack of preload. The Hct rises due to loss of fluid and concentration of the RBCs in the blood. This is termed an "Extracellular Volume Deficit." Patients come to cath NPO having drunk no fluids. Patients are encouraged to drink lots of water post-cath, but many need IV fluid replacement to prevent hypovolemia.

Low blood volume causes a compensatory pulling of tissue fluid into the vascular space by "transcapillary refill." However, in our example, the fluid loss through diuresis exceeds the "refill" so hypovolemia and polycythemia result. This can lead to hypovolemic shock. Retroperitoneal bleed leads to anemia with low Hct, not high.
See: Underhill, chapter on "Fluid and Electrolyte Balance." **Kewords:** diuretic hypovolemia following angiography increases Hct.

309. A patient with a hemoglobin of 22 gm% is suffering from:
 a. Hyperemia
 b. Hypervolemia
 c. Polycythemia
 d. Thrombocytopenia

ANSWER c. Polycythemia. Poly = many; cythemia = cell production. Any hemoglobin over 18 indicates an increased number of erythrocytes in the blood. This may be seen in response to prolonged hypoxemia or dehydration. The blood Hct level parallels the Hgb level, which is also elevated. Normal hemoglobin = 15, normal hematocrit = 45%. Hematocrit (Hct) measures the % by volume of RBCs in a centrifuged sample. Normal is 45%. This lab data is commonly used in invasive CV labs. **Don't use Hct for calculating O2 content, because Hgb is more accurately measured.**
See: Underhill, chapter on "Hemostasis." **Keywords:** polycythemia

310. Using the data in the box calculate this patient's Hgb arterial O2 content?

a.   8.4 vol.%
b.   10.8 vol.%
c.   12.5 vol.%
d.   15.0 vol.%

O2 DATA ON ANEMIC PATIENT

PaO_2 = 65 mmHg
SaO_2 = 90% by oximetry
Hgb = 12.0 gm%.
O_2 carrying capacity = 1.39 ml O2/gm Hgb.

ANSWER d. 15.0 vol.%. O2 content = Hgb. x carrying capacity x % sat.
$$C_aO_2 = 12 \times 1.39 \times .90 = 15.0 \text{ vol.}\%.$$
Note, that the S_aO_2 is changed into its decimal equivalent (90% = 0.90). Content of arterial O2 (C_aO_2) is the actual amount of O2 combined with Hgb in arterial blood. Physically dissolved O2 in the plasma can be calculated from the PO2 and a factor but is not usually figured because it is insignificantly small. Can you discriminate between useful and superfluous data? Here ignore the given PaO2. (Note: PaO2 = Partial Pressure of arterial blood Oxygen)
See: Grossman, chapter on "Cardiac Outputs." **Keywords:** Blood, O2 Content, Calc. C_aO_2

311. Most of the oxygen carried in the blood is in the:

a.   Dissolved form as plasma PO_2
b.   Hemoglobin as O_2 saturation
c.   Carboxyhemoglobin as CO saturation
d.   Met-hemoglobin as O_2 content

ANSWER b. Hemoglobin as O_2 saturation. Most of the O_2 is combined with hemoglobin to form oxyhemoglobin
$$C_aO_2 = \text{Hgb.} \times 1.39 \times S_aO_2.$$
The remainder is carried as dissolved in plasma. This small amount can be calculated by .004 X PO2 = dissolved in vol%. This amounts to approximately 0.4 vol.%. This is usually negligible, and ignored, except in patients receiving high level oxygen therapy. **E.g., 0.004 x PO2 of 500 = 2.0 vol%. Then, this amount becomes significant.**
See: Underhill, chapter on "Pulmonary Circulation and O2 transport."

312. What element in the hemoglobin molecule combines chemically with oxygen?

a.   Globulin
b.   Hydroxyl (OH-)
c.   Benzine ring (Carbon)
d.   Iron (Fe)

ANSWER d. The iron (Fe++) in the heme part of hemoglobin forms a loose bond with O2. This allows the O2 to bind to Hgb easily in the lung and be released easily in the tissues. Heme is the chelate of iron which combines with O_2. Like "rust" its oxide turns a reddish color.

Each molecule of hemoglobin contains one globin polypeptide chain and four heme groups. Each heme group can combine with one O2 molecule. If all 4 groups are oxidized, that molecule is 100% saturated. There are thousands of hemoglobin molecules in each RBC. The white discs on in this diagram are where the 4 oxygen molecules would combine to form oxyhemoglobin.
See: Guyton, chapter on "Blood Cells." **Keywords:** Blood, Heme, Iron , Fe

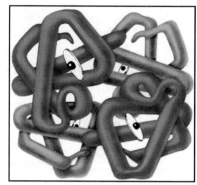
Hemoglobin molecule
(after Spence, chapter on Circ. System)

313. The percent of RBC's by volume in whole blood is known as:
   a.   **Hemolysis**
   b.   **Hematocrit**
   c.   **Hemoglobin**
   d.   **Oxygen content**

ANSWER b. Hematocrit (Hct) measures the % by volume of RBCs in a centrifuged sample. Normal is 45%. This lab data is commonly used in invasive CV labs. **Hgb is more accurately measured than Hct.**
See: Underhill, chapter on "Hemostasis." **Keywords:** hematocrit

314. A normal adult male hematocrit is:
   a.   **12-15 %**
   b.   **15-22 %**
   c.   **25-36 %**
   d.   **45-52 %**

ANSWER d. 45-52 %. Hematocrit is measured by centrifuging blood in a test tube until all the packed cells are spun to the bottom and plasma floats to the top. The ratio of packed cells to the total volume is the percent of the volume occupied by RBC's in the blood. A man's normal hematocrit averages 45%. This means that 55% of the test tube contains plasma. The average female Hct is 5% lower due to menses, around 40%. Hct and Hgb are increased in polycythemia and decreased in anemia.
See: Guyton, chapter on "Blood Cells." **Keywords:** Blood, Hct, male normal Hct.

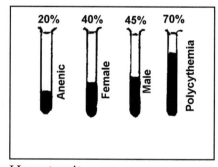
Hematocrits

315. Identify the oxygen abbreviation labeled #2 in the box.

a. Arterial blood O_2 saturation
b. Arterial blood O_2 content
c. Arterial blood O_2 content
d. Oxygen consumption rate
e. Inspired O_2 %

BLOOD GAS ABBREVIATION
1. V̇O_2
*2. SaO_2
3. CaO_2
4. FIO_2
5. PaO_2

ANSWER a. Arterial blood O_2 saturation. In blood abbreviations the first large capital letter represents the type of measurement taken. E.g.. Content, Saturation, Partial pressure... The second small letter, represents the type of blood sample taken E.g.. arterial, venous, mixed venous, capillary... The last part is obviously the gas measured e.g. oxygen, CO2... An initial capital V and F indicate Ventilation or Fraction.

MATCH THE OTHER BLOOD GAS ABBREVIATIONS SHOWN:

1. V̇O_2: Oxygen consumption rate in ml/min as used in the Fick CO technique (the dot above the V indicates rate/min)
2. SaO_2: Saturation of arterial Oxygen, as measured by oximetery
3. CaO_2: Content of arterial Oxygen, as calculated from O2 sat. & Hgb
4. FIO_2: Fraction of inspired Oxygen, normally 21% unless pt. is on O2.
5. PaO_2: Partial pressure of arterial oxygen, as in arterial blood gas PO2
Be able to match all answers above.
See: Underhill, chapter on "Hemostasis." **Keywords:** Blood O2 abbreviations

316. Gas exchange across the alveolar capillary membrane is accomplished by what mechanism?

a. Filtration
b. Diffusion
c. Osmosis
d. Active transport

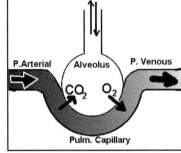

ANSWER b. Diffusion. Pulmonary gas diffuses across an alveolar capillary pressure gradient. O2 level in the alveolus exceeds that in the capillary blood, so O2 diffuses across the pulmonary capillary membrane into the blood. CO2 diffuses in the opposite direction. **See:** Tortora chapter on "Introduction to Chemistry." **Keywords:** diffusion

317. The primary drive to breathing comes from the patient's:

a. O2 level
b. CO2 level
c. pH level
d. Hemoglobin

ANSWER b. CO2 level in arterial blood is the primary stimulus used by the brain to regulate respiration. High PCO2 (hypercapnea) means the patient is hypo-ventilating and needs to breath deeper and faster. Hypocapnea indicates hyperventilation. It is normally much more sensitive than the O2 drive. But, the CO2 drive may be blunted in chronic lung patients with abnormal PCO2 and pH levels. **See:** Tortora, chapter on "Respiratory System" **Keywords**: CO2 =stimulates respiration

3. Clotting

318. **If red blood cells are placed in a hypertonic solution they will:**
   a.   **Swell**
   b.   **Sickle**
   c.   **Rupture**
   d.   **Crenate**

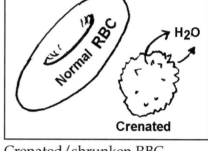

Crenated/shrunken RBC

ANSWER d. Crenate. Hypertonic solutions draw water out through the semipermeable membrane of the erythrocyte, making it shrink. Abnormal notches may appear at the edge+ of RBCs due to shrinkage. Desiccation implies complete drying of a sample.

   The opposite is when cells are placed in hypotonic solutions. They take on water. They continue to swell until the cell walls burst. This sample is then "hemolyzed." It releases free Hgb molecules into the plasma and turn it pink. **See:** Underhill, chapter on "Hemostasis."

319. **What is the shape of a normal red blood cell?**
   a.   **Biconvex disc**
   b.   **Biconcave disc**
   c.   **Spherical**
   d.   **Ameboid**
   e.   **Double helix**

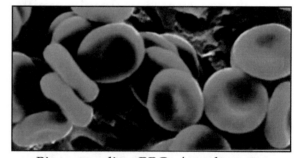

Biconcave discs RBCs / erythrocytes

ANSWER b. Biconcave disc. In cross section the RBCs look like dumbbells. This shape is the most efficient surface area for blood gas transfer. The RBC in this picture appear to stack-up. But, when they flow In the circulation they flow individually and are flexible enough to change shape depending on the shape of the vessel. **See:** Underhill, chapter on "Hemostasis."

320. **The chief receptor responsible for platelet aggregation is:**
    a.   **Alpha adrenergic**
    b.   **Beta adrenergic**
    c.   **GP Ib**
    d.   **GP IIb IIIa**

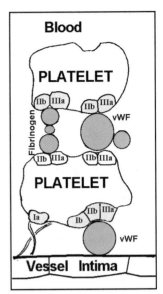

GP IIb/IIIa platelet aggregation

ANSWER d. GP IIb IIIa receptors on the platelet wall provide the final pathway for platelet aggregation and white clot. White clots occur through platelet aggregation. Platelets clump together via fibrinogen which bridges the GP IIb IIIa receptors on adjacent platelets.
      Platelets also interact with the vessel wall through GP Ia with a von Willebrand factor (vWF) protein bridge. These large vWF molecules provide the glue that makes the platelet adhere to damaged endothelium.
See: Apple, chapter on "Coagulation."

321. **The protein threads that form the basis of a clot are:**
    a.   **Fibrinogen**
    b.   **Globulin**
    c.   **Hemoglobin**
    d.   **Thrombin**
    e.   **Fibrin**

ANSWER e. Fibrin threads form a web that traps blood products and form a clot. The fibrin is formed from fibrinogen by the catalytic action of thrombin. Hemostasis, or the clotting, includes 3 phases: vasoconstriction, platelet phase, and coagulation phase.
See: Underhill, chapter on "Coagulation." **Keywords:** Blood, Coagulation, Fibrin, Clot

322. **What blood cells initiate clotting?**
    a.   **Erythrocyte**
    b.   **Fibrocyte**
    c.   **Platelet**
    d.   **Leukocyte**

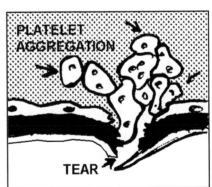

Platelets

ANSWER c. Platelet or thrombocyte. These disc shaped structures (2-4 μm in diameter), play a chief role in blood coagulation. They clump together (agglutination) and become entrapped in the thrombin net during coagulation. Specific drugs such as aspirin reduce this clumping tendency and thus act as anticoagulants. Platelets also lack a nucleus and DNA.
See: Guyton, Human Physiology. **Keywords:** blood, clotting, platelets

323. **A blood clot is a combination of which two proteins? (Select 2 below.)**
  a.   **Thrombin**
  b.   **Fibrinogen**
  c.   **Prothrombin**
  d.   **Calcium**
  e.   **Globulin**

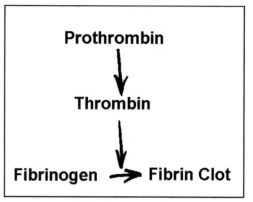

Clotting cascade

ANSWERS: a & b. Thrombin & Fibrinogen. Fibrin forms the essential portion of any blood clot. Fibrin is the insoluble protein formed from fibrinogen after the prothrombin is converted to thrombin which then converts fibrinogen to fibrin.
      This is a complicated series of enzymatic reactions. Twelve different clotting factors have been identified including thromboplastin and Ca++. First prothrombin must be converted to thrombin (heparin interferes with this step) and second this thrombin converts fibrinogen into fibrin. Note how the longer words convert into shorter words (prothrombin ➡ thrombin and fibrinogen ➡ fibrin).
See: Underhill, chapter on "Normal Hematopoiesis and Coagulation."

324. **Which process of hemostasis acts first to temporarily patch the inner walls of injured and/or bleeding vessels?**
  a.   **Fibrin clot**
  b.   **Thrombosis**
  c.   **Hematopoiesis**
  d.   **Platelet aggregation**

ANSWER d. Platelet aggregation. When platelets are exposed to injured vessel subintimal wall tissue, they form a soft white mass which quickly patches injured vessel walls. When they begin to adhere to the exposed/injured area, they liberate ADP which changes their shape. They become ameboid with pseudopod arms which enhance adhesion and entrap other clotting components within blood. This is termed the "white clot."
See: Underhill, chapter on "Normal Hematopoiesis and Coagulation." **Keywords:** blood, platelet aggregation

325. **Which factor below speeds and enhances blood clotting?**
  a.   **Hemophilia**
  b.   **Fibrinolysis**
  c.   **Laminar blood flow**
  d.   **Slow blood flow**

ANSWER d. Slow blood flow. The chief reason vein grafts clot off is reduced blood flow. When vein bypass graft flow falls below 20-30 ml/min stagnation of blood allows agglutination and clotting. This also is the basis for clots in fibrillating atrial appendages or in aneurysms. **See:** Underhill, chapter on "Coagulation."

326. **What is the fastest way to measure the extent of heparin anti-coagulation?**
a. PT
b. PTT
c. ACT
d. TPA time

ANSWER: c. The ACT test (activated clotting time) is used to monitor the effect of high-dose heparin before, during, and shortly after procedures that require intense anticoagulant administration, such as cardiac bypass surgery, cardiac angioplasty, and dialysis. It is ordered in situations where the partial thromboplastin time (PTT) test takes too long time. It should be measured about 5 minutes after the initial dose of heparin and every hour thereafter.

The partial thromboplastin time (PTT) or activated partial thromboplastin time (aPTT or APTT) measures both the "intrinsic" (now referred to as the contact activation pathway) and the common coagulation pathways. It is also used to monitor the treatment effects with heparin, not warfarin. It is used in conjunction with the prothrombin time (PT) which measures the extrinsic pathway. See:
https://labtestsonline.org/understanding/analytes/act/tab/test/

327. **Which anticoagulation lab value is best to evaluate a patient's Warfarin/Coumadin level?**
a. ACT (activated clotting time)
b. INR (international normalized ratio)
c. Platelet Count and Platelet activation time
d. aPTT (activated partial thromboplastin time)

ANSWER: b. INR (International Normalized Ratio). The prothrombin time (PT) and its derived measure INR are measures of the extrinsic pathway of coagulation. They measure blood clotting related to a patient's warfarin and vitamin K status. The INR is the ratio of a patient prothrombin time to a normal (control) sample. The normal range for the INR is 0.8–1.2. Post-myocardial infarction the prophylaxis target is INR 2.0-3.0. For mechanical heart valves the target is INR 2.5-3.5. New blood thinners that do not need frequent monitoring are Pradaxa (dabigatran), Xarelto (rivaroxaban), Eliquis (apixaban), and most recently, Savaysa (edoxaban).
See: https://labtestsonline.org/understanding/analytes/pt/tab/test/

4. Blood Types

328. **The expected blood volume of an average 70 Kg adult is:**
a. 2.8 Liters
b. 4.2 Liters
c. 5.6 Liters
d. 7.0 Liter

ANSWER c. 5.6 Liters. 8% of an adult body is blood. For a 70-kg adult this amounts to a 5.6 liter blood volume (70 x .08 = 5.6). Blood volume can also be approximated by the normal CO because an individual's total blood volume is circulated about once per minute. Remember, a normal CI = 3.5 L/min/M², so to get normal blood volume multiply CI by the patient's BSA. Since a gallon is approximately 4 liters, 5.6 L is a gallon and a half.
See: Underhill, chapter on "Hemostasis."

329. **In a child, what percent of the body weight is composed of the blood volume?**
    a.   **7%**
    b.   **15%**
    c.   **33%**
    d.   **50%**

ANSWER a. 7%.   The small percent of blood and the small size of a child make even small blood samples significant. Blood sampling in infants should be minimized. Large blood samples could lead to hypovolemic shock. In adults 8% of their body weight is blood. Thus, an large 100 Kg adult may have a blood volume of 8000 ml or 8 liters which is 92% water. But, a 5 Kg baby (11 lb), only has 350 ml of blood in its entire body. In infants IV administration may prevent hypovolemia.
See: Underhill, chapter on "Congenital Heart Disease." **Keywords:** child blood volume = 7% by weight, (adult 6 L.)

330. **Blood type "A" contains what factor on RBC membranes?**
    a.   **Antigen A**
    b.   **Antigen B**
    c.   **Antibody A**
    d.   **Antibody B**

ANSWER a. Antigen A. A person with type A blood has A antigens and forms anti-B antibodies. Note in the diagram how the antibodies (agglutinins B) are NOT shaped to fit over the antigen (Agglutinogen A) This person has no A antibodies (which would cover the A antigens), because these would attack and cover their own RBCs. So type A blood has type A antigens on the RBC and the opposite type of antibodies. This "opposite" type of antibody is true for all blood types.

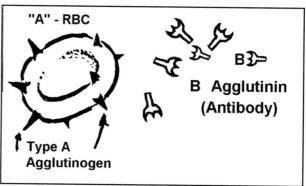

Blood "Type A" and antibody "B"

The suffix "-gen" means to produce. Antigens (agglutinogen) are the original stimuli for the antibody production.
See: Guyton, chapter on "Immunity and Allergy." **Keywords:** blood, type A, antigen A

331. "Type A" blood plasma contains only _____ iso-agglutinin antibodies.
   a.   Antibody O
   b.   Antibody AB
   c.   Antibody A
   d.   Antibody B

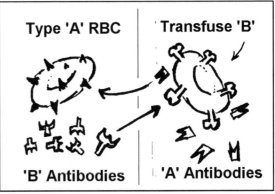

Type "A" transfused Type "B"

ANSWER d. Antibody B. A person with type A blood has A antigens present on the blood cell membranes. They form anti-B antibodies that circulate within the plasma to protect against B antigens. See the left side of the diagram. Note how the V shape of "A antibodies" can attach to the "A antigen" points on the RBC.

These B antibodies will cause a dangerous transfusion reaction if type B or AB blood is mistakenly transfused as shown in the right side of the diagram. This is because the anti-B antibodies react with the B antigens on the RBC in an "antigen-antibody" reaction. This shows the importance of accurate type and cross-match before surgery.
See: Guyton, chapter on "Immunity and Allergy." **Keywords:** blood type A, antibody B

332. Which type of "ABO plasma antibodies" (agglutinins) would a person with "type O" blood have?
   a.   A agglutinins
   b.   B agglutinins
   c.   A and B agglutinins
   d.   O agglutinins

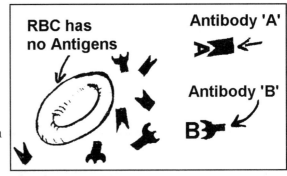

Blood type "AB"

ANSWER c. A and B agglutinins. There are both anti-A and anti-B agglutinins or antibodies present in the serum of the person with "type O" blood. These protect against both foreigners A and B. But these will be harmlessly diffused into the recipients blood. The important thing is that "type O" blood is a fairly safe "universal donor" because there are no antigens present on the transfused RBC membranes to be rejected.
See: Guyton, chapter on "Immunity and Allergy."

333. The "universal donor" blood type is:
   a.   A
   b.   B
   c.   AB
   d.   O

ANSWER d. O. Having no antigens (agglutinins). Type O blood can be given to either type A, B, or AB blood type recipients. This is because the recipient's plasma antibodies (anti-A and anti-B) will not find any foreign antigens to attack, hence no transfusion reaction.

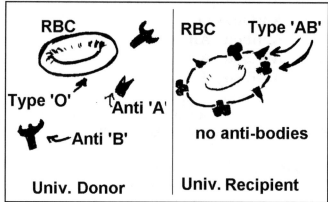

Universal Blood Donors / Recipients

Conversely, type AB blood recipients are sometimes called "universal recipients." They can theoretically receive any blood type because they have no antibodies (neither A nor B agglutinins).

See: Guyton, chapter on "Blood groups." **Keywords:** Blood type O, Universal Donor

334. **The Rh blood factor is a/an:**
   a.   **Antibody found on leucocytes**
   b.   **Platelet active in hemostasis**
   c.   **Antigen found on some blood cells**
   d.   **Natural anticoagulant secreted by vessel endothelium**

ANSWER c. Antigen found on some blood cells. The Rh factor is a genetically determined antigen present on the surface of erythrocytes. It is a standard factor evaluated during blood typing. Blood is either Rh+ or Rh-. This antigen was first discovered in Rhesus monkeys (where Rh comes from). If not carefully cross-matched to the donor, it can cause transfusion reactions.

See: Medical dictionary or Guyton, Human Physiology. **Keywords:** Blood, Rh factor

5. Acid Base

335. **The main organ responsible for regulating acid base and electrolyte balance in the body is the:**
   a.   **Kidney**
   b.   **Liver**
   c.   **Brain**
   d.   **Lung**

ANSWER a. Kidney regulates the bodies acid base and electrolyte balance by selectively eliminating some things in urine and retaining others. Being the main excretory organ they maintain the balance of water, pH, creatinine, and electrolytes, such as bicarbonate Na, K, and CA ions. When an acid base disorder is termed "metabolic" it is the kidney that is responsible, by retaining or excreting bicarbonate a strong base. **See:** Tortora chapter on "Urinary System" **Keywords:** Kidneys - electrolytes

336. **Oxygen chemically combined with hemoglobin for transport is termed:**
   a.   **Oxyhemoglobin**
   b.   **Oxyferroglobin**
   c.   **Carboxyhemoglobin**
   d.   **Carbamino hemoglobin**

ANSWER a. "Oxy" = Oxyhemoglobin = O_2 Hgb. This is measured by the standard oximeter O2 saturation. Some oximeters may measure carbon monoxide attached to Hgb. This carboxyhemoglobin may comprise as much as 10% of the Hgb in smokers. Obviously this would effect the O2 delivery to tissues.
   •Oxyhemoglobin is standard O2 + Hgb.
   •Carboxyhemoglobin (CO-Hgb.) is Hgb combined with carbon monoxide (CO).
   •Carbamino hemoglobin (CO2 Hgb.) is Hgb combined with CO2, as found in the venous blood.
See: Underhill, chapter on "Hemostasis." **Keyword:** Oxyhemoglobin ventilation.

pH	=	7.30
PCO2	=	52 mmHg
PO2	=	96 mmHg
HCO3	=	24 mEq/L

337. **Normal CO2 and O2 arterial blood gas tensions are:**
   a.   **PCO2= 20, PO2= 48 mmHg.**
   b.   **PCO2= 20, PO2= 80 mmHg.**
   c.   **PCO2= 40, PO2= 48 mmHg.**
   d.   **PCO2= 40, PO2= 80 mmHg.**

ANSWER d. PCO2= 40, PO2= 80 mmHg. Normal arterial blood gases are:
   pH=7.40 (range of 7.35-7.45)
   PO2=80-100 mmHg. (depending on altitude and age),
   PCO2= 40 (range of 35-45 mmHg)
See: Underhill, chapter on "Acid Base Balance." **Keywords:** normal PCO2 & PO2

338. **Bicarbonate functions as a base by:**
   a.   **Releasing CO_2 into solution**
   b.   **Removing free H+ ions from solution**
   c.   **Releasing hydrogen ions**
   d.   **Neutralizing OH- in solution**

ANSWER b. Removing free H+ ions from solution. A base is a substance that combines with and neutralizes acids (acids are high in H+ ions). The combination forms a neutral salt. This neutral salt is called a "buffer" because it stabilizes the pH making acidosis less likely. Eg. one common base $NaHCO_3$ (Bicarbonate) dissociates into Na+ and HCO_3^-. The HCO_3^- (base) combines with H+ ions (acid) decreasing the acidity of the solution.
See: Underhill, chapter on "Fluid and Electrolyte balance." **Keywords:** Blood, acid-base, bicarbonate, H+ ions

339. Respiratory failure allows which of the following acids to accumulate in the blood?
a. Carbonic acid
b. Oxalic acid
c. Pyruvic acid
d. Lactic acid

ANSWER a. Carbonic acid from CO_2 gas accumulation builds up during hypo-ventilation because it is inadequately "blown off." Any type of "failure" implies a "backing up" due to inadequate forward pumping. This could be "CHD" in cardiac patients or "COPD" in lung patients. In chronic pulmonary disease "COPD" patients, hypoventilation causes retention of CO2.
See: Underhill, chapter on "Fluid and Electrolyte balance." **Keywords:** blood, acid-base, resp. failure, carbonic acid

340. As acidosis increases in acute respiratory failure patients, the neural stimuli cause the respirations to:
a. Speed up in response to a neural stimulus
b. Become irregular in response to CO2 toxicity
c. Slow in order to blow off CO2
d. Become shallower in order to conserve CO2

ANSWER a. Speed up in response to a neural stimulus. CO_2 and PH receptors are the chief stimuli to respiration. Receptors in the brain's respiratory center increase ventilation. In some chronic respiratory diseases such as COPD the CO2 drive becomes blunted due to CO2 retention. When this primary respiratory drive fails, the O2 drive may take over. When O2 becomes the primary drive high dose O2 administration may be fatal. Nasal cannula flows in excess of 5 L/min should be used cautiously in chronic COPD patients.
See: Berne and Levy, Chapter on "Special Circulations." **Keywords:** blood, acid-base, respiratory failure, H_2CO_3

341. What does a high arterial PH (e.g., 7.60) indicate?
a. Excess of H+ ions
b. Deficiency of H+ ions
c. Excess of HOH molecules
d. Deficiency of HOH molecules

ANSWER b. Deficiency of H+ ions. Normal arterial pH is 7.40. Basic solutions have less H^+ ions (and thus more OH^- ions) than normal. PH is the relative balance between H^+ and OH^- ion concentrations as expressed by the Henderson-Hasselback equation PH $\propto HCO_3$ /PCO2. The H.H. equation states that as bicarbonate increases so does pH. And as PCO2 increases pH decreases. Administration of bicarbonate raises the PH because it combines with H^+ ions and turns them into H_2CO_3. Can you state and balance the chemical equation expressed here? $H^+ + HCO_3 = H_2CO_3$. HOH is simply H_2O water.
See: Underhill, chapter on "Fluid and Electrolyte balance." **Keywords:** blood, acid base,

acidosis, hydrogen ion excess

342. **During a "code" the nurse accidentally gives an overdose of bicarbonate (NaHCO3). After the patient stabilizes, this is likely to lead to:**
a. Metabolic acidosis
b. Metabolic alkalosis
c. Respiratory alkalosis
d. Respiratory acidosis

ANSWER: b. Metabolic alkalosis. Bicarb is a base that neutralizes acid. (You take bicarbonate of soda for an acid stomach.) Whenever you hear the term "metabolic" that means the bicarbonate and BE are causing a pH imbalance. Whenever you hear the term "respiratory" that means the respirations and PCO_2 are causing the pH imbalance. **See:** Underhill, chapter on "Fluid and Electrolyte Balance." **Keywords:** Metabolic alkalosis

343. **Kidneys affect arterial blood by controlling the:**
a. HC03 & Base Excess
b. HC03 & O2 Sat
c. pC02 & Base Excess
d. pC02 & O2 Sat

ANSWER: a. HC03 & Base Excess. Bicarbonate (HCO3-) is the base that neutralizes acid. E.g., You take bicarbonate of soda for an acid stomach. Base Excess or BE is how far from normal your patient's blood bicarbonate level is. E.g., A normal bicarbonate is 24. So if a patient has a bicarb of 26 his BE is +2. That is 2 mEq above normal. **See:** Underhill, chapter on "Fluid and Electrolyte Balance." **Keywords:** Kidneys = Bicarbonate (HCO_3^-) & BE (deviation from normal)

344. **One of the byproducts of ANAEROBIC metabolism is/are:**
a. Amino acid
b. Lactic acid
c. Citric acid
d. CO_2 and H_2O

ANSWER b. Lactic acid. The Krebs cycle requires oxygen to adequately metabolize nutrients. Normal aerobic metabolic byproducts are CO_2 and water. When O_2 is unavailable inefficient anaerobic metabolism results. One of the end products of anaerobic metabolism is lactic acid. It is commonly produced during cardiac arrest when oxygenation is poor. Its build up in the blood leads to "metabolic acidosis." The good form of metabolism is "aerobic" because it uses air. In aerobic metabolism O_2 oxidizes glucose with a byproduct of CO_2. Distinguish anaerobic from aerobic metabolism. **See:** Tortora chapter on "Metabolism." **Keywords:** lactic acid

345. **Metabolic acidosis may occur after acute MI due to:**
   a. Diabetic coma
   b. Lactic acidosis
   c. Aerobic metabolism
   d. CPR hyperventilation

ANSWER: b. Lactic acidosis is the main cause of metabolic acidosis. It may be due to a period of anaerobic metabolism where lactate is a byproduct, instead of CO2. Normal aerobic metabolism produces CO2 which can be quickly blown off by the lungs, but lactic acid takes time to be eliminated by the kidneys.

346. **After receiving 200 micrograms of preop fentanyl the patient's respiratory rate declines and O2 sat drops. What do you expect the arterial blood gases to show?**
   a. Decrease pCO_2, and low pH
   b. Increase pCO_2 and low pH
   c. Decrease HCO3 and high pH
   d. Increase HCO3 and high pH

ANSWER: b. Increased pCO_2, and low pH. A normal IV dose of Fentanyl is 25-50 mcg. This is respiratory acidosis induced by a narcotic overdose. Ventilation rate slows chiefly affecting the CO2 levels in arterial blood. Hypoventilation results in CO2 retention and excess carbonic acid in blood. This decreases the pH. The more carbon dioxide and carbonic acid, the lower the pH. Bag this patient.

   If bagging doesn't adequately raise the pH, you can give bicarb. NaHCO3. Bicarbonate is chiefly regulated by the kidneys, and takes a long time for the body to create. So, adding bicarb to the blood immediately raises the pH. It neutralizes the carbonic acid by buffering the hydrogen ion (acid) thus raising the pH. **See:** Grossman, chapter on "...Adjunctive Pharmacologic Therapy" **Keywords:** Fentanyl overdose = respiratory acidosis

6. Blood - Other

347. **The normal blood potassium electrolyte levels are:**
   a. 0.1-1 mEq/L
   b. .5-1 mg/L
   c. 3-5 mEq/L
   d. 10-22 mg/L

ANSWER c. 3-5 mEq/L. K^+ concentration dramatically affects cardiac cell repolarization. Remember K^+ is the most common ion found inside the resting cardiac cell. Normal K^+ = 3-5 mEq/L. Hypokalemia leads to dangerous arrhythmias. It may be recognizable on ECG as the "u" wave becomes enlarged. In contrast, hyperkalemia (High K^+) leads to peaked or tented "T" waves on the ECG.
See: Underhill, chapter on "The Effects of Electrolyte Imbalance on the CV System."

348. **Leukocytes function in which 2 processes below?**
    a.   **Transportation of oxygen**
    b.   **Phagocytosis**
    c.   **Meiosis**
    d.   **Antibody production**
    e.   **Thrombosis**

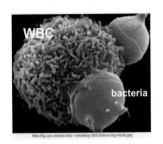

ANSWERS: b & d. Phagocytosis and antibody production. Phagocytosis means "cell eating." Leukocytes are the WBCs as distinguished from the erythrocytes (RBC's). Only erythrocytes transport O_2. WBCs fight infection. They eat up germs and foreign materials. Phagocytosis means "to eat." Note the WBC eating bacteria in the image. A special type of leucocyte, the β lymphocyte creates plasma cells that create antibodies. Be able to match all answers above. Meosis is creation of sperm or egg cells with only one set of chromosomes. **See:** Guyton, chapter on "Blood in Function of the Human Body." **Keywords:** blood, leukocytes, WBC

349. **In the adult, erythrocytes are produced in the:**
    a.   **Spleen**
    b.   **Kidney**
    c.   **Liver**
    d.   **Bone marrow**

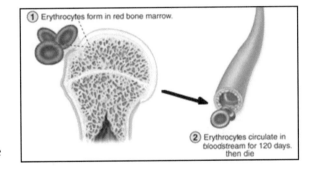

ANSWER d. Bone marrow. RBC's are produced in the red bone marrow from undifferentiated cells called "stem" cells. The spleen destroys old RBC's in the adult, and creates new RBC's only during fetal life in the newborn. (the word "erythrocytes" comes from "erythremia" which means a red flushing color). By the time the infant is born, red and white cell formation no longer occurs anywhere except the bone marrow. The marrow of the membranous bones (skull, vertebrae, ribs, ilia and sternum) produce more RBC's than the long marrow. **See:** Guyton, chapter on "Blood Cells."

350. **Each red blood cell lives approximately:**
    a.   **21 days**
    b.   **28 days**
    c.   **56 days**
    d.   **120 days**

ANSWER d. 120 days. Normal RBC's survive 120 days (4 months) with a half life of 60 days. Aspirin reduces the life-span of normal RBCs, thinning the blood. RBC survival times are important to valve replacement patients. Mechanical valves all "chew up" cells. Their survival time may be so short that anemia develops. This is termed "Hemolytic Anemia." **See:** Underhill, chapter on "Normal Hematopoiesis and Coagulation."

351. **The main function of the blood is:**
a.   **To fight infection**
b.   **Thermoregulation**
c.   **Transportation**
d.   **Carry oxygen to the lungs**

ANSWER c. Transportation. While blood is involved in all these, the best answer is transportation. Blood circulation transports nutrients and O_2 to the tissues and carries waste products(CO_2) away.
See: Tortora, chapter on "Blood." **Keywords:** Blood, function of blood, transportation

352. **Plasma contains what percent water?**
a.   **55%**
b.   **66%**
c.   **75%**
d.   **92%**
e.   **99.5%**

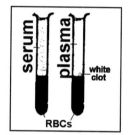
Plasma - Serum

ANSWER d. 92%.   Plasma consists of about 92% water. Plasma is what is left after centrifuging out all RBC's and WBC's. Serum can be made from plasma by liberating fibrinogen and forming a "white clot." The remaining fluid is called plasma.

The remaining 8% of blood is composed of solid solutes, chiefly proteins such as albumin and globulin. Albumins are plasma proteins largely responsible for the blood's thick viscosity. Along with the blood electrolytes these solutes help prevent water in the blood from diffusing into the tissues and causing edema. The globulins are the chief remaining solutes in plasma. They are the antibody proteins released by plasma cells which form antigen-antibody complexes.   **See:** Guyton, chapter on "Immunity and Allergy." **Keywords:** Plasma, % water, immune system, antibodies

353. **The average adult alveolar-capillary surface <u>area</u> in the lungs is:**
a.   **1-2 M²**
b.   **5-10 M²**
c.   **20-40 M²**
d.   **50-70 M²**

ANSWER d. 50-70 M². If the millions of spherical alveoli could be opened and stretched out flat. They would have the area of a "tennis court." This tremendous area is used for gas exchange, O_2 transport being a slow process (the slowest gas to diffuse). In lung disease such as COPD this surface area is drastically reduced. **See:** West, "Pulmonary Physiology."

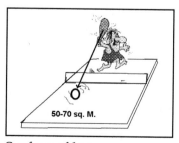
50-70 sq. M.

Surface of lung

354. A white blood count of 8,000 WBCs/mm^2 is termed _____ and usually indicates that the patient has a/an _____.
  a. Normal, normal blood count
  b. Leucopenia, infection
  c. Leucopenia, immune deficiency
  d. Leucocytosis, infection
  e. Leucocytosis, immune deficiency

ANSWER a. Normal, normal blood count. Leukocytes (WBCs) are 700 times less numerous than erythrocytes (RBCs). WBC counts normally range from 5,000 to 9,000 /mm^2. Counts over 9,000 usually indicate infection or inflammation. If the WBC count exceeds 10,000 /mm^2 a pathological condition probably exists.

A differential blood count is the percentage of each type of white cell. Normal range is given. Abnormally high counts may indicate:

TYPE OF WBC	NORMAL RANGE	ELEVATION INDICATES
Neutrophils	60-70%	Bacterial infection
Eosinophils	2-4%	Allergic reaction
Basophils	0.5-1%	Allergic reaction
Lymphocytes	20-25%	Antigen/antibody reaction
Monocytes	3-8%	Chronic infection

See: Tortora, chapter on "Components of Blood." **Keywords:** WBC count, normal range, differential

355. What does a WBC count of 21,000 indicate about an adult patient?
  a. Normal WBC
  b. Anemic patient
  c. Polycythemia
  d. Systemic infection

ANSWER d. Systemic infection. Normal blood leukocyte count averages 5000-10,000/mm^3. A patient's elevated WBC indicates infectious or inflammatory response. Invasive procedures should be postponed until the infection is resolved.
See: Tilkian & Conover, chapter on "The Complete Blood Count." **Keywords**: high WBC = infection

356. Where is insulin produced?
  a. Pancreas (beta cells in Isle of Langerhans)
  b. Adrenal cortex (outer portion of Suprarenal gland)
  c. Parathyroid gland (hypophysis)
  d. Liver (Kupffer's cells)

ANSWER a. Pancreas (beta cells in Isle of Langerhans) produce insulin. This hormone producing part of the pancreas secretes Insulin directly onto the blood stream when elevated sugar levels are detected in the blood. It reduces sugar levels in several ways:
  1. Accelerates the transport of glucose from blood into muscle cells
  2. Accelerates the conversion of glucose into glycogen (glycogenesis)

3. Stimulates the conversion of glucose or other nutrients into fatty acids (lipogenesis)

4. Stimulate protein synthesis

See: Tortora chapter on "Endocrine System." **Keywords**: insulin, pancreas Islets of Langerhans

357. **Insulin secretion causes a/an _____ by accelerating it's the absorption into the muscle cells and other tissues.**
   a.   **Increase in blood glucose**
   b.   **Increase in blood glycogen**
   c.   **Decrease in blood glucose**
   d.   **Decrease in blood glycogen**

ANSWER c. Decrease in blood glucose. The hormone insulin regulates the level of sugar in the blood. Once liberated in the blood it causes a decrease in blood sugar levels. Insulin accelerates transport of glucose from blood into cells - especially of muscle cells.

Diabetes mellitus results if insulin production is inadequate. In diabetes there is excess glucose in the blood and urine. Glucose is $C_6H_{12}O_6$. It is also called dextrose. Glycogen is $C_6H_{12}O_5$ and is largely stored in the liver to be liberated as needed. Glycogen is also termed hepatin.

See: Tortora, chapter on "The Endocrine System." **Keywords:** Insulin, blood sugar level

358. **Diabetic coma results from an excess accumulation in the blood of:**
   a.   **Sodium bicarbonate, causing alkalosis**
   b.   **Glucose from rapid carbohydrate metabolism, causing drowsiness**
   c.   **Nitrogen from protein metabolism, causing ammonia intoxication**
   d.   **Ketones from rapid fat breakdown, causing acidosis**

ANSWER d. Ketones from rapid fat breakdown for energy, this causes ketone acidosis. This occurs because the patient has inadequate insulin and cannot normally metabolize glucose to form glycogen. Glycogen is a main energy source

See: Spence, chapter on "Endocrine System" **Keywords:** Ketones acidosis, diabetic coma

Blood & Lymph Components

359. **Match the name of the formed blood cells to their common name.**
   1. Red blood cells _____
   2. White blood cells _____
   3. Platelets _____
      a. Leucocytes
      b. Erythrocytes
      c. Thrombocytes

ANSWER
1. Red blood cells (RBC) = b. Erythrocytes

2. **White blood cells (WBC)** = a. Leucocytes
3. **Platelets** = c. Thrombocytes
> There are many types of leucocytes or white blood cells (WBC): Granulocytes, neutrophils, eosinophils, basophils, monocytes, and lymphocytes.
See: Alexander, Human Anatomy and Physiology, chapter on "The Blood"

360. **The only blood component neither seen nor measured in a hematocrit is the:**
   a.   **Plasma**
   b.   **Leucocytes**
   c.   **Erythrocytes**
   d.   **Thrombocytes**

ANSWER d. Thrombocytes. Platelets do not normally separate out during the centrifuging process. Hematocrit (Hct) is determined by centrifuging blood and then noting the ratio of red blood cells (Erythrocytes) to total hematocrit blood volume. Between the red cells on the bottom and the plasma on top lies a thin white layer of leucocytes. The plasma contains the platelets (Thrombocytes). They can be clumped together with fibrinogen to form a "white clot" or platelet plug. After the plasma loses its fibrinogen it is termed "serum." **See:** Tortora, chapter on "Blood." **Keywords**: hematocrit, thrombocytes

361. **What is the most plentiful component of normal blood?**
   a.   **O2**
   b.   **Plasma**
   c.   **Erythrocytes**
   d.   **Leucocytes**

ANSWER b. Plasma comprises 55-60% if the blood hematocrit. Blood is mostly water. But, the next largest compound is comprised of erythrocytes (red blood cells) at 40-45% of the packed cell volume. **See:** Tortora, chapter on "Blood."

362. **Injured endothelium tends to collect a "white clot" formed from:**
   a.   **Fibrin and entrapped erythrocytes**
   b.   **Platelets or thrombocytes**
   c.   **Prothrombin and thrombin**
   d.   **White blood cells**

ANSWER b. Platelets or thrombocytes. Platelets are also called thrombocytes, because of their role in initiating thrombosis. When platelets are exposed to injured vessel subintimal wall tissue, they form a soft white mass which quickly patches injured vessel walls. This is termed the "white clot." These attract fibrin which entraps RBCs and forms a red clot or thrombus. **See:** https://www.verywell.com/how-the-blood-clots-how-to-prevent-abnormal-clotting-1745326

363. A microscopic blood exam that estimates the percentage of each type of white cell is called a:

    a.   White matter evaluation
    b.   Differential blood count
    c.   Phagocyte count
    d.   Leucocyte ratio

ANSWER b. Differential blood count involves staining a blood smear and then counting each type of leukocyte seen through the microscope. The differential count gives a percentage of each type of leukocyte. White cells are the bodies response to infection. Most are large phagocytic cells that devour foreign organisms, and remove debris such as dead tissue or injured cells. They are found in larger numbers in the lymphoid tissues and are capable of ameboid movement.
See: Allmers, Review for Surgical Tech. Exam, chapter on "Fundamentals"

Osmotic Pressure

364. When increased hydrostatic pressure pushes plasma out of the capillary it may enter the interstitial space and cause edema. What normally happens to this excess volume of plasma?

    a.   Massaged out by venous pump
    b.   Removed by thebesian veins
    c.   Removed by lymphatic system
    d.   Reabsorbed by renal tubules

ANSWER c. Removed by lymphatic system. Plasma and other materials that accumulate in the intercellular space diffuse may be picked by the venous capillary or absorbed into the blind ended lymph capillary. These are conducted up through the thoracic duct and back into the bloodstream. This process helps prevent edema from occurring. **See:** Tortora, chapter on "Blood."

365. What is the process by which water diffuses across a semipermeable membrane into an area of higher concentration?

    a.   Emesis
    b.   Osmosis
    c.   Active transport
    b.   Mediated transport

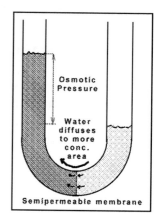

ANSWER b. Osmosis occurs across semipermeable membranes in an attempt to equalize the concentration gradient. Most solute molecules are too large to move across these membranes. Thus only the solvent (usually water) diffuses across the cell membrane and into the higher concentration area to dilute it. This is the basis for fluid shift and the rationale for low osmolar contrast agents in heart failure patients. **See**: Tortora chapter on "Introduction to Chemistry." **Keywords**: osmosis

366. **Compared to normal intracellular contents, a hypertonic solution will have a ___ solute concentration and a _____ osmolarity.**
   a.   **Higher, higher**
   b.   **Higher, lower**
   c.   **Lower, higher**
   d.   **Lower, lower**

ANSWER a. High solute concentration and high osmolarity. Tortora says, "A hypertonic solution has a higher concentration of solutes and a lower concentration of water than the red blood cells....The greater the solute concentration of a solution, the greater its osmotic pressure." Guyton says, "Because the amount of osmotic pressure exerted by a solute is proportional to the concentration of the solute in numbers of molecules or ions, expressing the solute concentration in terms of mass is of no value... To express the concentration in terms of numbers of particles, the unit called the *osmole* is used in place of grams."
See: Tortora, chapter on "Intro to Chemistry" Guyton, chapter on "Membrane Physiology"
Keywords: hypertonic, osmolarity, solute concentration

367. **Your CHF patient takes diuretic pills (water pills) for edema. The most important electrolyte serum level to monitor and watch is:**
   a.   **Calcium.**
   b.   **Chloride.**
   c.   **Potassium.**
   d.   **Bicarbonate.**

ANSWER c. Potassium. Usually, the patient receiving a diuretic loses large amounts of potassium through the urinary tract and will suffer from hypokalemia. To help prevent hypokalemia, a patient receiving a diuretic ordinarily has levels of potassium in blood serum monitored and receives potassium supplements as indicated. Signs of potassium deficit include cramping and weakness of muscles, an irregular pulse rate, postural hypotension, thirst, anorexia, and vomiting. There are new "potassium sparing" diuretics.
See: Lippincott's State Board Review for NCLEX-PN. **Keywords**: diuretic - watch K level

368. **A blood sample is obtained from your untreated CHF patient for determination of serum electrolytes. Her legs are puffy and you suspect that she is likely retaining excessive amounts of what electrolyte?**
   a.   **Calcium**
   b.   **Sodium**
   c.   **Potassium**
   d.   **Magnesium**

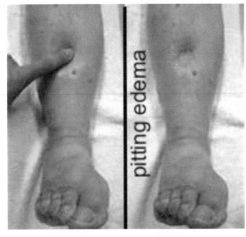
pitting edema

ANSWER b. Sodium. A patient with congestive heart failure tends to retain excessive amounts of sodium. And the sodium causes edema, which occurs when the body retains water. Water usually goes where salt is.
See: Lippincott's State Board Review for NCLEX-PN. **Keywords**: CHF retain sodium

REFERENCES

Berne, R. M. and Levy, M. N., *Cardiovascular Physiology*, 6th Ed., Mosby Year Book, 1992

Baim, D. S. and Grossman W., *Cardiac Catheterization, Angiography, and Intervention*, 7th Ed., Lea and Febiger, 2006

Braunwald, Eugene, Ed., *HEART DISEASE A Textbook of Cardiovascular Medicine*, 6th Ed., W. B. Saunders Co., 2001

Guyton, A. C., and Hall, J.E., *Textbook of Medical Physiology*, 9th Ed., WB Saunders Co., 1996

Spence, Alexander P., and Mason, Elliot B., Human Anatomy and Physiology, 3rd Ed., Benjamin/Cummings Publishing Co., 1987

Tilkian, S.S., Conover, M.B., & Tilkian, A.G., *Clinical Implications of Laboratory Tests*, 4th Ed., The C. V. Mosby Co., 1987

Tortora, G. J., *Introduction to the HUMAN BODY*, Harper and Row Pub., 1988

Underhill, S. L., Ed., *CARDIAC NURSING*, 2nd Ed., J. B. Lippincott Co., 1989

West, J. B/ Pappano & Wier, *Pulmonary Physiology - The Essentials*, 10th Ed., Williams and Wilkins Co., 2013

OUTLINE: B2 - Blood and Acid Base

1. LIPOPROTEINS
   a. Plasma lipoprotein types
      i. Hyperlipidemia
      ii. Chylomicron
      iii. Very-LDL
      iv. LDL (worst)
      v. HDL (best)
         (1) hyper-triglyceridemia
   b. Cholesterol
      i. hyper-cholesterolemia
      ii. normal < 200
   c. Triglycerides
      i. hyper triglyceride-emia
   d. APO-proteins
   e. Atherosclerosis
      i. athero-genesis theory
   f. Treatment for high lipids
      i. Diet
         (1) low caloric
         (2) low saturated fat
         (3) low cholesterol
      ii. Tobacco - stop
      iii. hypertension - control
      iv. exercise
      v. stress
      vi. familial causes

2. HGB. & O2
   a. O2 transport
      i. Hgb - most carried
         (1) Hgb - normal = 15 gm%
            (a) anemia
            (b) polycythemia
            (c) Hct normal = 45%
         (2) O2 content
         (3) O2 capacity, 1.34-1.39 x Hgb
         (4) O2 dissociation curve
            (a) arterial, venous location on
            (b) AV difference on
            (c) O2 loading - unloading
            (d) shifts in due to pH, PCO2, temp
            (e) P 50 = PO2 where O2 sat is 50-% (measures curve shift)
      ii. Blood Gases
         (1) PaO2
            (a) normal PaO2 = 70-100 mmHg
               (i) depends on age & altitude
         (2) O2 Saturation - normal >95%
            (a) red r depends on O2 saturation
         (3) PCO2

(a) normal Pa CO2 = 40 mmHg
(b) Carried in blood as:
   (i) Carbamino Hgb
   (ii) physically dissolved (PO2)
   (iii) Bicarbonate (HCO3⁻)
      1) normal = 24

3. CLOTTING
  a. Coagulation
    i. prothrombin changes to thrombin
    ii. thrombin changes to fibrinogen
    iii. fibrinogen changes to fibrin
    iv. fibrin threads trap platelets & RBCs
    v. predisposition to thrombus
      (1) slow blood flow
      (2) injury
      (3) platelet aggregation
    vi. Platelets - initiate clot

4. BLOOD TYPES
  a. Blood groups (ABO types)
    i. O
    ii. A
    iii. B
    iv. B
  b. Agglutination - tool for cross matching
    i. agglutinin
    ii. antibodies
    iii. antigens
  c. Rh factor
  d. Universal Donor = type O
  e. Universal Recipient = type AB

5. IMMUNE RESPONSE
  a. Antigens
  b. Antibodies
  c. Antigen-antibody reaction
  d. T cells
  e. Gamma-globulin

6. ACID BASE
7. Definitions
  a. Acid - pH < 7.35
  b. Base - pH > 7.45
  c. Hyperventilation PCO2 < 35
  d. Hypoventilation PCO2 > 45
  e. Hypoxemia PO2 < normal for age, alt.
  f. O2 saturation = O2 cont./O2 capacity
  g. Bicarbonate (= 24
  h. Henderson Hasselbach pH balance

8. Buffers
  a. Limit pH changes in blood
  b. H2CO3 > H20 + HCO⁻
  c. HCO⁻ administration, raises pH
  d. protein buffers
9. Respiratory Component = PCO2
  a. Normal PaCO2 = 40 mmHg
  b. Hyperventilation raises pH (alkalosis)
  c. hypoventilation lowers pH (Acidosis)
10. Renal Component
  a. HCO⁻ eliminated by kidneys in

hypercarbia
  b. H⁺ excretion by kidneys
  c. NAHCO3 reabsorbed
11. Acid base imbalances
  a. Respiratory Acidosis
    i. high PCO2, Low pH, normal HCO3
    ii. treat by ventilating more
  b. Respiratory Alkalosis
    i. low PCO2, high pH, normal HCO3
    ii. treat by ventilating less
  c. Metabolic Acidosis
    i. high HCO3, high pH, normal PCO2
    ii. treat by correcting original problem or by administration of bicarbonate (NaHCO3)
  d. Metabolic Alkalosis
    i. low HCO3, low pH, normal PCO2
    ii. respiratory component quickly tries to compensate with hyperventilation
  e. Treat original problem or by administration of KCl if diuretic caused
12. Bodies Compensation of pH imbalance
  a. Body tries to maintain 20:1 acid / base balance
  b. Chronic Respiratory Acidosis may be compensated with Metabolic alkalosis
  c. Chronic Respiratory Alkalosis may be compensated with Metabolic acidosis
  d. Metabolic Alkalosis may be - compensated with Respiratory acidosis
  e. Metabolic Acidosis may be - compensated with Respiratory alkalosis
  f. pH never returns completely back to normal

13. BLOOD - OTHER
  a. Leucocytes
    i. formation in bone marrow
    ii. CBC
      (1) WBC normal 5000-8000
        (a) elevated in infection
        (b) reduced in leukemia
  b. Erythrocytes
    i. formation erythropoiesis
    ii. plasma
      (1) 99.5% water
    iii. blood volume
      (1) 7-8% ob body weight
        (a) averages 6.00 L in adult
  c. Insulin
    i. secreted in pancreas, Isle of Langerhans
    ii. reduces blood sugar
    iii. deficiency = diabetes
  d. Osmotic pressure
    i. Solute- solvent
    ii. Hypertonic/hypotonic
    iii. Low osmolar contrast
    iv. Salt Na buildup in CHF

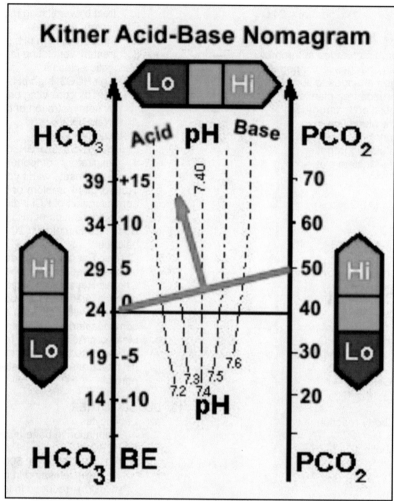

Kitner Diagram, shows acid-base balance
E.g., If PCO2 elevates to 50, tips the arrow to left= low pH
(Acidosis) See: Todd Blood Gas Game

Cardiac Anatomy

INDEX: B3 - Cardiac Anatomy

1. Cardiac X-ray Anatomy

BOTH QUESTIONS BELOW REFER TO THIS DIAGRAM.

369. In this lateral chest X-ray projection of the heart identify the most anterior structure labeled #1.
a. Interventricular septum
b. LV apex
c. RV
d. PA
e. LA

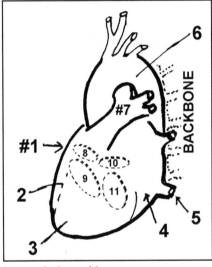
Lateral chest film

370. In the lateral chest X-ray, which structure is most posterior?
a. RV
b. IVC
c. Ascending AO
d. Coronary Sinus

BOTH ANSWERS LISTED BELOW CONSECUTIVELY:

369. ANSWER c. The RV is the most anterior structure. Here it is clearly seen anterior to the LV. This X-ray view is good for identifying RV dilation/hypertrophy since it shows the RV and RV outflow track in silhouette. **CORRECTLY MATCHED ANSWERS ARE:**

1. RV
2. Anterior IV Groove (LAD area)
3. LV apex
4. LA
5. PV
6. AO

7. PA
8. Pulmonic Valve
9. Tricuspid Valve
10. Aortic Valve
11. Mitral Valve

Be able to match all answers above. **See:** Netter's collection of medical illustrations, "The Heart." **Keywords:** Lateral X-ray view, RV

370. ANSWER d. Coronary Sinus. The LA is the most posterior cardiac chamber, and just below it lies the coronary sinus. The fact that coronary sinus (CS) is most posterior, is easily visualized in the lateral views. A catheter placed in the CS may mistakenly be thought to be in the RV. RV pacing catheter placement should always be checked in the lateral view to make sure it was not accidentally placed in the coronary sinus. You can tell that it is in the CS only by noting the posterior catheter tip near the backbone in the lateral view. **Note following diagram.**
See: Braunwald, chapter on "Radiologic Examination of the Heart." **Keywords:** Cor. Sinus, Posterior, PA Chest film

371. **Which structure forms the patient's right cardiac border? (Marked #1 on this posterior-anterior chest film.)**
   a.   RA
   b.   RV
   c.   PA
   d.   LV

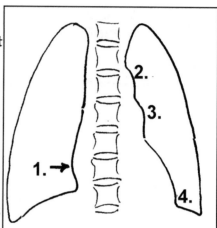
PA chest film

ANSWER a. RA. The right heart (left side of film) is formed by the vena cavae and RA borders. A Swan-Ganz catheter is easily seen to be in the RA as it is inflated. Identify all the borders of the cardiac silhouette.
   1. RA border
   2. AO knob
   3. PA border (exaggerated)
   4. LV apex
See: Braunwald, chapter on "Radiologic Examination of Heart." **Keywords:** PA Chest film, RA border

372. **What structure normally appears as a circle on the superior aspect of the cardiac silhouette in the PA chest radiograph? (Labeled #1 in the diagram.)**
   a.   Main PA bifurcation
   b.   Transverse aortic arch
   c.   Epiglottis
   d.   Calcified LA

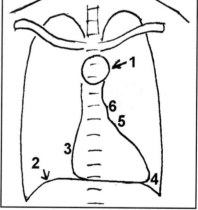
PA Chest film

ANSWER b. The transverse arch passes over the RPA and appears on end in PA and shallow RAO views. This circle is the column of blood passing over the arch. This circular appearance is often called the **"aortic knob"** because it looks like a gear shift knob sitting on top of the heart. Your ability to recognize the AO on X-ray will allow you to identify where a catheter is positioned. Landmarks shown are:
   1. AO Knob
   2. Diaphragm

3. RA border
4. LV Apex
5. LA appendage - seen here if dilated
6. PA border

Be able to match all answers above. **See:** Braunwald, chapter on "Radiographic Examination of the Heart." **Keywords:** AO Knob, PA Chest film

373. **When viewing the heart in a 60 degree LAO projection, which of the following structures form the <u>patient's</u> right cardiac border?**
a. **RA, RV**
b. **RA, PA**
c. **AO, RV**
d. **PA, RV**

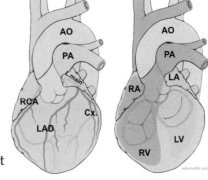

ANSWER: a. RA, RV. This is the short axis view. In this view you are looking down the LV barrel, with the RA & RV on your left, and the LA & LV on your right. The right cardiac border of the patient means the border on your left as you look at him.

374. **In this LAO projection of the heart identify the structure labeled #1.**
a. **Aortic valve**
b. **Pulmonary valve**
c. **Eustachian valve**
d. **Tricuspid valve**

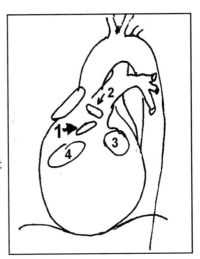

LAO Film

ANSWER a. Aortic valve. This view clearly shows the right and left sides of the heart in profile. The aortic valve is between the other three valves and tilted slightly toward the ascending aortic arch (patients rt.) This LAO view is the best view for identifying the arch vessels, and therefore is the preferred view for aortography.
CORRECTLY MATCHED ANSWERS ARE:
1. AO valve
2. PA valve
3. Mitral valve
4. Tricuspid valve

Note: The eustachian valve is a small flap of tissue at the junction of the IVC and the RA. It may occasionally be seen on echocardiography. It functions only in the fetus, to direct oxygenated placenta blood into the foramen ovale. Be able to match all answers above. **See:** Braunwald, chapter on "Radiographic Examination of the Heart." **Keywords:** LAO Film, AO valve

BOTH QUESTIONS BELOW REFER TO THIS DIAGRAM.

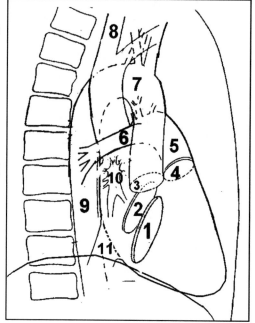

RAO Film

375. In this RAO projection of the heart identify the structure labeled at #6 ?
   a.   Right subclavian artery
   b.   Right pulmonary artery
   c.   Right pulmonary vein
   d.   Right main stem bronchus

376. In this RAO view identify the structure labeled at #1.
   a.   Aortic valve
   b.   Mitral valve
   c.   Pulmonic valve
   d.   Tricuspid valve

375. ANSWER. b. Right pulmonary artery. This view clearly shows the long axis of the heart. This RAO view is the best view for separating the atria and ventricles. The RV chamber and PA are the most anterior structures. Note the right PA beneath the aortic arch supplying the right lung. Be able to match all answers above.
CORRECTLY MATCHED ANSWERS ARE:

1. Tricuspid valve	7. Aorta
2. Mitral valve	8. SVC
3. AO valve	9. Descending AO
4. PA valve	10. Pulmonary veins
5. Main PA	11. IVC
6. Right PA	

See: Braunwald, chapter on "Radiographic Examination of the Heart." **Keywords:** RAO chest film structures

376. ANSWER d. Tricuspid valve. The tricuspid valve is larger and slightly lower than the mitral valve. It is lower partly because the heart is tilted at 60 degrees. But, the tricuspid attachment to the AV septum is slightly lower than the mitral valve attachment. The mitral valve is attached to the aortic valve. Be able to match all answers above.
See: Braunwald, chapter on "Radiographic Examination of the Heart." **Keywords:** RAO chest Film, tricuspid valve

BOTH QUESTIONS BELOW REFER TO THIS DIAGRAM.

377. In this view of the BACK of the heart identify the structure labeled at #11.
  a. Ascending AO
  b. Descending AO
  c. SVC
  d. IVC
  e. Right PA

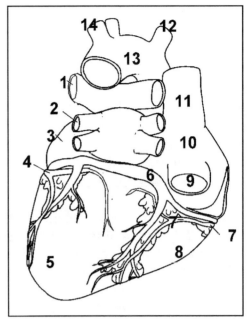

Posterior view of heart

378. Identify the structure labeled at #6.
  a. Left anterior descending coronary artery
  b. Circumflex coronary artery
  c. Posterior descending coronary artery
  d. Coronary sinus

BOTH ANSWERS ARE TOGETHER BELOW.

377. ANSWER c. SVC. This view clearly shows the vessels leading to and from the base of the heart.

CORRECTLY MATCHED ANSWERS ARE:

1. Left PA	8. Right ventricle (RV)
2. Left PV	9. Inferior vena cava (IVC)
3. LA	10. Right atrium (RA)
4. Circ. artery	11. Superior vena cava (SVC)
5. LV apex	12. Innominate (Brachiocephalic artery)
6. Cor. sinus	13. Aortic arch (AO)
7. Rt. coronary artery	14. Left subclavian artery

Be able to match all answers above. **See:** Braunwald, chapter on "Radiographic Examination of the Heart." **Keywords:** posterior view of heart, SVC

378. ANSWER d. Coronary Sinus. The coronary venous blood returns via the great cardiac vein (beneath the LA) and coronary sinus (#6). Here near the crux of the heart the CS dumps its black blood into the RA.
See: Netter's, Collection of Medical Illustrations or Braunwald, chapter on "Radiographic Examination of the Heart." **Keywords:** posterior view of heart, Coronary Sinus

2. Echocardiographic Anatomy

379. The diagram at the right represents five standard transducer imaging locations used in echocardiography. What imaging position is labeled at #3 on the diagram?

a. Parasternal
b. Apical
c. Subcostal
d. Suprasternal
e. Trans-esophageal

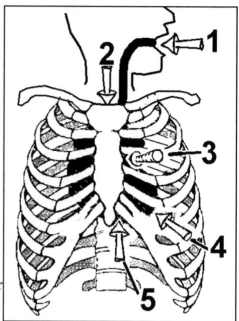
Imaging windows, echocardiography

ANSWER a. Parasternal = alongside the sternum, usually 2-4 intercostal space (ICS) to the left of the sternum. The heart can only be seen through echocardiographic windows, through soft tissue and between the bony part of the chest. When a transducer on an esophageal probe is swallowed by the patient, echograms may be taken from inside the chest.
CORRECTLY MATCHED ANSWERS ARE:
    1. Transesophogeal (TE)
    2. Suprasternal (above sternum)
    3. Parasternal (next to sternum)
    4. Apical
    5. Subcostal (below costal cartilage/rib cage)
See: Braunwald, chapter on "Echocardiography" The Heart. **Keywords:** Echo views

380. What standard echo transducer position is shown?

a. Parasternal
b. Apical
c. Subcostal
d. Suprasternal
e. Trans-esophageal

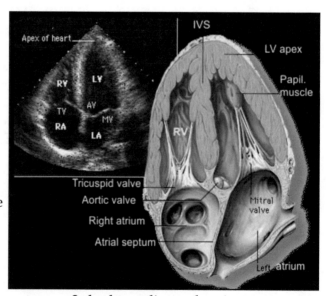
2-d echocardiography view

ANSWER b. Apical 4 chamber view. The transducer is place between the ribs at the LV apex. With the transducer imaging plane turned horizontal you see all 4 chambers of the heart. **See:** Braunwald, chapter on "Echocardiography" The Heart." **Keywords:** Apical echo view

THE NEXT TWO QUESTIONS REFER TO THIS DIAGRAM.

381. This is a diagram of the three orthogonal planes imaged in 2-D echocardiography. Name the plane labeled #1.
  a. Four chamber
  b. Two chamber
  c. Long axis
  d. Short axis

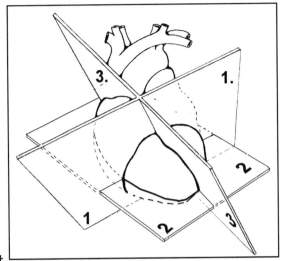

382. The appearance of the orthogonal 2-D echocardiographic planes or slices shown, are similar to standard angiographic equivalent views. The echo plane labeled #2 in the diagram at the right would result in a 2-D echogram looking like diagram _____ below?

Orthogonal 2-D echocardiography planes

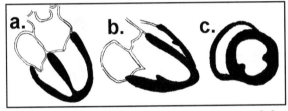

LAO cranial   RAO   LAO caudal

BOTH ANSWERS LISTED CONSECUTIVELY BELOW:
381. ANSWER d. Short axis = plane #1. These three orthogonal planes are perpendicular to each other.
CORRECTLY MATCHED ANSWERS ARE:
1. The short axis cuts the body in the horizontal plane. The image resembles the LAO caudal angiographic view. In this view the RV and LV are clearly outlined. It is viewed as if looking *down the barrel* of the ventricle. In the short axis view the LV is displayed in its shortest length and resembles a circle.

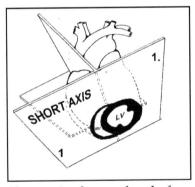

Short axis plane at level of the papillary muscles

2. The four chamber view cuts the body in a slightly tilted frontal plane. Note that all 4 chambers of the heart show as ellipses connected by the AV valves. The 4-chamber view resembles the LAO cranial or hepato-clavicular angiographic view shown here➔.

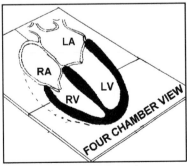

Four chamber echo plane

3. The long axis cuts the body in a tilted sagittal plane. This view resembles the RAO angiographic view with the RV on top of the LV. In any long axis view the LV is displayed in its longest length and resembles an ellipse.
See: Braunwald, chapter on "Echocardiography"
Keywords: Echo orthogonal views

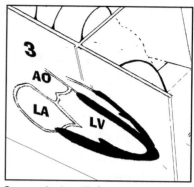

Long Axis - Echo Plane

382. ANSWER a. the four chamber view is imaged in plane #2. It resembles the LAO cranial angiographic view or "chin shot." Note that these 3 echo planes are similar to the standard angiographic views seen at cardiac catheterization. However, the angiographic view is shot perpendicular to the plane viewed, while the echo transducer is in the same plane and parallel to the plane viewed. Although the orientation from which you view both types of images is the same, the nature of the image is completely different. 2-D echo images display tissue interfaces in that plane. Whereas, an X-ray image is a composite *shadow* of all the structures between the X-ray tube and the film.

CORRECTLY MATCHED ANSWERS ARE:
    Plane #1 = Answer c. short axis.
    Plane #2 = Answer a. four chamber view
    Plane #3 = Answer b. long axis
    The accepted echo viewing screen orientation, positions the transducer at the top of the viewing screen, so that the pie shape fans-out below it. Each plane may be imaged by placing the transducer on any echogenic window within that plane.
    The displayed field cuts off anything outside of the pie shaped sector as shown. In addition to this, the pointer on the transducer indicates the right side of the displayed image. So, if you rotate the 2-D transducer head 180 degrees the image flips around the central scan line. With a little practice all cath lab professionals can make the transition to understanding these echocardiographic images.
See: Braunwald, chapter on "Echocardiography" **Keywords**: 3 echo planes, resemble angio equivalent views

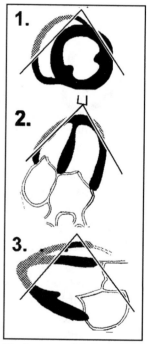

Orthogonal 2-D echos

383. The diagram at the right represents transducer positions for the 4 short axis views imaged in 2-D echocardiography. The echocardiographic plane labeled #2 in the diagram at the right would result in a 2-D echogram looking like diagram lettered _____ below ?

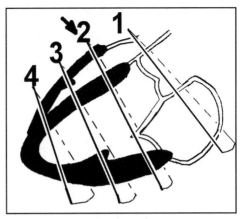
Cross sectional echo planes

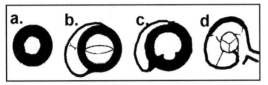
Short axis echo views of heart

ANSWER b. Short axis view at the level of mitral valve. Note the bicuspid valve within the round LV cavity. The RV appears as a "C" attached to the LV septum. With transducer angulation the tricuspid valve may occasionally be seen within the RV.
CORRECTLY MATCHED ANSWERS ARE:
1. **Base of heart** showing three right heart structures wrapped around the aorta.
2. **Short axis view** at the level of mitral valve. Note the anterior RV with tricuspid valve, and the round LV surrounding both mitral leaflets. In a 2-D echo the mitral valve resembles a "winking eye."
3. **LV at level of papillary muscles**. Note papillary muscles on inferior wall of LV.
4. **LV apex.** Note smaller LV chamber size below papillary muscles.
See: Braunwald, chapter on "Echocardiography" The Heart. **Keywords:** 2-D short axis echo

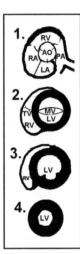
Short Axis

384. The diagram at the right represents a short axis 2-D echocardiographic view imaged at the base of the heart at the level of the great vessels. What chamber/structure is labeled at #3 on the diagram?
a. RA
b. Tricuspid valve
c. RV
d. Pulmonic valve
e. PA
f. Aorta

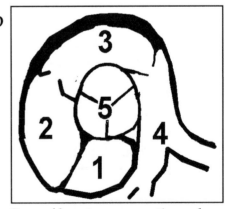
Base of heart - cross section echo.

ANSWER c. RV. The cross sectional view shows the base of heart with the right heart structures wrapped around the aorta. The PA divides into right and left PA posteriorly. With angulation all 3 right heart chambers and both valves may be visualized. There is no analogous angiographic view. The closed aortic valve is visible as an upside down

Mercedes Benz or Y Sign.
CORRECTLY MATCHED ANSWERS ARE:
   1. LA
   2. RA (note tricuspid valve between RA and RV)
   3. RV (note pulmonic valve between RV and PA)
   4. PA
   5. Aortic valve
See: Braunwald, chapter on "Echocardiography" The Heart." **Keywords:** 2-D short axis echo at base of heart

385. **The diagram at the right represents a parasternal M-mode echo scan from LV to AO. What valve or structure is labeled in the box at #5?**
   a.   **Mitral valve**
   b.   **Aortic valve**
   c.   **Papillary muscle**
   d.   **Interventricular septum**

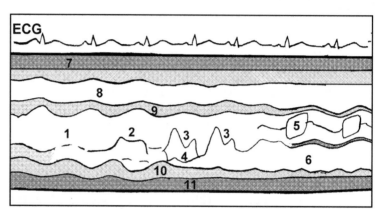

M-mode parasternal echo scan waveforms, with ECG

ANSWER b. Aortic valve. Note the box shape of the open aortic orifice in systole. As the aortic leaflets close in diastole their approximation is seen as a single down sloping line at the end of the tracing.
CORRECTLY MATCHED ANSWERS ARE:
   1. Papillary muscle/chordae
   2. Mitral chordae tendinea
   3. Mitral - anterior leaflet
   4. Mitral - posterior leaflet
   5. Aortic valve orifice
   6. LA
   7. Chest wall
   8. RV
   9. Interventricular Septum (IVS)
   10. Post. LV wall
   11. Lung, mediastinum

See: Braunwald, chapter on "Echocardiography" The Heart." **Keywords:** M-Mode echo parasternal scan

386. **The diagram at the right represents an M-mode echo scan of the LV and AO. What transducer location would be used to obtain the pattern labeled at #2?**

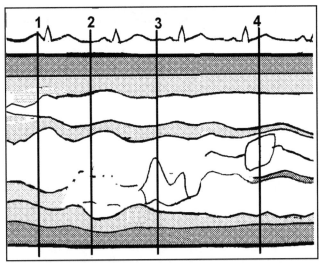

Four M-mode echo scan patterns- parasternal

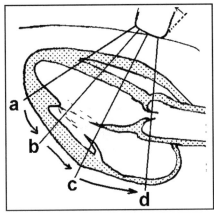

Transducer angles used for
M mode parasternal scan shown

ANSWER b. LV location. The M-mode transducer is pointed at the apex (#a) and slowly directed upward, towards the base of the heart (#d). This M-mode scan of the 4 areas results.

CORRECTLY MATCHED ANSWERS ARE:

1. LV apex - includes posterior papillary muscle
2. LV chamber above the papillary muscles. Ventricular diameter dimension are measured here.
3. Mitral valve position. The anterior leaflet is best seen. It appears with 2 diastolic "bumps": one for rapid LV filling, and a second as atrial contraction forces the last bit of blood through the open the mitral valve.

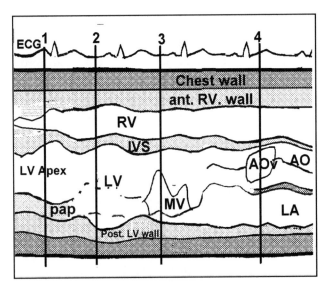

Four M-Mode echo scan patterns

4. Aortic position. Aortic opening appears as the leaflets separate in systole.

See: Braunwald, chapter on "Echocardiography" The Heart." **Keywords:** M-Mode echo parasternal scan

3. Cardiac Valve Anatomy

387. **Which heart valves are attached to the chordae tendinea?**

    1. Tricuspid
    2. Pulmonic
    3. Mitral
    4. Aortic
            a. 1 & 2
            b. 1 & 3
            c. 2 & 3
            d. 3 & 4

ANSWER b. 1 & 3 The tricuspid and mitral AV valves have chordae tendinea. These are cords (#2) attaching the valve leaflet to its papillary muscles (#1). The AV valves need this extra support and tethering because they must withstand the full ventricular systolic pressure without regurgitation. The AV valves have a large orifice size to allow adequate inflow with a small driving pressure.

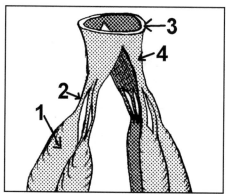

Chordae tendinea and papillary muscles (after Guyton)

    The other valves (the great vessel valves) are called "semilunar" valves, because each cusp is like a half moon or "lunar crescent" shape.
See: Underhill, chapter on "Functional Cardiac Anatomy." **Keywords:** Chordae Tendinea, semilunar valves

388. **Which valve (or valves) are open during ventricular systole?**
    a.   **Bicuspid valve**
    b.   **Tricuspid valve**
    c.   **A-V valves**
    d.   **Semilunar valves**

ANSWER d. Semilunar valves. Ventricular contraction causes systolic squeezing. This opens the aortic and pulmonary semilunar valves as shown in the right diagram. S, S, S = systole, squeezing & semilunar valves.

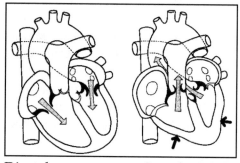

Diastole   Systole, S-S-S

    During diastole or relaxation, shown in the left diagram, the two AV valves open and the ventricles fill. See chapter on hemodynamics.
See: Underhill, chapter on "Cardiac Physiology."
Keywords: Blood flow, lungs→PV→LA

389. In this superior view of the cardiac valves the atria have been removed. The most anterior heart valve labeled #1 on the diagram is the:
a. Mitral
b. Tricuspid
c. Aortic
d. Pulmonic

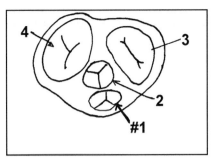
Base of heart - valves

ANSWER d. The pulmonary valve is the most anterior cardiac valve, nearly touching the sternum. It exists anteriorly and slightly left of midline. (You'd think it would be right-ward, since the RV is right-ward, but it's NOT!) For this reason pulmonary valve murmurs are usually heard to the left of midline and aortic valve murmurs to the right of midline. (Note the crossing of aorta and pulmonary vessels.)

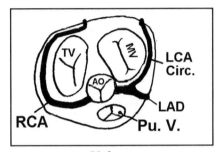
Valves

A superior view of the cardiac valves forms a kind of "cat face" shape - with the large AV valves forming the eye sockets, the AO the nose, and the PA valve the mouth. Note the two coronary arteries arise from the AO to form a moustache. **See:** Netter's Collection of Medical Illustrations, "The Heart." **Keywords:** pulmonic valve, location

390. Where is the fibrous skeleton of the heart or annuli fibrosi located?
a. Around the heart valves
b. At the IVC - SVC annuli
c. At the pericardial attachments
d. In the interventricular septum

ANSWER a. Around the heart valves. These four fibrous rings encircling the four valves at the base of the heart are called the cardiac skeleton. Except through the AV node area, there is no electrical conduction through this fibrous ring. These four rings are joined by triangular pads of fibrous tissue (trigones). This makes the AV rings a rigid structure into which the cardiac muscles are anchored. This ring may become calcified in old age and in valve disease blocking AV electrical conduction.
See: Grays anatomy. **Keywords:** Fibrous skeleton, annuli fibrosi

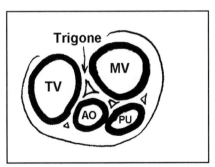
Fibrous rings skeleton

391. **The largest cardiac valve is the:**
a. **Mitral**
b. **Tricuspid**
c. **Aortic**
d. **Pulmonic**

ANSWER b. Tricuspid. Both AV valves are large 4-5 cm². But the tricuspid valve has a slightly larger orifice. It will admit three fingers, whereas the mitral will only admit two fingers. You can remember this because the mitral valve has two leaflets (two fingers) while the tricuspid has three leaflets (and admits three fingers). The RA does not normally generate as much pressure as the LA so the orifice area must be larger to admit the same amount of blood. **See:** Underhill, chapter on "CV Anatomy" **Keywords:** Tricuspid valve largest

4. Ventricular Anatomy

392. **The worm like muscle strands within the RV chamber are termed?**
a. **Chordae tendinea**
b. **Papillary muscles**
c. **Ligamentum arteriosus**
d. **Trabeculae carneae**

ANSWER d. Trabeculae carneae are irregular bundles and bands of muscle projecting from the inner surfaces of the ventricles - except in the conus arteriosus area. They are found chiefly in the RV where they provide a mesh in which to entrap trans-venous pacemaker leads and prevent dislodgement. The largest of the trabeculations - the moderator band - crosses the RV free wall and attaches to the septum where it strengthens RV contraction. It also acts to speed electrical conduction of the RV, and prevent the RV from overfilling. In congenital heart disease it is possible to

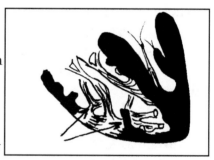

Trabeculations of RV

distinguish native RV from LV (sometimes difficult in transposition) based on how much trabeculation exists.
See: "Gray's Anatomy." or Netter, chapter on "Cardiac Anatomy "**Keywords**: Trabeculae Carneae, RV

393. **The His bundle divides into several main ventricular conduction branches which are the:**

    1. Right hemibundle
    2. Right bundle branch
    3. Kent bundle
    4. Left anterior fascicle
    5. Left posterior fascicle

        a. 1, 3
        b. 1, 4, 5
        c. 2, 3
        d. 2, 4, 5

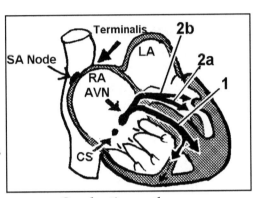

Conduction pathways

ANSWER d. Right bundle branch, left anterior fascicle, and left posterior fascicle. The 3 main conduction pathways from the AV node and His bundle are:

1. **The common right bundle branch**. It has one major branch crossing from the septum to the RV anterior wall through the moderator band.
2. **The left common bundle** has two main divisions which are:
    a. Left anterior fascicle (to anterior LV papillary muscle)
    b. Left posterior fascicle (to posterior LV papillary muscle).
    c. The septal fascicle (not shown) is a small 3rd branch of the left bundle.

When any two of these major fascicles are blocked it is called a *bifasicular* block. If all three are blocked it is a complete heart block. Block of either division of the *left bundle branch* is termed a *hemi-block*. The *Kent* bundle (not on diagram) is an abnormal accessory pathway between the atria and ventricles associated with pre-excitation and WPW syndrome. Note that the anatomy here is analogous to the coronary artery anatomy with two main divisions on the left side and one on the right.
See: Berne and Levy, chapter on "Electrical Activity of the Heart" **Keywords:** Conduction pathways, fascicles, HIS

394. **What cardiac valve is labeled at #1 in the schematic heart diagram?**
    a.   Mitral valve
    b.   Tricuspid valve
    c.   Semilunar valve
    d.   Aortic valve

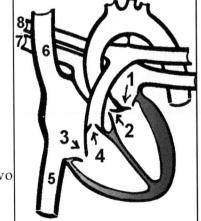

ANSWER a. Mitral valve, comes from the word "miter," a two pointed hat worn by bishops, which resembles the mitral valve shape (the only two cusp valve).
CORRECTLY MATCHED ANSWERS ARE:

Heart Valves

1. Mitral (Left AV) Valve   5. IVC
2. Aortic (Left semilunar) valve   6. SVC
3. Tricuspid (Right AV) Valve   7. RPV
4. Pulmonic (Right semilunar) Valve   8. RPA

Be able to match all answers above. **See:** Underhill, chapter on "Cardiac Anatomy." **Keywords:** Mitral Valve

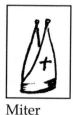

Miter

395. Which cardiac chamber normally has the thickest wall?
   a.   **Right atrium**
   b.   **Left atrium**
   c.   **Right ventricle**
   d.   **Left ventricle**

ANSWER d. The left ventricle (LV) generates the highest pressure, does the most work, and has the largest muscle mass (about 100 gm/M^2). When the RV is dissected away from the interventricular septum, an average LV mass is approximately three times the RV muscle mass.
See: Braunwald, chapter on "Assessment of Ventricular Function" and chapter on "Cor Pulmonale" **Keywords:** Thickest ventricle, LV

Ventricles

396. The diaphragmatic surface of the LV is also called the:
   a.   **Inferior wall**
   b.   **Lv free wall**
   c.   **Posterior lateral wall**
   d.   **Base**

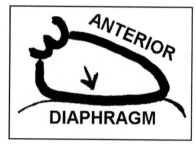

RAO, LV GRAM

ANSWER a. Inferior wall. The diaphragm supports the inferior wall of the heart - including both ventricles. The posterior descending coronary artery runs between both ventricles on this diaphragmatic surface. This is important because when the RCA or PDCA are infarcted it is termed an "inferior MI." Identify all heart walls.
See: Braunwald, chapter on "Radiologic Examination of the Heart." **Keywords:** Inferior wall, diaphragmatic wall

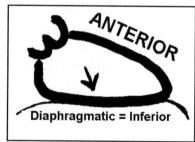

RAO, LV GRAM

397. The LV wall labeled #5 in the RAO diagram is termed the:
a. Inferior wall
b. Anterior basal wall
c. Posterior lateral wall
d. Infero-septal wall

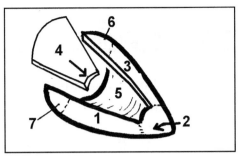

RAO, LV GRAM

ANSWER c. Posterior lateral wall. The posterior-lateral LV wall is sometimes termed the *LV free wall* because it only touches the left lung. This PA view shows the back wall of the heart (posterior-lateral) by removing the interventricular septum. The posterior lateral LV wall is normally fed by the posterior lateral branches of the right coronary artery as wall as circumflex branches of the left coronary artery.

Knowing the names of the LV walls is important to locate a myocardial infarction and coronary artery territory. Note that only the anterior, apical, and inferior walls are outlined during the RAO LV angiogram. The septal and posterior lateral walls are only outlined and seen during LAO LV angiography.

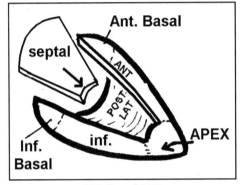

Walls of LV

WALLS SEEN ARE:
1. Inferior
2. Apical
3. Anterior
4. Septal
5. Posterior lateral
6. Anterior basal
7. Inferior basal

See: Braunwald, chapter on "Radiologic Examination of the Heart." **Keywords:** Inferior wall, diaphragmatic wall

398. The outflow tract of the RV inferior to the pulmonary valve is termed the:
a. Moderator band
b. Infundibulum
c. Pulmonary artery
d. Crista supra-ventricularis

ANSWER b. Infundibulum. The RV outflow above the crista supra-ventricularis is smooth with no trabeculae. It is termed the conus arteriosus (conus coronary artery feeds it), or the infundibulum. This infundibulum extension of the RV outflow tract makes the PA valve the most superior valve. RV subvalvular stenosis may also be termed *infundibular stenosis*. Infundibular stenosis is analogous to IHSS except that it occurs on the right side of the heart.

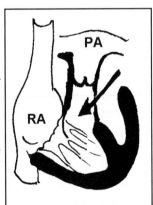

RV Outflow

See: Gray's Anatomy, chapter on "Heart." **Keywords:** RV outflow, infundibulum

5. Atrial Anatomy

399. The normal pacemaker of the heart is the:
   a.   SA node
   b.   AV node
   c.   His bundle
   d.   Purkinje fibers

ANSWER a. The SA or sino-atrial node normally initiates each heartbeat by virtue of its rapid intrinsic rate. It is located at the superior junction of the SVC and RA. An ectopic pacemaker site may take over this function (such as atrial, junctional or ventricular tissue) and escape if the SA node slows or stops functioning.
See: Underhill, chapter on "Cardiac Electrophysiology." **Keywords:** SA Node, pacemaker

400. The SA node lies at the junction of the ____.
   a.   Coronary Sinus and tricuspid valve
   b.   IVC and RA
   c.   SVC and RA
   d.   IVC and tricuspid valve

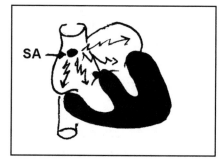

SA & AV Node

ANSWER c. SVC and RA. The SA node lies in the crista terminalis at the anterior junction of the SVC and RA. The AV node is near the orifice of the coronary sinus in the lower RA septal wall.
See: Hurst, "Atlas of the Heart." **Keywords:** SA node location, RA

401. In biventricular pacemaker lead placement, access to the coronary sinus is sometimes difficult due to obstruction by the:
   a.   Crista terminalis
   b.   Atrial appendage
   c.   Tricuspid valve
   d.   Thebesian valve

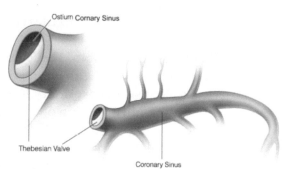

ANSWER: d. Thebesian valve. The valve of the coronary sinus (Thebesian valve) is a semicircular fold of the lining membrane of the atrium, at the orifice of the coronary sinus. The Thebesian valve may make it difficult to cannulate the coronary sinus. This valve may help prevent regurgitation into the coronary veins with atrial contraction. The eustachian ridge just above the tricuspid annulus may also form a barrier.
See: http://europace.oxfordjournals.org/content/11/9/1136.extract

See: Indian Pacing and Electrophysiology Journal, 2008; 8 (Suppl. 1): S105-S121

6. Micro-anatomy

402. **The basic contractile unit in myocardial tissue is called:**
a. Actin
b. Collagen
c. Sarcomere
d. Myosin

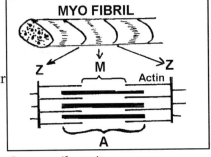

Contractile unit

ANSWER c. Sarcomere. Thousands of sarcomeres are connected in series within the myofibril bundles in the cardiac cell. Each sarcomere is made up of thin filaments (actin molecule) and thick filaments (myosin molecule). These filaments are connected to Z-lines or bands on either side. The thick filaments (myosin molecule) are surrounded by thin filaments. These two types of filaments slide together as the heart contracts. The elements of the sarcomere shown are:
- Actin = thin filaments
- Myosin = thick filaments
- A band = thick and thin overlap
- Z band = end plates of sarcomere
- M band = thick filament only

See: Underhill, chapter on "Physiology of the Heart." **Keywords:** Sarcomere, contractile unit

403. **What microscopic myocardial cell structure is labeled #1 on the diagram? This structure divides adjacent myocardial cells.**
a. Z line
b. M line
c. Sarcomere
d. Intercalated disc

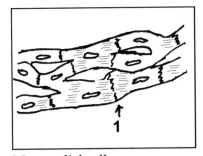

Myocardial cells

ANSWER d. Intercalated disc. These disks are like the joints between bamboo tubes (sarcomeres), which connect the long myocardial cells together. They form physical barriers between cells and rapidly transmit electrical impulses. Don't get cardiac cells and sarcomeres mixed up. The cells are separated by the intercalated discs while the sarcomere are separated by Z lines. Each cell contains thousands of sarcomeres.
See: Braunwald, chapter on "Mechanics of Cardiac Contraction..."
Keywords: Intercalated disc, cardiac cell, sarcomere

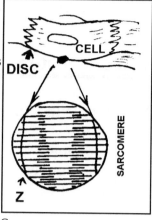

Sarcomere

404. **Cardiac cells contain both transverse tubules (TT) and longitudinal tubules (LT) for transfer of _____ ions to the sarcoplasmic reticulum.**
   a. CA^{++}
   b. Na^+
   c. K^+
   d. Cl^-

ANSWER a. CA^{++}. The intracellular networks of tubules are in contact with ventricular interstitial fluid. Electrical excitation of the cell is transmitted via the T tubules. CA^{++} enters the cell through the T tubules and triggers the sarcoplasmic reticulum (intracellular) to release more CA^{++}. This initiates excitation coupling between actin and myosin fibers.
See: Berne and Levy, chapter on "The Cardiac Pump."
Keywords: Ca++, T Tubules

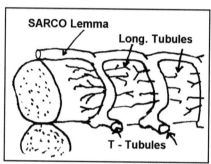

Sarcoplasmic reticulum

405. **What is the central anatomic structure of the sarcomere which is believed to have globular heads spiraling from its side, which facilitate cross-bridge linking between the two filaments?**
   a.   **Actin, thick filament**
   b.   **Actin, thin filament**
   c.   **Myosin, thick filament**
   d.   **Myosin, thin filament**

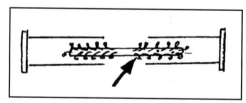

Sarcomere filament

ANSWER c. Myosin, thick filament. Myosin is the larger thick structure with the heads which act as oars. These heads form cross-bridges with the troponin when CA^{++} is present. The actin and myosin fibers slide together in systole. This is termed *interdigitation*. It is similar to the way the

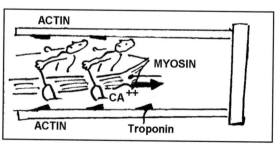

Sarcomere

fingers of your hands can slide together. .

Remember *myosis is the thick filament* because the prefix "myo" means muscle, and the muscled myosin has the oars which pull the actin strands inward.

See: Braunwald, chapter on "Mechanism of Cardiac Contraction." **Keywords:** Myosin, thick filament, oars

7. Other Cardiac Anatomy

406. **Identify the inner layer of the LV labeled #1 on the diagram.**
   a.   Epicardium
   b.   Endocardium
   c.   Myocardium
   d.   Pericardium
   e.   Pericardial fluid

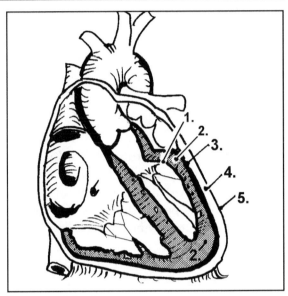
Layers of the heart

ANSWER b. endocardium.
CORRECTLY MATCHED ANSWERS ARE:
1. ENDOCARDIUM (endo means inside):
   It is composed of endothelial cells in continuation with the intima of the vessels.
2. MYOCARDIUM (myo means muscle):
   Inner layers of cardiac muscle cells of the atria and ventricles.
3. EPICARDIUM (epi means outside layer) also termed visceral pericardium:
   The external layer of the heart. It merges with the tunica Adventia of the great vessels.
4. PERICARDIAL FLUID within pericardial sack is:
   A potential space between the two layers of pericardium that contains 10-50 ml of fluid. This fluid is secreted by the serous lining of the tough pericardial sack.
5. PERICARDIUM or serous parietal pericardium is:
   The outer layer of the pericardial sack.
Be able to match all answers above. **See:** Underhill, chapter on "Cardiac Anatomy"
Keywords: heart layers and Pericardium

407. **What type of tissue grows over implanted valves and stents?**
   a.   Epicardium
   b.   Endocardium
   c.   Epithelium
   d.   Endothelium

ANSWER d. Endothelium is the inside lining of all organs. "Endo-" mean "inner." Stainless steel, Dacron, and other inert foreign implants are quickly overgrown with endothelial

tissue which makes the surface less thrombogenic.
See: "Medical Dictionary." **Keywords:** Endothelium

408. **The epicardial covering of the heart labeled at #3 in the diagram is the:**
   a.   **Outer myocardium**
   b.   **Fibrous pericardium**
   c.   **Visceral serous pericardium**
   d.   **Parietal serous pericardium**

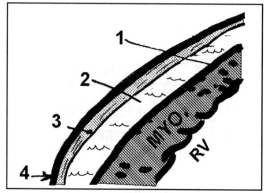
Ventricular wall layers

ANSWER d. Parietal serous pericardium forms the outer layer of the pericardial sack. The visceral pericardium (also called epicardium) forms the inner wall of the pericardial sack. It extends to the roots of the great vessels at which point it doubles over the heart as the parietal pericardium within which is the 10-50 cc of pericardial fluid. The outer pericardium has the fibrous and parietal layers.

   The pericardial sack is formed embryologically as the heart presses into a sack of fluid - like a fist pressing into a balloon. This balloon around the heart becomes the pericardial sack. **Labeled structures are:**

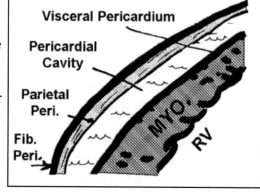
Ventricular wall layers

      1. Visceral pericardium (epicardium)
      2. Pericardial cavity
      3. Parietal pericardium
      4. Fibrous pericardium
Be able to match all answers above. See: Hurst, "Atlas of the Heart." **Keywords:** Parietal pericardium

409. **Which of the following refers to the walls of a body cavity?**
   a.   **Parietal**
   b.   **Pleural**
   c.   **Medial**
   d.   **Cranial**

ANSWER a. Parietal. The parietal pericardium is the outer layer of pericardium which touches the lung pleura. This is distinguished from the "visceral" pericardium which is in contact with the epicardium.
See: Medical Dictionary **Keywords:** parietal **Keywords:** Parietal.

410. **Parietal and visceral pericardial tissue are forms of:**
   a.   Cutaneous membranes
   b.   Synovial membranes
   c.   Mucous membranes
   d.   Serous membranes

ANSWER d. Serous membranes. Tortora says, "A serous membrane, or serosa, lines a body cavity that does not open directly to the exterior, and it covers the organs that lie within the cavity. . . . The membrane lining the heart cavity and covering the heart is the *pericardium*. The serous membrane lining the abdominal cavity and covering the abdominal organs and some pelvic organs is called *peritoneum*." Serous membranes are also called "tunica serosa." They consist of a mesothelial coating over tough connective tissue that secretes a watery exudate. **See**: Tortora chapter on " Tissues" **Keywords**: serous membranes

411. **Peritoneum:**
   a.   Surrounds all the organs in the chest
   b.   Lines the mediastinum
   c.   Surrounds the abdominal viscera
   d.   Is part of the pericardium
   e.   Is part of the pelvic cavity

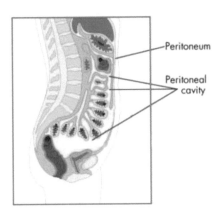

ANSWER c. Surrounds the abdominal viscera. Peritoneum is a serous membrane lining the abdominal pelvic walls (parietal peritoneum) and investing the viscera (visceral pericardium). It is a strong colorless membrane with a smooth surface, forming a double-layered sack. It is a potential space between the parietal and visceral peritoneum called the peritoneal cavity. It is used in "peritoneal" dialysis.
See: Medical Dictionary   **Keywords**: Peritoneum

412. **The main function of the pericardium and its fluid is to:**
   a.   Prevent pericardial effusion
   b.   Improve diastolic filling
   c.   Return plasma to the RA
   d.   Lubricate the heart surface

ANSWER d. Lubricate the heart surface with 10-50 ml of straw colored pericardial fluid. The pressure within the pericardial space is normally below 0 mmHg and varies with respiration. Pericarditis may scar the surface of the pericardium causing a friction rub. The pericardial fluid reduces friction within the pericardium by lubricating the epicardial surface allowing the membranes to glide over each other with each heart beat. It also cushions the heart against trauma.

BOTH QUESTIONS BELOW REFER TO THIS DIAGRAM.

413. Arterialized blood from the lungs flows through the ____ into the _____ . (Labeled #2 & 3 on the schematic diagram.)
a.   PA, RA
b.   PA, LA
c.   PV, RA
d.   PV, LA

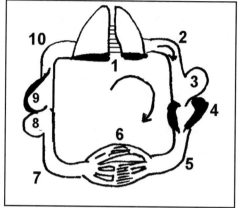

Blood Circuit

414. What cardiac chamber pumps deoxygenated blood to the lungs? (Labeled #9 on the schematic diagram.)
a.   RA
b.   RV
c.   PA
d.   LV

BOTH ANSWERS ARE TOGETHER BELOW.

413. ANSWER d. PV, LA. Arterialized (red) blood enters the LA through the four pulmonary veins. This is the only place in the adult where red-oxygenated blood flows in a "vein"

CORRECTLY MATCHED ANSWERS ARE:
      1. Lungs
      2. Pulmonary Veins (PV)
      3. Left Atrium (LA)
      4. Left Ventricle (LV)
      5. Aorta (AO)
      6. Peripheral Capillary Bed
      7. Inferior, Superior Vena Cava - IVC & SVC (not shown)
      8. Right Atrium (RA)
      9. Right Ventricle (RV)
      10. Pulmonary Artery (PA)
See: Underhill, chapter on "Cardiac physiology."
Keywords: Blood flow, PV→LA

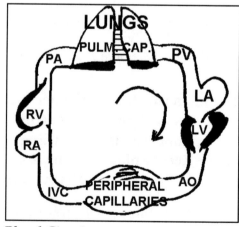

Blood Circuit

414. ANSWER b. RV. The RV receives venous blood from the RA and pumps into the PA and the lungs. This diagram clearly shows that the right and left heart, or the pulmonary and systemic circuits are connected in series.
See: Underhill, chapter on "Cardiac physiology." **Keywords:** Blood flow, PV→LA

415. Normally blood flows from the coronary veins into the_____and from there into the_____.
- a.   Coronary sinus, left atrium
- b.   Coronary sinus, right atrium
- c.   Sinus of Valsalva, left atrium
- d.   Sinus of Valsalva, right atrium

ANSWER b. Coronary sinus, right atrium. The cardiac and coronary veins parallel the coronary arteries and normally drain into the coronary sinus in the left AV groove and from there into the inferior RA between the IVC and tricuspid valve.
See: Berne and Levy, chapter on "Coronary Arteries." **Keywords:** Blood flow, Cor. sinus, RA

416. Which system of arteries and veins feeds the LV from the small endocardial channels, shown at #2, and dumps venous blood back into the ventricles - decreasing its O_2 saturation?
- a.   Bronchial
- b.   Anomalous
- c.   Anastomosis
- d.   Azygous
- e.   Thebesian

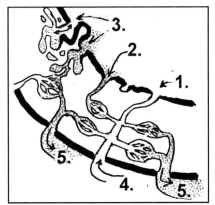
LV Endocardial channels

ANSWER e. Thebesian. There are three vascular communications which feed a chamber and dump right back into that chamber. They are:
     1. Arterio-luminal (arteries)
     2. Thebesian vessels (veins)
     3. Arterio-sinusoidal (cavities)
The Thebesian vessels are small veins which drain from coronary capillaries directly into the LV. This coronary venous blood should have returned via the coronary veins.

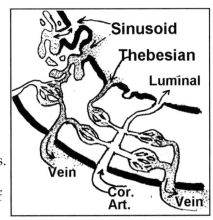
Thebesian Veins, etc.

     The sinusoids are tiny caves in the ventricle which feed the ventricular endocardium with minute amounts of blood passing in both directions. Note that the sinusoid and Thebesian veins constitute a small R-L shunt. This venous blood combined with the dark bronchial venous return from the lungs slightly reduce the LA O2 saturation. Although most noticeable in the LV, these small shunts can dump into any cardiac chamber.

     A new form of laser surgery termed "Transmyocardial Revascularization" utilizes this principle. The laser punches dozens of small holes through the LV myocardium. These provide endocardial channels for increased collateral flow to ischemic areas.

See: Berne and Levy, chapter on "Coronary Circulation." **Keywords:** Blood Flow, Thebesian veins, Sinusoids

417. **Considering the special drainage of the bronchial veins and Thebesian veins, which cardiac valve has slightly higher blood flow than the others?**
   a.   **Aortic valve**
   b.   **Tricuspid valve**
   c.   **Pulmonic valve**
   d.   **Eustachian valve**

ANSWER a. Aortic valve. About 1% more blood is pumped by the LV through the aortic valve. The bronchial arteries branch from the thoracic AO feed the lung bronchi and bronchioles with O_2 and nutrients. In addition, some coronary veins empty into the LA and LV instead of the coronary sinus. Both of these circulations are small anatomic shunts contaminating the red blood from the pulmonary veins. These normal small shunts prevent the arterial blood from ever attaining 100% saturation. See previous question.
See: Berne and Levy, chapter on "Special Circulations." **Keywords:** Blood flow, Bronchial Circulation

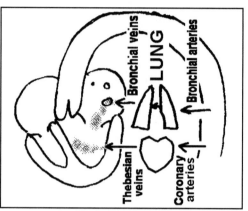

Bronchial & Thebesian Circulation

418. **The pericardium is normally filled with_____ml of clear serous fluid.**
   a.   **2-10 ml**
   b.   **10-50 ml**
   c.   **50-100 ml**
   d.   **100-200 ml**

ANSWER b. 10-50 ml. Braunwald quotes "less than 50 ml" as the normal pericardial contents. When the volume exceeds 150 ml acutely, the pericardial pressure rises and begins to compress the heart. This may reduce cardiac output by decreasing venous return. Pericardial centesis or drainage may relieve the pressure and be life saving.
See: Braunwald, chapter on "Pericardial Disease."
Keywords: Pericardial fluid, 10-50 ml.

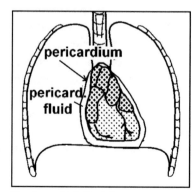

Pericardial fluid

419. The pouch like structures above the aortic valve from which the coronary arteries arise are termed the:
a. Coronary sinus
b. Sinus of Valsalva
c. Sinus venosus
d. Fossa ovalis

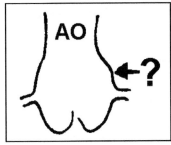
Pouches above AO valve

ANSWER b. Sinus of Valsalva. Between the aortic valve cusps and the aortic wall are dilated pockets called aortic sinus' or Sinus of Valsalva. The RCA originates from the right sinus of Valsalva and the left main coronary from the left sinus of Valsalva. Their shape aids to funnel coronary flow blood into the coronary arteries.
See: Gray's Anatomy chapter on "Heart." **Keywords:** Sinus Valsalva

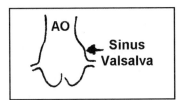
Sinus of Valsalva

420. Trace the normal flow of blood after it leaves the RA. (Note: PV = Pulmonary Valve, TV = Tricuspid...)
a. RA, TV, PA, PV, RV
b. RA, TV, RV, PV, PA
c. RA, PV, RV, TV, PA
d. RA, RV, TV, PV, PA

ANSWER b. Right atrium through tricuspid valve, to right ventricle, through the pulmonic valve into the pulmonary artery and finally the lungs. These forward flow patterns are important to know. They are also important in reverse because when a Swan-Ganz catheter is pulled back while pressure recording, it must pass through these same structures retrograde. Note special circulations seen in the diagram. The bronchial arteries supply the lung tissue and dump into PV. The coronary circulation dumps into the RA.
See: Underhill, chapter on "Cardiac Anatomy."
Keywords: Blood Flow, RA→TV→RV→PV→PA

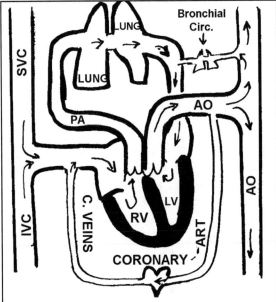
Blood flow circuit

BOTH QUESTIONS BELOW REFER TO THIS DIAGRAM.

421. **Identify the cardiac structure located anatomically between chambers labeled #4 & #6 on the schematic heart diagram.**
a.   Inter-Atrial Septum (IAS)
b.   Inter-Ventricular Septum (IVS)
c.   Ligamentum Arteriosus
d.   Ductus Venosis

422. **An O2 saturation drawn from chamber labeled #5 on the schematic heart diagram would normally be approximately _____ %.**
a.   55%
b.   75 %
c.   85%
d.   95%

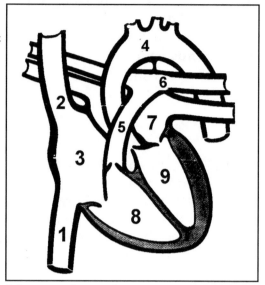
Schematic heart diagram

ANSWERS LISTED CONSECUTIVELY BELOW:

421. ANSWER c. Ligamentum arteriosus lies between the AO and PA. It is the residual ligament that is left over from the congenital ductus arteriosus.
CORRECTLY MATCHED ANSWERS ARE:

1. IVC	6. LPA
2. SVC	7. LA
3. RA	8. RV
4. AO	9. LV
5. PA	

See: Kern

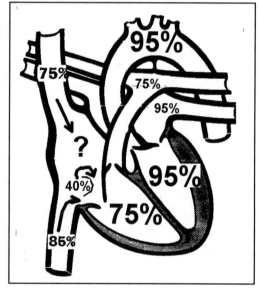
Blood flow circuit

422. ANSWER b. 75%. #5 is the PA. All right heart chambers will be approximately 75% saturated at rest. This number will drop on exercise as the tissues extract more O2 and the AV difference widens. However, the RA blood is poorly mixed between the SVC, IVC, and CS venous returns. Mixing occurs due to turbulence in the RV and the PA blood is considered "mixed venous." The entire left side of the heart will normally be red blood at approximately 95% O2 saturation.
See: Kern, The Cardiac Catheterization Handbook, chapter on "Hemodynamic and ECG data." **Keywords:** O2 sat

BOTH QUESTIONS BELOW REFER TO THIS DIAGRAM.

423. **Which cardiac chamber/vessel in the schematic heart diagram would normally have a blood pressure of approximately 130/0/9 mmHg?**
    a. #4
    b. #5
    c. #8
    d. #9

424. **What would be a normal blood pressure for chamber labeled #2?**
    a. 0/-5/-2 mmHg
    b. 4/5/3 mmHg
    c. 8/15/9 mmHg
    d. 10/13/8 mmHg

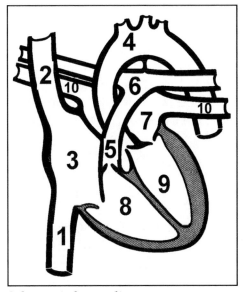

Schematic heart diagram

BOTH ANSWERS LISTED TOGETHER BELOW

423. ANSWER d. #9. LV pressure rises to full systole, then both beginning and end diastole are low. LV-EDP is the same as normal LA mean pressure. Kern quotes the following normal values:

#1=2=3=RA	6/5/3 mmHg	(a/v/mean)
#4 =AO	130/70/85	(s/d/mean)
#5=6 =PA	25/9/15	(s/d/mean)
#7 =LA	10/13/8	(a/v/mean)
#8 =RV	25/0/4	(s/bd/ed)
#9 =LV	130/0/9	(s/bd/ed)

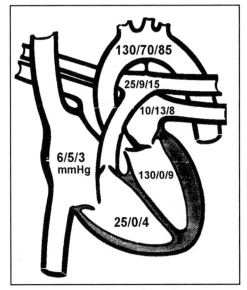

Schematic heart blood pressures

424. ANSWER b. = SVC = 4/5/3 mmHg the same as RA pressure. The right atrial pressure averages 3 mmHg, which is 5 mmHg lower than the LA pressures. Because of gravity in the upright patient, the SVC pressures would be slightly lower than the IVC. When the venous pressure reaches 0 mmHg, as it does in the neck veins of a sitting patient, the neck veins collapse. And although they still allow some venous return, they cannot transmit negative pressure upward, because they collapse so easily. In right heart failure jugular venous distension (JVD) is assessed by sitting the patient up in bed at 30 degrees. Engorged veins at this angle indicate the increased venous pressure associated with peripheral edema. The only pressure that might be below zero is the pericardium. Intracardiac pressures are always above zero.
See: Kern, chapter on Hemodynamic and ECG Data." **Keywords:** Normal pressures, LV

REFERENCES:

Berne, R. M. and Levy, M. N., *Cardiovascular Physiology*, 8th Ed., Mosby Year Book, 2001

Braunwald, Eugene, et al., Ed., HEART DISEASE A Textbook of Cardiovascular Medicine, 9th Ed., W. B. Saunders Co., 2012

Daily, E. K., and Schroeder, J. S., *Techniques in Bedside Hemodynamic Monitoring*, 4th Ed., C. V. Mosby Company, 1989

Gray, Henry, *ANATOMY OF THE HUM-AN BODY*, 77th Ed., Lea and Febiger, 1959

Hurst, J. W., and Logue, R. B., et. al., *THE HEART Arteries and Veins*, 3rd Ed., McGraw-Hill Book Co., 1974

Hurst, J.W., Ed., *ATLAS OF THE HEART*, Gower Medical Publishing, 1988

Kern, M. J., Ed., *The Cardiac Catheterization Handbook*, 6th Ed., Mosby-Year Book, Inc., 2016

Rushmer, R. F.,*CARDIOVASCULAR DYNAMICS*, W. B. Saunders Co., 1976

Underhill, S. L., Ed., *CARDIAC NURSING*, 2nd Ed., J. B. Lippincott Co., 1989

Netter, *CIBA Collection of Medical Illustrations*, "The Heart", CIBA Pharmaceuticals

Tortora, G. J., *Introduction to the HUMAN BODY*, Harper and Row Pub., 1988

OUTLINE: B3 - Cardiac Anatomy

1. CARDIAC X-RAY ANATOMY
   a. Frontal View = PA Chest film
      i. Aorta, AO knob
      ii. PA
      iii. LA appendage
      iv. LV, apex
      v. RV
      vi. IVC
      vii. RA
      viii. SVC
      ix. Pulmonary vasculature (Pulmonary edema - hypertension)
   b. Lateral View
      i. AO arch
      ii. PA (PA Window)
      iii. RV (most anterior)
      iv. Apex
      v. LA, Pulm. veins (most posterior)
      vi. Esophagus
      vii.
   c. RAO view
      i. long axis
      ii. valves on edge
   d. LAO
      i. short axis
      ii. septum on edge
      iii. valve locations

2. ECHOCARDIOGRAPHIC ANATOMY
   a. Transducer positions
   b. Imaging planes
      i. cross section views of heart
   c. M-mode scans
3. CARDIAC VALVES

   a. Fibrous skeleton
      i. trigone
      ii. valve rings
   b. AV valves
      i. Open is diastole
      ii. Tricuspid (largest valve)
         (1) 3 cusps
      iii. Mitral Valve (Mitre - hat)
         (1) bicuspid
      iv. Chordae tendinea
      v. Papillary Muscles
      vi. Arrangement in base
   c. Semilunar Valves
      i. Open in systole
      ii. Aortic (smallest thickest valve)
         (1) noncoronary cusp
         (2) Rt. & Left Cor. cusps
            (a) Sinus Valsalva
            (b) Main Left coronary
            (c) Right Coronary
      iii. Pulmonic
      iv. Arrangement in view of base

4. VENTRICLES
   a. Epicardium = visceral pericardium
      i. Parietal pericardium (sack)
         (1) contains 50 ml fluid
         (2) Myocardium
   b. Endocardium
   c. LV = thickest chamber
      i. spiral arrangement
      ii. syncytium (all cells connected)
      iii. LV Walls
         (1) Anterior

        (2) Post lateral
        (3) Inferior
        (4) Septal
        (5) Apical

- d. RV
  - i. most trabeculations
  - ii. infundibulum = outflow tract
- c. Conduction system
  - i. AV node
  - ii. His bundle (common bundle)
  - iii. Rt. & Left Bundles
    - (1) Anterior and Post fascicle

5. ATRIA
   - a. Appendage
   - b. Conduction system
     - i. SA node - near SVC
     - ii. Interatrial pathways
     - iii. Bachman's bundle
     - iv. AV node - near CS
   - c. Pulmonary veins
     - i. Normally 4 enter LA
   - d. SVC
   - e. IVC

6. MICRO-ANATOMY
   - a. sarcomere
     - i. Actin = thin filament
     - ii. Myosin = thick filament (oars)
     - iii. A-line
     - iv. M line
     - v. Z line
     - vi. Intercalated disks (joints)
     - vii. Transverse tubules
     - viii. Longitudinal tubules

7. OTHER ANATOMY
   - a. Coronary arteries
     - i. collateral circulation
   - b. Coronary veins - to CS
   - c. Coronary Sinus - Cor. Art. to RA
   - d. Thebesian veins - lungs to LA
   - e. Bronchial veins
   - f. Sinusoid, luminal
   - g. Endothelium grows over artificial valves
   - h. Layers of heart
     - i. endo
     - ii. myo
     - iii. epi
     - iv. pericardium
       - (1) function is lubrication
       - (2) prevents rapid expansion
       - (3) contains 10-50 ml fluid
   - i. Great vessels
     - i. Aorta
       - (1) red, Arteriolized blood
     - ii. PA
       - (1) dark, unarteriolized blood
   - j. The Flow Circuit
     - i. trace flow of blood
   - k. Schematic diagram of heart
     - i. valves
     - ii. chambers
     - iii. great vessels
     - iv. venous return
     - v. septum

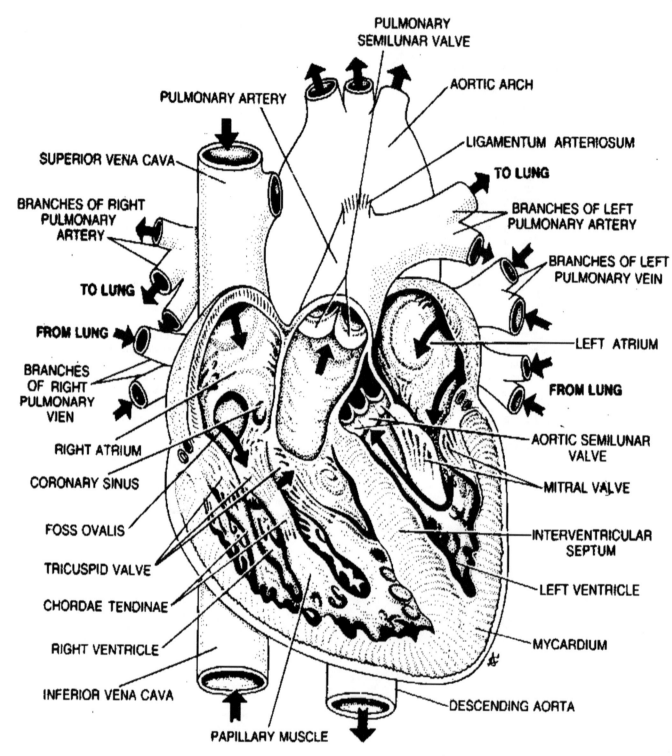

PULMONARY
SEMILUNAR VALVE

AORTIC ARCH

PULMONARY ARTERY

LIGAMENTUM ARTERIOSUM

SUPERIOR VENA CAVA

TO LUNG

BRANCHES OF RIGHT
PULMONARY
ARTERY

BRANCHES OF LEFT
PULMONARY ARTERY

TO LUNG

BRANCHES OF LEFT
PULMONARY VEIN

FROM LUNG

LEFT ATRIUM

BRANCHES
OF RIGHT
PULMONARY
VIEN

FROM LUNG

AORTIC SEMILUNAR
VALVE

RIGHT ATRIUM

CORONARY SINUS

MITRAL VALVE

FOSS OVALIS

INTERVENTRICULAR
SEPTUM

TRICUSPID VALVE

LEFT VENTRICLE

CHORDAE TENDINAE

RIGHT VENTRICLE

MYCARDIUM

INFERIOR VENA CAVA

DESCENDING AORTA

PAPILLARY MUSCLE

after tutornext.com, online tutoring

Coronary Anatomy and Physiology

1. Coronary Anatomy: Views

425. Identify the three major coronary arteries of the heart. (Select 3 below.)
   a.   RCA
   b.   LAD
   c.   Circumflex
   d.   PDA
   e.   Diagonal
   f.   Left Main

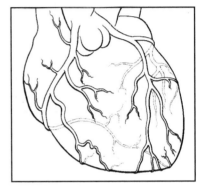

Three main coronary arteries

ANSWERS: a, b, & c. Because the LAD is usually the largest coronary artery, it is called "the artery of life." It runs down the front of the heart between the two ventricles. The RCA and circumflex are the other two major arteries. These two run around each side of the heart in the right and left AV grooves.
BE ABLE TO MATCH ALL ANSWERS:
   1. RCA
   2. LAD
   3. Circumflex

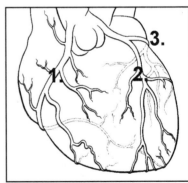

Three Main Coronaries

The PDA is NOT normally called a separate coronary artery, but a branch of the RCA. Even so, it is vital since it runs on the inferior & posterior wall of the heart from base to apex, in the inferior interventricular groove.
See: Grossman, chapter on "Coronary Arteriography."

426. **What angiographic view is shown in this coronary angiogram?**
   a.   AP
   b.   Shallow RAO
   c.   Shallow LAO
   d.   Steep RAO
   e.   Steep LAO

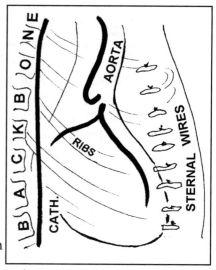

Left Cor. Angio. Landmarks

ANSWER d. Steep RAO.   This is a steep, almost lateral, right anterior oblique view. The backbone is seen on the left - the sternum and LV apex on the right. The oblique must be an RAO because of the following three landmarks. The backbone and ascending catheter are seen on the left. The ribs can be seen descending from the backbone on the left downwards toward the sternum which shows surgically placed sternal wires. Often the apex of the heart can also be discerned and the direction which it points usually names the view (points Rt. In RAO views). To distinguish the LAD from the Circumflex artery, you can utilize the rule **"Circumflex nearest the backbone"**.
See: Braunwald, chapter on "Coronary Arteriography."

427. **Which branch of the left coronary artery is nearest the backbone in most oblique X-ray views?**
   a.   LAD
   b.   RAD
   c.   LAO
   d.   Circumflex
   e.   PDCA

ANSWER d. Circumflex. In coronary angiography it is often difficult to distinguish the 2 major branches of the left coronary; the LAD and the circumflex. Anatomically the circumflex runs around the base of the heart near the backbone. A few generalities help:

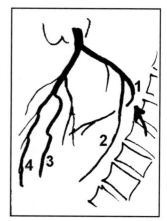

Circumflex coronary artery nearest backbone

   •In all oblique views the **"CIRCUMFLEX is nearest the backbone."** It may be off the screen, so clues listed below will help you locate it.
   •In oblique views the **"LAD and LV apex are nearest the sternum."**
   •In oblique views **"the sternum and backbone appear on opposite sides of the frame."** In RAO views the backbone appears on the left and on the right the cardiac apex, sternum and LAD. In LAO views the backbone is on the right side of the frame and the apex and LAD to the left.
Main coronary arteries shown are:
   1. Circumflex

2. Obtuse Marginal
3. Diagonal
4. LAD

See: Braunwald, chapter on "Coronary Arteriography." **Keywords:** Cor. Views, Cx., nearest backbone

428. **In this posterior view of the base of the heart, what coronary vessel is labeled at #5?**
a. **Proximal right coronary**
b. **Distal right coronary at crux**
c. **Left anterior descending**
d. **Mid circumflex coronary**
e. **Posterior lateral branches RCA**
f. **Sinus node branch RCA**
g. **Left atrial branch of circumflex**

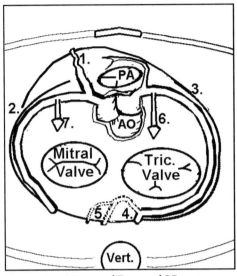

Posterior View of Base of Heart

ANSWER e. Posterior Lateral branches RCA. This posterior view shows both atria, great vessels and venous returns. This is a short axis view that shows the "C" shaped RCA and Circumflex vessels. These vessels encircle the base of the heart and form the rim of the coronary "crown." Note the backbone with the aorta descending to its left and the IVC ascending to its right.

BE ABLE TO MATCH ALL ANSWERS:

1. LEFT ANTERIOR DESCENDING: Descends to the left of the PA in the interventricular groove.

2. MID CIRCUMFLEX CORONARY: Follows the left AV groove around the left atria.

3. PROXIMAL RIGHT CORONARY: Follows the right AV groove around the RA.

4. DISTAL RIGHT CORONARY AT CRUX: As the distal RCA goes under the IVC (shown dotted) and approaches the backbone, it reaches the crux of the heart. The "crux" is where the two atria and ventricles meet. Here the RCA usually makes a "jog" shown as another dotted line. This "jog" often shows up in coronary arteriogram and marks where distal right coronary artery trifurcates into the: AV node artery, PDCA, and posterior lateral branches.

5. POSTERIOR LATERAL BRANCHES RCA: The distal RCA usually continues past the crux into the area of the LV. These are the posterior and lateral branches of the RCA.

6. SINUS NODE BRANCH RCA: Normally arises from the proximal RCA to the RA and SVC, SA node area.

7. LEFT ATRIAL BRANCH OF CIRC. or SA NODE BRANCH: Atrial branches arise from the circumflex (and RCA) to supply the atria and/or SA node.

Be able to match all answers above. **See:** Braunwald, chapter on "Coronary Arteriography." **Keywords:** Base of heart showing coronary arteries

429. **Which coronary arteries arise near the "crux?" (Crux = The intersection of the RA, RV, LA and LV walls at the base of the heart.)**
    1. **Posterior descending coronary origin**
    2. **Diagonal branch origin**
    3. **Acute marginal branch origin**
    4. **AV nodal branch origin**
        a. 1,3
        b. 1,4
        c. 2,3
        d. 2,4

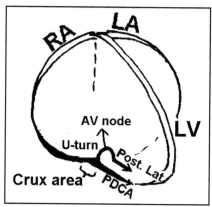
Cardiac Grooves

ANSWER b. Posterior descending coronary origin and AV node branch origin. The crux is the intersection of all four chambers on the inferior base of the heart. Here the RCA makes a U turn. Here the RCA normally branches into the PDCA, AV node artery and posterior LV (or posterior lateral) branches. Be able to match all answers above.
See: Grossman, chapter on "Coronary Arteriography."
Keywords: RCA, crux, PDCA, AV node

430. **What radiologic view is usually best to image the origin of the LCA ostium?**
    a.   20 degree RAO
    b.   45 degree RAO
    c.   20 degree LAO
    d.   45 degree LAO

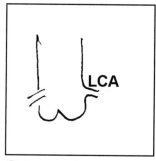
Coronary Ostia

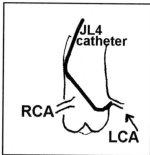
20 degree LAO

ANSWER c. 20 degree LAO. When the coronary ostia is being catheterized the LAO view shows these vessel origins on the aortic border. This is usually the starting angle for placement of coronary catheters. 20-30 degrees LAO is preferred for the LCA ostium.
    Note how the RCA origin arises anteriorly to the LCA origin. It is almost anterior. So a steeper LAO 30-40 degrees bring the RCA ostia into a better profile.
See: Grossman, chapter on "Coronary Arteriography." **Keywords:** Cor. Views, imaging LCA Ostia

431. **In patients who have had coronary bypass surgery, which branch of the left coronary artery is nearest the sternal wires in most oblique X-ray views?**
  a. LAD
  b. RAD
  c. LAO
  d. Circumflex
  e. PDCA

ANSWER a. LAD. Since they often overlap in angiography, it is often difficult to distinguish the LAD from the circumflex coronary artery. Anatomically the Left Anterior Descending (LAD) runs down the front of the heart, closest to the sternum. The trick of distinguishing LAD from circumflex is to find the backbone or the sternum. In RAO views the backbone appears on the left, the sternum on the right. In LAO views these are reversed.
See: Braunwald, chapter on "Coronary Arteriography." **Keywords:** Cor. Views, LAD nearest sternum

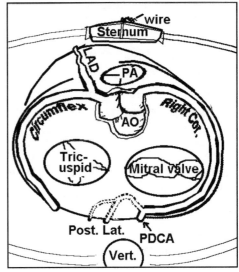
Coronary artery nearest sternum

432. **In the aortic root angiogram shown, the vessels labeled at #10 are the:**
  a. Left Main
  b. Left Anterior Descending (LAD)
  c. Diagonal
  d. Anterior Septal
  e. Obtuse Marginal

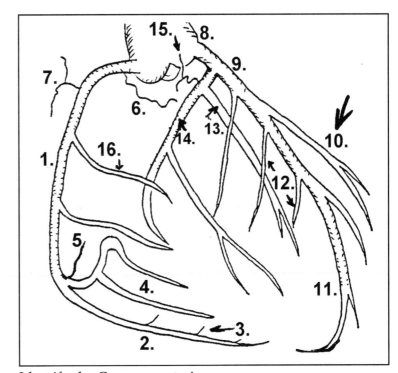
Identify the Coronary arteries

ANSWER c. Diagonal. This is an RAO view of both coronary arteries. Diagonal branches arise from the LAD. They supply the anterior LV free wall and arise from the left side of the LAD while septal branches arise from the right (septal) side.

BE ABLE TO MATCH ALL ANSWERS:

1. Right Coronary	9. Left Anterior Descending (Lad)
2. Posterior Descending	10. Diagonal
3. Inferior Septal	11. Distal Lad
4. Posterior Lateral	12. Anterior Septal
5. AV Node Branch	13. Obtuse Marginal
6. Conus Branch	14. Mid Circumflex
7. S.A. Node	15. Left Atrial
8. Left Main	16. Acute Marginal

See: Grossman, chapter on "Coronary Angiography." **Keywords:** RAO view AO root angio. Identify all coronaries

433. **Identify the coronary artery labeled #6 in this aortic root angiogram.**
a. **Obtuse marginal**
b. **AV node**
c. **Acute marginal (RV)**
d. **Conus**
e. **SA node**

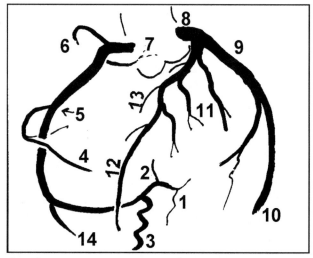

Aortic root - coronary arteries

ANSWER d. Conus. In this LAO view both right and left coronary arteries are shown. The conus is usually the first vessel to arise from the RCA, and in this view travels to the left (anteriorly) over the PA outflow tract (infundibulum). Note that the conus and SA node arteries arise from opposite sides of the RCA. They appear to switch positions depending on whether you're looking at an RAO or LAO view. Test yourself with our coronary anatomy game on our CD & USB interactive programs.

BE ABLE TO MATCH ALL ANSWERS:

1. Posterior Lateral LV	8. Main Left
2. AV Node	9. Circumflex
3. Posterior Descending	10. Obtuse Marginal
4. RV Branch or 1st Acute Marginal	11. Diagonal
5. Mid RCA	12. LAD
6. Conus	13. Septal Perforators
7. SA Node	14. Acute Marginal Branch

This is a normal right dominant system where the PDCA arises from the RCA.

See: Grossman, chapter on "Radiologic technique." **Keywords:** LAO coronary anatomy, PDCA

434. **What coronary artery normally supplies the right bundle conduction branch?**
   a.   RCA
   b.   LAD
   c.   PDCA
   d.   Circumflex

ANSWER b. LAD. The LAD runs in the anterior interventricular groove near the conduction bundles. The left bundle branches may be supplied by either the IV groove branches (PDCA or LAD).
See: Goss, Grays Anatomy, chapter on "CV System" **Keywords:** RBB supplied by LAD

435. **At the crux of the heart the posterior descending coronary artery begins:**
   a.   By following the right interatrial groove
   b.   By following the anterior interventricular groove
   c.   With a 45 degree inferior turn
   d.   Near a "U" turn

ANSWER d. Begins with a "U" turn. Whichever coronary supplies the crux of the heart, it penetrates the heart with a deep "U" shaped turn between the two AV valves. The PDCA then courses down the posterior interventricular sulcus toward the apex and supplies the inferior IV septum. Normally the RCA continues past the crux, onto the posterior lateral surface of the LV and gives off several branches parallel posterior lateral branches. This distinctive "U" turn marks the crux, intersection of AV and IV grooves, and origin of PDCA and AV note arteries.
See: Thomas, Chapter on "AV node artery" **Keywords**: U-turn of PDCA at crux

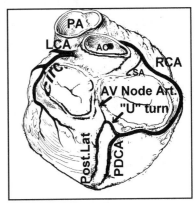

"U" turn of PDCA at crux

436. **With the X-ray detector near the patient's left clavicle as shown in these diagrams, estimate the radiographic position indicated?**
   a.   30° RAO, 60° cranial
   b.   60° RAO, 30° caudal
   c.   30° LAO, 60° cranial
   d.   60° LAO, 30° cranial

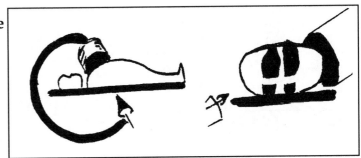

Side view   Inferior view
Identify Image intensifier position

ANSWER d. 60° LAO, 30° cranial. Cranial angulation of an X-ray system tilts the image intensifier (I.I.) toward the head (cranium). However much it is tilted from vertical is the degree of angulation.

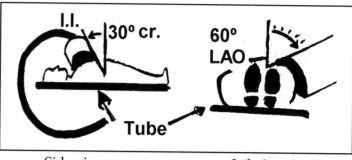

Side view   Inferior view

Oblique views are measured the same way only in the horizontal plane. Vertical - straight above the patient being zero (0° =AP view). Left lateral oblique (LAO) is an oblique angle to the left of the midline (90° = lateral).

See: Grossman, chapter on "Radiologic technique." **Keywords:** cranial angulation, 60 degree LAO

---

437. **The X-ray angulated view labeled #5 on the diagram at the right would result in a left coronary angiogram looking like the angiogram lettered at__ below.**

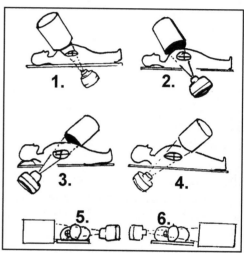

Angulated X-ray positions (different views)

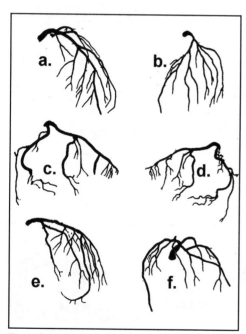

Resulting LCA angiogram

ANSWER d. Left lateral view shows LAD on the left and circumflex on the right. This diagram shows six angulated X-ray views of the LCA.
BE ABLE TO MATCH ALL ANSWERS.

1. RAO CRANIAL = a: Image intensifier (I.I.) positioned on patient's right side and toward his head (cranial). Resulting angiogram shows LAD & apex to your right with the LAD and its branches well shown (Diagonals & Septals). Circumflex is poorly seen behind LAD.

2. LAO CRANIAL = b: I.I. positioned on patient's left side and cranial. The resulting angiogram shows LAD and apex to your left. Fine view of LAD - Circ. bifurcation and diagonal branches between them.

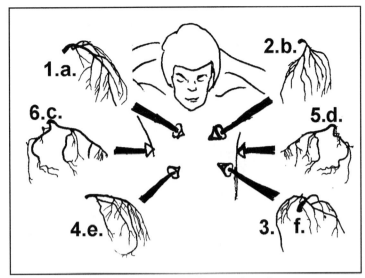
Left coronary angiograms with angulated views

3. LAO CAUDAL = SPIDER VIEW = f: I.I. positioned on patient's left side and caudal. The resulting angiogram shows LAD and apex to your left, circumflex to your right. This is the short axis view of the LV, looking down the LV barrel.

4. RAO CAUDAL = e: I.I positioned on patient's right side and caudal. Distal circumflex artery flows toward you on the bottom. LAD on top. LAD and diagonal branches overlap.

5. LEFT LATERAL = d: I.I. positioned on patient's far left side. Resulting angiogram shows LAD to your left and circ. to your right.

6. RIGHT LATERAL = c: A mirror image of #5 the other lateral. Since it gives no more information than the left lateral the right lateral is seldom shot.

Be able to match all answers above.

See: King, chapter on "angulated views." **Keywords:** ID angulated views LCA

2. Coronary Anatomy: RCA

USE THIS CORONARY ANGIO DIAGRAM FOR BOTH QUESTIONS BELOW.

438. What coronary angiographic view and major coronary artery is shown in this diagram?
   a.   RAO - RCA
   b.   RAO - LCA
   c.   LAO - RCA
   d.   LAO - LCA
   e.   LAO - LAD

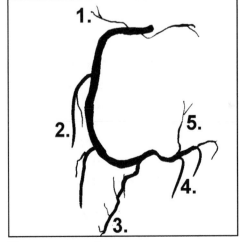
Coronary angiogram

439. What coronary artery branch is labeled at #3 in the box?
- a.   Conus C.A.
- b.   Posterior lateral LV branch
- c.   AV node branch
- d.   RV branch
- e.   PDCA

ANSWERS LISTED CONSECUTIVELY BELOW.

438. ANSWER c. LAO - RCA This is the LAO view of the RCA. The apex of the LV is pointing at you. This must be the RCA (not left CA) because only 1 major vessel is seen. The RCA takes a "C" shape as it travels around the right AV groove.
See: Braunwald, chapter on "Coronary Arteriography." **Keywords:** Cor. View, RAO-RCA

439. ANSWER e. PDCA = Posterior Descending Coronary Artery.
BE ABLE TO MATCH ALL ANSWERS:
       1. Conus C.A. = 1st branch off the main RCA to RV infundibulum.
       2. RV branch = several branches to RV free wall.
       3. PDCA = Posterior Descending Coronary Artery. Supplies the inferior interventricular septum.
       4. Posterior lateral branch to inferior LV.
       5. AV node branch = arises near the crux and supplies the AV node.
See: Braunwald, chapter on "Coronary Arteriography." **Keywords:** RAO-RCA branches, PDCA

BOTH QUESTIONS BELOW REFER TO THIS DIAGRAM.

440. What coronary artery and angiographic view is seen in this coronary angiogram?
- a.   RCA seen in RAO view
- b.   RCA seen in LAO view
- c.   LCA seen in RAO view
- d.   LCA seen in LAO view
- e.   LCA seen in PA view

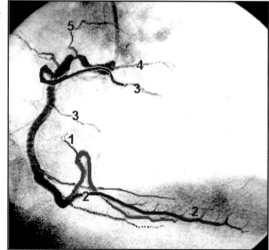

Coronary Arteriogram

441. What branch of the coronary system is labeled at #1 in this coronary angiogram?
- a.   Conus branch
- b.   Acute marginal
- c.   Obtuse marginal
- d.   PDCA branch
- e.   AV node artery

BOTH ANSWERS BELOW:
440. ANSWER a. RCA seen in RAO view. The apex of the LV is pointing down toward the

right (RAO). This must be the RCA (not left CA) because only 1 major vessel is seen. In the RAO view the RCA takes an "L shape as it changes planes from the AV groove to the IV groove. The PDCA travels toward the apex supplying the inferior IV septum. Note the critical stenosis in the proximal RCA just after the SA node artery (#5).
See: Braunwald, chapter on "Coronary Arteriography." **Keywords:** Cor. View, LAO-RCA

441. ANSWER e. AV node artery. In this RAO view of the RCA the posterior lateral branches make a sharp U turn at the crux. From this U turn, the AV node artery is shown coursing up to the AV node. Note how the SA node artery (#5) and the conus artery (#4) lead in opposite directions. The SA heading up to the RA and SA node while the conus heads to the right ventricular outflow track. Be able to match all answers above.
BE ABLE TO MATCH ALL ANSWERS.
    1. AV node
    2. PDCA
    3. RV branch also termed acute marginal
    4. Conus
    5. SA node
See: Braunwald, chapter on "Coronary Arteriography." **Keywords:** RCA, AV node

442. **This coronary arteriogram shows a:**
    a.   **RAO view of a nondominant RCA**
    b.   **LAO view of a dominant RCA**
    c.   **RAO view of a nondominant LCA**
    d.   **LAO view of a dominant LCA**

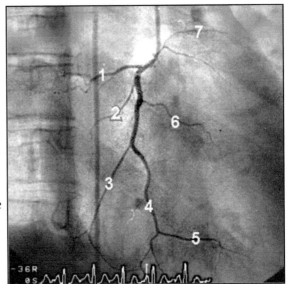

ANSWER a. RAO view of a nondominant RCA. This small RCA does not reach the crux, PDCA or inferior LV wall. It is probable that the LCA has a large dominant circumflex branch. Be able to match all answers below.
  CORRECTLY MATCHED VESSELS ARE:
    1. SA node branch of RCA
    2. RA branch of RCA
    3. RA branch of RCA
    4. Distal RCA
    5. RV branch of RCA
    6. RV branch of RCA
    7. Conus branch of RCA

Coronary arteriogram

See: Braunwald, chapter on "Coronary Arteriography." **Keywords:** ID dominant RCA

443. **Which coronary artery normally supplies the AV node?**
    a.   **Proximal Right**
    b.   **Distal Right**
    c.   **Proximal Circumflex**
    d.   **Distal Circumflex**

ANSWER b. Distal right coronary artery. At or near the crux (where all 4 chambers intersect in the back of the heart) the dominant artery gives rise to the AV node artery which passes upward to the AV node. Since the RCA is usually dominant, it normally gives rise to the AV node artery.

Which artery supplies the **SA node**? Proximal RCA= 54% or Proximal Cx. = 42%.
See: Braunwald, chapter on "Coronary Angiography."
Keywords: RCA, AV node

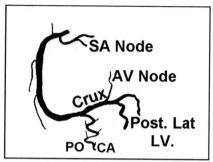
AV Node branch

444. **Occlusion of the mid RCA would normally cause infarction of the LV:**
  a.   **Anterior wall and anterior interventricular septum**
  b.   **Lateral wall**
  c.   **Apex (tip of the heart)**
  d.   **Inferior wall (diaphragmatic surface)**

ANSWER d. Inferior wall (diaphragmatic surface). The RCA normally supplies the RV, inferior IV septum, and posterior & inferior walls of the LV. Since the PDCA will be occluded, the inferior septal perforator arteries will effect the inferior IV septum. Be familiar with all the LV walls as seen on ventriculogram and what vessels supply each.
See: Braunwald, chapter on "Coronary Angiography."
Keywords: RCA, RCA infarction, Inferior wall

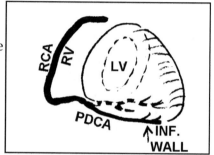
RCA-PDCA Inferior Septum

445. **Which of these coronary occlusions results solely in a RV myocardial infarction?**
  a.   **PDCA occlusion**
  b.   **Diagonal occlusion**
  c.   **Obtuse marginal occlusion**
  d.   **Acute marginal occlusion**

ANSWER d. Acute marginal occlusion. The acute marginal arteries feed the RV. See question on next page. Acute marginals are sometimes simply called "RV branches." RV infarctions may not be as serious as LV infarctions, since only RV hemodynamics are normally affected. However, many RCA infarctions are commonly associated with inferior LV wall infarctions. Note that there are two types of "marginal" arteries - acute and obtuse. Acute marginals always arise from the RCA. These are near the "right acute margin" of the heart - where the RV meets the diaphragm and chest wall. Obtuse marginal arteries arise from the circumflex artery. In each case "marginals" arise from a coronary in the AV ring towards the apex - like the points of a crown (corona).
See: Braunwald, chapter on "Myocardial Infarction." **Keywords:** RCA, RV Infarction, Acute marginal

446. Which small coronary artery frequently originates from a separate ostia within the right sinus of Valsalva?

a.   Conus coronary artery
b.   1st acute marginal coronary artery
c.   SA node coronary artery
d.   Ramus medianus coronary artery

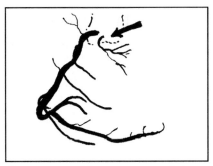

Coronary with separate origin

ANSWER a. Conus coronary artery. The conus is usually the 1st branch off the right coronary. However, in 50% of normal individuals it has its own separate origins off the sinus of Valsalva - next to the right coronary ostia. This makes it difficult to visualize without either a separate aortic root angiogram or dye reflux into the root.

The RCA conus branch normally supplies only the RV outflow tract sometimes called the "infundibulum of the RV." Be cautious and gentle when injecting right coronaries until you are sure your catheter is in the **main RCA** and **NOT the conus artery**.
See: Hurst and Logue, chapter on "Anatomy of the Heart" **Keywords:** RCA, SA Node artery

447. Normally the second branch off the RCA (after the conus branch) is the:

a.   AV node
b.   SA node
c.   Acute marginal
d.   Obtuse marginal

ANSWER b. SA node. The second branch is normally the SA node artery. This artery is directed into the RA and SA node. The SA node artery is outside the "L" of the RCA ring in the RAO view, but within the C of the RCA in the LAO view. The SA node artery usually travels in the opposite direction from the AV node artery, especially in the RAO view.

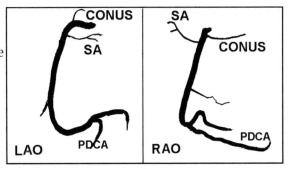

SA Node artery

About ½ the time the SA node artery originates from the circumflex coronary artery on the left side. If the SA node artery arises from the circumflex it must travel over the top of the LA to the SVC and SA node area.
See: Braunwald, chapter on "Coronary Angiography." **Keywords:** RCA, SA node, 2nd branch of RCA

448. **What small branches of the coronary system are shown at label #5 on the diagram?**
   a. **Conus branch**
   b. **Acute marginal**
   c. **PDCA**
   d. **Septal perforator**
   e. **SA node**
   f. **RA branch**

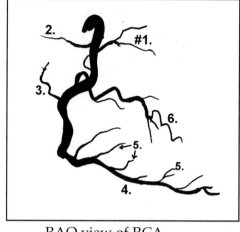

RAO view of RCA

ANSWER. d. Septal perforator. This is the RAO view of the RCA. It is in this view the atrial branches are all up and left-ward, while ventricular branches all course downwards toward the apex. This is an excellent view to distinguish atrial from ventricular branches. In the RAO view everything coming off the right side of the prox RCA goes to the ventricle (conus, RV, acute marginals, & PDCA). Everything arising to the left of the prox RCA goes to the atrium (SA node). Note the easy separation of SA node and conus vessels.

BE ABLE TO MATCH ALL ANSWERS:
   1. Conus (infundibular)
   2. SA node
   3. RA branch
   4. PDCA
   5. Septal perforators
   6. RV, acute marginal

See: Braunwald, chapter on "Coronary Arteriography." **Keywords:** LCA, Conus

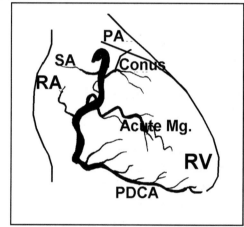

RAO view showing how the RCA separates atria from ventricle

3. Coronary Anatomy: LCA

449. **What is the name of the coronary arteries which normally branch off the circumflex artery toward the apex of the heart?**
   a. **Diagonal branches**
   b. **Obtuse marginal branches**
   c. **Acute marginal branches**
   d. **Posterior descending branches**

ANSWER b. Obtuse marginal branches. Marginal branches all come off AV groove coronary arteries. The left-sided AV groove artery contains the circumflex, and its branches

are termed "obtuse marginal." Whereas, "acute marginal" branches arise from the right coronary near the "acute margin." The acute margin is the sharp angle the RV makes as the chest wall RV folds under and becomes the diaphragmatic RV.
See: Kern, chapter on "Angiography." **Keywords:** Obtuse marginal branches off Circ.

450. **In the aortic root angiogram shown, the vessel labeled at #18 is the:**
  a. **Mid circumflex**
  b. **Distal circumflex**
  c. **1st obtuse marginal**
  d. **2nd obtuse marginal**
  e. **1st acute marginal**
  f. **2nd acute marginal**

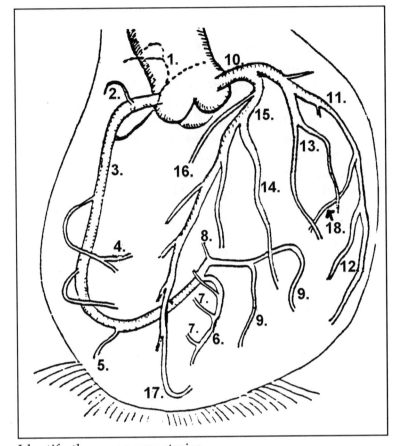

ANSWER b. Distal circumflex in the AV groove. **This is the same view as in our coronary anatomy game.**
BE ABLE TO MATCH ALL ANSWERS:

Identify the coronary arteries

1. S.A. Node	10. Left Main
2. Conus Branch	11. Mid Circumflex
3. Right Coronary	12. 2nd Obtuse Marginal
4. RV Branches	13. 1st Obtuse Marginal
5. Acute Marginal	14. Diagonal (1st)
6. Posterior Descending	15. Left Anterior Descending (LAD)
7. Inferior Septal	16. Anterior Septal (1st)
8. AV Node Branch	17. Distal LAD
9. Posterior Lateral	18. Distal Circumflex

See: Grossman, chapter on "Coronary Angiography." also Malincrodt handout
Keywords: LAO view AO root angio. Identify all coronaries

451. **The dotted line in the drawing shows a:**
- a. **IMA graft to LAD**
- b. **IMA skip graft to circumflex and LAD**
- c. **CABG skip graft to circumflex and LAD**
- d. **CABG skip graft to diagonal and LAD**

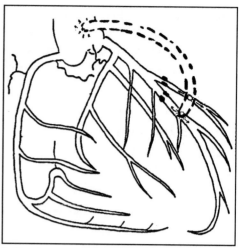

ANSWER d. CABG skip graft to diagonal and LAD. This is a standard RAO view of both coronary arteries. The dotted line is an saphenous vein bypass graft from the aorta to the diagonal branch of the LAD. Then it "skips" over to the LAD and supplies it also. This is the type of drawing made following bypass surgery to document the location of grafts.

See: Braunwald, chapter on "Coronary Arteriography." ? Graft ➜ to coronary

Keywords: CABG to Diag. & LAD

452. **Identify the coronary vessel labeled #5 in this "spider" angiographic view.**
- a. **Ramus medianus**
- b. **Obtuse marginal**
- c. **Left main**
- d. **Circumflex**
- e. **Diagonal**
- f. **Distal LAD**
- g. **LAD**

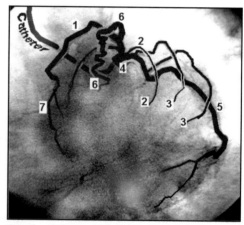

Spider View of LCA

ANSWER d. The circumflex comes off the left main coronary in the left AV groove.

   This "spider" or LAO caudal view (the view from down under) is like looking at a spider from below. The arteries radiating from the left main are: the LAD down and to the left, diagonal up to the left and circumflex to the right.

BE ABLE TO MATCH ALL ANSWERS.
   1. LAD
   2. Ramus medianus
   3. Obtuse marginal
   4. Left main
   5. Circumflex
   6. Diagonal
   7. Distal LAD

See: Grossman, chapter on "Coronary Angiography." also Malincrodt handout
Keywords: Spider view coronaries

BOTH QUESTIONS BELOW REFER TO THIS DIAGRAM.

453. What coronary arteriography view is shown in this diagram?
   a.   Steep RAO, no cranial
   b.   RAO caudal
   c.   RAO cranial
   d.   LAO cranial
   e.   LAO caudal

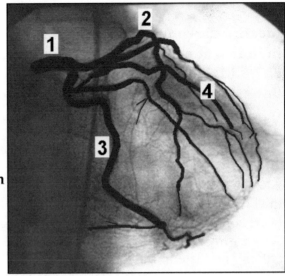

454. The coronary artery shown on the diagram at #3 is a:
   a.   Proximal circumflex
   b.   Distal LAD
   c.   PDCA
   d.   RCA
   e.   Obtuse marginal

Coronary arteriogram

BOTH ANSWERS LISTED TOGETHER BELOW.
453. ANSWER b. RAO caudal. The apex is tilted up and to the right as if looking at the heart from below. The aortic catheter is seen rising near the backbone, near #3. Remember "the circumflex is nearest the backbone." The circumflex coronary is large and shows well because it is perpendicular to the X-ray beam. At least one obtuse marginal can be seen arising from the circ. The caudal views are best for the circumflex because the LAD is moved up out of the way.
See: Braunwald, chapter on "Coronary Arteriography."

454. ANSWER a. Proximal circumflex. This large circumflex branch moves around the back of the heart and supplies the LV posterior lateral wall.
   BE ABLE TO MATCH ALL ANSWERS:
       1. Main LCA
       2. LAD
       3. Circumflex
       4. Obtuse marginal
See: Braunwald, chapter on "Coronary Arteriography."

455. RAO caudal angulation helps prevent overlapping coronary segments and improves imaging of the:
   a.   LAD and its septal branches
   b.   LAD and its diagonal branches
   c.   PDCA and its septal branches
   d.   Circumflex and its marginal branches

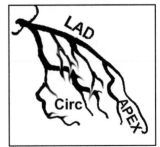

RAO view of LAD

ANSWER d. Circumflex and its marginal branches. In the diagram , note how the circumflex is below and behind the LAD and its branches. Caudal angulation lets you look under those LAD branches to uncover the circumflex and its branches. **See:** Braunwald, chapter on "Coronary Arteriography."

456. **Identify the coronary artery shown indicated at #1 on the coronary angiogram.**
a.   **Main LCA**
b.   **Obtuse marginal**
c.   **Circumflex**
d.   **Diagonal**
e.   **LAD**

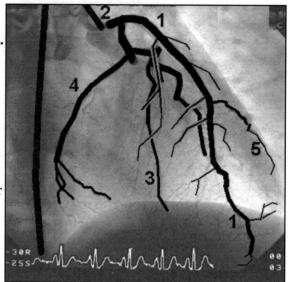
Coronary Angiogram

ANSWER e. LAD. In this RAO caudal view of the LCA, the LAD is oriented along the anterior heart border. Small diagonal branches can be seen arising from the LAD (#5) and feed the anterior and lateral wall of the LV. Septal perforators can be seen (not labeled) beneath the LAD. The circumflex artery arises from the main coronary artery (#2) and travels in the AV groove around the back of the heart (#4). This is a large dominant circumflex artery with a large obtuse marginal branch (#3). Note how the circumflex is covered by the LAD. Caudal angulation would help uncover the circumflex.

BE ABLE TO MATCH ALL ANSWERS:
    1. LAD
    2. Main-stem LCA
    3. Obtuse marginal branch of Cx.
    4. AV groove branch of Cx.
    5. Diagonal branch of LAD
See: Grossman, chapter on "Coronary Arteriography."

457. **The coronary artery shown on the diagram at #3 is a:**
a.   **Circumflex**
b.   **LAD**
c.   **SA Node**
d.   **Diagonal**
e.   **Catheter**

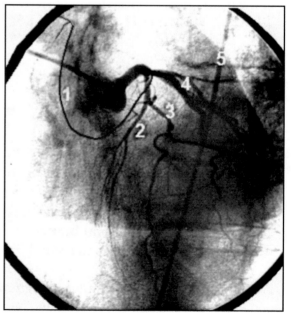
Coronary arteriogram

ANSWER d. Diagonal. This is a shallow LAO cranial view of the left coronary system. The main LCA branches into the LAD (#2) and circumflex (nearest backbone #4). The LAD give off a large diagonal branch on the anterior wall of the LV. The long SA node artery (#1 highlighted) arises from the proximal circumflex artery. It comes off the circumflex, like this, about 45% of the time. However, most of the

time it arises from the RCA.
BE ABLE TO MATCH ALL ANSWERS:
     1. SA Node
     2. LAD
     3. Diagonal
     4. Circumflex
     5. Catheter
See: Braunwald, chapter on "Coronary Arteriography."

458. **Identify the coronary artery labeled #1 on the coronary angiogram.**
   a.   **1st diagonal**
   b.   **LAD**
   c.   **1st septal**
   d.   **Obtuse marginal**

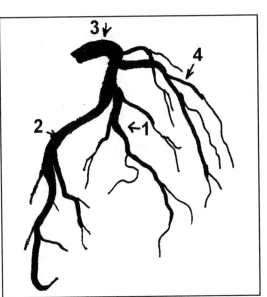

ANSWER a. 1st diagonal. This is an LAO view, because the LV apex is pointing to our left. It is an LCA in configuration. The large diagonal branch is seen between the LAD and circumflex. There are usually 2-4 diagonals all arising from the LAD and supplying the anterior lateral free wall of the LV.
BE ABLE TO MATCH ALL ANSWERS:
     1. Diagonal
     2. LAD
     3. Main-stem LCA
     4. Circumflex

Coronary Angiogram

See: Braunwald, chapter on "Coronary arteriography."

459. **What two types of arteries normally branch from the LAD coronary artery?**
     1. Septals
     2. Marginals
     3. SA Node
     4. Diagonals
        a. 1,2
        b. 1,4
        c. 2,3
        d. 2,4

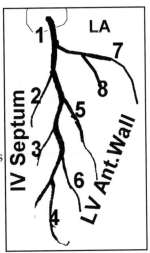

ANSWER b. Septals & diagonals. The LAO view nicely separates the septal and diagonal branches of the LAD. As you look at the LAO (cranial may help) the septals can be seen branching leftward down into the IV septum. The two large diagonal arteries branch down onto the anterior lateral wall of the LV. **BE ABLE TO CORRECTLY MATCH ALL ANSWERS BELOW:**
     1. Main-stem LCA

LAO cranial angio - LCA

2. 1st Septal Perforator
3. 2nd Septal Perforator
4. LAD - Distal
5. 1st Diagonal Branch
6. 2nd Diagonal Branch
7. Circumflex (in AV groove)
8. Obtuse Marginal Branch of Circumflex

Be able to match all answers above. **See:** Braunwald, chapter on "Coronary Arteriography."

460. **What coronary artery normally supplies the anterior aspect of the interventricular septum?**
   a.   **LAD**
   b.   **Circumflex**
   c.   **PDCA**
   d.   **Obtuse marginal**
   e.   **Acute marginal**

ANSWER a. The LAD runs down the anterior interventricular groove, and sends down septal perforators which normally supply the anterior 2/3 of the IV septum. The LAD sends down septal perforators at right angles. The RCA supplies the inferior 1/3 of the IV septum. The diagram shows the 4 anatomical grooves in the heart where the main epicardial coronary vessels run.

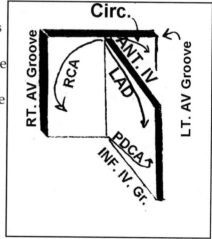

   1. Anterior IV groove (LAD)
   2. Inferior IV groove (PDCA)
   3. Right AV groove (RCA)
   4. Left AV groove (Circumflex)

See: Braunwald, chapter on "Coronary Arteriography."

461. **The "widow-maker" lesion is a stenosis in the _____ AV & IV GROOVES coronary artery.**
   a.   **LAD**
   b.   **Diagonal**
   c.   **Circumflex**
   d.   **Main stem left**
   e.   **Main right coronary**

ANSWER d. Main stem left. This is the most serious coronary lesion since this main vessel feeds the LAD (usually the largest coronary artery) and the circumflex. Widow-maker lesions of 50% or more are especially critical and usually require IABP insertion and immediate CABG surgery. **I have also heard some Drs. call the LAD a widowmaker.**

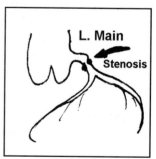

Widow-maker

See: Braunwald, chapter on "Coronary Arteriography."

462. The coronary artery shown on the diagram at #6 is a:

a.   Proximal circumflex
b.   Distal LAD
c.   PDCA
d.   RCA
e.   Obtuse marginal

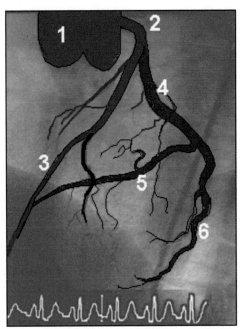

ANSWER e. Obtuse marginal branch of circumflex. This is an LAO view of the left coronary system. The main circumflex (#4) divides, sending off a large obtuse marginals branch (#6) to the lateral LV and the distal circumflex in the AV groove (#5). Note how the distal circumflex is covered by the LAD. Caudal angulation would help uncover the circumflex.
BE ABLE TO MATCH ALL ANSWERS:

1. Aortic root
2. Main left coronary
3. LAD
4. Proximal circumflex
5. Distal circumflex - in AV groove

30° LAO cr. Coronary arteriogram

See: Braunwald, chapter on "Coronary Arteriography."

463. Which coronary artery normally supplies the apex of the LV?

a.   RAD
b.   LAD
c.   PDCA
d.   Circumflex

ANSWER b. The LAD or its diagonal branches usually supply the apex. They are is especially well seen in the RAO view where the LAD runs across the top of the heart silhouette to the apex. The LAD is the largest of the 3 coronary arteries. (There is no "RAD" artery.) When they overlap, identifying the artery at the apex helps distinguish LAD from circumflex arteries.
See: Braunwald, chapter on "Coronary Arteriography."

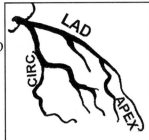

LAD to LV APEX

464. Which coronary artery normally supplies the anterior lateral wall of the LV?

a.   Diagonal branches of LAD
b.   LV branches of RCA
c.   Obtuse marginal
d.   Acute marginal

ANSWER a. Diagonal branches of LAD. The LAD runs in the anterior lateral wall of the LV.

In the 30 degree RAO view the wall segments are:
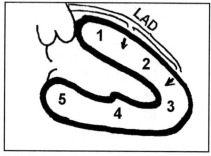

30° RAO - LV gram

1. Anterior basal
2. Anterior lateral
3. Apical
4. Diaphragmatic (inferior)
5. Posterior basal

Normally the "anterior" walls and "apex" are supplied by the LAD and diagonal branches. The "diaphragmatic" is supplied by the PDCA branch of the RCA. The "posterior basal" is composed mainly the mitral valve apparatus. The only 2 walls not shown are: the septal wall (in front in this view), and posterior-lateral wall (on the back side in this view). These two walls must be viewed in the orthogonal or RAO view.
See: Braunwald, chapter on "Coronary Arteriography."

465. **A trifurcation branch of the main left coronary artery that arises between the LAD and circumflex is called the:**
    a.   **Septal perforator**
    b.   **Acute marginal**
    c.   **Conus branch**
    d.   **Ramus medianus**

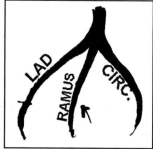

Ramus Medianus

ANSWER d. Ramus medianus. In 37% of the patients the LCA has a trifurcation instead of a bifurcation. In these cases a "ramus medianus" arises between the LAD and the circumflex arteries. The ramus is often called the "intermediate artery" since it is the middle.
See: Braunwald, chapter on "Coronary Arteriography."

4. Coronary Physiology and Flows

466. **Left coronary blood flow occurs primarily during the _____ phase of the cardiac cycle because _____.**
    a.   **Systolic, coronary driving pressure is greatest**
    b.   **Systolic, systolic ejection opens the aortic valve**
    c.   **Diastolic, semilunar valves cover the coronary ostia in systole**
    d.   **Diastolic, diastole releases compressed endocardial capillaries**

ANSWER d. Diastolic, in diastole the ventricle relaxes and releases the compressed endocardial capillaries. Most flow occurs in diastole due to the compression of LV capillaries in systole. This is why the IABP is so effective at augmenting diastolic coronary flow. Although the left coronary capillaries obstruct flow during systole, the low pressure RV capillaries are less occluded because of the lower RV pressure. A common misconception is that the open aortic leaflets occlude the coronary ostia and inhibit flow. They do not.
See: Berne and Levy, chapter on "Coronary Artery Physiology."

467. **Which coronary artery normally has steadiest flow even throughout systole?**
  a.   LAD
  b.   Circumflex
  c.   RCA
  d.   LCA

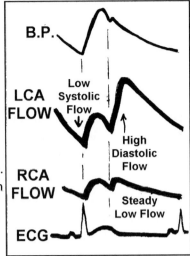

Right and left coronary flows

ANSWER c. RCA. In both right and left coronary arteries the limit on coronary flow is the coronary resistance. The LV compresses the sub-endocardial capillaries in systole - the RV not so much. Since the right coronary supplies the lower pressure chambers (RV) it has less dramatic resistance change.

 This compression makes it hard to force blood through LV capillaries in systole. As a result, **the left coronary has almost no flow during systole**. This is because of extreme LV capillary compression during the systolic phase.
See: Berne and Levy, chapter on "Coronary Circulation."

468. **Considering the branching anatomy of coronary arterial perforators which area of the heart is most susceptible to heart attack and injury?**
  a.   Pericardial
  b.   Epicardial
  c.   Sub-endocardium
  d.   SA node
  e.   AV node

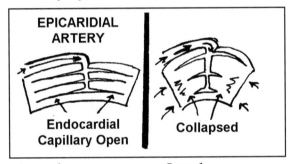

Diastole   Systole

ANSWER c. Sub-endocardium. During systole the sub-endocardial arteries collapse due to increased wall tension and compression there. This makes the sub-endocardium more susceptible to ischemia.

 The branching patterns of coronary arteries penetrate from "epi" to "endo"-cardium. An occlusion anywhere in this branch is potentially most damaging to the inner sub-endocardium because:
  •It is the furthest downstream
  •It receives less blood because of sub-endocardial compression
  •Its branches fan out to supply a large area of sub-endocardial wall
These are called sub-endocardial infarctions. Sub-endocardial infarction do NOT usually cause Q waves. They are not usually as serious as the transmural infarctions, because all heart layers are not involved. **See:** Grossman, chapter on "Coronary Arteriography."

469. When lactic acid or lactate is found in excessive amounts in the coronary sinus, it is an indication for:
   a. Coronary ischemia
   b. RV infarction
   c. Excessive preload
   d. Excessive afterload

ANSWER a. Coronary ischemia. Lactate is a byproduct of anaerobic metabolism indicating lack of O_2 availability or ischemia. A similar process occurs in extreme exercise of skeletal muscle where lactate builds up causing muscle pain. Normal aerobic coronary metabolic by-products are CO_2 and water. **See:** Berne and Levy, chapter on "Coronary Arteries."

470. The lowest blood oxygen saturation normally found in the heart is in the:
   a. Coronary sinus
   b. Pulmonary artery
   c. Inferior vena cava
   d. Superior vena cava

ANSWER a. Coronary sinus. Normal coronary sinus O2 saturation is 30% - 40%. This is compared to 60% - 80% in the rest of the body's veins. CS blood is the blackest blood anywhere in the body. The heart extracts more O_2 from each cc of blood than any other organ. There is virtually **no coronary extraction reserve.**

   The CS is one reason why RA blood is so poorly mixed. Depending on where you draw a sample, you could get saturations from 30% to 80%. And this causes uneven mixing of venous blood. Considerable streaming occurs in the Rt. Ht. the PA is the only right heart chamber where the blood is "well mixed." That is why mixed venous blood samples are usually taken from the PA. **See:** Braunwald, chapter on "Coronary Physiology."

471. Resting coronary sinus O2 saturation is normally around:
   a. 10%
   b. 40%
   c. 70%
   d. 95%

ANSWER b. 40% O2 sat. The heart extracts almost all the O2 from the coronary blood. This is why the coronary O2 saturation is so low, around 40%. This blood is so black that there is no oxygen reserve in it. It can't go much lower. Compare this with the normal 70% O2 sat in the PA.

   This means that to increase cardiac work (MVO_2), coronary flow must increase in direct proportion to the heart's workload. When the heart needs to increase its blood supply, any significant stenosis will cause myocardial ischemia.
See: Braunwald, chapter on "Coronary Physiology."

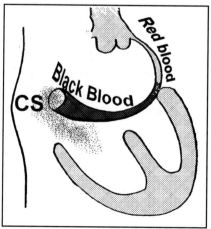

HIGH coronary O2 extraction

5. Other Coronary

472. The _____ returns deoxygenated blood from the myocardium to the ___ .
   a.   Azygous vein, RA
   b.   Azygous vein, LA
   c.   Coronary sinus, RA
   d.   Coronary sinus, LA

ANSWER c. Coronary sinus, RA. The CS drains the coronary veins, runs between the LA and LV in the AV groove, and enters the lower RA near the IVC entrance. It can be entered with a catheter for pacing or electrophysiology sensing. Small amounts of coronary venous blood may drain into other chambers via the small Thebesian veins.
See: Underhill, chapter on "Cardiac Anatomy"

473. A major coronary artery which passes beneath a segment of contracting myocardium may be obstructed during systole. This is termed a:
   a.   Myocardial bridge
   b.   Myocardial tunnel
   c.   Coronary spasm
   d.   Epicardial coronary

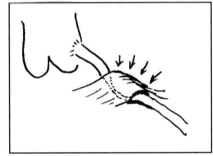
What is this?

ANSWER a. A myocardial bridge is contracting myocardium that encircles a coronary artery. It may pinch the artery, and obstruct it during systole. Then it may relax and open up in ventricular diastole. Significant myocardial bridges cause angina, especially during tachycardia - when diastolic coronary flow is limited. Surgery may relieve the problem.
See: Grossman, chapter on "Coronary Arteriography."

474. Where is this Amplatz catheter tip directed?
   a.   RCA
   b.   LAD
   c.   Circumflex
   d.   CABG bypass graft

ANSWER d. CABG bypass graft. Sternal wire loops are on the right. Three circular graft markers are clearly seen on the left. The Amplatz catheter is in the aorta and pointed directly into one of the graft origins. The PCI balloon is seen in the lower right corner. **See:** Grossman, chapter on "Coronary Arteriography."

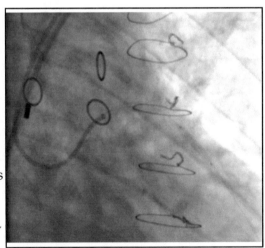
Amplatz catheter in bypass graft

Dominance

BOTH QUESTIONS BELOW USE THIS DIAGRAM.

475. This coronary angiogram demonstrates that this patient has a dominant_____ with the _____ arising from the circumflex artery.
   a.   RCA, PDCA
   b.   RCA, RCA
   c.   LCA, PDCA
   d.   LCA, RCA

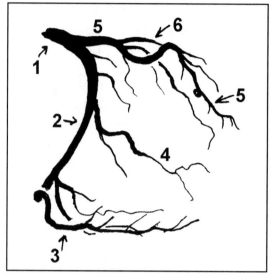

Coronary Angiogram

476. In this coronary arteriogram identify the branch labeled #6?
   a.   Obtuse marginal
   b.   LAD
   c.   Diagonal
   d.   Main-stem LCA
   e.   Circumflex in AV groove
   f.   PDCA, arising from Cx.

BOTH ANSWERS ARE TOGETHER BELOW.

475. ANSWER c. LCA, PDCA. This is a huge left coronary artery shown in the RAO view. In a dominant LCA like this, the LCA supplies all of the LV coronary supply. The RCA is small and does NOT supply the inferior septum. The dominant LCA does that here. This places great importance on the left coronary system. A main-stem LCA infarction would be fatal. Fewer than 20% of patients have this dominate LCA system. The branch which indicates dominance is #3 the PDCA branch in the inferior interventricular groove. If the PDCA arises from the RCA it is called right dominance, if from the LCA it is called left dominance. **See:** Grossman, chapter on "Coronary Arteriography."

476. ANSWER c. Diagonal coronary artery. Dominant LCA system shown in the RAO view.
BE ABLE TO MATCH ALL ANSWERS:
   1. Main-stem LCA
   2. Circumflex in AV groove
   3. PDCA, arising from Cx.
   4. Obtuse marginal
   5. LAD
   6. Diagonal
See: Grossman, chapter on "Coronary Arteriography."

477. **This RAO view coronary angiogram suggests what type of "coronary dominance"?**
   a.   RCA dominance
   b.   LCA dominance
   c.   LAD dominance
   d.   Balanced dominance

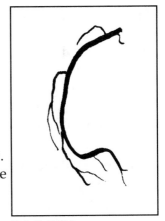
RAO-RCA

ANSWER b. LCA dominance. The RCA is shown in the RAO view. No PDCA branch is seen. The RCA is small and does not supply the inferior IV septum. The LCA angiogram should show a large Circumflex branch leading to a PDCA. This is an uncommon "left dominant" coronary system. Note that "dominant" does not necessarily mean that artery is "largest" - just that it supplies the inferior IV septum. Often dominant RCA's are not especially large.
See: Grossman, chapter on "Coronary Arteriography." Also, see previous question.

478. **In this LAO view of the aortic valve and arch, identify the structure labeled #3.**
   a.   Non-coronary cusp
   b.   Left coronary artery
   c.   Left sinus of Valsalva
   d.   Ascending aorta
   e.   Right sinus of Valsalva
   f.   Right coronary artery

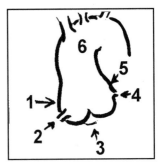
Aortic Root

ANSWER a. Non-coronary cusp.   The posterior or non-coronary aortic cusp. The RCA originates from the right sinus of Valsalva and the left main coronary from the left sinus of Valsalva. **BE ABLE TO MATCH ALL ANSWERS:**

1. Right sinus of Valsalva	2. Right coronary artery
3. Non-coronary cusp	4. Left coronary artery
5. Left sinus of Valsalva	6. Ascending aorta

See: Gray's Anatomy chapter on "Heart."

479. **The right or left coronary system is called dominant, depending on which one supplies the heart's:**
   1. Anterior IV septum
   2. Posterior IV septum
   3. RV lateral wall
   4. LV Lateral wall
   5. Diaphragmatic LV wall
        a. 1,4
        b. 2,4
        c. 2,5
        d. 3,5

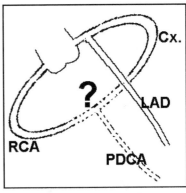
Coronary artery Dominance

ANSWER c. Posterior IV septum & diaphragmatic LV wall. The entire diaphragmatic (inferior) heart is supplied by the dominant coronary vessel. (Usually the RCA). Other landmarks indicating which artery is dominant are:

      1. Identify the artery that supplies the "crux" (where all 4 heart chambers meet at the back of heart).

      2. Identify the artery that supplies the PDCA and AV node arteries.

See: Braunwald, chapter on "Coronary Arteriography."

480. **What percentage of the population has a right dominant coronary circulation?**
- a.   **80%-90%**
- b.   **50%-70%**
- c.   **20%-40%**
- d.   **10%-30%**

ANSWER a. 80%-90%. Most hearts have a right dominant coronary supply (77-90%). The remainder are either left dominant or balanced. Remember that right dominance means the RCA supplies the crux, PDCA, and inferior IV septum.

See: Braunwald, chapter on "Coronary Arteriography."

481. **In this anterior view of the heart what structure connects the LAD and acute marginal arteries?**
- a.   **AV anastomosis**
- b.   **CAB graft**
- c.   **Collateral**
- d.   **Great coronary vein**
- e.   **Myocardial bridge**

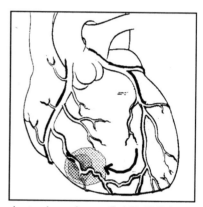

Anterior view - LAD-RCA collateral

ANSWER c. Collateral circulation often develops to feed an ischemic area of the heart. Blood flow then proceeds across the collateral "bridge" and retrograde up the blocked vessel to the ischemic area. For example this patient may have a partially occluded acute marginal RCA for which the LAD grew collateral vessels, to provide additional blood supply.

    Epicardial collaterals like this are unusual. Most collateral supplies are tiny capillary networks often invisible on angiography. These small collaterals develop over an extended period in response to ischemia.

See: Medical Dictionary **Keywords:** Collateral

482. **Which below is most likely to potentiate coronary vasoconstriction in CAD patients?**
- a.   **IV adenosine**
- b.   **IV nitric oxide (NO)**
- c.   **IV magnesium (MG^{++})**
- d.   **Ice applied to skin**
- e.   **Hypoventilation**

ANSWER d. Ice applied to skin. In CAD patients ice packs on the skin may cause a "COLD PRESSOR" response. They may occasionally be applied as a cold pressor test to potentiate spasm via the sympathetic nervous system. It increases the coronary resistance and coronary O2 extraction. For this reason Darovic says to keep CAD patients warm, and avoid cold temperatures. A cold pressor coronary response is apparently rare in normal people.

Actions of listed coronary dilators and pressors are:
1.   IV adenosine: Coronary vasodilator drug - now used as antiarrhythmic drug
2.   Nitric oxide (NO): Normally occurring local coronary vasodilator is also termed ERF- (endothelial relaxation factor)
3.   Magnesium (MG++): Coronary vasodilator - now used in code 55
4.   Ice applied to skin: May potentiate coronary spasm
5.   Hypoventilation: May enhance O2 carrying - HYPERventilation may potentiate spasm

See: Darovic, chapter on "CV Anatomy and Physiology."

483. **Your patient is right coronary dominant. Which of the following LV segments would MOST likely be affected by a significant distal RCA stenosis past the crux?**
a.   **Apex**
b.   **Inferior LV wall**
c.   **Anterior LV wall**
d.   **Posterior-lateral LV wall**

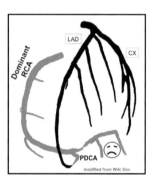

ANSWER: d. Posterior-lateral LV wall. The posterior-lateral branches of the RCA arise past the crux and supply the posterior-lateral wall of the LV. The distal circumflex artery may also supply that general area depending on the patient's coronary distribution. If the stenosis had been in the PDCA(which arises at the crux) then the inferior wall would be effected.

REFERENCES:

Baim, D. S. and Grossman W., Cardiac Catheterization, Angiography, and Intervention, 7th Ed., Lea and Febiger, 2006
Braunwald, Eugene, et al., Ed., HEART DISEASE A Textbook of Cardiovascular Medicine, 9th Ed., W. B. Saunders Co., 2012
Underhill, S. L., Ed., *CARDIAC NURSING*, 2nd Ed., J. B. Lippincott Co., 1989
Hurst, J. W., and Logue, R. B., et. al., *THE HEART Arteries and Veins*, 3rd Ed., McGraw-Hill Book Co., 1974
Kern, M. J., Ed., *The Cardiac Catheterization Handbook*, 4th Ed., Mosby-Year Book, Inc., 2016
King, S.B. III and Yeung, Alan, *Interventional Cardiology*, McGraw-Hill, 2007
Berne, R. M. and Levy, M. N., *Cardiovascular Physiology*, 8th Ed., Mosby Year Book, 2001
Darovic, G.O., *Hemodynamic Monitoring: Invasive and Noninvasive Clinical Applications*, 2nd Edition, W.B. Saunders Co., 1995
Thomas, N.J., *Anatomy of the Coronary Arteries*, Paul B. Hoeber, Inc. publisher, 1961
http://askdrwiki.com/mediawiki/index.php?title=Coronary_Angiography

OUTLINE: B4 - Coronary Anatomy and Physiology

1. CORONARY ANATOMY
   a. Surface Anatomy
      i. Rt. AV groove (RCA)
      ii. Left AV groove (Circ.)
      iii. Anterior IV groove (LAD)
      iv. Inferior IV groove (PDCA)
      v. Acute margin
      vi. Base, Atria, venous return
      vii. Apex, base
      viii. Ventricles
      ix. Great - Outflow vessels
      x. LV & RV free walls
      xi. Infundibulum RV
      xii. Coronary Sinus/veins
      xiii. Pericardial attachments
      xiv. Crux
      xv. Thebesian
      xvi. Arterio-Sinusoid vessels
      xvii. arterio-luminal vessels

   b. VIEWS
      i. RAO
         (1) Supplies what myocardium?
            (a) RV, inferior septum, Inferior LV, Posterior lateral LV
         (2) LCA = Backbone - Circ. - LAD
         (3) RCA = "L" shape
      ii. LAO
         (1) Supplies what myocardium?
            (a) Ant. LV, Lateral LV, Ant. IV Septum
         (2) LCA = LAD - Circ. - Backbone
         (3) RCA = "C" shape
         (4) Left Main angle = 20°
      iii. RAO Cranial
         (1) Mid & distal LAD
         (2) Origins LAD septals & Diagonal
      iv. RAO Caudal
         (1) L. main bifurcation
         (2) Prox. LAD
         (3) Prox-mid Cx.
         (4) View of choice for unstable angina pts.
      v. LAO Cranial
         (1) Intermedius
         (2) lst diagonal
         (3) Prox LAD
      vi. LAO Caudal
         (1) "Spider view"

         (2) main (esp. horiz.ht.)
         (3) LAD
         (4) prox Cx.
      vii. PA View
         (1) L main os.
      viii. LATERAL
         (1) Prox. Cx.
         (2) Prox & dist. LAD (esp. with cranial)
         (3) Mid RCA
      ix. RAO cine =LPO cut film view
      x. RPO cine =LAO cut film view

2. CORONARY ANATOMY - RCA
   a. Conus
      i. may have separate origin
   b. SA node
      i. usually 2nd vessel to take-off RCA
   c. RV Branches
   d. Acute Marginal branches
   e. Rt. Atrial
   f. AV node
   g. PDA
      i. Inf. Septal perforators
   h. Posterior Lateral (LV

3. CORONARY ANATOMY - LCA
   a. Main Left = Widowmaker
      i. Widowmaker MI = 90% mortality
   b. Medianus (Ramus)
   c. LAD
      i. Diagonals
      ii. Ant. Septal perforators
   d. Circumflex (nearest Backbone)
      i. Obtuse marginal
      ii. LA branches
      iii. AV node branch (if not off RCA)
      iv. PDCA (if not off RCA)

4. CORONARY PHYSIOLOGY - FLOWS
   a. Diastolic flow predominates
      i. RCA has more steady flow
      ii. Perfusion pressure
      iii. Endocardial vascular compression
         (1) Subendocardial MI & ischemia more common
   b. Neurological factors
      i. alpha, beta receptors
   c. Hormonal factors
      i. metabolic (O2 demand)
      ii. Lactic Acid in CS = ischemia
   d. Cardiac Work - VO_2

i. Coronary Sinus = lowest O2 sat (40%)
e. O2 Extraction
    i. Coronary Sinus extracts 12-14 vol% O2 (leaves 30-50% O2 sat. in CS)
f. Cardiac Efficiency
g. Substrate utilization
    i. aerobic metabolism

5. OTHER CORONARY
   a. CORONARY ARTERIOGRAMS
       i. Orifice adequacy
       ii. Lesions
           (1) eccentric plaque
       iii. concentric plaque
           (1) % area and diameter reduction
           (2) Widowmaker
       iv. Associated Ventricular function
           (1) RAO view LV identify:
               (a) Ant, Apical, Inf., Post. Lat.
           (2) LAO view LV identify
               (a) Lateral, Septal walls
       v. Washout
       vi. Missing branches (occlusions)
       vii. Bypass grafts
           (1) IMA, Skip, Y

viii. Collateral
ix. Congenital malformations
x. Coronary Fistulas

b. PITFALLS IN CORONARY ANGIOGRAMS
    i. Absent L. main
    ii. Total occlusion
    iii. Myocardial bridges
    iv. Aneurysms/ectatic/enlargement
    v. Foreshortening/overlapping
    vi. Spasm
    vii. Inadequate number of projections
    viii. Pulsatile injection
    ix. Superselective injection

c. Coronary DOMINANCE.
    i. Right Dominance
        (1) 80-90% have = most common
    ii. Left Dominance
        (1) Less than 20% have (rare)
    iii. Determine which coronary supplies the:
        (1) Crux
        (2) PDA
        (3) Inferior septum

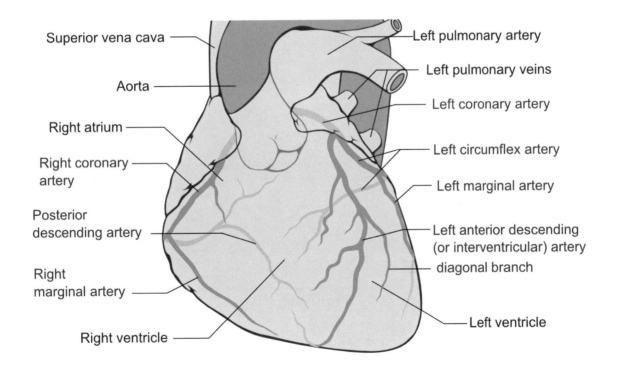

Superior vena cava — Left pulmonary artery — Aorta — Left pulmonary veins — Right atrium — Left coronary artery — Right coronary artery — Left circumflex artery — Posterior descending artery — Left marginal artery — Right marginal artery — Left anterior descending (or interventricular) artery — diagonal branch — Right ventricle — Left ventricle

AUTONOMIC CNS and ECG Basics

INDEX: B5 - Autonomic CNS and ECG Basics

1. General Autonomic

484. What area of the brain regulates heart rate and peripheral vascular resistance?

    a.   Pneumotaxic center in the hypothalamus
    b.   Reticular system in the cerebral cortex
    c.   Nucleus tractus solitarius area in the medulla
    d.   Vasomotor center in the cerebellum

ANSWER c. Nucleus Tractus Solitarius (NTS) area is a primitive regulatory center in the medulla oblongata at the base of the brain. The medullary regulatory center receives input from the pressor-receptors, chemoreceptors and other afferent nerves. After processing this information, the medulla sends efferent impulses out the sympathetic and parasympathetic nerves to regulate the heart rate, contractility, and vasomotor tone, etc. **See:** Berne & Levy, chapter on "Regulation of the Heartbeat." **Keywords:** Medulla (NTS) controls vasomotion

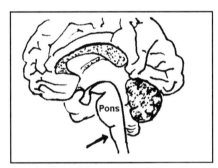

Medulla Oblongata

485. The anatomy of the two autonomic nervous systems differ. The sympathetic system originates mostly from the _____ , and the parasympathetic (vagal) system originates from _____.

    a.   L1-L8,   Sacral 1-2
    b.   Sacral 1-2,   L1-L8
    c.   T1-T12,   10th cranial
    d.   10th cranial,   T1-T12

ANSWER c. T1-T12, 10th cranial. The sympathetic system originates from the thoracic spinal nerves at T1-T12. They lead to a ganglionic chain near the spine where the first sympathetic synapse occurs. The post-ganglionic nerves then carry the signal to the heart (or other visceral organs) and terminate near sympathetic receptor sites (alpha or beta). They liberate norepinephrine (NE) which is the actual chemical mediator. Sympathetic nerves generally speed the SA node, AV node, and myocardial muscle.

The parasympathetic system originates in the medulla at the base of the brain. The parasympathetic nerves that effect the heart exit the medulla in the 10th cranial nerve termed the "vagus." These nerves follow the neck and esophagus to the heart. There they synapse within a ganglion and terminate at the parasympathetic receptors (cholinergic) within the heart. They liberate acetylcholine (ACh) which is the chemical mediator. Parasympathetic tone slows the SA node, AV node, and depresses myocardial muscle. Part of the parasympathetic system also originates from the lumbo-sacral region to innervate the viscera.

Remember all 12 thoracic vertebra are "sympathetic" - to each other. The parasympathetic (vagal) is a short word - has only 1 vagal nerve from brain stem.
See: Tortora, chapter on "Autonomic CNS." **Keywords:** Sympathetic neurotransmitters, Norepinephrine

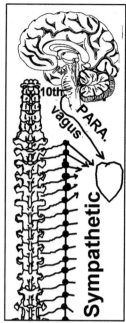

Autonomic nerves: Sympathetic & Parasympathetic

486. **Sympathomimetic medications work by stimulating specific receptor sites. Match these adrenergic receptor sites with where they are located?**
I. Alpha 1 _____
II. Beta 1 _____
III. Beta 2 _____
     a. Vascular smooth muscle
     b. Heart muscle & AV node
     c. Lung bronchioles

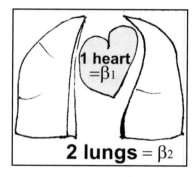

ANSWER
I. Alpha 1 = a. Vascular smooth muscle, arteriolar vasoconstriction
II. Beta 1 = b. Heart muscle & AV node, heart rate stimulation
III. Beta 2 = c. Lung bronchioles, bronchodilation
The adrenergic autonomic nervous system is the "fight or flight" system that excites the heart. The adrenergic system has three important types of receptors: alpha (α) adrenergic, beta-1 (β_1) and beta-2 (β_2). The effects of each respectively are: vasoconstriction, cardiac stimulation, and lung bronchodilation. Remember the acronym "1 heart 2 lungs." **See:** Pappano, chapter on Regulation of the Heartbeat

487. Stimulation of what autonomic receptor sites primarily result in #4 (cardiac depression)?

a. **Alpha adrenergic**
b. **Beta-1 adrenergic**
c. **Beta-2 adrenergic**
d. **Cholinergic**

> 1. Lung broncho-dilation
> 2. Cardiac stimulation
> 3. Vasoconstriction
> *4. Cardiac depression

BE ABLE TO MATCH ALL ANSWERS
ANSWER d. Cholinergic. The parasympathetic autonomic nervous system is the "vegetative" system which liberates acetyl choline. Thus the term "cholinergic." Parasympathetic stimulation depresses the heart rate and contractility. The main drug in this category is atropine, which blocks the cholinergic or parasympathetic system. Atropine thus stimulates the heart rate.

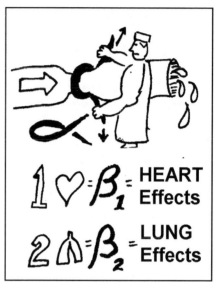

Adrenergic receptors

The adrenergic system has three important types of receptors: alpha (α) adrenergic, beta-1 (β1) and beta-2 (β2). The effects of each respectively are: vasoconstriction, cardiac stimulation, and lung broncho-dilation.

Remember alpha (α) adrenergic as follows: the Greek letter (α) alpha looks like a knot in a suture tied around a vessel - constricting it.

To remember the 2 types of beta receptors say the acronym "We have one heart, two lungs." To remind us that beta 1 (one heart) causes cardiac stimulation, and beta 2 (2 lungs) causes bronchial dilation and some vascular dilation of skeletal muscle.

Cholinergic = parasympathetic = vagal bradycardia/hypotension = (opposite of adrenergic). **Be able to match all answers above.**
See: Underhill, Chapter on "Pharmacologic Management of Patient with Coronary Artery Disease" **Keywords:** sympathetic, beta

488. Identify the class of autonomic drug at #2 in the box.

a. **Sympathomimetic**
b. **Cholinergic**
c. **Vagal blocker**
d. **Beta blocker**

> AUTONOMIC DRUGS
> 1. Atropine
> *2. Metoprolol (Lopressor)
> 3. Norepinephrine
> 4. Acetylcholine

BE ABLE TO MATCH ALL ANSWERS
ANSWER d. Beta Blocker - **Metoprolol (Lopressor)** is a common anti-hypertensive (all beta blocker drugs end in -lol). It blocks norepinephrine/epinephrine at the sympathetic nerve endings. This causes slowing of the heart and lowering of the BP.

AUTONOMIC DRUGS and their CLASS
1. Atropine . . Vagal Blocker (blocks vagal discharge)

2. **Metoprolol (Lopressor).**   Beta Blocker (blocks sympathetic discharge)
3. Norepinephrine.   .   Sympathomimetic (causes fight or flight)
4. Acetylcholine.   .   Cholinergic (causes depression of heart)
See: Underhill, Chapter on "Pharmacologic Management of Patient with CAD."

489. **Which regulatory system plays the predominant role in the regulation of cutaneous flow?**

a.   Motor nerves
b.   Sympathetic nerves
c.   Parasympathetic nerves
d.   Local hormonal control

ANSWER b. Sympathetic nerves.   AV anastomoses shunt blood from arterioles to venules & hence bypass the cutaneous capillary bed. Most skin resistance vessels are under sympathetic and local regulation. Parasympathetic nerves do not supply the skin and have no skin effects.
See: Berne and Levy, chapter on "Regulation of the Heartbeat" **Keywords:** Sympathetic

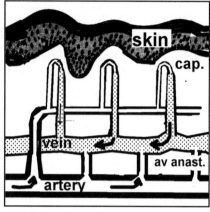
AV Anastomosis

490. **What is the chief effect of stimulating the autonomic receptor sites labeled #2 in the box (β_1 adrenergic)?**

a.   + Chronotropic and + inotropic
b.   - Chronotropic
c.   Arteriolar vasoconstriction
d.   Bronchodilation (lung)

AUTONOMIC RECEPTORS
1. Alpha$_1$ adrenergic
*2. Beta $_1$ adrenergic
3. Beta $_2$ adrenergic
4. parasympathetic

ANSWER a. + Chronotropic and + inotropic. The adrenergic autonomic nervous system is the "fight or flight" system that excites the heart. The adrenergic system has three important types of receptors: alpha (α) adrenergic, beta-1 (β_1) and beta-2 (β_2). The effects of each respectively are: vasoconstriction, cardiac stimulation, and lung bronchodilation.

<u>MATCH THE ANSWERS</u>

1. Alpha$_1$ = α_1, Arteriolar vasoconstriction (increase arterial blood pressure)
2. Beta$_1$ adrenergic, + chronotropic and + inotropic (speed HR and contractility)
3. Beta$_2$ adrenergic, bronchodilation (lung)
4. Parasympathetic, -chronotropic (slow HR)
Remember alpha (α) adrenergic as follows: the Greek letter (α) alpha looks like a knot in a suture tied around a vessel - constricting it.

To remember the 2 types of beta receptors say the acronym "We have one heart, two lungs". To remind us that beta 1 (one heart) causes cardiac stimulation, and beta 2 (2

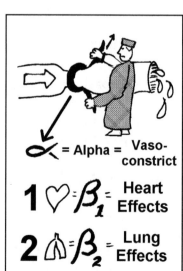
Adrenergic receptors

lungs) causes bronchial dilation and some vascular dilation of skeletal muscle. Stimulation of these receptors can come either from a sympathetic neural discharge or from circulating norepinephrine stimulating the heart. Thus, a total sympathetic discharge would prepare you for "fight or flight" by stimulating these receptors. These are important because the actions of many of the cardiac drugs effect these receptor site. **Be able to match all answers above.**
See: Underhill, Chapter on "Pharmacologic Management of Patient with Coronary Artery

491. **Cardiovascular alpha-adrenergic receptors are associated with the _____ nervous system and are primarily in the _____.**
a.   **Sympathetic,**   **SA and AV nodes**
b.   **Sympathetic,**   **Peripheral resistance vessels**
c.   **Parasympathetic,**   **Myocardium**
d.   **Parasympathetic,**   **Peripheral resistance vessels**

ANSWER b. Sympathetic, peripheral resistance vessels. Alpha adrenergic receptors are chiefly in the arteriolar sphincters of the skin, mucosa, intestine, and kidney. When stimulated they cause vasoconstriction, reduced blood flow to those organs, and raise the peripheral resistance and the blood pressure. Most vasopressors (constrictors)work this way. Sympathomimetic amine drugs like "dopamine" mimic catecholamines through stimulation of these alpha receptors.
See: Underhill, chapter on "Pharmacologic Management of Patient with Coronary Artery Disease." **Keywords:** Sympathetic, alpha adrenergic

2. Sympathetic

492. **Stimulation of sympathetic nerves liberates _____ as an end-site chemical mediator.**
a.   **GP IIb/IIIa**
b.   **Acetylcholine**
c.   **Dobutamine**
d.   **Norepinephrine**

ANSWER d. Norepinephrine. Sympathetic nerves when stimulated liberate norepinephrine as a synaptic mediator. This catecholamine speeds all heart activity. As shown in the diagram, it is liberated at the SA node, the AV node and in the ventricular muscle.
    The ganglia are also shown: sympathetic on the left (high up near the spine), parasympathetic on the right (in the organ). The terminal junction of each system is shown as a Y, almost touching the node. Instead of touching electrically, each system liberates a special chemical transmitter. Norepinephrine (NE)(shown as • in the diagram) is characteristic of the sympathetic system. Acetylcholine (ACh) (shown - in the diagram) is liberated

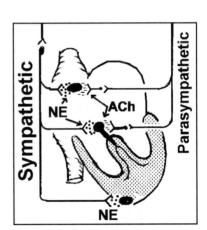

Autonomic nerves & synapse neuro-humoral transmitters

by the parasympathetic system terminal junctions end plates. ACH (shown as a - in the diagram) is liberated by the parasympathetic. It chiefly slows down the SA and AV conduction. The parasympathetic system has few receptors in the ventricular muscle. **Be able to match all answers above. See:** Berne and Levy, chapter on "Regulation of the Heartbeat"

493. **Which 3 answers are associated with stimulation of the SYMPATHETIC AUTONOMIC nervous system? (Select 3 below.)**

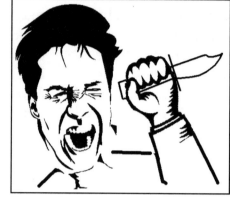

Sympathetic nervous discharge

       1. Adrenergic
       2. Cholinergic
       3. Vegetative response
       4. Fight or flight response
       5. Sacral - bowel nerve stimulation
       6. Acetylcholine end plate mediator
       7. Increase dP/dT
           a. 1, 4, 7
           b. 2, 5, 6
           c. 3, 4, 6
           d. 4, 6, 7

ANSWER a. 1,4, 7.   Sympathetic responses are mediated by norepinephrine & epinephrine (adrenalin) - thus the term "adrenergic." This sympathetic response affects people with a "fight or flight" sensation. These all result in increased contractility or increased dP/dT. The greatest sympathetic discharge occurs at orgasm. True!
      1. **YES: Adrenergic - comes from "adrenalin"**
      2. **NO:** Cholinergic - comes from "acetyl<u>choline</u>"
      3. **NO:** Vegetative response - associated with parasympathetic
      4. **YES: Fight or Flight response - fear, anger,**
      5. **NO:** Sacral - bowel nerve stimulation - associated with parasympathetic
      6. **NO:** Acetylcholine mediator - liberated at parasympathetic nerve synapse
      7. **YES: Increase dP/dT - muscles intrinsically more contractile**
Be able to match all answers above. See: Berne and Levy, chapter on "Regulation of the Heartbeat"

494. **Sympathetic nervous over-stimulation may be seen in acute massive myocardial infarction as:**
a.   **Warm, sweaty skin**
b.   **Cold, sweaty skin**
c.   **Warm, dry skin**
d.   **Cold, dry skin**

ANSWER b. Cold, sweaty skin. The typical acute MI patient is "cold and sweaty-clammy". He is vasoconstricted, has high sympathetic tone and high epinephrine levels. In cutaneous tissue epinephrine only causes vasoconstriction, since cutaneous blood vessels have no

parasympathetic fibers. Local factors also affect the skin's vasodilation and color. For example cold skin temperature has a direct local effect of constricting cutaneous blood vessels. Cold fingers often blanch and turn white. "Local" effects are those not regulated by nerves but by direct effect on the vessels.
See: Berne and Levy, chapter on "Regulation of the Heartbeat" and chapter on "Special Circulations, Cutaneous." **Keywords:** Sympathetic, Cold

495. **During exercise, the sympathetic fibers produce VENOUS _____ which _____ cardiac filling pressure.**
  a.   **Venodilation,**   **Increases**
  b.   **Venodilation,**   **Decreases**
  c.   **Venoconstriction,**   **Increases**
  d.   **Venoconstriction,**   **Decreases**

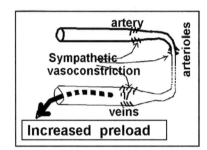

ANSWER c. Venoconstriction, increases. The veins store up to 60% of the blood volume and can liberate this through venoconstriction. This natural "transfusion" will increase preload and filling pressures. Increased preload will then increase the force of contraction and stroke volume through Starling's mechanism. Don't get venous vasoconstriction (increased circulating volume and preload) confused with arteriolar vasoconstriction that primarily increases resistance and BP (increased afterload). Nitroglycerin is one drug that causes both arterial and venous vasodilation.
See: Berne and Levy, chapter on "Regulation of the Heartbeat"

3. Parasympathetic

496. **Alterations in heart rate evoked by changes in blood pressure are dependent upon the baroreceptors located in the:**
  a.   **Circle of Willis**
  b.   **Vertebral arteries**
  c.   **Aortic arch and carotid sinuses**
  d.   **Coronary sinuses and abdominal aorta**

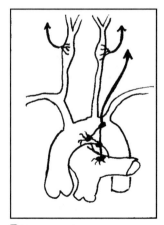

ANSWER c. Aortic arch and carotid sinuses. "Baro" means pressure. Pressure receptors in the carotid sinus' and aortic arch regulate the blood pressure by sensing the pulsations regardless of body position, blood volume, or contractility, etc. .

    The chemoreceptors (O2, CO2, & pH) are located in the same general areas as the baroreceptors - the carotid and aortic bodies. See section on "Chemoreceptors" in this chapter.
See: Berne & Levy, chapter on "Regulation of the Heartbeat."

Baroreceptors

497. **The main parasympathetic nerve that innervates the heart is the:**
   a.   Phrenic
   b.   Vagus
   c.   Cardiac plexus
   d.   Brachial plexus

ANSWER b. The vagus is the largest parasympathetic nerve of the heart. When a patient has a vaso-vagal response or VAGAL discharge, this depressant system "bradys" the patient's heart rate down.
See: Berne and Levy, chapter on "Regulation of the Heartbeat"

498. **The naturally occurring neurotransmitter liberated at the parasympathetic nerve junctions is:**
   a.   Adrenalin
   b.   Norepinephrine
   c.   Atropine
   d.   Acetylcholine

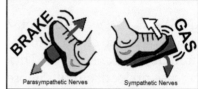
Todd CD, Meds Game

ANSWER d. Acetylcholine is the naturally occurring neurotransmitter liberated at parasympathetic neural junctions. From the word "ACETYLCHOLINE" comes the word "CHOLINERGIC" which refers to parasympathetic system of depressant nerves. Cholinergic sites are also termed: "muscarinic." Acetylcholine's effect is to stimulate the parasympathetic receptors that decrease the heart rate and as a result lower BP. Overstimulation of the vagal nerve leads to over-secretion of acetylcholine, overstimulation of the cholinergic/muscarinic receptors, and finally a "vaso-vagal reaction." Remember the

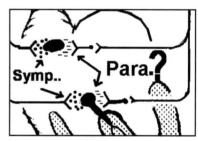
Parasympathetic transmitter

sympathetic system is the GAS pedal which speeds the heart, parasympathetic is the brake pedal that slows it. Play my meds game to practice with these medications
See: Berne and Levy, chapter on "Regulation of the Heartbeat" Acetylcholine

499. **The two primary cardiac responses associated with a PARASYMPATHETIC neural discharge are ____ heart rate and _____ .**
   a.   Increased HR,   Increased AV conduction
   b.   Increased HR,   Reduced AV conduction
   c.   Reduced HR,   Increased AV conduction
   d.   Reduced HR,   Reduced AV conduction

ANSWER d. Reduced HR, reduced AV conduction. The vagus nerve inhibition is mainly supraventricular. It depresses the SA node, atrial myocardium, & AV conduction. It's depressing effect on ventricular myocardium is less pronounced. That is why a vagal response usually appears initially as bradycardia and only later as

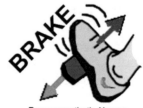
Parasympathetic Nerves

low BP or hypotension. Remember the parasympathetic system slows the heart like a car brake.
See: Berne and Levy, chapter on "Regulation of the Heartbeat."

500. **Which of the following would be most likely to cause the vasovagal reaction shown? (Select 2.)**
      1. Pain
      2. Patient anxiety
      3. Dyspnea
      4. Cyanosis
          a. 1, 2
          b. 1, 4
          c. 2, 3
          d. 3, 4

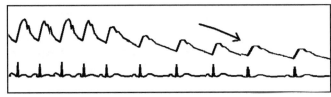

vaso vagal reaction

ANSWER a. Pain & patient anxiety. An anxious patient is ripe for a vaso-vagal or bradycardia reaction. Relaxing and preparing most patients for invasive procedures includes premedication with sedatives and/or hypnotics. The first painful needle sticks (before lidocaine has taken effect) or holding pressure at the arterial puncture site may trigger this bradycardia. **Be able to match all answers above.**
See: Braunwald's paragraph on "vagal reactions" in his chapter on "Heart Catheterization" & Todd, Ch. F6 **Keywords:** Parasympathetic, cholinergic

501. **What is the primary effect of vagal nerve stimulation on the heart?**
    a.   **Increases rhythmicity**
    b.   **Decreases rhythmicity**
    c.   **Increases automaticity**
    d.   **Decreases automaticity**

ANSWER d. Decreases automaticity. Automaticity is the automatic rate of the heart (normally SA rate). Vagal nerves (parasympathetic) depress and slow cardiac function. Remember that Vagal = parasympathetic = cardiac inhibitor. The <u>vagus</u> nerve is the "vegetative" nerve (both start with a "V"). It depresses all cardiac function: rate, contractility, and conduction. Rhythmicity relates to steady rhythm - not how fast, but how regularly it beats.
See: Berne and Levy, chapter on "Electrical activity of the heart" & Todd, Ch. F6,

502. **Increased vagal tone causes: (Note: + indicates increasing, - indicates decreasing.)**
    a.   **+ Inotropism, + Chronotropism**
    b.   **+ Inotropism, - Chronotropism**
    c.   **- Inotropism, - Chronotropism**
    d.   **- Inotropism, + Chronotropism**

ANSWER c. - Inotropism, - chronotropism. The vagal system is the depressor or vegetative system. When vagal nerve tone increases all cardiac function parameters decrease. The heart slows (- chronotropism), conducts slower (- dromotropism), and the

atria decreases their force of contraction (- inotropism). The ventricular contractility does not change much because there are very few parasympathetic receptors there. These result in lower CO and BP. The balance between these two opposing systems (sympathetic and parasympathetic) determines the HR, PR interval, and dP/dT.
See: Berne and Levy, chapter on "Regulation of the Heartbeat" & Todd, Ch. F6

503. **What is atropine's effect on the autonomic nervous system?**
   a.   **Sympathetic stimulant (adrenergic)**
   b.   **Sympathetic blocker (adrenergic blocker)**
   c.   **Parasympathetic stimulant (cholinergic)**
   d.   **Parasympathetic blocker (anti-cholinergic)**

ANSWER d. Parasympathetic blocker (anti-cholinergic). Atropine (Belladonna) increases all cardiac parameters - rate, contractility, and AV conduction. It does this by blocking the parasympathetic system. Remember the parasympathetic system slows everything, so if it is blocked - things speed up. It's like having one foot on your cars gas (sympathetic) and another on the brake (parasympathetic). The balance of the two determines whether you are speeding or slowing.

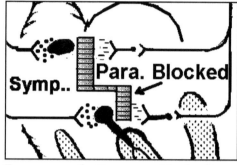
Parasympathetic nerves blocked

See: Berne and Levy, chapter on "Regulation of the Heartbeat" & Todd, Ch. F6, **Keywords:** Parasympathetic, Atropine

504. **What is the standard adult dosage for atropine given IV?**
   a.   **0.5 mg. bolus every 3-5 min. to a maximum of 3 mg.**
   b.   **0.5 mg. bolus every 1-2 min. to a maximum of 2 mg.**
   c.   **2-5 mg. bolus every 5 min. to a maximum of 5-10 mg.**
   d.   **2-5 mg. bolus every 2 min to a maximum of 10-20 mg.**

ANSWER a. 0.5-1.0 mg. bolus every 3-5 min. to a maximum of 3 mg. or 0.04 mg/Kg. ACLS guidelines say, "If perfusion is poor, move quickly through the following actions: Prepare for transcutaneous pacing. Do not delay pacing. If no IV is present pacing can be first. Consider administering atropine 0.5 mg IV if IV access is available. This may be repeated every 3 to 5 minutes up to 3mg or 6 doses. If the atropine is ineffective, begin pacing. Consider epinephrine or dopamine while waiting for the pacer or if pacing is ineffective. Epinephrine 2 to 10 μg/min. Dopamine 2 to 20 μg/kg per minute " AHA, ACLS Guidelines 2017

505. **What autonomic neural effect would result in the greatest tachycardia?**
   a.   **Sympathetic stimulation & parasympathetic stimulation**
   b.   **Sympathetic stimulation & parasympathetic blocked**
   c.   **Sympathetic blocked & parasympathetic stimulation**
   d.   **Sympathetic blocked & parasympathetic blocked**

ANSWER b. Sympathetic stimulation & parasympathetic blocked - for example, if both epinephrine and atropine were given together. Both stimulate the heart rate, but by different mechanisms. Epinephrine stimulates the sympathetic system (fight or flight response) and may result in tachycardia. In contrast, parasympathetic nerve stimulation slows the heart rate (vaso-vagal effect). But when atropine is

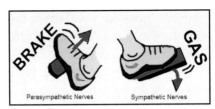
Todd, Meds game

given, this depressor system is blocked, resulting in exaggeration of the tachycardia. In contrast, sympathetic blocking & parasympathetic stimulation would result in bradycardia. It is the balance of these two systems in a push-pull relationship that determines the overall autonomic effect. Using the car analogy, the car goes faster when you release the brake and step on the gas.

See: Alexander, Human Anatomy and Physiology, chapter on "Nervous System"

506. **What autonomic neural effects would result in the most profound bradycardia?**
   a.   **Sympathetic stimulation & parasympathetic stimulation**
   b.   **Sympathetic stimulation & parasympathetic blocked**
   c.   **Sympathetic blocked & parasympathetic stimulation**
   d.   **Sympathetic blocked & parasympathetic blocked**

ANSWER c. Sympathetic blocked & parasympathetic stimulation - for example, if both beta-blockers and acetylcholine were given together. Both depress the heart rate, but by different mechanisms. Beta-blockers depress the sympathetic system and may result in bradycardia. Parasympathetic nerve stimulation slows the heart rate further by stimulating the vagal nerve. In contrast, sympathetic stimulation & parasympathetic

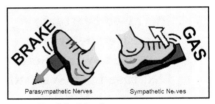
Todd, Meds game

blocking would result in profound tachycardia. It is the balance of these two systems in a push-pull relationship that determines the overall autonomic effect. Using the car analogy, the car slows when you press the brake and release the gas pedals.

See: Alexander, Human Anatomy and Physiology, chapter on "Nervous System"

4. Baroreceptors

507. **Stretch receptors in the aortic arch are termed:**
   a.   **Alpha receptors**
   b.   **Beta receptors**
   c.   **Baro-receptors**
   d.   **Chemo-receptors**

ANSWER c. "Baro" is a prefix for "pressure" as in the term "barometer." These receptors are located in the AO arch and carotid sinuses. Physicians may gently rub the carotid sinus in

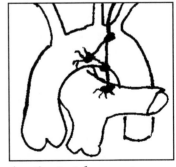
Aortic stretch receptors

a patient's neck to "fake" these baro-receptors into sensing an elevated BP. This increases vagal tone and drops HR. Carotid sinus massage may trigger the baroreceptor reflex and block or slow supraventricular tachycardia. The Valsalva maneuver has a similar effect.

Chemoreceptors (O2, CO2, pH) are located in the aortic and carotid bodies in the same areas as the baroreceptors.

See: Berne and Levy, chapter on "Regulation of the Heartbeat." **Keywords:** Baroreceptor

508. **Baro-receptors are most sensitive to:**
   a.   **Blood velocity**
   b.   **Blood pressure**
   c.   **Venous pressure**
   d.   **Blood flow**

ANSWER b. Blood pressure.   Baro-receptors sense arterial BP in the carotid sinus and AO and transport this as negative feedback to the SA node. Increased BP reduces contractility and HR, as in a carotid sinus massage.
See: Berne and Levy, chapter on "Regulation of the Heartbeat" and chapter on "Peripheral Circulation and its Control." **Keywords:** Baroreceptor

509. **When increased blood pressure is sensed in the arteries, the baroreceptor reflex causes:**
   a.   **Increased heart rate**
   b.   **Decreased heart rate**
   c.   **Increased sympathetic tone**
   d.   **Decreased parasympathetic tone**

ANSWER b. Decreased heart rate. Over a wide range of arterial blood pressure (70 - 160 mmHg) the sympathetic and parasympathetic systems have opposite effects; sympathetic - speeds, parasympathetic - slows. Like your cars gas pedal (speeds) and brake (slows). When your reflexes tell you to stop, you remove your foot from the gas and hit the brake. In the same way, the sympathetic and parasympathetic systems provide a push/pull control.

High blood pressures triggers the baroreceptor reflex to decrease the sympathetic tone and increase the parasympathetic tone. This decreased sympathetic stimulation pushes the heart rate and BP down. Then the added increased parasympathetic discharge pulls it down even more. This dual push/pull nature of the autonomic system, gives it a double control over involuntary organs. What counts is the balance between the two systems. **See:** Berne and Levy, Chapter on "Regulation of the Heartbeat.". **Keywords:** Baroreceptors

510. **Increased baroreceptor stimulation _____ sympathetic tone and _____ parasympathetic neural activity.**
   a.   **Increases, Increases**
   b.   **Increases, Decreases**
   c.   **Decreases, Decreases**
   d.   **Decreases, Increases**

ANSWER d. Decreases, increases. Activated baroreceptors stimulate the cholinergic (vagal) system and decrease tone in the adrenergic system (more brake, less gas). The overall effect is to depress the heart rate and BP.

Baroreceptors provide negative feedback to the heart. If BP increases, they tell the heart, through the autonomic nervous system to "Slow down! My BP is too high." Or if BP is low they tell the heart to "Speed up! I need more Cardiac Output."
See: Berne and Levy, chapter on "Regulation of the Heartbeat"

511. **What is the effect of pressing on the neck at the junction of the internal and external carotid arteries (carotid sinus massage)?**
a.   **+ Chronotropic**
b.   **- Chronotropic**
c.   **- Cholinergic**
d.   **+ Adrenergic**

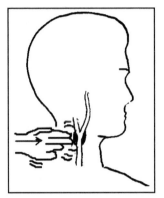
Carotid Massage

ANSWER b. - (Negative) Chronotropic. "Chronus" means "time" (as in chronometer). Thus "negative chronotropic" means slowing of heart rate. Pressure on the baroreceptor in the neck *fakes* them into thinking the blood pressure is high. This stimulates a parasympathetic vagal response and slows the heart rate. For this reason vagal maneuvers may be used to break supraventricular tachycardias. Other activities that increase vagal tone are: eye rubbing, carotid sinus massages, Valsalva, nausea, vomiting and endotracheal intubation. These maneuvers may depress the SA & AV node enough to break supraventricular tachycardia - sometimes a desired side effect.
The prefixes used mean:

Chrono...	**= Heart rate or speed**
Dromo...	**= AV conduction or PR interval**
Ino...	**= Contractility or dP/dT**

See: Braunwald's paragraph on "Vagal Reactions" in his chapter on "Heart Catheterization."

5. Chemoreceptors

512. **Which of the following are the result of mild depression in ventilation (hypoventilation)? (Select 3 below.)**
a.   **+ Chronotropic**
b.   **+ Inotropism**
c.   **Decreased pCO_2**
d.   **Decreased pH**
e.   **Decreases HCO3 (bicarbonate)**

ANSWERS: a, b, & d.
a.   + Chronotropic - YES
b.   - Inotropism - YES
c.   Decreased pCO2 - NO

d.   Decreased pH - YES
Breath holding or hypoventilation causes a buildup of CO2 a drop in pH and O2 in the
lungs and systemic blood. Both low PO2 and low pH stimulate chemoreceptors to speed
the heart rate (chronotropism), increased contractility (inotropism) and speed AV
conduction (dromotropism). **See:** Darovic, chapter on "Intro. to CV and Pulm. Anatomy
and Physiology."

513. **How do acidemia and hypoxemia effect the two vascular systems? In the systemic
circulation they cause _____, and in the pulmonary system they cause
_____.**

a.   **Vasodilation,   Vasodilation**
b.   **Vasodilation,   Vasoconstriction**
c.   **Vasoconstriction,   Vasodilation**
d.   **Vasoconstriction,   Vasoconstriction**

ANSWER b. Vasodilation, vasoconstriction.
The **systemic vasodilator** effect is opposite
to the potent **pulmonary vasoconstrictor**
effect. Remember that in the lungs,
nonventilated areas become ischemic and
need to be shut down or cyanosis may
result. Thus, blood flow is diverted away
from atelectatic (collapsed) alveoli. Whereas,
in the tissues, ischemic areas need more
perfusion and thus vasodilate.
See: Darovic, chapter on "Intro. to CV and
Pulm. Anatomy and Physiology."

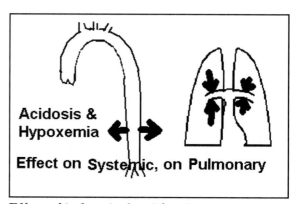

Effect of ischemia & acidemia

514. **Pulmonary hypertension increases with inhalation of_____gas.**
a.   **15% O2**
b.   **100% O2**
c.   **0% CO2**
d.   **5% CO2**

ANSWER a. 15% O2.   Low PO2 in the lung causes vasoconstriction of the pulmonary
arterioles. Low O2 levels in an area of the lung cause pulmonary blood flow to be
redirected (shunted) toward O2 rich areas and away from the poorly ventilated areas. This
optimizes arterial O2 saturation. Since 15% O2 is below the normal 21% O2 in room air, it
will cause general pulmonary vasoconstriction. High O2 levels will do the opposite, it
relaxes constricted pulmonary arterioles. Although CO2 is normally the chief drive for
respiration - it has little effect on the PA pressure. This is similar to high-altitude
pulmonary hypertension. **See:** Berne and Levy, chapter on "Special Circulations -
Pulmonary,"

515. **Persistent pulmonary hypertension in the newborn may be reduced with:**
  a.   Inhalation of 100% O2 & nitrous oxide (N2O) gas
  b.   Inhalation of 100% O2 & nitric oxide (NO) gas
  c.   IV indomethacin
  d.   IV prostaglandin E1

ANSWER b. Inhalation of 100% O2 & nitric oxide (NO) gases act as a local vasodilator. In the cath lab it may be diagnostic to give 100% O2 to patients in pulmonary hypertension. Adding small amounts of nitric oxide also has a local vasodilating effect. This is especially true in the cyanotic child, where low O2 levels increase PVR and R-L shunting. If their hypertension is due to low O2 and poorly ventilated areas of the lung, administering high O2 levels will relax the constricted pulmonary arterioles and reduce shunting. If they do not relax and PVR remains high, then inoperable fixed high pulmonary arteriolar resistance is suspected.

Merck Manual says, "Persistent pulmonary hypertension is a serious disorder in the newborn, where the arteries to the lungs remain narrowed (constricted) after delivery, thus limiting the amount of blood flow to the lungs and therefore the amount of oxygen in the bloodstream."

"Treatment involves opening (dilating) the arteries to the lungs by giving oxygen, often while supporting the newborn's breathing with a ventilator. To help dilate the arteries in the lungs, sometimes nitric oxide is added to the gas that the newborn is breathing. Extracorporeal membrane oxygenation (ECMO) is sometimes used."

Nitrous oxide is laughing gas for anesthesia. Prostaglandin dilates a PDA, and indomethacin closes a PDA. See: http://www.merckmanuals.com/professional/pediatrics/respiratory-problems-in-neonates/persistent-pulmonary-hypertension-of-the-newborn

516. **The endocrine gland that secretes the "fight or flight" hormone is the:**
  a.   Adrenal medulla (suprarenal)
  b.   Renal medulla (kidney)
  c.   Hypophysis (pituitary)
  d.   Pancreas (Isle of Langerhans)

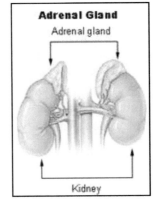

Adrenal Gland
Adrenal gland
Kidney

ANSWER a. Adrenal medulla (suprarenal). One adrenal gland sits on top of each kidney. Tortora says, "The two principal hormones synthesized by the adrenal medulla are *epinephrine* and *norepinephrine*, also called adrenalin and noradrenalin, respectively . . . Both hormones are sympathomimetic, that is, they produce effects that mimic those brought about by the sympathetic division of the autonomic nervous system. To a large extent, they are responsible for the fight-or-flight response."
Epinephrine (also known as adrenaline) is a hormone and neurotransmitter, which increases heart rate, contracts blood vessels, dilates air passages and participates in the fight-or-flight response of the sympathetic nervous system. **See**: Tortora chapter on "Cardiovascular System: Blood Vessels."

6. Basic ECG & Heart Rate

517. **When the heart is insensitive to stimuli and cannot be depolarized by stimulation (such as pacing), it is said to be:**
a. Aberrant
b. Blocked
c. Arrested
d. Refractory

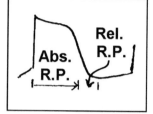
Refractory Pd.

ANSWER d. Refractory. This is the period of the cardiac cycle when the myocardium **cannot** respond to a second impulse because it has not fully recovered. That is why a ventricular pacing impulse in the ST segment (refractory period) is ineffective. The refractory period has two parts: absolute and relative refractory periods. Absolute refractory period includes the entire action potential plateau (ST segment) as shown. However, during the relative refractory period the heart is sensitive to extrastimuli. An extrastimuli or PVC here may initiate V. tach. or V. fib. This is how electrophysiologists induce ventricular tachycardia during EP studies.
See: Berne and Levy, chapter on "Electrical activity of the heart."

518. **Purkinje and ventricular cells have their own rhythmicity and intrinsic rate. These lower pacemaker rates are usually suppressed as long as:**
a. Enough calcium is available
b. The AV node conduction rate is normal
c. The SA node rate is fast enough
d. The conduction system is normal

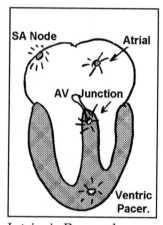
Intrinsic Pacemakers

ANSWER c. The SA node pacemaker rate is normally the fastest in the heart. Only when the SA rate slows or another pacemaker speeds up, does it relinquish its control of the heart rhythm.
　　Pacemaker control goes to the one with the fastest rate.
　　These lower pacemakers with slower intrinsic rates are found in the atrium (60), junctional (50), & ventricular tissue (30-40). They are normally suppressed until they escape the control of the SA node - and pace the heart at their own intrinsic rate (60, 50, or 30-40 ppm respectively). **See:** Dubin, chapter on "Heart Rate."

519. **Sympathetic nervous stimulation of the heart primarily affects the heart rate by altering what phase of the SA node action potential?**
a. Phase 1
b. Phase 2
c. Phase 3
d. Phase 4

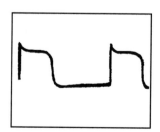
Action Potential, NSR

ANSWER d. Phase 4. A mechanism to speed the sinus rate is to increase the slope of phase 4, so that the cell reaches firing threshold sooner. The other mechanisms that change the heart rate are altered threshold and resting potential. NSR is Normal Sinus Rhythm. **See:** Berne and Levy, chapter on "Electrical activity of the heart."

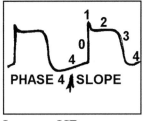

Increase HR

520. **Changes in heart rate of the TRANSPLANTED heart are due only to: (Select 2.)**
        1. **Sympathetic effects**
        2. **Parasympathetic effects**
        3. **Motor nerve effects**
        4. **Humoral - circulating catecholamine**
        5. **Neural - autonomic dromotropic effects**
        6. **Starling's intrinsic mechanism**
           a. 1,4
           b. 2,6
           c. 3,5
           d. 4,6

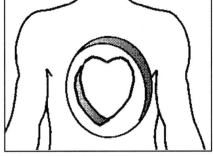

Transplanted heart rate changes

ANSWER d. Humoral (circulating catecholamines) and Starling's intrinsic mechanism. Since transplants have no neural connections, transplanted hearts are completely unaffected by nervous tone. So the only things that will change cardiac output are circulating humors like adrenalin or intrinsic responses like preload (Starling effects). **See:** Berne and Levy, chapter on "Regulation of the Heartbeat" **Keywords:** HR, denervated heart, transplanted heart

521. **Inspiration normally causes _____ heart rate and _____ RV stroke volume.**
    a.   **Increased HR, Increased SV**
    b.   **Increased HR, Decreased SV**
    c.   **Decreased HR, Decreased SV**
    d.   **Decreased HR, Increased SV**

ANSWER a. Increased heart rate and increased RV stroke volume. Marked cyclic variation in heart rate with breathing is termed "sinus arrhythmia." With inspiration

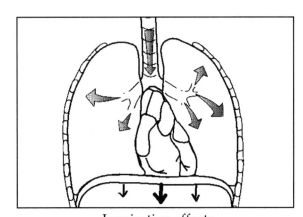

Inspiration effects

more blood is sucked into the RA, thus increasing venous return. The Bainbridge stretch receptors in the RA then cause reflexive drop in vagal tone which speeds the heart rate. This is easily seen while monitoring PA pressures. Remember, inspiration causes both the diaphragm and blood pressures to drop. Within seconds venous return, HR and CO increase.

    Deep inspirations drop the negative pressure in the thorax and may **double** venous return. The Starling mechanism then stimulates the heart to pump harder and increase the

RV stroke volume. This respiratory pump is termed the "auxiliary venous pump." Inspiration thus dramatically increases both the rate and output of the heart.

This effect reverses on expiration. Heart rate and stroke volume drop. The venous valves prevent reflux of blood back into the veins. **See:** Berne and Levy, chapter on "Electrical activity of the heart." **Keywords:** HR, Inspiration

522. **What medication is potentially dangerous to asthmatics who rely on bronchodilators?**
a.   **Atropine**
b.   **Beta-blockers**
c.   **Calcium channel blockers**
d.   **ACE inhibitors**

ANSWER b. Beta-blockers may render an asthmatic patient's bronchodilators ineffective in a asthmatic crisis. Opie says: "Pulmonary absolute contraindications are severe asthma or bronchospasm. . . . No patient may be given a beta-blocker without questions for past or present asthma. Fatalities have resulted when this rule is ignored. "
See: Opie, chapter on "Beta-blockers"

523. **Concerning the ion transfer across myocardial cell membranes, throughout systole (QT interval):**
a.   **Sodium seeps in**
b.   **Sodium rushes in**
c.   **Potassium leaks out**
d.   **Potassium seeps in**

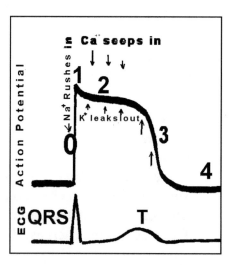

ANSWER c. Potassium leaks out. Throughout systole the K+ ions slowly exit and Ca^{++} ions slowly enter. The positive ions pass each other making the voltage change approximate zero during this phase 2 plateau period. After the Ca stops seeping in, phase 3 or repolarization is due to K continuing to leak out of the cell. These slow currents follow the rapid in-rushing of sodium during rapid depolarization. **See:** Fogoros, chapter on "The Cardiac Electrical System."

524. **What ion rushes across the myocardial cell membrane during phase 0 of the action potential?**
a.   **Sodium seeps in**
b.   **Sodium rushes in**
c.   **Potassium leaks out**
d.   **Potassium seeps in**

ANSWER b. Sodium rushes in during phase zero which is the time of the ECG QRS complex. This is termed a fast current, because it happens quickly as the cell wall suddenly becomes permeable to the Na+ ion. Cardiac muscle cells are different from purkinje and automatic tissues in that their rapid upstroke (phase 0) is due to Na+ rushing in through the fast channel. Automatic cells don't have this rapid channel; and their phase zero is a slow upstroke. The slope of the phase zero also influences conduction velocity. E.g., Nodal tissue has slow upstroke and slow conduction velocity. **See:** Fogoros, chapter on " The Cardiac Electrical System."

525. What cardiac tissue has the fastest electrical conduction velocity?
   a.   **SA node**
   b.   **Atrial muscle**
   c.   **AV node**
   d.   **Purkinje fibers**
   e.   **Ventricular muscle**

ANSWER d. Purkinje fibers rapidly conduct the electrical signal to the ventricles 2-3 M/sec. That is a factor of 20 times faster than the other cardiac tissues. Thus, the normally narrow QRS complex. By comparison, the node and muscle fibers conduct slowly 0.1-.5 M/sec (broad QRS). **See:** Braunwald, chapter on "Arrhythmias, Sudden death, and Syncope"

526. The impulse's principal delay in the passage from the SA node to the ventricular myocardial cells occurs in the:
   a.   **Atrial muscle**
   b.   **Specialized atrial conduction fibers**
   c.   **AV node (upper regions AN-N)**
   d.   **AV node (lower region -NH)**

ANSWER c. The AV node (upper region) is where the principal AV delay occurs. The slowed conduction occurs in the upper ("AN" and "N") regions of the node. The conduction velocity here is 10 times slower than in the ventricular Purkinje cells. The proper AV delay (PR interval) allows the atrial kick to pack the ventricle with just enough blood (preload) before contraction to optimize systole. **See:** Underhill, chapter on "ECG" also, Todd, Vol. II, chapter on "ECG."

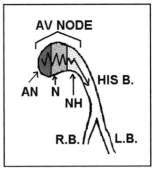

ECG Activation

527. Which of the following is the heart's normal conduction sequence to the His bundle?
   a.   **SA node, RA atrial muscle, LA muscle, AV node**
   b.   **SA node, LA atrial muscle, RA muscle, Purkinje fibers, AV node**
   c.   **AV node, atrial muscle, SA node**
   d.   **AV node, Bachman's bundle, atrial muscle, SA node**

ANSWER a. SA node, RA atrial muscle, LA muscle, AV node. The SA node normally initiates right atrial contraction. The impulse then travels through 3 specialized atrial conduction fibers to the AV node, and through Bachman's bundle across the atrial septum into the LA. The RA contracts first, then the LA. As the RA completes its contraction the impulse enters the AV node where it is delayed to allow ventricular filling. **See:** Braunwald, chapter on "Electrocardiography." also, Todd, Vol. II, chapter on "ECG."

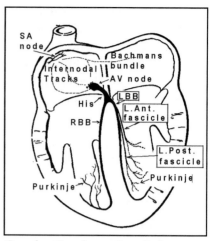

Conduction branches in heart
- after Rushmer fig. 3-9

528. **Which of the following is the normal conduction sequence after an electrical impulse has traveled through the AV node?**

a.   **Bundle branches, Bachmann's bundle, Purkinje fibers**

b.   **Bundle branches, bundle of His, Purkinje fibers**

c.   **Bundle of His, bundle branches, Purkinje fibers**

d.   **Purkinje fibers, His bundle, AV junction**

ANSWER c. Bundle of His, bundle branches, Purkinje fibers. The sequence is:
- SA node
- Inter-atrial tracts (including *Bachmann's bundle)
- AV Node
   AN = Transitional tissue between atria and AV Node.
   N = Mid AV nodal tissue (most of the AV time delay occurs in these upper 2 regions of the AV node)
   NH = Region where nodal fibers gradually merge with bundle of His tissue.
   His = The upper portion of ventricular conduction tissue
- Bundle of HIS
- Right and left bundle branches (Left has 2 fascicles, anterior & posterior)
- Purkinje System - to myocardium

See: Underhill, chapter on "Cardiac Electrophysiology"

529. **Normal interventricular conduction proceeds from the bundle of HIS through 3 major fascicles. Identify these three fascicles. (Select 3 below.)**

a.   **Right bundle branch**

b.   **Right posterior fascicle**

c.   **Left anterior fascicle**

d.   **Left posterior fascicle**

e.   **Circumflex related fascicle**

ANSWERS: a, c, & d. The 3 branches of the conduction system are the: Right bundle branch, left anterior fascicle, and left posterior fascicle. The 2 branches of the left bundle go to the 2 papillary muscles attached to the anterior and posterior mitral valve leaflets. This division of the left bundle into 2 is analogous to the way the main left coronary divides into 2 major branches to supply the LV. There is also a common main left bundle between the His and left fascicle division analogous to the main left coronary artery. As with the right coronary, the right bundle branch supplies the RV. When one of these 3 fascicles is blocked, it is termed a fascicular block. **See:** Davis, chapter on "IV Conduction Abnormalities" also, Todd, Vol. II, chapter on "ECG."

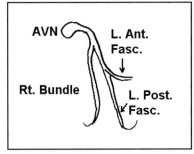

Vent. Conduction

530. **Non-compensated pauses are most often seen after a _____ and compensatory pauses are seen after a/an _____.**
   a.   PAT, PVC
   b.   PVC, PAC
   c.   PJC, PAC
   d.   PAC, PVC

ANSWER d. PAC, PVC. Since PACs (Premature Atrial Complexes) originate in the atria they often penetrate and "reset" the SA node. The SA pacemaker then starts over and resumes firing at the set rate. PVCs (Premature Ventricular Contractions) are not usually conducted retrograde into the atria and may not reset the SA node. The normal "P" wave usually falls in the refractory period of the AV node and is not conducted. This makes the long compensatory pause following most PVCs. **See:** Dubin, chapter on "Rhythm."

531. **How does a PVC normally effect the blood pressure? The systolic BP associated with the PVC will _____ in pressure, and the following sinus beat will _____ in pressure.**
   a.   Increase,   Decrease
   b.   Increase,   Increase
   c.   Decrease,   Decrease
   d.   Decrease,   Increase

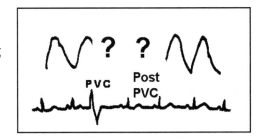

ANSWER d. PVC BP decreases, post PVC BP increases. The long compensatory pause following the PVC allows for more LV filling and thus a stronger ejection. Patients normally don't feel PVCs - but instead the large surge of blood pumped during the post-PVC beat.
See: Braunwald, chapter on "Electrocardiography."

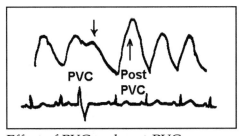

Effect of PVC and post-PVC

ECG Tracings and Equipment

532. This calibration signal on an ECG machine is
termed:
a.   Underdamped
b.   Overdamped
c.   Normal
d.   Resonant
e.   Increased high frequency response

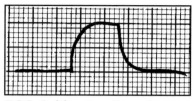
ECG Calibration Signal

ANSWER b. Overdamped. This ECG pen responds too
SLOW. Damping slows things. This will reduce the
recorder's frequency response and impair recording of
rapidly occurring waves such as the QRS. Underdamping
is the opposite. Underdamping is shown in the first half of
this diagram. The second half of the diagram shows only
slight underdamping (up to 10% overshoot), which is
acceptable, since it increases the high frequency response
of the recorder. **See:** Equipment manuals also, Todd, Vol. II, chapter on "ECG."

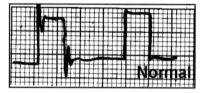
Underdamped Calibration
Signal

533. If the 1 mV calibration signal deflects as shown on the ECG
paper, what adjustment should be made?
a.   Nothing, it should only go up .5 cm
b.   Turn up the position control
c.   Turn down the position control
d.   Turn down the sensitivity control
e.   Turn up the sensitivity control

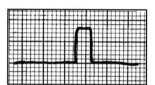
ECG 1 mv Calibration
X1

ANSWER e. Turn up the sensitivity (gain) control. The gain sets
the relative size of the QRS and other complexes in cm/mV.
Standard gain is 1 cm/mV. Gain may be halved if the QRS
complex goes off the paper (E.g., in high voltage V leads).
Calibration signals (1 mV) should appear on every ECG for
accurate voltage measurements. **See:** Underhill, chapter on "ECG."

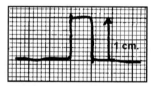
ECG 1 mv Calibration
X1

534. How is the QRS complex labeled at #5?
a.   QR
b.   QRS
c.   QRSR'
d.   QS
e.   RS

Label the ventricular complexes

ANSWER d. QS wave. Being all
negative with no "R" wave, it is
considered a large "Q" or "S" wave, or
together a "QS." The "Q" wave is the first negative deflection. The "S" wave is the second.

"R" is the first positive deflection, R' the second, R" the third, etc. In addition, some authors use upper and lower case letters to indicate the relative size of the complexes. Classic rSR' is termed "rabbit ears" and is seen in RBBB. **CORRECTLY MATCHED** answers are:

1. RS
2. QR
3. QRS
4. QRSR'
5. QS

See: Davis, chapter on "IV Determination of HR and Normal Heart Rhythms."

535. **Which unipolar ECG lead is recorded from a unipolar chest level electrode placed at the left mid-axillary line at the the 4th intercostal space, labeled as #4 in the diagram.**

a. V1
b. V2
c. V3
d. V4
e. V5
f. V6

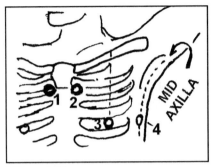
V Lead Placement

ANSWER f. V6. V6 is labeled as #4 in the diagram. Know how to place all 12 ECG leads using proper land marks.

    1. V1 - V1 is placed at the RSB 4th ICS.
    2. V2 - V2 is at the LSB 4th ICS. V2 is at the LSB 4th ICS. The second intercostal space can be located just below the "angle of Louis" at the Junction of manubrium and sternum.
    (V3 -V3 goes between V2 and V4.)
    3. V4 - V4 is placed in the 5th intercostal space (mid-clavicular line - marked in dotted line).
    (V5 - V5 goes between V4 and V6.)
    4. V6 - V6 is placed at the same level as V4 - marked in the dotted line. This not actually in the 5th ICS. Since, as you move around the left side, the ribs more up - V6 is nearer the 5th intercostal space in the mid axillary line (armpit). **See:** Braunwald, chapter on ECG.

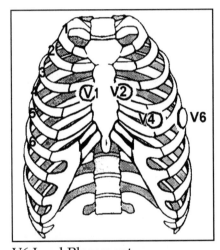
V6 Lead Placement

536. **After having applied the 12 lead ECG electrodes to a young asymptomatic patient, you notice large negative QRS complexes in Lead I. The cause of this is usually:**

a. **Athletic heart (LVH)**
b. **Unipolar pacemaker spikes**
c. **Right arm & left arm electrodes reversed**
d. **Right leg ground electrode loose or disconnected**

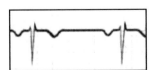

ANSWER: c. Right arm & left arm electrodes reversed. This is an easy mistake to make. Lead I is the voltage measured between the two arms, with the left arm being positive. Lead I normally has an upright R wave configuration, but if the arm lead wires are reversed, where the left arm is incorrectly connected to the right arm electrode, the reading will be inverted. P waves and QRS will deflect downward, instead of upward. It's very easy to recognize. To remember which lead goes to the right arm say, "White is right!" **See:** Dubin, "Rapid Interpretation of EKGs"

537. **How many lead wires or electrodes are used in taking a 12 lead EKG? Count them.**

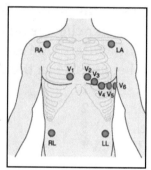

    a.   2
    b.   6
    c.   10
    d.   12
    e.   20

ANSWER: c. 10: RA, LA, RL, LL, V1-2-3-4-5-& V6. These are the 10 wires and electrodes on the skin - four limb leads and 6 chest leads. Various combinations of these give us the standard 12 lead ECG. **See:** Dubin, "Rapid Interpretation of EKGs"

ECG Artifacts

538. **You observe a muscle tremor artifact on ECG leads I and II, but NOT on lead III. Which ECG electrode is probably causing this artifact?**
    a.   **Left arm**
    b.   **Left leg**
    c.   **Right arm**
    d.   **Right leg**

ANSWER c. Right arm. The electrode resistance is probably increased on the right arm electrode. The RA is the only electrode common to lead I and II. Draw an Einthoven triangle and note how lead I and II intersect at the right arm. Try re-prepping that electrode to improve the artifact. Poor skin prep is the usual cause of ECG artifacts. With a roughening of the skin, and application of electrode paste, good ECGs can even be obtained during exercise. Also, move the electrodes up to the shoulders, where arm motion will not be sensed. **See:** Phillips, The Cardiac Rhythms, chapter on "The Electrocardiogram" also, Todd, Vol. II, chapter on "ECG"

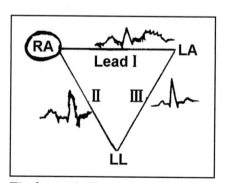

Einthoven's Triangle

539. **How could you reduce the artifacts seen on this ECG?**

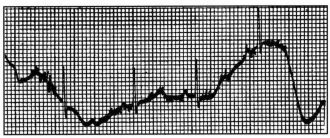

Monitoring Lead II ECG

a. Relax and quiet the patient

b. Check for electric motors & improper ground

c. Increase the damping on the machine

d. Reapply the ECG limb electrodes more distally

ANSWER a. Relax and quiet the patient. This artifact is a somatic muscle tremor with wandering baseline due to motion. Make the patient comfortable and ask him to relax all over. If this fails to eliminate the noise, the electrodes should be moved more proximally, onto the shoulders and hips after thoroughly prepping the skin. This kind of noisy ECG signal can interfere with ECG interpretation.
See: Davis, chapter on "12 Lead ECG Interpretation." also, Todd, Vol. II, chapter on "ECG."

540. **A patient's monitor alarm has just sounded. You come running and see this ECG. What do you do?**

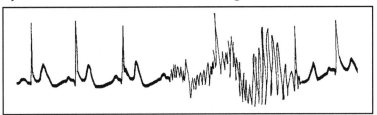

Monitoring Lead II ECG

a. Defibrillate

b. Call for help and begin CPR

c. Awake the patient by shaking and shouting

d. Check ECG electrodes and leads

ANSWER d. Check ECG electrodes and leads. This is a normal sinus rhythm disturbed by motion artifact. Noisy ECG artifacts may occur due to patient motion or a loose electrode. Although this artifact resembles ventricular fibrillation it returns to sinus rhythm at the end of the strip. No patient should be resuscitated or treated, based on the ECG alone. *Treat the patient, not the monitor.* **See:** ACLS Manual also, Todd, Vol. II, chapter on "ECG." **Keywords:** ECG artifact, check patient 1st

541. **The irregularity seen in the baseline of the ECG tracing below is:**

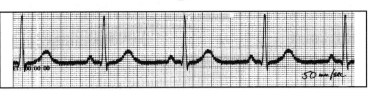

Baseline ECG artifact - recorded at 50 mm/sec

a. DC interference

b. AC (60 Hz) interference

c. Muscle tremors

d. Wandering baseline

ANSWER b. AC (60 Hz) interference. This is due to 60 cycle interference from such appliances as: electric motors(beds), transformers (fluorescent lights), or improper electrical ground. Turn off all electrical appliances close to the patient and check all machine grounding. On slower paper speeds this may appear as a very wide regular baseline. But if you look closely there are tiny sine wave vibrations within the baseline. **See:** Davis, chapter on "12-Lead ECG Interpretation" also, Todd, Vol. II, Chapter on "ECG."

Measurements

542. **On this ECG identify the segment, wave or interval labeled at #2 in the diagram.**
a.   "P" wave
b.   ST segment
c.   PR interval
d.   "R" wave
e.   RS (QRS)
f.   QT interval
g.   "T" wave
h.   "S" wave

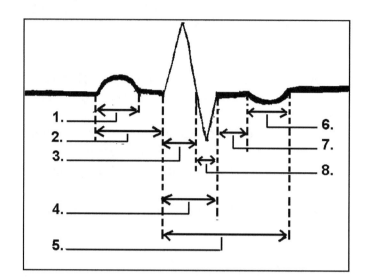

ANSWER c. PR interval. The PR interval is from the beginning of the P wave to the beginning of the QRS complex. It is the sum of the P wave duration (atrial contraction) and the PR segment (AV conduction time). Be able to match all answers.

     1. "P" wave
     2. PR interval
     3. "R" wave
     4. RS (QRS)
     5. QT interval
     6. "T" wave
     7. ST segment
     8. "S" wave

See: Davis, chapter on "IV Determination of HR and Normal Heart Rhythms" also, Todd, Vol. II, chapter on "ECG." **Keywords:** ECG intervals, segments & waves

543. **Determine the heart rate.   HR = ?/min**
a.   40-50
b.   50-65
c.   65-75
d.   75-85

Measure heart rate variation on this ECG

ANSWER c. 65-75 beats/min. Remember the quick "box counter" method: 300-150-100-75-60-50 beats/min. The first beat R-R interval measures 5 large boxes = just over 60/min. The last R-R interval is 4 large boxes = 75/min. This example shows how you need a regular R-R interval to use this method for an overall average heart rate.

Another method is to calculate the RR interval by counting the number of small boxes between QRS complexes. Remember, the normal ECG paper speed is 25 mm/sec., so each small box is .04 sec. Count the number of boxes, multiply times .04 sec/box and then divide that time into 60 sec/min, for beats/min where HR = 60/RR int.
See: Dubin, chapter on "Rate." also, Todd, Vol. II, chapter on "ECG."

544. **Calculate the heart rate (HR) if the R-R interval is 920 msec.**
   a. 42 bpm
   b. 51 bpm
   c. 65 bpm
   d. 72 bpm

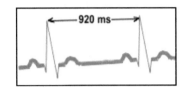

ANSWER c. 65 bpm
Use the basic formula (you should memorize): HR = 60/RR, or HR = (60,000 msec/min)/(r-r interval in msec). It is just under 1 sec. so, the rate us just over 60 bpm.
   (60,000 msec/min)/ 920 msec = 65/min.
EP study and pacemaker rates are now calculated not with ECG boxes, or seconds but in milliseconds. Since there are 1000 msec/sec, the standard HR formula uses 60,000 in the numerator. Note how the units cancel to give beats / min. **See:** Braunwald, chapter on "Electrocardiography."

USE THIS ECG COMPLEX BELOW FOR THE NEXT 3 QUESTIONS.

545. **On this magnified ECG, measure the PR interval.**
   a. 0.06 sec
   b. 0.10 sec
   c. 0.14 sec
   d. 0.18 sec

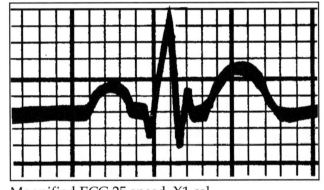

Magnified ECG 25 speed, X1 cal

546. **On this magnified ECG measure the QRS duration.**
   a. .08 sec
   b. .12 sec
   c. .16 sec
   d. .24 sec

547. **On this magnified ECG measure the "R" wave voltage.**
   a. 0.6 mV
   b. 1.0 mV
   c. 1.6 mV
   d. 3.2 mV

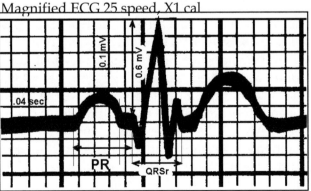

Magnified ECG 25 speed, X1 cal

ALL THREE ANSWERS LISTED CONSECUTIVELY BELOW:

545. ANSWER c. 0.14 sec. Measure from the beginning of the "P" wave to the beginning of the QRS and find 3.5 boxes. Each box is .04 sec. Interval = 3.5 x .04 = .14 sec. PR interval is key to evaluating AV node conduction. Normal adult PR interval = .12 - 0.20 sec.
See: Davis, chapter on "IV Determination of HR and Normal Heart Rhythms." **Keywords:** measure PR interval

546. ANSWER b. 0.12 sec. From the beginning of the "q" wave to the end of the r' wave it is 3 boxes (leading edge to leading edge). Interval = # boxes x .04 sec/box = 3 x .04 = .12 sec. QRS duration is key to evaluating abnormally conducted ventricular complexes. Normal range for QRS duration in the limb leads is 0.04 - .10 sec.
See: Davis, chapter on "ECG Graph Paper and Measurements." **Keywords:** measure QRS duration

547. ANSWER a. 0.6 mV. Voltage is measured vertically. Remember the calibration signal is 1 mV = 1 cm. Each small box is 0.1 mV. The "R" wave deflects 6 boxes above the baseline or 0.6 mV. R wave voltage is key to evaluating hypertrophy of a chamber.
See: Davis, chapter on "ECG Graph Paper and Measurements" also, Todd, Vol II, chapter on "ECG."

548. If an idioventricular pacemaker "escapes" it will usually fire at a rate of:

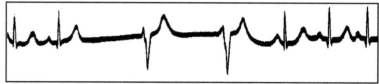

a.   10-20 bpm
b.   30-40 bpm
c.   60-80 bpm
d.   100-200 bpm

ANSWER b. 30-40 bpm. The ideoventricular pacemaker is the slowest escape rhythm. It is the heart's last resort when all other pacemakers fail. Our hearts have different levels of automatic - "escape" pacemakers to prevent asystole. These "potential" escape pacemakers and their usual rates are:
- Junctional (nodal) = 40-50 bpm
- Ventricular   = 30-40

The SA node is like a teacher in control of the class. Myocardial cells are like student's, they only pay attention to the fastest leader. When the teacher speaks at a normal rate (SA node rate around 60 bpm) everyone follows. But if a fast jazz band were to prance through the hall it would take the student's attention, like an ectopic focus. The teacher then loses control.

Also, if the teacher is too slow, he loses the class' attention - as in sinus bradycardia. A quicker student may stand up and take over. This is analogous to a lower pacemaker that "escapes" at a rate faster than the SA node. A junctional rate of 50 can take over when the sinus node rate falls below 50

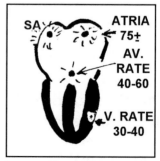

Latent Pacer Rates

bpm. **See:** Dubin, chapter on "Rate"

7. Other Reflexes

549. **The pharmo-mechanical response to any substance secreted into the blood stream by an endocrine gland is termed:**
   a.   **Humoral**
   b.   **Antagonistic**
   c.   **Autonomic**
   d.   **Intrinsic**

ANSWER a. Humors are secreted by endocrine glands. Most of them circulate in the blood stream. For example, the adrenal cortex secretes epinephrine, which has the same effect as injecting IV "Epi.".

    The heart is controlled by both intrinsic and extrinsic sources. Circulating humors like adrenalin cause an "extrinsic response." These come from areas other than the heart (CNS, endocrine glands). An example of the heart's "intrinsic response" would be Starling's preload mechanism because it is "inherent" in the heart muscle. **See:** Berne and Levy, chapter on "Regulation of the Heartbeat"

550. **An increased RA filling pressure leads to increased heart rate and diuresis. This is termed the_____ reflex.**
   a.   **Bainbridge**
   b.   **Natriuretic**
   c.   **Chemoreceptor**
   d.   **ACE inhibitor**

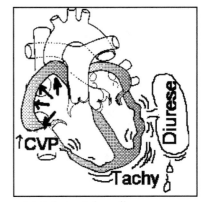
Atrial stretch reflex

ANSWER a. Bainbridge. At slow HR, increases in blood volume evoke the Bainbridge reflex which increases HR. Stretch receptors in both atria send afferent impulses to the brain and from there efferent impulses go to the SA node to increase HR. The atrial stretch receptors also increase urine production principally through "vasopressin" secretion and "Anti-Diuretic Hormone" (ADH). This reflex is also termed the "atria-pressor reflex."
See: Berne and Levy, chapter on "Regulation of the Heartbeat."inhibitors

References

Braunwald, Eugene, Ed., *HEART DISEASE A Textbook of Cardiovascular Medicine*, 9th
    Ed., W. B. Saunders Co., 2012
Underhill, S. L., Ed., *CARDIAC NURSING*, 2nd Ed., J. B. Lippincott Co., 1989
Hurst, J. W., and Logue, R. B., et. al., *THE HEART Arteries and Veins*, 3rd Ed.,
    McGraw-Hill Book Co., 1974
American Heart Association, *Textbook of ADVANCED CARDIAC LIFE SUPPORT*,, 2010
Pappano & Wier, *Cardiovascular Physiology*, 10th Ed., Mosby Year Book, 2013
Dubin, Dale, *RAPID INTERPRETATION of EKG's*, 3rd Ed., Cover Publishing Co., 1982

Darovic, G.O., *Hemodynamic Monitoring: Invasive and Noninvasive Clinical Application,*
WB Saunders, 1995

OUTLINE: B5 - Autonomic CNS and ECG Basics

1. SYMPATHETIC
   a. Location
      i. ganglia, stellate
      ii. higher centers
      iii. Heart innervation: nodes, myocardium, Coronary
   b. Physiology
      i. Mediator: Nor-Epi, Epi., (Adrenalin)
      ii. Adrenergic response = fight/flight
      iii. Receptors
         (1) Alpha (α1) = Arterial vasoconstriction
         (2) Beta (β1) = Cardiac Stimulation
            (a) + HR automaticity (chronotropism)
            (b) +AV conduction (Dromotropism)
         (3) Beta (β2) = Bronchodilation
         (4) Venoconstriction (capacitance)
         (5) Blocker (Beta blocker - Inderal)
      iv. Other adrenergic effects
         (1) Cutaneous regulation
         (2) Overstimulation = cold sweat
2. PARASYMPATHETIC
   a. Location:
      i. Vagus
      ii. Cardiac Innervation
   b. Physiology
      i. Mediator=Acetylcholine
      ii. Responses
         (1) Vegetative
         (2) -Heart rate (-chronotropism)
         (3) -AV Conduction (-dromotropism)
         (4) -automaticity
         (5) Lung effects, Sinus Arrhythmia
         (6) gut effects
      iii. Vasovagal Reaction
         (1) Causes
            (a) pain
            (b) anxiety
            (c) Carotid Sinus Massage
         (2) Blocker (Atropine)
         (3)

3. BARORECEPTORS
   a. Pressure (stretch) Receptor Locations -
      i. Carotid sinus
      ii. AO
      iii. PA
   b. Baro-reflex
      i. HR inversely related to BP
      ii. Carotid sinus Massage

4. CHEMORECEPTORS
   a. Ventilation effects
      i. CO2 drive
      ii. Hypoxic (O2) drive
         (1) Pulmonary Hypertension
      iii. pH

5. EP, HR
   a. Automaticity - Intrinsic pacers
      i. SA, Atria, Junction, Ventricle
   b. Heart Rate
      i. Action Potential
         (1) HR relation to Slope of phase 4
         (2) Refractory Period
   c. ECG
      i. AV Block
      ii. Transplanted heart

      iii. hormonal response
         (1) Starling response
      iv. Overdrive suppression
      v. Sinus Arrhythmia
6. OTHER
   a. Humoral effects
      i. Circulating catecholamines
      ii. Renin-Angiotensin System
         (1) ACE inhibitors
   b. Bainbridge Reflex (atria-Pressor)
      i. Anti-Diuretic effect
         (1) ADH
         (2) Vasopressin
   c. Starlings reflex/Law
      i. preload

Hemodynamics and Pressure Basics

1. The Circuit

THE NEXT 5 QUESTIONS REFER TO THIS DIAGRAM. It shows the relative values of 4 hemodynamic measurements as the systemic blood moves from the aorta, arterioles, through the capillaries and venules, and into the vena cavae.

551. The principal level at which the vascular RESISTANCE (vasoconstriction) develops is in the:
    a. Venules
    b. Arterioles
    c. Large veins
    d. Large arteries

552. At what level is blood flow through the systemic vessels SLOWEST?
    a. Veins
    b. Arteries
    c. Capillaries
    d. Arterioles

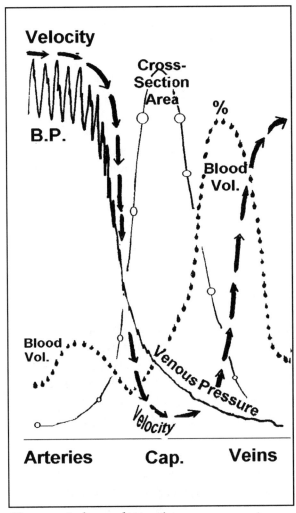

Changes in hemodynamic measurements - As blood passes through vascular system

553. When considered together, which vessels have the greatest cross-sectional area?
- a.   Arteries
- b.   Veins
- c.   Capillaries
- d.   Arterioles

554. As blood passes through the vascular system where does the largest mean blood pressure (gradient) drop occur?
- a.   Aorta
- b.   Venules
- c.   Vena Cava
- d.   Arterioles

555. Which class of vessels has the capacity to store the largest volume of blood?
- a.   Pulmonary veins
- b.   Systemic veins
- c.   Pulmonary capillaries
- d.   Arteries

ANSWERS TO THE ABOVE 5 QUESTION LISTED BELOW.

551. ANSWER b. Arterioles contain the precapillary sphincters which pinch off the pressure. Constricted arterioles are the chief resistance to blood flow. Thus, vasoactivity dramatically affects vascular resistance, blood pressure and flow. BP is directly proportional to the cardiac output and the Resistance. BP = CO x SVR
See: Berne & Levy, chapter on "The Circuit." **Keywords:** Arterioles, Resistance

552. ANSWER c. The huge capillary cross sectional area slows blood flow to its slowest flow. This allows time for O_2, CO_2 and nutrient exchange within the tissue. **See:** Berne & Levy, chapter on "The Circuit." **Keywords:** Flow, Capillaries

553. ANSWER c. The tremendous number of capillaries (3 billion) provide a cross-sectional area of over one square meter. This tremendous cross-sectional area slows blood flow and allows time for O_2, CO_2, and nutrient transport between the blood

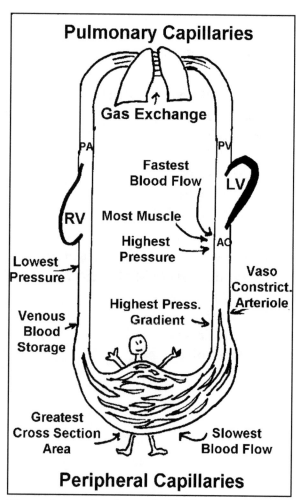

Hemodynamics through CV System

and the tissues.
See: Berne & Levy, chapter on "The Circuit." **Keywords:** cross section of capillary bed

554. ANSWER d. Arterioles are the "resistance vessels." They have precapillary sphincters that pinch off blood flow in response to intrinsic and extrinsic regulatory factors. Because these sphincters act as a stenosis, the pressure gradient is greatest across the arterioles.
See: Berne & Levy, chapter on "The Circuit." **Keywords:** Arterioles, Resistance

555. ANSWER b. Systemic veins are called the "capacitance vessels." When dilated the systemic veins can store 2/3 of the total blood volume. This tremendous reservoir can be liberated with exercise or vasoconstrictors. Venoconstriction is like a transfusion that provides more blood for the heart to pump. Excessive venodilation may rob blood from the heart and can pool enough blood to result in hypovolemic or neurogenic shock.
See: Berne and Levy, chapter on "The Circuit." **Keywords:** veins, blood storage

556. **Which of the following is primarily responsible for changing the pulsatile output of the heart into continuous smooth flow to the periphery?**
  a. **Low vascular resistance**
  b. **High vascular resistance**
  c. **Elastic recoil of the veins**
  d. **Elastic recoil of the arteries**

ANSWER d. The elastic recoil of the arteries absorbs the pulsatile ejection of blood out of the aorta. Its compliance acts to smooth out the arterial pressure, reduces the work of the heart, and assures continuous arterial flow during diastole. The vascular resistance at the arteriolar level drops the pressure and regulates the flow.
See: Berne & Levy, chapter on "Arterial System."
Keywords: smooth arterial flow due to elastic recoil of the arteries

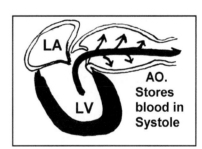

Aortic compliance

557. **Identify the hemodynamic characteristic of the area in the peripheral vascular system labeled at #2 (large arteries).**
  a. **Most pressure drop**
  b. **Largest cross section area (slowest flow)**
  c. **Capacity to store most blood**
  d. **Lowest blood pressure**
  e. **Fastest blood flow**
  f. **Most smooth muscle**

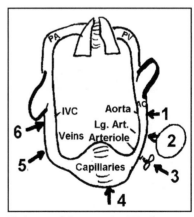

Points of Systemic Circ'n.

ANSWER f. Most smooth muscle. Large arteries have more smooth muscle than any other vessel. This gives them the strength they need to contain the high systemic blood pressure. **BE ABLE TO MATCH ALL ANSWERS.**
1. AO valve = fastest blood flow
2. Large arteries = most smooth muscle
3. Arterioles = most pressure drop
4. Capillary bed = largest cross section area (slowest flow)
5. Small and large veins = capacity to store most blood
6. IVC =SVC = lowest blood pressure

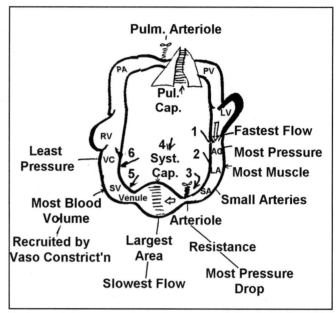

Points of Systemic Circulation

558. **In the supine individual, the lowest mean vascular blood pressure will be found in the:**
  a. Systemic arterioles
  b. Peripheral capillaries
  c. Pulmonary venules
  d. Superior vena cava

ANSWER d. Superior vena cava. Capillaries, venules and vena cava all normally have very low pressures. The highest BP is found in the AO. Pressures drop rapidly and become less pulsatile as the lumen size decreases. Arterioles drop the BP from around 70 mmHg in the small arteries to around 15 in the capillaries. For all venous blood, CS blood, and plasma to return to the IVC, SVC, and RA the mean pressure in these chambers must be the lowest. **See:** Berne and Levy, chapter on "The Circuit." **Keywords:** Arterioles, SVC, Lowest Pressure

2. Phases of Systole and Diastole (Wiggers)

559. **What phase of the cardiac cycle immediately follows closure of the AV valves and precedes the opening of the semilunar valves? All valves are closed as shown.**
  a. Atrial contraction
  b. Isometric contraction
  c. Isometric relaxation
  d. Systolic ejection period

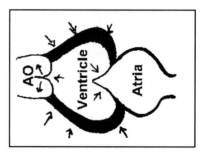

LV systole, valves closed

ANSWER b. Isometric contraction is the first part of systole. It starts at the peak of the ECG "R" wave. At the beginning of phase #1 the mitral valve snaps shut and the LV pressure builds up against closed valves (isometric contraction). Between #1 and #2 the semilunar valves open and systolic ejection occurs. Phases shown are:

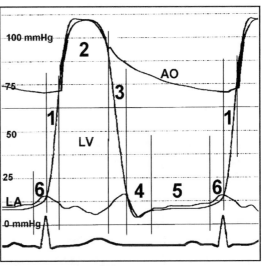
Wiggers Diagram

1. Isometric contraction
2. Systolic ejection
3. Isometric relaxation
4. Rapid diastolic filling
5. Diastasis or slow passive filling
6. Atrial contraction
Note: Diastolic filling is composed of phases #4, 5, & 6 above.
Be able to match all answers above.
See: Underhill's chapter on "The Cardiac Cycle"
Keywords: Isometric contraction follows AV valve closure

560. **On this Wiggers diagram identify the valve event labeled at #3.**

a. **Systolic ejection**
b. **AO valve opens**
c. **Diastolic filling**
d. **Mitral valve closure**
e. **Isometric contraction**
f. **AO valve closes**
g. **Isometric relaxation**
h. **Mitral valve opens**

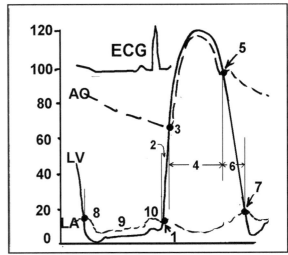
Wiggers Diagram: LV, LA, AO

ANSWER b. The aortic valve opens when the LV has built up enough pressure to equal or exceed aortic pressure. Note that all pressure crossover points are marked with a ●.
BE ABLE TO MATCH ALL ANSWERS.
   ● 1. MITRAL VALVE CLOSES.
          The QRS wave "fires" the ventricle and systole begins.
          Increasing LV pressure closes the mitral valve and -
      2. Isometric contraction builds up the LV pressure against closed valves.
          When the LV pressure equals the aortic pressure -
   ● 3. THE AORTIC VALVE OPENS
      4. Systolic ejection begins.
          When the LV begins relaxing the pressure falls until
   ● 5. THE AORTIC VALVE CLOSES.
      6. Isometric relaxation
          allows the LV pressure to fall to atrial level - at which point

- 7. THE MITRAL VALVE OPENS
  8. Rapid filling or *suction cup* filling occurs
  9. Diastasis is a slow or passive filling phase.
        Blood returning form lungs flows through the open mitral valve.
  10. Atrial contraction or kick
        When the ventricle is full, The QRS fires the ventricle and -
- 1. MITRAL VALVE CLOSES - and it start again...

This cycle is simultaneously occurring in the right heart. Just change the names of the chambers and valves. This cycle is the key to understanding pressure hemodynamics. **See:** Berne and Levy, Chapter on "Cardiac Pump." **Keywords::** Wiggers, AO Open

561. **Which of the following events begins isometric ventricular diastole?**
  a.   **Isometric contraction**
  b.   **Closing of semilunar valves**
  c.   **Opening of semilunar valves**
  d.   **Opening of AV valves**

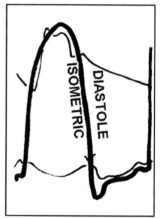

Ventricular diastole

ANSWER b. Closing of semilunar valves causes the dicrotic notch. Iso=constant, metric=measurement (volume). Isometric phases of the ventricle occur when both inlet and outlet valves are closed. The ventricle may contract (isometric contraction) or relax (isometric relaxation) but NO blood moves. These are the short phases of rapid ventricular pressure increase or decrease. The best way to study these phases is to memorize and be able to describe all phases on a Wiggers diagram. Be able to identify all cardiac phases. **See:** Underhill, chapter on "The Cardiac Cycle." **Keywords:** Isometric diastole begins with semilunar valves closing

562. **Identify the phase of LV diastole labeled at #3 on the diagram.**
  a.   **Atrial contraction**
  b.   **Isometric relaxation**
  c.   **Slow filling**
  d.   **Rapid filling**
  e.   **Closure mitral valve**
  f.   **Opening mitral valve**

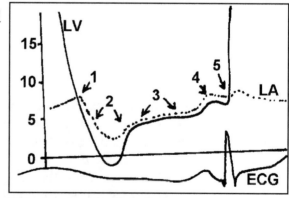

LV pressures in diastole

ANSWER c. Slow filling. As blood slowly returns from the lungs and LA it enters the LV through the open mitral valve. Slow filling is static. The term *diastasis* suggests no contraction or valve events.
BE ABLE TO MATCH ALL ANSWERS.
        1. The mitral valve opens
        2. The rapid filling phase "suction cup effect,"
        3. Slow filling (diastasis)

4. Atrial contraction (active filling)
5. The firing of the ventricle causes closure of the mitral valve.
Be fluent in all cardiac phases as shown in the Wiggers diagram.
See: Berne and Levy, chapter on "The Cardiac Pump." **Keywords:** Wiggers, diastolic phases

---

563. **The "Systolic Ejection Period" for the aortic valve area calculation is measured between the:**
   a.   **AO dicrotic notch to next AO upstroke**
   b.   **AO upstroke to next dicrotic notch**
   c.   **ECG "R" wave to next AO dicrotic notch**
   d.   **AO dicrotic notch to next ECG "R" wave**

ANSWER b. AO upstroke to next dicrotic notch. Systolic ejection time is measured between aortic valve opening and aortic valve closure. This time is measured after shifting the aortic pressure so that it is superimposed accurately on the LV tracing as shown. The SEP should be precisely measured horizontally between LV and AO pressure crossover points. This time interval must be measured accurately for the Gorlin aortic valve area formula.
See: Grossman, chapter on "Valve Area Calculation."
Keywords: Identify SEP

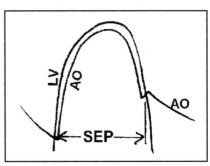
Systolic Ejection Phase

BOTH QUESTIONS BELOW REFER TO THIS DIAGRAM.

564. **This recording shows LA and LV pressures recorded simultaneously. What intracardiac event occurs at the pressure crossover point indicated at the arrows?**
   a.   **Mitral valve closes**
   b.   **Mitral valve opens**
   c.   **Diastolic filling begins**
   d.   **Systolic ejection begins**

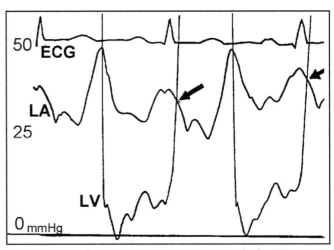
Simultaneous pressures recorded X50

565. **This simultaneous pressure tracing recorded above on x 50 shows:**
   a.   **Atrial fibrillation with pure mitral stenosis (MS)**
   b.   **Sinus rhythm with pure mitral regurgitation (MR)**
   c.   **Sinus rhythm with combined MS and MR**
   d.   **Atrial fibrillation with combined MS and AS**

BOTH ANSWERS APPEAR TOGETHER BELOW.

564. ANSWER a. Mitral valve closes. Immediately following the QRS complex, contraction begins. The LV pressure increases rapidly until it crosses and exceeds the LA pressure. Here the mitral valve closes. Valve events always occur at these crossover points. Mitral closure usually causes a "c" or "closure" wave on the atrial pressure curve - poorly seen here. Note the 20-30 mmHg LA-LV pressure gradient.
See: Kern, chapter on "Hemodynamics." **Keywords:** mitral closure at pressure crossover

565. ANSWER c. Combined MS and MR. Mitral stenosis is present because of the large 30 mm diastolic pressure gradient between LV and LA. Mitral regurgitation is probably present because of the 50 mm "V" waves. It is common for valves to show signs of both regurgitation and stenosis. This ECG shows sinus rhythm because "P" waves precede each QRS, and they result in an atrial "a" wave just before the first arrow.
See: Kern, chapter on "Hemodynamics." **Keywords:** Combined mitral stenosis and mitral regurgitation.

566. **The ending of the hearts isometric contraction phase is associated with:**
   a.   **Closure of mitral valve**
   b.   **Closure of AO valve**
   c.   **Opening of mitral valve**
   d.   **Opening of AO valve**

ANSWER d. Opening of AO valve. Isometric contraction elevates the ventricular pressure with the valves closed. As the LV pressure rises and exceeds aortic pressure the aortic valve opens - just as any swinging door opens when the pressure on one side is higher than on the other side. Each of the four pressure crossover points is associated with a valve opening or closing. Know the associated valvular events.
See: Berne and Levy, chapter on "Cardiac Pump." **Keywords:** Wiggers, Mitral Closure

567. **In the LV pressure - volume curve drawn in the box, what cardiac event occurs at #7 in the diagram?**
   a.   **Systolic ejection**
   b.   **AO valve opens**
   c.   **Diastolic filling**
   d.   **Mitral valve closure**
   e.   **Isometric contraction**
   f.   **AO valve closes**
   g.   **Isometric relaxation**
   h.   **Mitral valve opens**

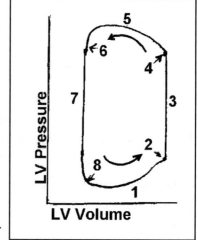

LV P-V Loop

ANSWER g. Isometric relaxation is the beginning of diastole. The heart relaxes after the AO valve closes. So the LV is relaxing without changing its volume - against closed valves. This rapid down slope of the LV pressure curve is termed "isotonic" or "isometric", because the volume is constant. LV pressure is still too high to allow the mitral valve to open. At point #8 the mitral valve opens and allows diastolic filling.

The pressure - volume loop is an X-Y plot of the LV pressure on the Y-axis against LV volume on the X-axis. The loop progresses counterclockwise representing all phases of LV hemodynamics. This graph may look foreign to you, but study it. Note how it resembles systole of an LV pressure (drawn on the right). The aortic valve opens in the upper right corner. If you reverse the systolic ejection phase of a pressure curve, it begins to resemble the top of the PV curve. Each corner is associated with a valvular event (marked with a •). Systolic ejection occurs in a right-left direction across the top of the box. **BE ABLE TO MATCH ALL ANSWERS.**

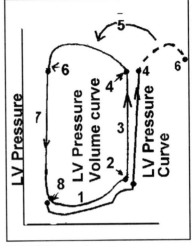

    1. Diastolic filling
    2. Mitral valve closure
    3. Isometric contraction
    4. AO valve opens
    5. Systolic ejection
    6. AO valve closes
    7. Isometric relaxation
    8. Mitral valve opens
See: Berne & Levy, chapter on "Cardiac Pump."
Keywords: Wiggers, PV Loop

LV PV loop & pressure

3. Arterial

568. **The arterial blood pressure wave shown at #4 in the drawing is termed the _____ wave/phase.**

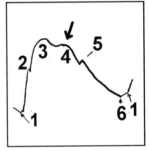

    a.   **Percussion wave (rapid systolic ejection)**
    b.   **Tidal wave (slow systolic ejection)**
    c.   **Dicrotic notch**
    d.   **Diastolic**
    e.   **Beginning systole**
    f.   **Anacrotic notch**

Arterial BP

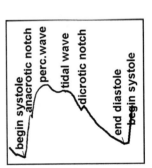

ANSWER b. Tidal wave. MATCH THE OTHER COMPONENTS OF THE ARTERIAL WAVE with their name below. **BE ABLE TO MATCH ALL ANSWERS.**

    1. Beginning systole: Initial upstroke of the pulse associated with opening of the aortic valve
    2. Anacrotic notch: occasionally seen on the upstroke of the arterial wave, associated with aortic stenosis and slowed ejection.
    3. Percussion wave (rapid systolic ejection)
    4. Tidal wave (slow systolic ejection) The tidal wave is the reflected percussion pulse returning after bouncing off the aorto-iliac bifurcation
    5. Dicrotic notch: The dicrotic notch or "incisura" is the slight back-flow of aortic blood that occurs with aortic valve closure, resulting in a rebound in aortic pressure when the back-flow of blood bounces off the slammed aortic valve. This notch is the

Arterial BP

critical landmark for inflation of aortic counter pulsation devices.

6. End diastole: ends ventricular filling associated with closure of AV valves. On the arterial waveform it occurs immediately before the beginning of systole. This is occasionally seen on pulse tracings as a slight dip just prior to the up stroke.

See: Kern's Chapter on "Pressure measurement." **Keywords:** Arterial, BP

569. The aortic dicrotic notch marks the beginning of ventricular:
   a.   RV systole
   b.   RV diastole
   c.   LV systole
   d.   LV diastole

ANSWER d. LV diastole. The dicrotic notch marks the beginning of diastole when the aortic valve closes. The first phase of diastole after the aortic valve closes is "isometric relaxation." The LV relaxes with diastole. Nevertheless, its pressure is not low enough yet to open the mitral valve and begin filling. The PA dicrotic notch would mark the beginning of RV diastole.

See: Kern, chapter on "Hemodynamics." **Keywords:** Dicrotic notch begins diastole

570. An arterial pulse which is felt as two distinct impulses during systole is termed pulsus _____ .
   a.   Alternans
   b.   Paradoxicus
   c.   Bisferiens
   d.   Bigeminus

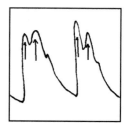
Double pulse

ANSWER c. Pulsus Bisferiens. This is a double systolic pulse (bi = 2). Both bumps occur before the dicrotic notch, which may look like a third hump. Pulsus Bisferiens is associated with both IHSS and AR. In IHSS/HOCM it is due to a double outflow of systolic blood where the subvalvular obstruction closes mid systole. (IHSS = Idiopathic Hypertrophic Subaortic Stenosis, or the modern term HOCM = Hypertrophic Obstructive CardioMyopathy). Aortic insufficiency has a characteristic water-hammer pulse (E.g. 180/50) which tends to overshoot systole and resonate in the aorta creating a double pulse. See arterial pulses in chapter B1.

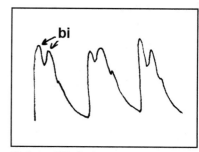
Pulsus Bisferiens

See: Braunwald chapter on "Physical Exam." **Keywords:** Pulsus Bisferiens

571. Closure of the aortic valve is associated with a hemodynamic:
   a.   "C" wave
   b.   "V" wave
   c.   Anacrotic notch
   d.   Dicrotic notch

ANSWER d. The dicrotic notch or "incisura" is the notch on the down slope of the great vessel pressures. It is sometimes called the "incisura." The incisura results from back flow of blood in the great vessel as each semilunar valve closes. The dicrotic notch (incisura) begins ventricular diastole. **See:** Braunwald, chapter on "Heart Sounds and Murmurs." **Keywords:** dicrotic notch = closing semilunar valves

572. **The dip in the downstroke shown at #1 on the arterial blood pressure curve is associated with _____.**

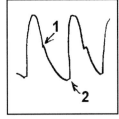

Arterial BP

    a.   **closure of semilunar valves**
    b.   **Closure of AV valves**
    c.   **Opening of semilunar valves**
    d.   **Opening of AV valves**

ANSWER a. Closure of semilunar valves. The "dicrotic notch" or "incisura" is the slight back-flow of aortic blood that occurs with aortic valve closure. It results in a rebound in aortic pressure when the back-flow of blood slams shut the aortic valve. This notch is the critical landmark for inflation of aortic counter-pulsation devices. #2 is the end diastolic point where the aortic valve opens and ejection begins.
See: Kern, chapter on "Pressure Measurement." **Keywords:** Arterial, BP

573. **Which arterial blood pressure is most typical of <u>normal</u> hardening of the arteries in an 80 year old American? (Assume a normal and constant CO.)**

    a.   **95/50 mmHg.**
    b.   **130/70 mmHg.**
    c.   **160/90 mmHg.**
    d.   **180/110 mmHg.**

ANSWER c. 160/90 mmHg. The systolic BP is very dependent on the compliance/stiffness of the aortic vessels. Rigid calcified arteries (as in ASHD) create a water hammer effect and dramatically raise systolic BP. Isolated systolic hypertension like this may be normal. After age 40 the normal systolic BP of 120 rises about 10 mmHg every 10 years of age. Thus an 80 year old's systolic BP will normally be 120 + 40 = 160 mmHg ± 10 mmHg. The diastolic and mean levels do not rise as much with age. They are more dependent on the arteriolar resistance. A normal ratio of systole to diastole about is 3:2. Thus, 120/80 mmHg is the normal ratio.

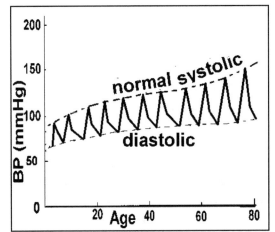

Normal range of BP with age
(After Guyton fig 15-8)

See: Berne and Levy, chapters on the "Arterial System" and Guyton, chapter on "Vascular Distensibility." **Keywords:** Arterial, BP, ASHD, Compliance

574. **Arterial PULSE PRESSURE is defined as the:**
a. **Difference between arterial and venous pressures**
b. **Difference between systolic and diastolic pressures**
c. **Highest point in the pulse wave**
d. **Average blood pressure**
e. **Peak to peak pressure gradient**

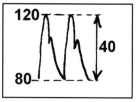

AO Pulse Pressure

ANSWER b. Difference between systolic and diastolic pressures. In a BP of 120/80 the pulse pressure is 120-80 or 40 mmHg. When we palpate a pulse, it is the pounding of this *pressure difference* we feel. Thus, a BP of 140/100 may be harder to palpate than a BP of 120/60 because the pulse pressure is lower - 40 verses 60 mmHg. **See**: medical dictionary. **Keywords**: Arterial, Pulse Pressure

575. **What is the PULSE PRESSURE of a recorded arterial pressure of 140/65,90?**
a. **50 mmHg**
b. **65 mmHg**
c. **75 mmHg**
d. **90 mmHg**

ANSWER c. 75 mmHg is the difference between systole and diastole. 140 - 65 = 75 mmHg pulse pressure. 90 is the mean BP.

4. Veins and Venous Return

576. **Identify the venous wave (trough) labeled #5 in this RA tracing.**
a. **"a" wave**
b. **"c" wave**
c. **"v" wave**
d. **"x" wave**
e. **"y" wave**

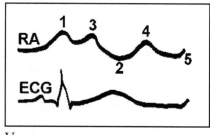

Venous pressure waves

ANSWER e. "y" wave. The positive waves are a, c, & v in alphabetic order. The negative waves are "x" and "y" again in alphabetic order. These negative waves are sometimes called "dips" or "troughs." Note that the pressures are normally slightly delayed from the ECG. Be able to match all venous waves to their letter. **BE ABLE TO MATCH ALL ANSWERS.**
   1. "a" positive wave - follows ECG "p" wave
   2. "x" negative wave - follows ECG "p" wave
   3. "c" positive wave - follows ECG "QRS" wave
   4. "v" positive wave - follows ECG "T" wave
   5. "y" negative wave - follows ECG "T" wave
See: Kern, chapter on "Hemodynamics." **Keywords**: Venous waves: a, c, v, x, y

577. **Identify the CAUSE of the positive venous wave labeled #1 in this PAW tracing.**
    a.   **Atrial contraction**
    b.   **Closure of mitral valve (beginning LV contraction)**
    c.   **Filling of ventricle against closed valve**
    d.   **Atrial relaxation & pulling down AV groove**
    e.   **Early rapid diastolic filling of LV (suction cup effect)**

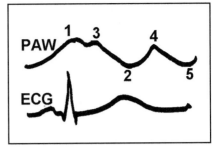

Venous pressure waves

ANSWER a. Atrial contraction. Remember the positive waves are a, c, & v and the negative waves are "x" and "y." Be able to identify these in comparison to the simultaneous LV pressure or ECG. **BE ABLE TO MATCH ALL ANSWERS.**
    1. "a" positive wave - follows ECG "p" wave, (Due to atrial contraction.)
    2. "x" negative wave - follows ECG "p" wave, is sometimes labeled the x' wave. (Due to atrial relaxation and pulling down of AV ring with ventricular systole.)
    3. "c" positive wave - follows ECG "QRS" wave, (Due to closure of the AV valve and ventricular contraction.)
    4. "v" positive wave - follows ECG "T" wave. It rises due to atrial filling against a closed AV valve. (It peaks at AV valve opening.)
    5. "y" negative wave - follows ECG "T" wave, (Due to earlY rapid diastolic filling)
Note that the wedge pressure is slightly delayed (0.1 sec) from the ECG (electrical always precedes mechanical). Be able to match all venous waves to their letter.
See: Kern, chapter on "Hemodynamics." **Keywords:** Venous waves: a, c, v, x, y

578. **This is a normal pulmonary artery wedge tracing (PAW). Significant elevation of the venous wave labeled #1 (following P wave) is associated with:**
    a.   **A "stiff heart" (noncompliant LV)**
    b.   **A-V valve stenosis (slow Y descent)**
    c.   **AV valve insufficiency**
    d.   **"Fusion" of atrial and ventricular contractions (cannon waves)**

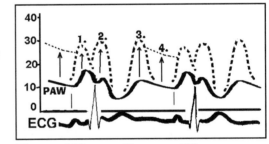

Elevated Venous Pressure Waves

ANSWER a. Elevated "a" wave associated with a "stiff noncompliant LV." When the LV begins to fail, the atrium comes to the rescue of the LV. The LV may need a good stiff "atrial kick" to give adequate preload. MATCH THE OTHER LABELED WAVES with their name. **BE ABLE TO MATCH ALL ANSWERS:**
    1. ELEVATED "A" WAVE = "STIFF NONCOMPLIANT HEART."
    Also, associated with LV hypertrophy, CHF, MS, MI, or other diseases that stiffen the heart.
    2. ELEVATED "C" =FUSION OF ATRIAL AND VENTRICULAR CONTRACTION (CANNON WAVES). Fusion of atrial and ventricular contractions during systole causes a large "cannon wave" which is evident in the

jugular pulse. This can also occur with heart block or fixed rate pacing when the atrial and ventricular complexes are dissociated.

3. ELEVATED "V" = AV VALVE INSUFFICIENCY: Here the atria fills antegrade from normal venous inflow and retrograde from a leaky AV valve. Pressure rises upstream to the leak.

4. ELEVATED OR GRADUAL DESCENT OF "Y" = A-V VALVE STENOSIS: The early ventricular filling is impaired because of A-V stenosis so the "y" descent (runoff) is slowed. This slow drop in atrial pressure or flow can be measured as the "pressure half time." A prolonged ½ time indicates A-V stenosis. This ½ time measurement on mitral flow is now routinely done by Doppler echocardiography to evaluate MS. Be able to match all abnormal venous waves to their letter.

See: Kern, chapter on "Hemodynamics." **Keywords:** Elevated venous waves: a, c, v, y descent

5. Preload and Wedge Pressure

579. The majority of ventricular filling results from:
  a. Closure of the AV Valves
  b. Opening of the semilunar valves
  c. Active atrial contraction
  d. Initial rapid inflow

ANSWER d. Initial rapid inflow. Most (60%) of the filling volume enters due to diastolic recoil of the ventricle. This rapid filling is termed the "suction cup effect." Although the pressure does not actually go negative, the ventricle recoils like the release a suction cup, drawing in blood from the atria.

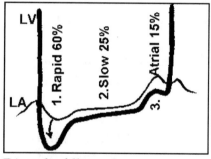

The phases of diastolic filling are:
  1. Rapid inflow: Suction cup effect, 60%
  2. Diastasis: Slow inflow, 25%
  3. Atrial kick: Active filling, 15-20%

Diastolic filling phases

See: Braunwald, chapter on "Cardiac Catheterization -Pressures." **Keywords:** Most diastolic filling is PASSIVE

580. When a patient goes from sinus rhythm into atrial fibrillation (as shown) and the heart rate stays the same, the cardiac output is expected to:
  a. Increase 5-10%
  b. Increase 15-25%
  c. Stay the same
  d. Decrease 5-10%
  e. Decrease 15-20%

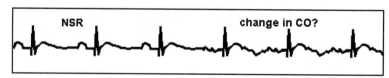

Sinus rhythm changing to atrial fibrillation

ANSWER e. Decrease 15-20% with loss of atrial kick. During diastole, atrial contraction kicks 15-20% more blood into the filling ventricle. Loss of P waves and atrial kick drops the cardiac output by the same amount. When a patient suddenly goes into atrial fibrillation and loses atrial kick, the stroke volume and cardiac output will drop 15-20%.

This phenomenon is seen in sinus bradycardia in ventricular pacemaker patients. When the pacemaker begins firing, the heart rate may increase. Because the patient loses atrial kick these patients may actually feel worse with VVI pacing. This is termed *pacemaker syndrome*. These patients benefit from modern DDD pacemakers which assure AV synchrony.

See: Underhill, chapter on "The Cardiac Cycle." **Keywords:** Preload, Atrial Kick

581. **At rest the mean PA Wedge pressure can be evaluated by monitoring the PA-EDP through a deflated Swan-Ganz catheter. This is possible because the PA end diastolic pressure at rest is normally and consistently _____ the mean wedge pressure.**
   a.   **1-4 mmHg lower than**
   b.   **10-15 mmHg lower than**
   c.   **Exactly equal to**
   d.   **1-4 mmHg higher than**
   e.   **20-15 mmHg higher than**

ANSWER d. 1-4 mmHg higher than. When evaluating LV preload with a Swan Ganz catheter it is often inconvenient to inflate the balloon each time you want a LV-EDP. It has been found that the blood flow through the pulmonary capillaries is so slow at the end of diastole that a small pressure gradient exists (normally, 1-4 mm Hg) between PA and LA. So, normally PA-EDP is 1-4 mmHg higher than the PA wedge. This is consistent for any one patient. So measure the PA-EDP and subtract that difference to get the estimated mean wedge pressure.

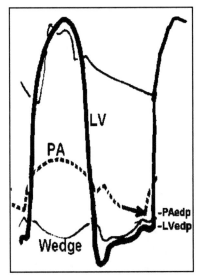

Diastolic equalization of LV, PA, & PAW

There are two exceptions to the 1-4 mmHg rule: lung disease and high CO. This small pressure difference elevates with high pulmonary vascular resistance as in chronic lung disease or ARDS. This happens because the tight arterioles/capillaries may act as a stenosis and create a pressure gradient across the lung bed. Normally the resistance in the lung bed is small. Second, the PA--wedge pressure difference may be elevated in high cardiac output states. The increased flow increases the pressure gradient across normal vasculature. This may occur in exercise, pregnancy, and when the HR is over 130 bpm. Both exceptions prove the truth of the equation:

Pressure gradient = CO x Resistance.
This is a form of Ohm's Law: V = I x R. Just remember Ohm's law then you won't have to memorize P = CO x R. CO is analogous to current flow (I) and Voltage is analogous to the fluid driving pressure or gradient (P) in (mmHg).

> ΔP = CO x Resistance
> Ohms Law: V = I x R

This insignificant normal difference between PA and wedge pressure is why cardiologists often record simultaneous LV-PA pressures. As shown in the diagram a

minimal gradient between PA-EDP and LV-EDP proves there is **no mitral stenosis.**
See: Daily chapter on "PA Pressure monitoring." **Keywords:** Wedge, PA pressure

582. **Which hemodynamic parameter best evaluates ventricular preload?**
a. **Cardiac output**
b. **Peripheral vascular resistance**
c. **Mean aortic pressure**
d. **LV end-diastolic pressure**

ANSWER d. LVEDP is a measure of LV preload. Like a balloon, the more you put into it, the higher the filling pressure gets. LA pressure, wedge pressure, and LV-EDV are also measures of preload. They quantitate how full the LV is packed with blood at the end of diastole. This preload level determines how hard the ventricle will contract based on Starling's Law.
See: Daily chapter on "PA Pressure monitoring." **Keywords::** Preload, LV-EDP

583. **PA wedge (or pulmonary capillary wedge) pressure normally reflects: (Select 2.)**
1. **Right ventricular end-diastolic pressure**
2. **Left atrial pressure**
3. **Left ventricular end-diastolic pressure**
4. **Pulmonary artery systolic pressure**
a. 1 & 2
b. 1 & 4
c. 2 & 3
d. 2 & 4

ANSWER c. Left atrial pressure (LA) and Left ventricular end-diastolic pressure (LV-EDP) are reflected in a wedge. This is a classic question. The wedged catheter cuts off PA flow and measures pressures through the capillary bed into the LA. Since the mitral valve is open in diastole, PAW also measures LV-end diastolic pressure. **See:** Daily, chapter on "Right heart catheterization." **Keywords::** Preload, Wedge, LA, PA-Edp

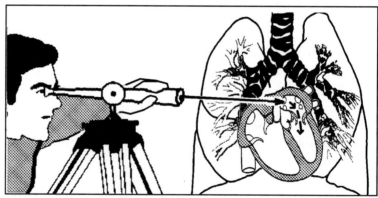
Wedge pressure looks through the lungs into LA & LV

6. Normal Heart Sounds

584. Which heart sound component, shown at the arrow, is normally delayed and splits off during inspiration?
a.   S1A (also termed A1)
b.   S1P (also termed P1)
c.   S2A (also termed A2)
d.   S2P (also termed P2)

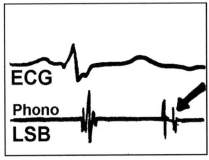
ECG and heart sounds

ANSWER d. S2P (also termed P2). The last component of the second heart sound is due to closure of the pulmonic valve. ("S" for sound, "2" for 2nd heart sound, "P" for pulmonary component) With inspiration more blood is sucked into the right heart and pulmonary ejection takes longer. **See:** Braunwald, chapter on "Heart Sounds and Murmurs." **Keywords:** S2P (also termed P2)

585. The second heart sound is caused by closure of what 2 valves?
a.   **Mitral and Tricuspid**
b.   **Mitral and Aortic**
c.   **Aortic and Pulmonic**
d.   **Pulmonic and Tricuspid**

ANSWER c. Aortic and Pulmonic. The closure of semilunar valves is the main cause of the second heart sound. Each semilunar valve has a distinct component of the second heart sound. Understand the cause and components of all 4 heart sounds.
See: Braunwald chapter on "Heart Sounds and Murmurs." **Keywords:** S2 = closure AO and pulmonic valve

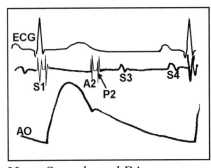
Heart Sounds and PA pressure

586. What valvular event is most closely associated with the dicrotic notch on the PA pressure tracing?
a.   Opening of aortic valve
b.   Opening of tricuspid valve
c.   Closure of tricuspid valve
d.   Closure of pulmonic valve
e.   Atrial contraction

ANSWER d. Closure of pulmonic valve. The PA dicrotic notch is similar to the aortic incisura, except it occurs after aortic closure, this normal delay in closure of the pulmonary valve accounts for the normal splitting of S2 with inspiration. The 2nd sound is normally A2 followed by P2.

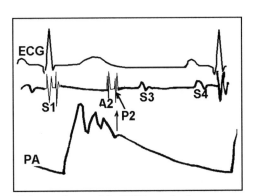
PA tracing with ECG and phono-

See: Braunwald, chapter on "Physical exam (auscultation)." **Keywords:** Arterial, PA, PV Closure

587. **Which heart valve is normally the first to open in systole and the last to close at the end of systole?**
  a.   Aortic
  b.   Mitral
  c.   Pulmonic
  d.   Tricuspid

ANSWER c. Pulmonic. In the beginning of systole the mitral valve closes 1st (MC) but it takes a long time to build up the LV pressure to aortic levels where the aortic valve opens (AOo). By the time it gets there, the pulmonic valve has already opened (Po), because the pressure does not have to rise as far. Pulmonary ejection takes longer because of the lower driving pressure.

At the end of systole the aortic valve closes 1st and the pulmonic 2nd - accounting for the normally split second heart sound (A_2-P_2) .

Understand thoroughly this Wiggers diagram of cardiac pressure interrelationships.
See: Kern, chapter on "Hemodynamics," diagram of simultaneous pressure happenings of all cardiac chambers. **Keywords**: Wiggers, AO open/close

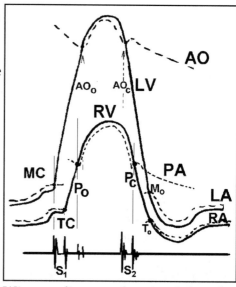

Wiggers diagram showing left and right side pressures with phono...

588. **This is a diagram of LV diastolic pressure, a phonocardiogram, and the ECG. Identify the heart sound labeled #4. It is associated with rapid LV filling.**
  a.   S1
  b.   S2
  c.   S3
  d.   S4
  e.   SC (systolic click)

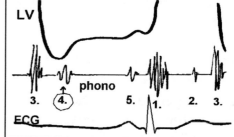

ECG, Heart Sounds and LV diast.

ANSWER c. S3 is also called proto-diastole (early diastole), rapid filling sound, or an S3 GALLOP sound. S3 occurs in the ventricle's early "Rapid filling phase." This sudden relaxation of the LV causes it to hit the chest wall and the sudden in rushing of blood through the mitral valve causes this low frequency filling sound.

S3 is associated with the y descent of the atrial pressure curve and the beginning diastolic dip in the LV pressure curve. The LV pressure may go negative and actually suck in blood from the LA - a "suction cup effect." Although normal in young individuals, it is abnormal in adults. Here a loud S3 is associated with diastolic overload and impaired LV

function. **MATCH THE OTHER HEART SOUNDS WITH THEIR NAME.**
1. S1 = 1st sound. Closure AV valves and systolic contraction.
2. SC = Systolic click due to tensing/prolapsing of chordae tendinea, associated with mitral valve prolapse.
3. S2 = 2nd sound. Closure Semilunar valves and dicrotic notch.
4. S3 = 3rd sound. Rapid filling sound due to rapid inflow of blood into LV. Suction cup effect.
5. S4 = 4th sound. Atrial contraction causes final rush of blood into LV just before LV contraction.
See: Braunwald, chapter on "The Physical Examination." **Keywords::** S3, Rapid fill.

589. Closure of the AV valves produces the:
a. First heart sound - S1
b. Second heart sound - S2
c. Third heart sound - S3
d. Forth heart sound - S4

ANSWER a. The first heart sound (S1) begins in systole. The AV valves snap shut. This is followed immediately by the semilunar valves opening. Be able to label and describe all 4 phases of the heart sounds, as well as the abnormal murmurs, valvular clicks and snaps. Relate each to the phases of the cardiac cycle.
See: Braunwald's chapter on "Heart Sounds." **Keywords:** Closure AV valves = S1

590. During the isometric phases of the left ventricle's heart cycle:
a. Only the mitral valve is open
b. Only the aortic valve is open
c. Both valves are open
d. Both valves are closed

ANSWER d. Both valves are closed. During isometric contraction, both valves are closed as the LV contracts to build it pressure up to that of the aorta. No blood enters or is ejected from the LV during this short period of time. Isometric means no change in volume. It is sometimes called the iso-volumetric period. During isometric relaxation, again both valves are closed as the LV relaxes. The pressure falls from aortic level to atrial level.
See: Todd's, CV Review Book: Vol. I, chapter on "Hemodynamics" **Keywords:** isometric

591. Match each heart sound to its cause:
1. Closing semilunar valves _____
2. Closing AV valves _____
3. Rapid LV filling _____
4. Atrial contraction _____
a.   S1
b.   S2
c.   S3
d.   S4

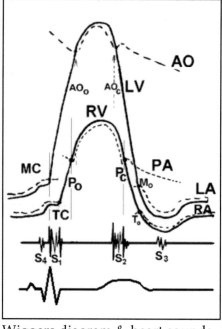

ANSWERS Be able to match all answers.
1. Closing semilunar valves = b. S2
2. Closing AV valves   = a. S1
3. Rapid LV filling   = c. S3
4. Atrial contraction   = d. S4

Wiggers diagram & heart sounds

S1 = 1st sound. Closure AV valves and systolic contraction.
S2 = 2nd sound. Closure semilunar valves and dicrotic notch.
S3 = 3rd sound. Rapid filling sound due to rapid inflow of blood into LV. Suction cup effect.
S4 = 4th sound. Atrial contraction causes final rush of blood into LV just before LV contraction. Be able to match all answers.
See: Braunwald, chapter on "The Physical Examination." **Keywords:** S1, S2, S3, S4

592. Splitting of the S2 sound during inspiration is due to a delay in:
a.   Opening of mitral valve.
b.   Closure of the mitral valve.
c.   Closure of the pulmonary valve.
d.   Opening of the tricuspid valve.

ANSWER c. Delay in closure of the pulmonary valve. The 2nd sound normally consists of aortic closure (A2) followed by pulmonary valve closure (P2). This normal delay in closure of the pulmonary valve accounts for the normal splitting of S2 with inspiration. It may be even further delayed in cases of volume overload of the RV as in ASD. Note in the diagram on previous page, how the S2p sound comes after the S2a sound. Pulmonary valve closure is later than **aortic closure. Note in the previous question the diagram shows the PA dicrotic notch following the aortic dicrotic notch. Thus P2 is normally split off from and follows A2. See:** Braunwald, chapter on "The Physical Examination."
Keywords: split S2, delayed pulmonary closure

593. The blood flow through the inferior vena cava and superior vena cava is termed the:
  a. Cardiac output
  b. Venous return
  c. Peripheral supply
  d. Regurgitant volume

ANSWER b. Venous return. The IVC and SVC return blood from the periphery to the RA. This return accounts for most of the cardiac output, with the exception of the coronary return, which is 5-10% of the CO. You can think of the heart as a single pump by ignoring the pulmonary circulation. Here the dark venous blood returns to the RA (venous return) and red arterial blood is pumped out the aorta (cardiac output). Of course these two normally match. Returning blood = outgoing blood.
See: Guyton, chapter on "Cardiac Output" **Keywords**: venous return

7. Pressures: Normal, Recording, Etc.

594. Cardiac pressure waveforms are normally read at three points. What three points are read on the right heart pressure labeled #1 in the diagram (PAW)?
  a. A wave, V wave, mean
  b. Systolic, begin diastolic, end-diastolic
  c. Systolic/diastolic, mean

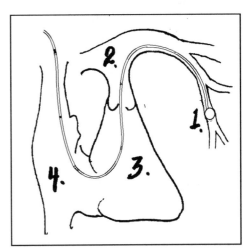

Right heart pressure sites

ANSWER: a. PAW = A wave, V wave, Mean. These three pressure points are read and reported on all atrial pressures PAW (LA) and RA.
MATCHED ANSWERS ARE:
  1. **PAW = A wave, V wave, Mean** - Read on all atrial pressures: (PAW, LA, and RA)
  2. **PA = Systolic/Diastolic, Mean** - Read on all arterial pressures (PA and AO)
  3. **RV = Systolic, Begin diastolic, End diastolic** - Read on all ventricular pressures (RV and LV)
  4. **RA = A wave, V wave, Mean** - Read on all atrial pressures (PAW, LA, and RA)
  Be able to match all answers above.
See: Company Literature **Keywords**: Read three pressure numbers

595. What are the average normal RA and LA pressure means respectively?
  (RA=_____ and LA=_____ in mmHg)
  a. 0, 2 mmHg
  b. 3, 8 mmHg
  c. 5, 15 mmHg
  d. 8, 20 mmHg

ANSWER b. 3, 8 mmHg. According to Kern, mean RA pressure is 2.8 mmHg (range 1-5) while mean LA pressure is 8 mmHg (range 2-12). This LA mean is the same as PA wedge pressure of 8 mmHg. Also memorize great vessel mean pressures (PA=15, AO=85). **See:** Kern or Grossman, normal pressure chart in their appendix. **Keywords:** Pressures, atrial

596. **What is the normal pressure found in the cardiac chamber labeled #2 in the diagram?**
a.   6/5/3 mmHg
b.   130/0/9 mmHg
c.   130/70/85 mmHg
d.   25/0/4 mmHg
e.   25/9/15 mmHg
f.   10/13/8 mmHg

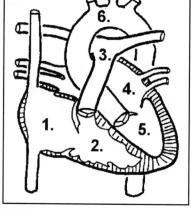

CV Pressures

ANSWER RV = d = 25/0/4 mmHg (systolic/begin diastolic/end diastolic). **BE ABLE TO MATCH ALL ANSWERS.**
    1. RA = 6/5/3 mmHg   (a/v/mean)
    2. RV = 25/0/4 mmHg   (s/bd/ed)
    3. PA = 25/9/15 mmHg   (s/ed/mean)
    4. LA = 10/13/8 mmHg   (a/v/mean)
    5. LV = 130/0/9 mmHg   (s/bd/ed)
    6. AO = 130/70/85 mmHg   (s/ed/mean)
See: Kern or Grossman, normal pressure chart in their appendix. **Keywords:** Pressures, RV pressure

597. **What normal cardiovascular pressure is recorded at #2 on the pullback shown?**
a.   RA
b.   RV
c.   PA
d.   PAW

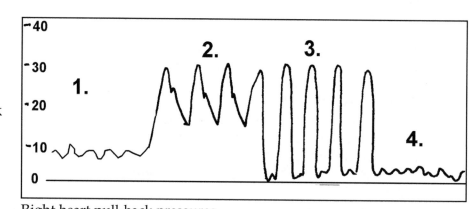

Right heart pull-back pressures

ANSWER c. PA
This sequence shows normal pressures recorded as a Swan-Ganz catheter pulls out of the right heart. **BE ABLE TO MATCH ALL ANSWERS:**
    1. = PAW (5-10 mmHg) pulmonary venous pressure reflecting LA
    2. = PA (25/10 mmHg) arterial triangular waveform
    3. = RV (25/5 mmHg) ventricular square waveform
    4. = RA (0-5 mmHg) systemic venous pressure
See: Grossman, chapter on "Balloon-tipped Flow-directed catheters" **Keywords:** Identify Swan pullback pressures ➔ PA

598. **Central venous pressure (CVP) is the same as _____ pressure.**
   a.   Left atrial pressure (LA)
   b.   Right atrial (RA)
   c.   Diastolic blood pressure (BP$_d$)
   d.   Left ventricular end-diastolic pressure (LV-EDP)

ANSWER b. CVP = RA or peripheral venous pressure. CVP can be measured by a water manometer in cm of water, or in mmHg by a transducer through the proximal port of a Swan-Ganz catheter. It is determined by the balance of blood volume, venous return and RV cardiac output. If venous return exceeds CO, the CVP increases. High CVP is associated with hypervolemia. Low CVP is associated with hypovolemia.
See: Underhill, chapter on "Hemodynamic Monitoring." **Keywords:** CVP = RA pressure

599. **A normal MEAN PA blood pressure is approximately:**
   a.   15 mm Hg
   b.   25 mm Hg
   c.   50 mm Hg
   d.   80mm Hg

ANSWER: a. 15 mm Hg. Kern gives normal PA values of 25/9/15 mm Hg. Remember the diastolic PA is close to the mean wedge pressure. This pressure is needed to calculate pulmonary vascular resistance. The higher the resistance, the higher the PA mean pressure.
See: Kern, chapter on "Hemodynamic Data" **Keywords:** nml. PA =25/9/15 mm Hg.

600. **On which of the following chambers is a mean pressure NEVER recorded?**
   a.   PAW
   b.   LV
   c.   AO
   d.   Femoral artery
   e.   None of the above

ANSWER b. LV. Ventricular pressures are never recorded with a mean. With ventricular pressures we only use the systolic and diastolic numbers. The "mean" of atrial and arterial pressures are essential for accurate calculation of vascular resistance. Note that mean is not one of the numbers read for ventricles, only systolic, beginning and end diastolic pressures. Whereas, with the inlet and outlet vessels the last number displayed is the always the "mean."
See: Kern, chapter on "Hemodynamics" **Keywords:** no ventricular mean pressure read

601. **Match the cardiac chamber or vessel labeled #4 in the diagram at the right with its usual pressure waveform shown below.**

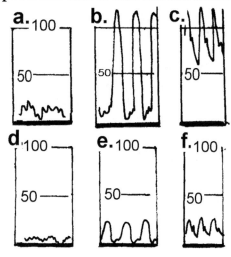

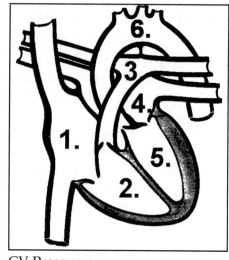

CV Pressures

Cardiac pressure waveforms x 100

ANSWER: a. #4 is the sinusoidal shaped LA or PAW pressure. It normally has the same pattern as the RA pressure, except it is about twice as high. The PAW pressure = 10 mmHg instead of 5 mmHg for the RA. These are the only 6 pressure waveforms normally found in the heart. You should be able to identify them by their shape, range, readings, and pullbacks. **BE ABLE TO MATCH ALL ANSWERS.**

1. RA = Sine wave shaped low pressure (0-5 mmHg)

2. RV = Rapidly rising and falling pressure, systolic pressure around 25 mmHg

3. PA = Triangular waveform with dicrotic notch, systolic pressure around 25

4. LA (PAW) = Sine wave shaped low pressure (5-10 mmHg)

5. LV = Rapidly rising and falling pressure, systolic pressure usually over 100

6. AO = Triangular waveform with dicrotic notch, systolic pressure usually over 100

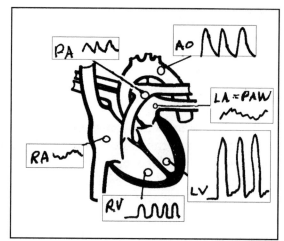

CV Waveforms

THE NEXT 2 QUESTIONS REFER TO THIS DIAGRAM.

602. What is the normal pressure found in the cardiac chamber labeled #5 in the diagram?

a. 6, 5, 3 mmHg
b. 130 / 0, 9 mmHg
c. 130 / 70, 85 mmHg
d. 25 / 0, 4 mmHg
e. 25 / 9, 15 mmHg
f. 10, 13, 8 mmHg

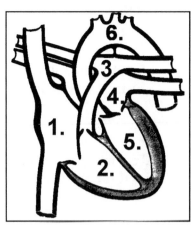
CV Pressures

ANSWER: b. 130 / 0, 9 mmHg (s/bd, e d)
BE ABLE TO MATCH ALL ANSWERS.
   1. RA = 6,5,3 mmHg (a, v, mean)
   2. RV = 25/0,4 mmHg (s/bd, ed)
   3. PA = 25/9,15 mmHg (s/ed, mean)
   4. LA = 10,13,8 mmHg (a, v , mean)
   5. LV = 130/0,9 mmHg (s/bd, e d)
   6. AO = 130/70,85 mmHg (s/ed, mean)
Know all the normal values for every cardiac chamber.
See: Todd, Vol 1, chapter on "Hemodynamics", also Kern, chapter on "Hemodynamics"
Keywords: normal pressure

603. Match the normal mean pressure range with the chamber labeled #3 (PAW) in the box.

a. 1-5 mmHg
b. 5-13 mmHg
c. 9-19 mmHg
d. 70-105 mmHg

MEAN PRESSURES
1. RA
2. PA
*3. PAW
4. AO

ANSWER: b. 5-13 mmHg. According to Kern, mean LA or PAW pressure is 5-13 mmHg (average 9 mmHg). This diagram shows the normal range of pressures in the four chambers where "means" are recorded. [low mean - (average mean) - high mean range]. The average mean numbers (in parentheses or with lines over them) are the most important numbers to remember.
BE ABLE TO MATCH ALL ANSWERS:
<u>NORMAL MEAN PRESSURE RANGES</u>
1. RA = 1-(3)-5 mmHg
2. PA = 9-(15)- 19 mmHg
3. PAW = 5-(9)- 13 mmHg
4. AO = 70-(80) -105 mmHg
See: Kern or Grossman, normal pressure chart in their appendix **Keywords:** atrial pressures

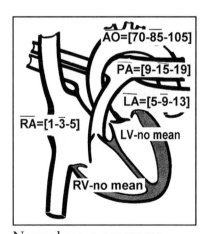
Normal mean pressures

604. **PA wedge (or pulmonary capillary wedge) pressure readings are normally the same as the:**
   a. **Right ventricular diastolic pressure**
   b. **Left atrial pressure**
   c. **Central venous pressure**
   d. **Pulmonary artery systolic pressure**

ANSWER b. Left atrial pressure. This is a classic question found on every hemodynamic exam. The wedged catheter cuts off PA flow and measures pressures through the capillary bed to the LA. Since the mitral valve is open in diastole, PAW and LA both measure the important LV-end diastolic pressure. LV-EDP is one of the best indicators of left sided preload.
See: Daily, chapter on "Right Heart Catheterization" & Todd Vol 1   **Keywords:** preload, wedge, LA, PA-EDP

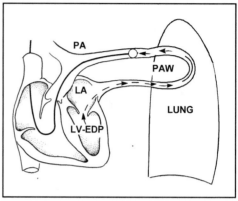

PA Wedge pressure = LA = LV-EDP

605. **This diagram shows normal pressures from a Swan-Ganz catheter insertion. What pressure is recorded at #2 on the diagram?**
   a. **RA**
   b. **RV**
   c. **PA**
   d. **PAW**

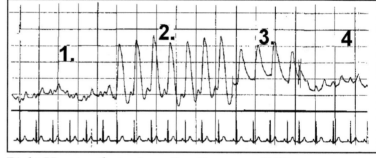

Right Heart catheter insertion Pressures X 50

ANSWER: b. RV   This sequence shows normal pressures recorded as a Swan-Ganz catheter is inserted into the right heart. Balloon insertion sequence is RA➔RV➔PA➔PAW. Note how the tracing begins and ends with a venous tracing. Be able to identify all right heart pressures on insertion or pull back.

BE ABLE TO MATCH ALL ANSWERS.
1. = RA (5 mmHg) also termed CVP
2. = RV (23/5 mmHg)
3. = PA (20/10 mmHg)
4. = PAW (10 mmHg) also termed PCW or just "Wedge"
See: Grossman, chapter on "Balloon-tipped Flow-directed Catheters" **Keywords:** identify Swan pullback pressures

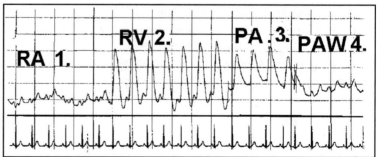

Right Heart catheter insertion Pressures X 50

8. Other

606. **The greatest expenditure of O2 during the cardiac cycle is used to:**
a.   Build up LV pressure (isometric contraction)
b.   Eject blood out of the LV and into the AO
c.   Open the mitral valve (diastolic filling)
d.   Overcome the friction of blood viscosity and muscle compliance

ANSWER a. Build up LV pressure. Most of the work of the LV is to build up enough pressure to open the aortic valve (isometric contraction). This isometric "pressure" work accounts for 90% of the work done by the LV. The remaining 10% is the "volume work" of ejecting the stroke volume.

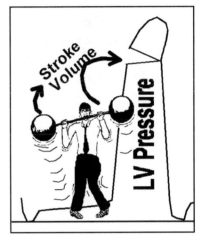
Pressure work: building up LV pressure prior to ejection

It's like lifting a 100 lb. weight, and then dropping it into a high net. All the work is in lifting the weight. The work of pushing a stoke volume across the aortic valve is small compared to the work of raising the pressure high enough to open the aortic valve.

To help reduce pressure work the balloon pump is often used. It lowers the aortic diastolic pressure just before the aortic valve opens. This is analogous to lowering the net in the diagram. **See:** Quall, chapter on "Myocardial Excitation" **Keywords:** greatest expenditure of O2 during isometric contraction

607. **The amount of blood pumped from each ventricle during a single systole is the:**
a.   Cardiac output
b.   Cardiac index
c.   Stroke volume
d.   Stroke index

ANSWER c. Stroke volume is the amount of blood the heart pumps with each beat. This can be calculated from the Cardiac Output (CO) and Heart Rate (HR)

    SV = CO/HR
    E.g. (4900 ml/min) / (70 beats/min) = 70 ml/beat.
It can also be calculated from the LV angiographic volumes as the difference between the full ventricle (EDV) and the almost empty ventricle (ESV).

    SV = EDV - ESV
    E.g. 150 ml - 80 ml = 70 ml

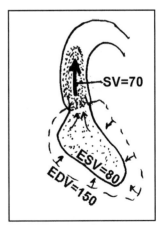
SV = EDV - ESV

Stroke volume adjusted to body size is termed "Stroke Index". It is stroke volume divided by the person's body surface area.

    SI = SV/BSA
These essential terms and formulas must be memorized.
See: Kern, chapter on "Hemodynamics." **Keywords:** Define stroke volume

608. **The formula to calculate cardiac output from hemodynamic data is:**
   a.   CO = (LVEDP) x SVR
   b.   CO = SV / EDV
   c.   CO = SV x HR
   d.   CO = HR x mean BP

ANSWER c. CO = SV x HR. Stroke volume times heart rate. Since SV is the amount pumped per beat, and HR is the number of beats/min, the product is amount pumped/min. SV is usually measured in ml/beat, HR in beats/min.
   CO = SV ml/beat x HR b/min = ml/min
   To change into L/min, divide by 1000 ml/L
E.g. CO = SV x HR = (70 ml/beat) x (70 beats/min) / (1000 ml/L) = 4.9 L/min.
Cardiac Output adjusted to body size is termed "Cardiac Index". It is cardiac output divided by the person's body surface area.
   CI = CO/BSA
See: Braunwald, Chapter on "Evaluation of LV Function." **Keywords**: LV Performance, dP/dt

609. **Calculate the ejection fraction of the patient above, where EDV = 150 ml and ESV = 80 ml.**
   a.   47%
   b.   53%
   c.   56%
   d.   70%

ANSWER a. 47%. Ejection fraction is the ratio of stroke volume to end-diastolic volume. It is the ratio of the amount pumped to the total filled volume. Because the denominator EDV is dependent on body size, it need not be adjusted to BSA. Normal is 70-85%. When it falls below 50%the heart is probably in failure. EF is the most important measure of LV function, and a vital number to know before heart surgery is performed. It may be measured by angiographic, ultrasound, or nuclear methods.
The ejection fraction calculation is made as follows:

$$EF = SV/EDV$$

   SV = EDV - ESV = 150-80 = 70 ml
   EF = SV/EDV   = 70/150 = .466 = 47% (below normal)
See: Braunwald, chapter on "Evaluation of LV Function." **Keywords**: calculate EF

610. **The maximum slope of the LV pressure curve is termed:**
   a.   Ejection fraction
   b.   LV-EDP
   c.   PEP/LVET
   d.   dP/dT

ANSWER d. The dp/dt comes from delta P/delta T or change in pressure over time. It is a good index of LV contractility but must be measured with catheter tip manometers (Millar brand) to be accurate. Maximum LV dp/dt is measured at the steepest slope occurring in isometric contraction. It should be over 1200 mmHg/sec. This means that theoretically, if the LV was pressed to contract at its maximum for one second, the resulting BP would be 1200 mmHg.
See: Braunwald, chapter on "Evaluation of LV Function."
Keywords: LV performance, dp/dt

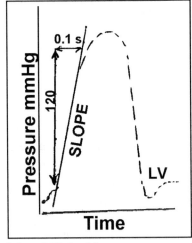

Max. LV dp/dt

611. **Inspiration normally results in an immediate _____ in intracardiac pressure and a/an _____ in venous return.**
    a.   Increase,   Increase
    b.   Increase,   Decrease
    c.   Decrease,   Increase
    d.   Decrease,   Decrease

ANSWER c. Decrease, Increase. The intracardiac pressures all drop immediately by the amount of the negative inhalation. Pressures drop with the diaphragm. This negative pressure sucks blood into the thorax and RA with inspiration and increases venous return. It also reflexively increases the heart rate. Within a few seconds the increased venous return will increase the output of the left heart and BP (unless followed immediately by another inspiration). **See:** Braunwald, chapter on "Auscultation."
Keywords: Venous Return, Inspiration

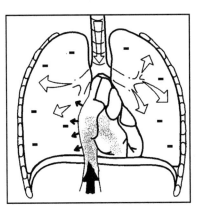

Inspiration sucks in venous return

612. **How does mechanical ventilation and positive pressure breathing affect a patient's hemodynamics?**
    a.   Decreased venous return
    b.   Increased contractility
    c.   Increased preload
    d.   Decreased afterload

ANSWER a. Decreased venous return. Any increase in lung pressure will reduce venous return from the extra thoracic veins and may impair CO. Lung pressure is normally negative, but mechanical ventilation makes it POSITIVE. IPPB, and PEEP all push gases into the lungs, bypassing the normal mechanisms. Positive pressure

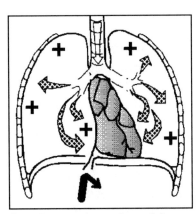

Positive pressure breathing

breathing may actually compress the RA and RV impairing venous return. This becomes especially important in CHF patients who already have high venous pressures and reduced venous return. One new form of CPR actually uses a suction cup on the chest to pull the thoracic pressure negative with inspiration.
See: Daily, chapter on "Intensive Care Monitoring." **Keywords::** Venous return, IPPB

613. **What is the result of a sustained Valsalva maneuver (bearing down) on the heart? It _____ the blood pressure by _____ venous return.**
  a.   **Increases,   Increasing**
  b.   **Increases,   Decreasing**
  c.   **Decreases,   Increasing**
  d.   **Decreases,   Decreasing**

ANSWER d. Decreases, Decreasing. Straining as during coughing and defecation is termed the Valsalva's maneuver. Sustained expiratory efforts increase intra-thoracic pressure and thereby impede venous return reducing CO

Cough CPR acts as an auxiliary pump in cardiac arrest. Here blood is propelled to the brain and extra-thoracic tissues because the increased intrathoracic pressure is transmitted to the arteries - but not the veins. **See:** Berne & Levy, chapter on "Cardiac Output." **Keywords:** Other, Valsalva, venous return, CO

614. **This is a BP recorded during Valsalva straining and release in a normal person. What causes the phase labeled at #3 in the box?**
  a.   **Thoracic pressure drops**
  b.   **Venous return increases with inspiration**
  c.   **Increased thoracic pressure**
  d.   **Venous return is impeded.**

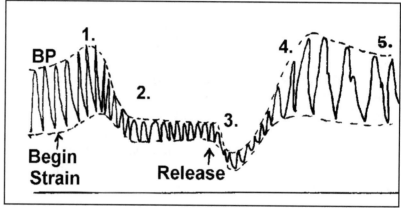
Effect of Valsalva maneuver on BP

ANSWER a = BP drops as thoracic pressure drops with Valsalva release and inspiration. Phases #1 and #3 are not reflexes, but only a reflection of the thoracic pressure.

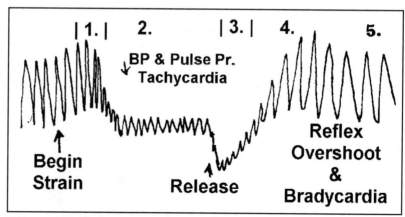
Effect of Valsalva maneuver on BP

Phases #2 and #4 are reflexes due to altered venous return (Starling's effect). In severe LV dysfunction disease the Valsalva response is relatively flat. Valsalva does not drop BP but increases it slightly in a "square wave response."

BE ABLE TO MATCH ALL ANSWERS:
 1. BP reflects increased thoracic pressure (straining)
 2. Venous return is impeded. BP and CO fall (Starling's law)
 3. BP drops as thoracic pressure drops suddenly with release and inspiration
 4. Reflexive overshoot of BP and bradycardia as venous return increases with inspiration
 5. BP normalizes

See: Berne & Levy, chapter on "The Circuit." **Keywords:** Valsalva phases

615. **"Indexed" hemodynamic parameters like "Stroke Index" are corrected for the patient's:**
 a. Age and sex
 b. Ideal body weight
 c. Height in cm.
 d. Body surface area

ANSWER d. Body surface area is what many cardiac parameters are "indexed" to, because it has been found to be the most closely correlated with body size. Thus, cardiac index and stroke index are the parameters divided by BSA. A normal adult males's BSA is about 2.0 square meters. Normal BSA can be found by plotting the patient's height and weight on a nomogram or using the Du Bois formula: $0.007184 \, Wt^{.425} \times Ht^{0.725}$.
See: Tortora, chapter on "Cardiovascular System: Blood Vessels." **Keywords:** BSA

616. **Most physiologic measurements are adjusted to a patient's body size (indexed) by:**
 a. Multiplying it times body surface area (BSA)
 b. Dividing it the body surface area (BSA)
 c. Multiplying it times body weight in Kg.
 d. Dividing it by body weight in Kg.

ANSWER b. By dividing by the body surface area (BSA). Then it is *indexed*. Most physiological measurements increase as the size of the person increases. Indexing adjusts the measurement so that it can then be compared to a normal population of people irrespective of body size. For example, cardiac output (CO) adjusted to body size is termed cardiac index (CI). It is simply cardiac output divided by the person's body surface area: CI = CO / BSA.

 BSA is read from a nomogram or formula after plotting the person's height and weight. BSA is a more accurate index of body size than just weight alone. Any term with the word "index" behind it means it has been divided by BSA. Some hemodynamic measures are not indexed, such as: HR, BP, and ratios such as Qp/Qs. **See:** Braunwald, chapter on "Evaluation of LV Function." **Keywords:** CI, index adjusts for body size

617. The normal resting cardiac output varies with age, position, and BSA. Estimate the normal resting cardiac index (CI) for patient #3 (reclining 70 year old adult) in the box.

1. Reclining 7 year old child
2. Standing 7 year old child
*3. **Reclining 70 year old adult**
4. Standing 70 year old adult

    a.   2.0 L/min/M^2
    b.   2.5 L/min/M^2
    c.   3.5 L/min/M^2
    d.   4.5 L/min/M^2

ANSWER b. 2.5 L/min/M^2. Grossman says, "The normal cardiac output appears to vary with age, steadily decreasing from approximately 4.5 L/min/M^2 at age 7 to approximately 2.5 L/min/M^2 at age 70... In addition to age, cardiac output is affected by posture, decreasing approximately 10% when rising from a lying to a sitting position and approximately 20% when rising (or after being tilted) from a lying to a standing position. Also, body temperature, anxiety, environmental heat and humidity, and a host of other factors influence the normal resting cardiac output."

    Normal reclining CI declines with age from 4.5. to 2.5 L/min/M^2. Thus the overall average CI for a reclining middle aged individual is around 3.5 L/min/M^2.
BE ABLE TO MATCH ALL ANSWERS BELOW.
    1. Reclining 7 year old child = 4.5 L/min/M^2 (children have high metabolic rate)
    2. Standing 7 year old child = 3.5 L/min/M^2 (reduced 20% from reclining CI)
    3. Reclining 70 year old adult = 2.5 L/min/M^2
    4. Standing 70 year old adult = 2.0 L/min/M^2 (reduced 20% from reclining CI)
See: Baim and Grossman, chapter on "Blood Flow Measurement." **Keywords:** normal CI declines with age from 4.5 to 2.5 L/min/M^2.

618. Which normal individual would be expected have the highest cardiac index?
    a.   **Reclining 6 year old child**
    b.   **Standing 6 year old child**
    c.   **Reclining 60 year old adult**
    d.   **Standing 60 year old adult**

ANSWER a. Reclining 6 year old child normally have a CI of 4.5 L/min/M^2. Children have higher metabolic rates than older individuals. Also, reclining elevates CO about 20% from the standing position.

    Remember CI is indexed to body size by M^2 which is supposed to adjust heart performance to the size of the person. In this way changes in cardiac performance can be more fairly compared among individuals. Thus, resting CI should not change between large and small normal people, but will change with disease, posture, age, drugs, etc.
See: above question **Keywords:** normal CI highest in reclining child

619. The normal male adult (70 years old) reclining cardiac output is:
    a.   2-4 L/min
    b.   4-5 L/min
    c.   1.0 Mets
    d.   3.5 Mets

ANSWER b. 4-5 L/min. Grossman gives a normal adult resting supine CI is 2.5 L/min/M^2. Using normal body BSA's between 1.5 - 2. M^2 and multiplying times the normal CI of 2.5 yields an average CO of 3.75 - 5 L/min. or approximately 4-5 L/min. The resting reclining CO would be higher for younger individuals. See previous question.

A met is a basal metabolic rate based on individual size. One met is equal to a unit of resting oxygen consumption measuring approximately 3.5 O2/Kg/min. Mets are used to evaluate exercise level not resting CO.

See: Braunwald's, Heart Disease chapter on "Assessment of Cardiac Function" and Baim and Grossman, chapter on "Blood Flow measurement." **Keywords:** normal CI

620. **The formula for stroke volume (SV) is:**
   a.   **CO/HR**
   b.   **HR/CO**
   c.   **CO/BSA**
   d.   **CO x HR**

ANSWER a. CO/HR = SV. The stroke volume is the amount of blood ejected by the ventricle in one beat. Since Cardiac Output = Stroke Volume x Heart Rate the formula can be rearranged to give SV=CO/HR. Eg., if CO = 4900 ml/min and HR = 70/min; SV = 4900/70 = 70 ml/beat.

See: Tortora, chapter on "Cardiovascular System: Heart." **Keywords:** stroke volume

621. **The formula for arterial compliance is:**
   a.   **dP/dV**
   b.   **dV/dP**
   c.   **dP/Q**
   d.   **Q/dP**

ANSWER b. dV/dP. Soft compliant balloons blow up easily. Stiffness is the reciprocal of compliance. Compliance of the ventricle decreases during acute myocardial infarction. This makes LV filling more difficult. The filling pressure must increase to get the same volume of preload - thus high PA wedge pressures. Know the formula: Compliance = ΔV/ΔP, or dV/dP. Don't confuse this with the LV contractility measure dP/dT. **See:** Medical Dictionary **Keywords:** compliance

622. **What phases of the LV cardiac cycle normally have the fastest blood flow? Forward systolic flow is greatest immediately after the _____, and inward diastolic filling is greatest following the_____:**
   a.   **Isometric contraction, Isometric relaxation**
   b.   **Isometric contraction, P wave**
   c.   **Dicrotic notch, Isometric relaxation**
   d.   **Dicrotic notch, P wave**

ANSWER a. Isometric contraction, Isometric relaxation. First the QRS fires, then the LV pressure builds up during isometric contraction. Then the aortic valve opens and blood is rapidly ejected during the first phase of systole. When the T wave initiates relaxation, isometric relaxation allows the LV pressure to drop to atrial level. Then the mitral valve opens and allows rapid diastolic filling. This is also termed the suction cup effect because the LV is squeezed down and ready to suck in blood from the LA. Then there is a slow period of filling, followed by the p wave and the atrial kick which pushes another 25% more blood into the ventricle. **See:** Underhill's chapter on "The Cardiac Cycle." and http://library.med.utah.edu/kw/pharm/hyper_heart1.html **Keywords:** Greatest flow follows isometric phases

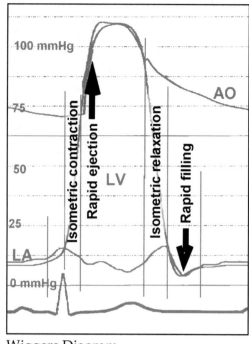

Wiggers Diagram

623. **End diastolic volume, end diastolic pressure and the length of the resting sarcomere are all measures of:**
   a.   **LV contractility**
   b.   **LV preload**
   c.   **Afterload**
   d.   **Valve competence**

ANSWER b. LV preload. The resting sarcomere fiber length can be stretched with increased preload. The end diastolic volume (EDV) fills the LV. This increases the end-diastolic pressure (EDP). The LV-EDP is most commonly measured as mean PA wedge pressure. Increased filling of the LV increases resting fiber length and preload. According to Starling's Law, the greater the preload or stretch - the greater is the force of contraction. **See:** Todd's, CV Review Book: Vol. I **Keywords:** preload

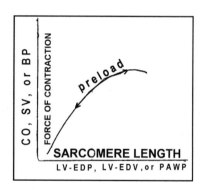

624. These Starling curves are from a patient in CHF. He is at point A and is experiencing symptoms of mild dyspnea. Which management regimen below would move him to point #1 on the curve?

a. VOLUME EXPANSION: or increased salt intake
b. DECOMPENSATION: continued deterioration
c. DIURETIC: or Na restricted diet
d. DIGITALIS: or other inotropic drug

Starling curves in CHF

ANSWER d. DIGITALIS: or other inotropic drug such as dobutamine. These curves can be divided into 4 quadrants called the "Forrester Subsets" described below.

BE ABLE TO MATCH ALL ANSWERS BELOW.

1. DIGITALIS - Increased Contractility: or other inotropic drug such as a catecholamine. This will move him to a higher contractile state - a whole higher "supercharged" curve. Dig. will move up the CO and down the wedge pressure which will help the dyspnea.

2. VOLUME EXPANSION - Increased Preload: or increased salt intake, veno-constriction, continued IV infusions. These do not move him to a new contractile state - only moves up the preload along the same curve to point #2. May increase CO slightly but also moves up the wedge pressure above the acute pulmonary edema point.

3. DECOMPENSATION - Decreased contractility: continued deterioration - no therapy. The patient deteriorates to a lower LV function curve.

4. DIURETIC - decreased preload: or Na restricted diet or veno-dilator to pool venous blood away from the main circulating volume. Moving down the same contractility curve will reduce wedge pressure and CO. The patient will breathe better, but may feel more tired.

Note how the best therapy may be to combine #one (Digitalis) with #4 (Diuretic). This would move the patient to the higher curve and move him down that curve to a new point not shown on the diagram, but on the far left of the upper curve. Know these abnormalities of the Starling curve, as therapy is based on it.

See: Underhill, chapter on "Heart Failure", also, Todd, Vol. I,   **Keywords:** Rx for acute CHF, Starling curves

REFERENCES

Baim, D. S. and Grossman W., Cardiac Catheterization, Angiography, and Intervention, 7th Ed., Lea and Febiger, 2006

Pappano & Wier, Cardiovascular Physiology, 10th Ed., Mosby Year Book, 2013

Braunwald, Eugene, et al., Ed., HEART DISEASE A Textbook of Cardiovascular Medicine, 8th Ed., W. B. Saunders Co., 2012

Daily, E. K., and Schroeder, J. S., *Techniques in* Darovic, G.O., *Hemodynamic Monitoring: Invasive and No Bedside Hemodynamic Monitoring,* 4th Ed., C. V. Mosby Company, 1989

Darovic, .O., Hemodynamic Monitoring, *Ininvasive and Noninvasive Clinical Application,*WB Saunders, 1995

Kern, M. J., Ed., The Cardiac Catheterization Handbook, 6th Ed., Mosby-Year Book, Inc., 2016

Quall, S. J., *Comprehensive Intra-aortic Balloon Pumping,* CV Mosby Co., 1984

Taylor, E. J. Ed., *Dorland's Medical Dictionary,* 27th ed., W. B. Saunders Co.,1988

Tortora, G. J., *Introduction to the HUMAN BODY,* Harper and Row Pub., 1988

Underhill, S. L., Ed., *CARDIAC NURSING,* 2nd Ed., J. B. Lippincott Co., 1989

Wiggers diagram: http://library.med.utah.edu/kw/pharm/hyper_heart1.html

OUTLINE: B6 - Hemodynamics & Pressures Basics

1. **THE CIRCUIT**
   a. Pulmonary Circulation
   b. Systemic Circulation
      i. Arteries
         (1) Highest Blood velocity (AO)
         (2) Most Elastic Tissue (AO)
         (3) Thickest smooth muscle
      ii. Arterioles
         (1) highest resistance
         (2) highest pressure gradient
      iii. Capillary bed
         (1) Blood velocity, slowest
      iv. veins
         (1) Capacitance
         (2) Highest blood storage
2. **WIGGERS, PHASES**
   a. Wiggers pressure interrelationships
      i. Mitral valve closure
      ii. Isometric contraction
      iii. AO valve opens
      iv. Systolic ejection period
      v. AO valve closes
      vi. Isometric relaxation
      vii. Mitral valve opens
      viii. Diastolic filling period
      ix. Phases of diastole
      x. Isometric Relaxation
      xi. Mitral valve opens
      xii. Rapid filling phase
         (1) "suction cup effect,"
      xiii. slow filling (diastasis)
      xiv. atrial contraction (active filling)
      xv. closure of the Mitral valve
   b. Atrial kick
      i. 15-25% of preload
   c. Pressure volume curve
      i. Mitral valve closure
      ii. Isometric contraction
      iii. AO valve opens
      iv. Systolic ejection
      v. AO valve closes
      vi. Isometric relaxation
      vii. Mitral valve opens
      viii. Diastolic filling
3. **ARTERIAL**
   a. Arterial Waves
      i. Percussion wave (rapid systolic ejection)
      ii. Tidal wave (slow systolic ejection)
      iii. Dicrotic notch = incisura
      iv. Diastolic
      v. Beginning systole
      vi. Anacrotic notch

   b. Pulse Pressure = syst. - diast.
   c. Arterial elastic recoil
      i. Windkessel, hydraulic filter
   d. Arterial waveform abnoralities
      i. Bisferiens,
      ii. Bigeminal
      iii. Pulsus paradox
      iv. Pulsus alternans
   e. Blood pressure
      i. Rises with age 10 mmHg/10yr
4. **VEINS, VENOUS RETURN**
   a. Venous pressure waves
      i. a, c, v x, y
      II. Abnormal venous waves
      iii. Pathology of elevated a, c or v
   b. Capacitance vessels
      i. venodilation
      ii. blood storage
      iii. compliance
   c. Pressure (lowest in SVC/IVC)
   d. Venous return, to rt. Ht.
      i. muscular pump
      ii. inspiration (increased return)
5. **WEDGE, PRELOAD**
   a. Normal:
      i. EDV
      ii. LVEDP
         (1) Relationship to LA
         (2) Wedge
         (3) PA-EDP
   b. Preload
      i. Starlings Law
      ii. Measured as PAW
      iii. Filling pressures
6. **Normal Heart Sounds**
   a. Identify S1, S2, S3. S4
   b. components of S1 & S2
   c. causes of heart sounds & gallops
   d. associate sounds, pressures, ECG
7. **PRESSURES: NORMALS,**
   a. Normal
      i. LA, LV, AO
      ii. IVC, RA, RV, PA, PAW
   b. Pullback pressures
      i. Right heart pullback
         (1) PAW, PA, RV, RA
      ii. Left heart pullback
         (1) LV, AO
8. **OTHER**
   a. Valsalva Effects on BP
   b. dP/dT
   c. IPPB effect on venous return

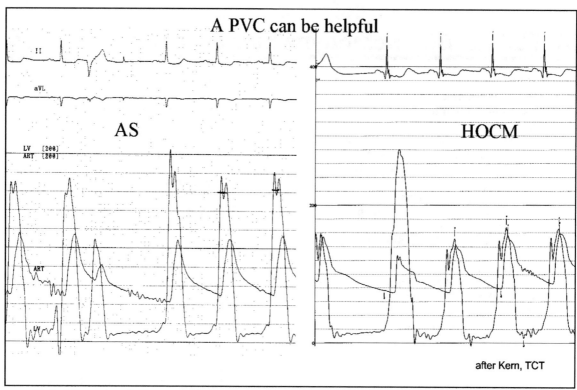

A PVC can be helpful

AS

HOCM

after Kern, TCT

FYI: Note the different effects of a PVC on aortic stenosis verses HOCM.

Contractility and Frank Starling Law

1. Sarcomere

---

625. What ION enters the sarcomere in systole and combines with the troponin-C molecule? This then allows actin and myosin cross-bridges to form. The sarcomere then contracts.

    a. Na^+
    b. K^+
    c. Mg^{++}
    d. Ca^{++}

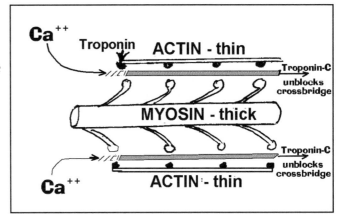

Sarcomere: Actin/Myosin

ANSWER d. Ca^{++} enters the cell through calcium channels (of calcium blocker fame). This triggers release of large amounts of calcium stored in the sarcoplasmic reticulum. This Ca^{++} combines with troponin-C to uncover these troponin activation sites (beads shown on the actin molecule). The troponin then couples with myosin molecules to form cross-bridges. This causes systolic contraction. The heads of the myosin molecules are like little oars that pull against the actin beads and slide the sarcomere filaments together.

See: Berne and Levy, chapter on "Cardiac Pump." and Underhill, chapter on "Physiology of Heart. **Keywords:** Sarcomere, actin, myosin, Ca ion, troponin

626. The normal resting sarcomere length is:

    a.   1 - 12 μ (microns)
    b.   2 - 2.2 μ
    c.   4 - 7.5 μ
    d.   8.3 - 17.7 μ

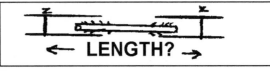

Sarcomere

ANSWER b. 2 - 2.2 μ. This sarcomere length is the average stretch at end diastole. It allows efficient cross bridge coupling in the sarcomere and is comparable to a LV-EDP of 5-10 mmHg. Increasing the stretch to 2.4 microns is comparable to an LV-EDP of 12-18 mmHg. Above 20 mmHg the LV over-stretches and cross-bridge coupling in the sarcomere becomes inefficient on the downslope of the curve more blood is being returned to the LV than it can pump. The LV contractions are weaker and congestion sets in.
See: Berne Levy, chapter on, "The Cardiac Pump." **Keywords:** Sarcomere, Preload, 2 microns, LV FUNCTION

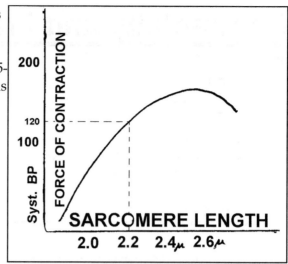

Frank Starling Curve

627. **Stroke volume is determined by what mechanical properties of the myocardium? (Select 3.)**
a.   Preload
b.   Afterload
c.   Heart rate
d.   Ejection fraction
e.   Contractility
f.   Elasticity

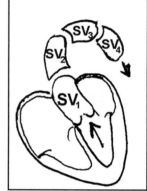

Stroke Volume

ANSWERS: a, b, & e. Preload, Afterload, and Contractility. The balance of these 3 properties predetermine the force of contraction and stroke volume of each heart beat. They are the three determinants of ventricular performance. Increasing preload and contractility increase SV, while increasing afterload decreases SV. Although, HR is an important determinant of CO it is neither a "property" of the myocardium, nor a determinant of stroke volume. **See:** Braunwald on "Assessment of Cardiac Function." Keywords: SV

628. **-The velocity of myocardial contraction increases with increasing _____**
a.   Afterload and preload
b.   Afterload and contractility
c.   Preload and contractility
d.   Preload, afterload and contractility

ANSWER c. Increasing preload and contractility make the heart beat faster and harder. The more you pack the ventricle full (preload) and hype its contractility up (epi.), the faster it will contract (velocity). Besides making the heart beat faster, increasing preload and contractility also increase the stroke volume and cardiac output. On the other hand, afterload is a form of friction that drags on the ejection of blood and reduces the velocity of contraction. Systemic resistance (SVR) is the chief form of afterload.
See: Underhill chapter on CV Physiology. **Keywords**: LV function, velocity contraction

2. Preload

629. **End-diastolic filling or stretching of the ventricle is termed:**
   a.   **Preload**
   b.   **Afterload**
   c.   **Inotropism**
   d.   **Chronotropism**

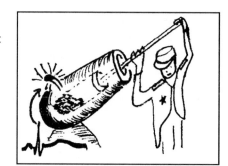

Starling preloading his cannon.

ANSWER a. Preload refers to the filling of the ventricular chambers in diastole. The more you stretch it (like a rubber band) the harder it will contract. This relationship is called "Starling's Law." Preload is like "loading" a cannon. The more powder you put in the harder it contracts. In this analogy:
    • **Preload** = amount of powder loaded before firing
    • **Afterload** = Resistance = resistance to cannon ball velocity after firing, such as: gravity, air resistance, and barrel resistance, etc.
    • **Dromotropism** = AV conduction = length of fuse
    • **Inotropism** = contractility = explosiveness of powder
    • **Chronotropism** = HR = rate of cannon fire (machine gun)
See: Underhill, chapter on "CV Physiology." **Keywords:** preload = stretch

630. **LV preload occurs entirely during:**
   a.   **Atrial systole**
   b.   **Atrial diastole**
   c.   **Ventricular systole**
   d.   **Ventricular diastole**

ANSWER d. Ventricular diastole. Diastolic filling in the heart is **preload**. How much the LV is stretched determines how hard it will contract. Just like a rubber slingshot - the more it's stretched the harder it shoots. The LV filling occurs throughout diastole. Atrial kick contributes only a fraction of the LV filling volume, and occurs only during the last part of ventricular filling.
See: Medical Dictionary. **Keywords:** preload, diastolic filling

631. **-Cardiac filling pressure (CVP) increases with: (Select 3.)**
   a.   **Contracting the calf muscles**
   b.   **Sympathetic vasomotor activity**
   c.   **Standing to an upright position**
   d.   **Hemorrhage**
   e.   **Exercise**

ANSWERS: a, b, & e. Anything that increases venous return back into RA increases central venous pressure (CVP) and preload. CVP is the same as RA mean pressure.

a. TRUE - The calf muscle pump shifts venous blood into the thorax, rasing CVP.

b. T RUE - Sympathetic venoconstriction in periphery shifts flood into the central veins and thorax, rasing CVP.

c. FALSE - By standing upright, gravity distends the veins in the lower body, thereby shifting blood out of the thorax into the legs and lowering CVP.

d. FALSE - Blood volume is a major determinant of CVP, because 2/3 of the blood is in the venous system. A fall in blood volume therefore reduces CVP.

e. TRUE - The calf muscle pump, sympathetic discharge, and peripheral venoconstriction together increase the central blood volume, which increases the diastolic filling pressure. This increases cardiac output according to Starlings law.

See: Berne and Levy, chapter on "Cardiac Pump." **Keywords:** calf muscle pump > CVP

632. **What three measurements evaluate LV preload?**

1. dP/dT	**6. Systolic BP**
2. Inotropic state	**7. EDP**
3. Resting fiber length	**8. SVR**
4. EDV	**9. PVR**
5. ESV	

a. 1, 2, 4
b. 3, 4, 7
c. 4, 7, 9
d. 5, 7, 8

ANSWER b. 3, 4, & 7 (Resting fiber length, EDV, and EDP.) The resting sarcomere fiber length can be stretched with increased preload. The end diastolic pressure (EDP) stretches the filling LV to its largest volume the end diastolic volume (EDV). The LV-EDP is most commonly measured as PA wedge pressure. Anything that stretches the LV at the end of its filling cycle increases resting fiber length and preload. These preload parameters are strictly related to diastolic filling of the ventricle. According to Starling's Law, the greater the preload or stretch - the greater is the force of contraction.

See: Berne and Levy, chapter on "Cardiac Pump." **Keywords:** Preload, LV function.

633. **The Frank Starling law shows how diastolic tension affects the force of LV contraction. What clinical parameter measures this resulting force of contraction?**

a. Systolic ejection period
b. LV-end diastolic volume
c. Diastolic filling pressure
d. Stroke volume

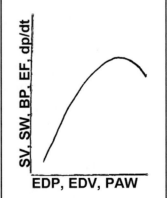

Frank Starling Law

ANSWER d. Stroke volume. The force of LV contraction may be measured by: stroke volume, stroke work, systolic BP, ejection fraction and dP/dT. These may be used as the vertical coordinates of the axis of Starling's curve. They are a result of the ventricular preload as measured by: LV-EDV, LV-EDP, and

wedge pressure. The Starling law plots force of systolic contraction on the vertical axis against diastolic preload on the horizontal axis. This is the famous Frank-Starling curve. Force continues to rise until the heart "max's out" at the top of the curve. There it reaches its contractile limit. Beyond this point more stretching is harmful. It begins to pull apart sarcomeres and the curve falls. **See: Todd Ch C4 on heart failure.**
See: Braunwald chapter on "Assessment of Cardiac Function." **Keywords:** Preload, Starling

634. **This classic live cat muscle experiment is used to study myocardial function. The weight that the muscle picks up and lifts when it contracts is the muscles: (shown on the diagram at #1)**
a. **Preload**
b. **Afterload**
c. **Isometric load**
d. **Filling load**

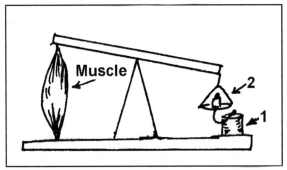
Cat muscle preparation - Diastole
(After Underhill fig. 4.2)

ANSWER b. Afterload is the force opposing ventricular ejection. In the drawing weight #2 is the preload or diastolic stretch on the muscle. Then in systole the larger weight #1 is picked up and lifted. This is analogous to ejecting a certain cardiac stroke volume into the aorta. This heart's real work begins "after" systole begins. Thus, it is termed afterload. Afterload is the "resistance the heart is pumping against" or in this picture "lifting." Some of these "afterload resistance factors" are: aortic blood pressure, aortic valve resistance

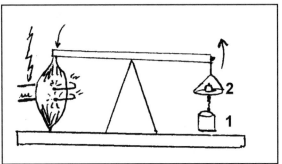
Cat muscle preparation: systole
(After Underhill fig. 4.2)

(especially in aortic stenosis), and peripheral arteriolar resistance due to viscosity.
See: Underhill, chapter on "CV Physiology" **Keywords:** afterload, cat muscle

635. **The Starling law says that (at a given SVR) THE HEART HAS THE CAPACITY TO VARY ITS _____ AS A FUNCTION OF _____.**
a. **End diastolic pressure, preload**
b. **End systolic pressure, afterload**
c. **Force of contraction, preload**
d. **Force of contraction, afterload**

ANSWER c. Force of contraction, preload. Starling law says that (at a given SVR) THE HEART HAS THE CAPACITY TO VARY ITS **(force of contraction, or velocity)** AS A FUNCTION OF **(preload)**. Diastolic preload fills the LV. The more

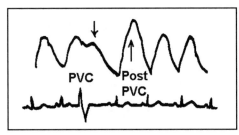
Effect of PVC and post-PVC

it is filled the harder the force of contraction. This effect occurs in all cardiac muscle on a beat by beat basis. Thus, the compensatory pause following a PVC increases filling time and the force of the post-PVC beat by the Frank-Starling mechanism. Note that the systemic resistance (SVR) must be held constant to isolate this preload effect.
See: Quall, chapter on "Physiologic Fundamentals". **Keywords:** Preload, Starling's law, EDP.

636. Two days after an anterio-lateral myocardial infarction a patient develops cool clammy skin and the signs shown in the box. How should this patient's preload be optimized?

| Pathologic S3 and S4 gallop |
| Sinus Tachycardia HR=124 |
| BP = 80/50 mmHg |
| PCW = 12 mmHg |

a.   Morphine to drop PCW to 4 mmHg
b.   Diuretics to drop PCW to 9 mmHg
c.   IV fluids to raise PCW to 18
d.   Whole blood to raise PCW to 25

ANSWER c. Give IV fluid to raise the PCW to around 18 mmHg. This is usually considered the average optimal wedge for cardiac failure patients. Raising preload this much increases BP and cardiac output to perfuse the vital core organs according to the Frank-Starling mechanism. Although 18 mmHg is an above normal PCW, this additional preload can usually be given without causing excessive pulmonary edema. There are however, more accurate ways to determine optimal fluid challenge (See Chapter C. Pathology of CHF).
See: Daily **Keywords:** optimal wedge = 18 mmHg.

637. Venous blood pressure, the rate of venous return and blood volume mainly effect _____.
a.   LV contractility
b.   LV preload
c.   Afterload
d.   Valve competence

ANSWER b. LV preload. Preload is affected by venous blood pressure and the rate of venous return. These are affected by venous tone and volume of circulating blood. Preload is related to the ventricular end-diastolic volume; a higher end-diastolic volume implies a higher preload. According to Starling's Law, the greater the preload or stretch - the greater is the force of contraction. **See:** Todd's, CV Review Book: Vol. I, chapter on "Hemodynamics." **Keywords:** preload

638. The intrinsic ability of the heart to contract with a particular intensity is termed:
a.   Inotropism
b.   Dromotropism
c.   Chronotropism
d.   Psychotropism

ANSWER a. Inotropism. Positive inotropic effect defines this state of "hyped up" chemical contractility that can be induced by cardiotonic and catecholamine drugs. E.g., digitalis, epinephrine, and dobutamine. Remember the term "contractility" is reserved for these chemical effects. Increased preload increases the force of contraction but not the "contractility" because it is not a chemical effect. **See:** Todd's, CV Review Book: Vol. I chapter on "Hemodynamics." **Keywords:** inotropism

639. **The intrinsic ability of heart muscle and automatic tissue to generate its own depolarization is termed:**
    a.   **Inotropism**
    b.   **Chronotropism**
    c.   **Rhythmicity**
    d.   **Automaticity**

ANSWER d. Automaticity causes heart tissue to beat regularly. Even when removed from the heart, and placed in a nutrient bath heart tissue regularly depolarizes itself. Normally the sinus node tissue beats the fastest (60 bpm) and cardiac muscle tissue the slowest (40 pbm). Occasionally an ectopic focus will trigger a tachycardia - all due to automaticity. **See:** Braunwald, chapter on "Electrocardiography" **Keywords:** Automaticity

3. Afterload

640. **If all other factors are held constant, INCREASING _____ will DECREASE cardiac output. (Note: inverse relationship)**
    a.   **Preload**
    b.   **Afterload**
    c.   **Contractility**
    d.   **Heart rate**

ANSWER b. Afterload. These all increase CO except afterload. The higher the afterload the lower the stroke volume. Afterload is the force **opposing** the ejection of blood. Note the inverse relationship - the heavier the load the slower it moves.

Nitroglycerin and other vasodilators relax the arterioles and reduces the load on the LV (usually by lowering BP). This allows the heart to work less. Whereas, vasoconstrictor drugs such as Neo-Synephrine and Dopamine increase the load on the LV and thus increase cardiac work (usually by raising BP). SVR is calculated from BP and CO. The systemic vascular resistance equation shows this inverse relationship between afterload (resistance) and CO.

$$SVR = BP/CO$$

Note that this equation is similar to Ohm's law R = V/I.
See: Underhill, chapter on CV Physiology (role of afterload).
Keywords: Afterload, CO

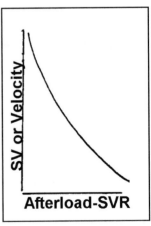

Afterload

641. In a normal patient with a fixed cardiac output the mean arterial blood pressure is determined chiefly by:
- a. Preload
- b. Afterload
- c. Contractility
- d. Heart rate

ANSWER b. Afterload. If CO is constant the only thing that determines what the mean BP will be is the resistance to flow. Resistance is best expressed by the resistance equation:

Mean BP = CO x SVR.

This shows that as vasoconstriction doubles the SVR the BP doubles as a result. The formula is analogous to Ohm's law in electricity: V= I x R. Most of this resistance to blood flow occurs in the precapillary sphincters. When vasoconstriction occurs, the BP goes up. The distractors are wrong answers mainly because they chiefly affect cardiac output. E.g. CO = SV x HR

See: Quall, chapter on "Physiologic Fundamentals" **Keywords:** Afterload, CO, SVR

642. Afterload is best measured by applying which formula?
- a. FICK = O_2 cons / (a-v diff.)
- b. Stroke Work = SV x BP / BSA
- c. Pulse Output = (systolic AO - diastolic AO) / CO
- d. SVR = (mean AO - mean RA) / CO
- e. SI = CO / HR / BSA

ANSWER d. Afterload resistance is measured by the systemic vascular resistance (SVR) formula SVR = (AO-RA) / CO. Note: SVR (Systemic Vascular Resistance) is sometimes also termed PVR **"Peripheral"** **V**ascular **R**esistance - often confused with **"Pulmonary"** **V**ascular **R**esistance." (AO-RA) is the difference between the mean aortic and right atrial pressures. This is the driving pressure across the peripheral capillary bed. For simplicity we often leave out mean RA pressure because it is usually negligible. Then the equation becomes simply:

SVR = $\overline{AO}$/CO   where $\overline{AO}$ = mean Aortic BP

See: Braunwald, chapter on "Assessment of Cardiac Function." **Keywords:** Afterload, SVR

643. Which hemodynamic measurement most directly reflects left ventricular afterload?
- a. Wedge pressure
- b. Mean BP
- c. End-diastolic volume
- d. LV contractility

ANSWER b. Mean blood pressure measures the amount of pressure the LV works against in **systole**. If the BP is low the heart has a light load. The afterload in a gun is the recoil you feel after it fires. Afterload is ejection resistance. Note this in the direct proportionality of SVR to AO pressure in the SVR formula: SVR=(AO-RA)/CO.

See: Braunwald chapter on "Assessment of Cardiac Function." **Keywords:** Afterload, BP

644. **The "impedance" against which the ventricle must work is defined as:**
   a.   Preload
   b.   Afterload
   c.   Isometric resistance
   d.   Viscous resistance

ANSWER b. Afterload. Impedance is a fancy word for resistance. 90% of the LV's work is against the aortic pressure during isometric contraction - the remaining 10% is the volume work ejecting each stroke volume out of the aortic valve during systolic ejection.
See: Quall, chapter on "Cardiac Physiology." **Keywords:** Afterload, impedance

4. Inotropism

645. **An increase in the contractile state of the sarcomere, usually caused by a stimulant such as epinephrine (adrenalin), is termed:**
   a.   - Inotropism
   b.   + Inotropism
   c.   - Preload
   d.   + Preload

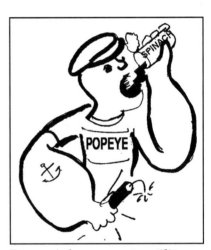

ANSWER b. + Inotropism. Cardiotonic and catecholamine drugs induce a state of augmented cardiac contractility. E.g., digitalis, epinephrine, and dobutamine. Contractility represents the performance of the heart at a given preload and afterload. Positive inotropic effect defines this increased "hyped up" chemical state of contractility. **I liken this "hyped up state" to Popeye's super-powers when he eats his can of spinach.**
See: Berne and Levy, chapter on, "Cardiac Pump."
Keywords: Inotropic, contractility

Popeye's hyper-contractility

646. **LV contractility is a measure of the heart's_____ state.**
   a.   Chronotropic
   b.   Barotropic
   c.   Chemotropic
   d.   Inotropic
   e.   Dromotropic

ANSWER d. Inotropic. This is another way to ask the above question. The inotropic state is the intrinsic ability of the heart to contract harder. Contractility is occasionally misinterpreted to mean increased force or velocity of contraction. Many things influence the force of contraction (preload, afterload...) but only the inotropic state influences myocardial contractility.

It is said that a frightened mother can lift a huge car off her child because she is super-charged with adrenalin. In the same way the heart beats intrinsically harder when charged with an inotropic drug.

See: Braunwald, chapter on "Assessment of Cardiac Function." **Keywords:** Inotropic, contractility

647. **Which medications are inotropic agents used in the treatment of heart failure? (Select 3.)**
a.   **Digitalis (Lanoxin, Digoxin...)**
b.   **Dobutamine (Dobutrex)**
c.   **Milrinone (Primacor)**
d.   **Verapamil (Isoptin)**

ANSWERS: a, b, & c.

The positive inotropic agents listed (Digitalis, Dobutamine, Milrinone) are used in the treatment of heart failure because they enhance myocardial contractility. An entirely new and higher Starling curve is created as shown. This will increase cardiac performance, cardiac output. But by increasing myocardial oxygen consumption this may also exacerbate existing ischemia.

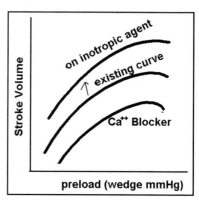
Cardiac function curves

Milrinone is an "ino-dilator" because it not only increases contraction (inotropic), it also increases vasodilation thereby reducing both preload and afterload. It is a short term IV medication for CHF.

Verapamil (Isoptin) has a negative inotropic effect - to decrease the force of contraction. It would NOT be used in heart failure because it would decrease the cardiac contractility even further. Calcium channel blockers like verapamil, nifedipine, and diltiazem block the excitation contraction coupling of smooth muscle. They depress the hearts function and relax it. Calcium channel blockers like verapamil cause vasodilation and are used to treat high blood pressure.

See: Underhill, chapter on "Pharmacologic Management." **Keywords:** Inotropic agents, Not Verapamil

648. **Cardiac contractility is best assessed by measuring:**
a.   **LVEDP**
b.   **Aortic EDP**
c.   **LV dP/dT**
d.   **Aortic dP/dT**

ANSWER c. LV dP/dT. The term dp/dt comes from delta P/delta T. It is the maximum change in pressure over time, or slope of the pressure curve. It is a good index of LV contractility. A failing heart has poor contractility and a slow upstroke. When an inotropic agent such as dobutamine is given; contractility, slope and dp/dt increase as shown.

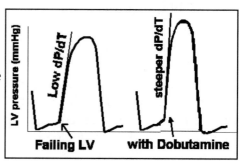
LV dp/dt increase with inotrope

See: Braunwald, chapter on "Evaluation of LV Function." **Keywords:** LV performance, dp/dt .

5. Other Reflexes

649. **The rate induced regulation of the force of contraction, sometimes called the staircase, Treppe or Bowdich effect is defined as:**
   a.   **Rapid HR increases the force of contraction**
   b.   **Slow HR increases the force of contraction**
   c.   **PVC beats show increased force of contraction**
   d.   **Post PVC beats show increased force of contraction**

ANSWER a. Rapid HR increases the force of contraction. The **faster** the heart beats, the **harder** it beats. This **up-staircase** phenomenon is a progressive increase in the force of muscular contraction following a sudden increase in heart rate. This effect plateaus after the rapid heart rate stabilizes. Similarly, sudden bradycardia results in a gradual decrease in the force of contraction over a period of several beats. This is like going **down** the staircase.

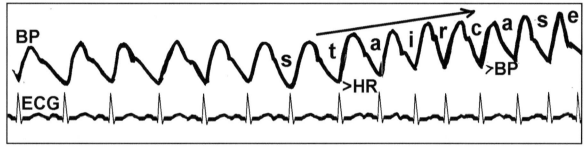

Staircase phenomenon: Increases in HR increase contractility

See: Berne and Levy, chapter on, "Cardiac Pump." **Keywords:** Other reflexes, HR, staircase

REFERENCES

Braunwald, Eugene, et al., Ed., HEART DISEASE A Textbook of Cardiovascular Medicine, 8th Ed., W. B. Saunders Co., 2008
Underhill, S. L., Ed., *CARDIAC NURSING*, 2nd Ed., J. B. Lippincott Co., 1989
Berne, R. M. and Levy, M. N., Cardiovascular Physiology, 8th Ed., Mosby Year Book, 2001
Quall, S. J. *Comprehensive Inta-aortic Balloon Pumping*, CV Mosby Co., 1984

OUTLINE: B7 - Contractility & Frank Starling Law

1. SARCOMERE
   a. Thick filament - Myosin
   b. Thin filament - Actin
   c. Resting length - 2.2 uM
   d. Properties myocardium
      i. Preload
      ii. Afterload
      iii. Contractility
      iv. (HR?)

2. PRELOAD
   a. Definition
      i. Compliance of Ventricle
         (1) Stiff hearts
   b. measurements of Preload
      i. LVedv
      ii. LVEDP, PAW
      iii. resting sarcomere length (stretch)
   c. Starling's Law
      i. Preload
      ii. Force of Contraction
      iii. Starlings Curve
         (1) optimal stretch

   (2) Failure on downslope

3. AFTERLOAD
   a. Definition = impedance to systolic ejection
   b. Impedance = Systemic Resistance
      i. Arteriolar Vasoconstriction
   c. Relation to BP
      i. BP= CO x Resistance
   d. Relation to CO
      i. inversely relate
      ii. CO = BP/Resistance

4. INOTROPISM
   a. Contractile state of myocardium
   b. Inotropic drugs
      i. Catecholamines
      ii. Digitalis

5. OTHER REFLEXES
   a. Staircase, Treppe, Bowdich effect
      i. Increased HR increases contractility

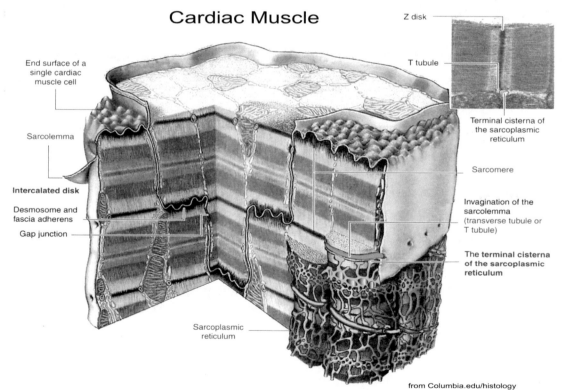

Cardiac Muscle

End surface of a single cardiac muscle cell

Sarcolemma

Intercalated disk

Desmosome and fascia adherens

Gap junction

Sarcoplasmic reticulum

Z disk

T tubule

Terminal cisterna of the sarcoplasmic reticulum

Sarcomere

Invagination of the sarcolemma (transverse tubule or T tubule)

The terminal cisterna of the sarcoplasmic reticulum

from Columbia.edu/histology

Drawing from Kelly DE, Wood RL, Enders AC. Textbook of Microscopic Anatomy. 18th ed. Baltimore. Williams & Wilkins. 1984.

Vascular Anatomy

INDEX: B8:

1. General Vascular Anatomy

650. What anatomic position is labeled #5 in the box?
a. Distal
b. Dorsal
c. Lateral
d. Proximal
e. Ventral
f. Cephalic
g. Caudal

ANATOMIC POSITIONING TERMS
1. Superior or cranial
2. Inferior
3. Anterior
4. Posterior
*5. Farther from the midline
6. Nearer to the point of origin
7. Farther from the point of origin

ANSWER c. Lateral. When a football is tossed "lateral" it is thrown to the side - away from the middle. **BE ABLE TO CORRECTLY MATCH ALL BELOW:**
1. **Cephalic** = superior = cranial = toward the head.
2. **Caudal** = inferior = away from the head.
3. **Ventral** = anterior = near the front of the body
4. **Dorsal** = posterior = near the back of the body
5. **Lateral** = farther from the medial plane or midline
6. **Proximal** = nearer to the point of origin
7. **Distal** = farther from the point of origin
Be able to match all answers above. **See:** Tortora, chapter on "Organization of the Human Body." **Keywords:** positioning, lateral

651. The body position numbered at #1 in the box is:
a. Horizontal
b. Vertical
c. Prone
d. Supine

BODY POSITIONING TERMS
*1. Reclining face down
2. Reclining face up
3. Reclining parallel to the earth
4. Standing perpendicular to the earth

ANSWER c. Prone is the reclining position face down, on your stomach. Supine is lying flat on your back. **BE ABLE TO CORRECTLY MATCH ALL BELOW:**
BODY POSITIONING TERMS

1. Reclining face down.	.	Prone
2. Reclining face up.	.	Supine
3. Reclining parallel to the earth.	.	Horizontal
4. Standing perpendicular to the earth.		Vertical

Be able to match all answers above. **See:** Tortora, Chapter on "Organization of the Human Body." **Keywords:** positioning, prone 7

652. **The abbreviation used in vascular procedures labeled at #10 is:**

a.   **CFA**
b.   **DSA**
c.   **SMA**
d.   **PTA**
e.   **DVT**
f.   **IVP**
g.   **DP**
h.   **V/Q**
I.   **BUN**
j.   **PFA**
k.   **NG**
l.   **KUB**

VASCULAR ABBREVIATIONS
1. Kidney function test
2. Artery punctured for AO-gram
3. Feeding tube to stomach
4. Artery supplying femur
5. Computerized digital X-ray imaging
6. Thrombosis of leg veins
7. X-ray of kidneys excreting dye
8. Artery to front of foot
9. Artery of the intestine
*10. Radio-isotope scan of lung
11. Vascular Angioplasty
12. X-ray of Kidneys excreting contrast

ANSWER h. V/Q scan.   This radio-isotope
scan evaluates the relative distribution of Ventilation (V)to blood Perfusion (Q). Pulmonary emboli typically cause a reduced perfusion to one area of the lung, seen on the scan as a "cold spot."
BE ABLE TO CORRECTLY MATCH ALL BELOW:
VASCULAR ABBREVIATIONS
1. BUN = Blood Urea Nitrogen = Kidney function test
2. CFA = Common Femoral Artery = Artery punctured for AO-gram
3. NG = Nasogastric = Feeding tube to stomach
4. PFA = Profunda Femoral Artery = Artery supplying femur
5. DSA = Digital Subtraction Angiography = Computerized digital X-ray imaging
6. DVT = Deep Vein Thrombosis = Thrombosis of leg veins
7. IVP = Intravenous Pyelogram = X-ray of kidneys excreting contrast
8. DP = Dorsalis Pedis = Artery to front of foot
9. SMA = Superior Mesenteric Artery = Artery of the intestine
10. V/Q = Ventilation/Perfusion Scan = Radio-isotope scan of lung
11. PTA = Percutaneous Transluminal Angioplasty = Vascular Angioplasty
12. KUB = Kidneys, Ureters, and Bladder film (If taken immediately after angiography a
        KUB film normally verifies excretion of contrast via the kidneys and ureters)
        Be able to match all answers above. See: CCI lists of approved abbreviations.

653. **What artery is palpated at #1 in the diagram?**

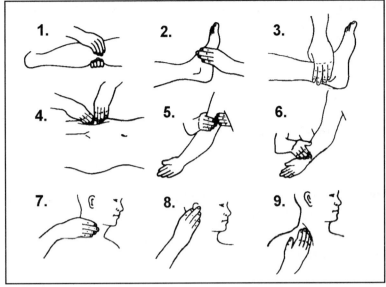

a.   Femoral
b.   Popliteal
c.   Dorsalis Pedis
d.   Posterior Tibial
e.   External Carotid (temporal)
f.   Common Carotid
g.   Subclavian
h.   Brachial
I.   Radial

ANSWER b. The popliteal artery is palpated behind the knee. It is best done on the supine patient by placing

Palpation of which systemic arteries?(after Anderson 14.1)

both hands around the knee and lifting it slightly while pressing up under the knee with your fingers. **BE ABLE TO CORRECTLY MATCH ALL BELOW.**

    1. Popliteal
    2. Dorsalis Pedis
    3. Posterior Tibial
    4. Femoral
    5. Brachial
    6. Radial
    7. Common Carotid
    8. External Carotid (temporal)
    9. Subclavian

See: Anderson, chapter on "Arteries." **Keywords:** Locations to palpate all arteries

654. **When you feel an arterial pulse, its amplitude is graded on a scale from zero (absent pulse) to ___ (normal pulse).**

a.   2
b.   4
c.   10
d.   100

ANSWER b. +4 out of 4, (4/4) is a normal pulse amplitude. When feeling these pulses use your index and middle fingers to palpate directly over the location where the artery is closest to the surface. They are evaluated manually according to intensity or amplitude of the pulse, with +4 being a normal strong pulse. Sometimes marked as ++++.

    0 = completely absent pulse
    +1 = markedly impaired pulse
    +2 = moderately impaired pulse
    +3 = slightly impaired pulse
    +4 = normal strong pulse

Grading allows follow up nurses to evaluate changes in the pulse over time. E.g. If you find a +3 pedal pulse after establishing hemostasis, and later the floor nurse measures it to be +1, the artery may be occluding with thrombus or by hematoma. This grading scale is analogous to grading the intensity of murmurs, with the loudest murmur being 6/6. The 4+ grading scale is most common. However, other grading scales exist, some that rate 2+ as normal, and 4+ as a bounding pulse. Be sure everyone in your institution agrees on the same pulse grading scale. See: Underhill, chapter on "History and Physical Examination." also, Cannobbio, *CV Disorders*

655. **What is the name of the artery that supplies organ/limb #1 (kidneys) in the box?**

a.	**Mesenteric**
b.	**Renal**
c.	**Bronchial**
d.	**Carotid**
e.	**Iliac**
f.	**Phrenic**
g.	**Portal/Hepatic**
h.	**Subclavian**

ORGANS
*1. **Kidneys**
2. Lungs
3. Intestines
4. Liver
5. Diaphragm
6. Brain
7. Legs
8. Arms

BE ABLE TO CORRECTLY MATCH ALL BELOW.

ORGANS		
1. **Kidneys**	b.	Renal
2. **Lungs**	c.	Bronchial
3. **Intestines**	a.	Mesenteric
4. **Liver**	g.	Portal/Hepatic
5. **Diaphragm**	f.	Phrenic
6. **Brain**	d.	Carotid
7. **Legs**	e.	Iliac
8. **Arms**	h.	Subclavian

ANSWER b. kidney = Renal. Be able to match all these terms. See: Medical Dictionary

656. **When palpating pedal pulses the posterior tibial artery is located (see diagram):**

a.	**Behind the lateral ankle bone**
b.	**In front of the lateral ankle bone**
c.	**Behind the medial ankle bone**
d.	**In front of the medial ankle bone**

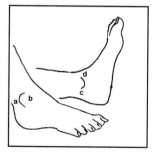

ANSWER c. Behind or posterior to the medial malleolus ankle bone. In fact it is sometimes called the medial malleolar branch of the posterior tibial artery. This artery arises from the popliteal artery behind the knee, which arises from the femoral artery. If the femoral becomes partially occluded, these pedal pulses will be diminished. There are 4 locations commonly palpated in the lower extremity:

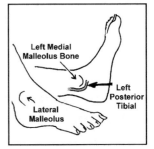

- •Femoral artery (above the femoral head in each groin)
- •Popliteal artery (posterior aspect of leg behind each knee)
- •Dorsalis pedis artery (on the anterior aspect of the foot between the first and second metatarsal)
- •Posterior tibial artery sometimes called the medial malleolar artery (behind or posterior to the medial malleolus ankle bone)

Post. Tibial Artery

See: Snopek, chapter on "Femoral Angiography." Keywords: post. tibial location

657. The anatomic term "axilla" or "axillary fossa" refers to the:
   a.   Central axis of the body (columna vertabis)
   b.   Suprasternal notch or jugular fossa
   c.   Antecubital fossa anterior to the elbow
   d.   Armpit under the shoulder

ANSWER d. Axilla refers to the ARMPIT. The axillary artery is normally accessible here. The "mid-axillary line" is also the reference point for placing the V6 ECG electrode. See: Medical Dictionary Keywords: Axilla

658. Which vessel would contain valves?
   a.   SVC
   b.   Pulmonary vein
   c.   Saphenous vein
   d.   Profunda femoralis

ANSWER c. Saphenous vein. The large veins (> 2 mm ID) contain valves especially in the lower extremity. These allow the "muscular pump" to move venous blood back to the heart on exercise. Diseased and dilated valves may be incompetent, and are associated with varicose veins and venous congestion.

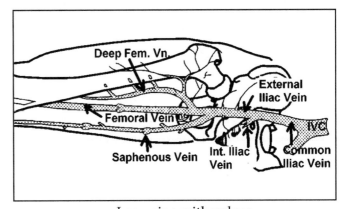

Leg veins with valves

   The valves in the saphenous veins may pose problems during vein bypass surgery. They have to be aligned in the right direction during CABG surgery or they will block arterial blood flow. Also, valves in "in-vivo" or "side-by-side' fem-pop grafts must be "cut" to allow

blood to bypass a femoral stenosis. This is because the bypass vein lies alongside the diseased artery and is not taken out or turned around. The femoral vein is anastomosed to the artery above and below the arterial stenosis. But the venous valves must be removed because they were designed to prevent flow in this new direction. Then arterial blood is directed into the vein to bypass the stenosis.
See: Gray's Anatomy, chapter on "Blood Veins". Keywords: venous valves in saphenous vein

659. **Which of the following venous problems is most likely associated with varicosities?**
a.   Blood clots in the venous system
b.   An inflammation of walls in the veins
c.   A thickening of the walls of the veins
d.   An incompetency of the venous valves

ANSWER d. An incompetency of the venous valves. Unlike arteries, most veins have one-way valves that function to allow blood to flow in only one direction. These valves become incompetent and the veins then become dilated and tortuous when varicosities are present. Veins are thinner when compared with comparable arteries. They do not tend to thicken or fill with plaque deposits as arteries do. Blood clots themselves and inflamed veins do not predispose patients to varicose veins.
See: Medical dictionary

660. **The descending aorta is divided into which 2 areas?**
a.   Parietal, abdominal
b.   Parietal, inguinal
c.   Thoracic, abdominal
d.   Thoracic, inguinal

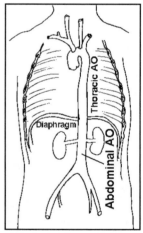
Abd. & Thor. Aorta

ANSWER c. Thoracic, abdominal aorta. After exiting the aortic valve blood flows up the ascending aorta and over the aortic arch into the descending aorta. The descending aorta is divided into 2 parts separated by the diaphragm, the thoracic aorta above and the abdominal aorta below the diaphragm.
See: Medical dictionary

2. Vascular Micro-anatomy

661. **How many peripheral capillaries does a normal adult have?**
a.   100,000
b.   600,000
c.   1,000,000
d.   3,000,000,000

ANSWER d. 2.7-3.0 billion peripheral capillaries exist with a cross sectional area of 1357 cm^2 (just over 1 square meter). The same number of pulmonary capillaries exists with the same cross section area. Compare this with the aorta whose cross section is 2.8 cm^2. Since Q=VA the velocity in the aorta is 500 times faster than in the capillaries.
See: Berne and Levy, chapter on "The Circuit."

662. **Which type of muscle tissue appears non-striated under the microscope and is located in the walls of hollow internal structures (viscera, ducts, vessels...)?**
    a.   **Skeletal muscle**
    b.   **Cardiac muscle**
    c.   **Smooth muscle**
    d.   **Flexor muscle**

ANSWER c. Smooth muscle is so named because they are not have the striated appearance of skeletal and cardiac muscle cells. It is found in the media of most blood vessels. Each cell is smooth and tapered at each end, and can migrate into plaque during the atherosclerotic process. See: Alexander, chapter on "Tissues" **Keywords**: Smooth muscle

663. **The tunica media of an artery is composed primarily of:**
    a.   **Elastic tissue**
    b.   **Smooth muscle**
    c.   **Connective tissue**
    d.   **Epithelium**

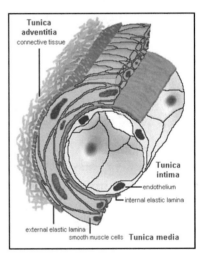

ANSWER b. Smooth muscle. The smooth muscle runs concentrically around the arteries and arterioles. When stimulated with sympathetic nerves or norepinephrine, these vessels constrict. The smooth muscle in the coronary arteries may cause coronary vasospasm and Prinzmetal angina. See: Underhill, chapter on "Cardiac Anatomy" Keywords: tunica media = smooth muscle

664. **Veins differ from arteries in that venous walls:**
    a.   **Are thicker**
    b.   **Are more compliant**
    c.   **Can withstand more pressure**
    d.   **Have more muscle**

ANSWER b. Veins are more compliant (stretchable). This is because veins have less elastic tissue than arteries. This makes veins 20 times more compliant than arteries. For this reason they can expand more and hold larger volumes of blood than arteries.

     The arterial walls are thicker with more muscle then veins of the same diameter. Veins are poorly suited to withstand arterial pressure, even though vein grafts do tolerate the arterial pressure for many years. And of course, the valves in vein grafts must point in the direction of flow.
See: Berne & Levy, chapter on "The Circuit." Keywords: artery, vein, differences

665. **Systemic veins function differently than arteries - in that veins:**
  a.   Carry blood away from the heart
  b.   Carry blood rich in oxygen
  c.   Lack innervation by the sympathetic nervous system
  d.   Contain venous valves.

ANSWER d. Contain venous valves. Most veins have valves which normally serve to prevent reflux of blood. These usually consist of two semi-lunar shaped valves. They are most numerous in the veins of the lower extremities, and absent in the vena cava and very small veins. Like arterial walls the veins are supplied with vaso-vasorum (nutrient vessels).
See: Gray's Anatomy, chapter on "The Heart" Keywords: veins have valves

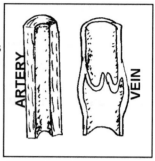
Artery Vein

666. **Arteries differ from veins in that arteries always carry:**
  a. O_2 rich blood (high O_2 sat)
  b. O_2 poor blood (low O_2 sat)
  c.   Blood toward the heart
  d.   Blood away from the heart

ANSWER d. Blood away from the heart. All arteries lead away from the heart. Veins all lead to the heart. The systemic arteries carry red oxygenated blood, but the venous arteries (PA) carries dark (75%) blood.
See: Underhill, chapter on "Systemic and Pulmonary Circulation." Keywords: arteries always carry blood AWAY from heart

667. **These two vessels run alongside each other and in opposite directions. Identify the layer of the vessel indicated with a #1 on the diagram.**
  a.   Venous media
  b.   Venous intima
  c.   Venous adventitia
  d.   Arterial media
  e.   Arterial intima
  f.   Arterial adventitia

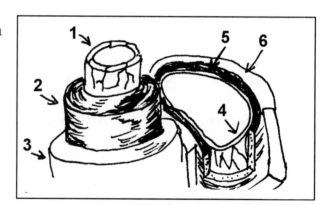
Arterial and venous walls

ANSWER e. Arterial intima. Arteries and veins have 3 layers. The intima is the thin inside layer - easy to remember because of the "in-". The media is the thick middle muscular layer - easy to remember because it is in the middle (media or median). The outside covering is the adventitia or tunica externa. The much thicker arterial media contains chiefly smooth muscle. The larger diameter veins (on the right side of diagram) are much thinner, more compliant, and have less smooth muscle. That is why veins pool blood. These outer layers are sometimes called the "tunica" for coat after the root "tunic" (e.g. tunica media). Remember the sequence -intima, media, & adventitia

MATCH THE LABELED VASCULAR LAYERS TO THEIR NAME BELOW.
> **1.** Arterial intima
> **2.** Arterial media
> **3.** Arterial Adventitia
> **4.** Venous intima
> **5.** Venous media
> **6.** Venous Adventitia.

Be able to match all answers above. See: Underhill, chapter on "Systemic and Venous Circulations." Keywords: vessel layers, intima, media, & adventia

668. **The larger blood vessel layer labeled at #5 in the diagram contains chiefly:**
> a.   **Endothelium**
> b.   **An internal elastic membrane**
> c.   **Smooth muscle and elastic fibers**
> d.   **Collagen and elastic fibers**

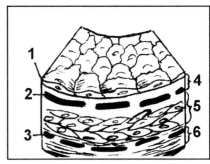

Normal vessel walls

ANSWER c. Smooth muscle and elastic fibers. The media is the only layer containing smooth muscle. This is most pronounced in arterioles which proportionately have the most muscle because they regulate the flow of blood to tissues. The veins also have a thin muscular media which makes them "capacitance" vessels. When dilated these "capacitance" vessels pool blood and reduce cardiac preload.
CORRECTLY MATCHED ANSWERS ARE:
> 1. Endothelium (intima)
> 2. Internal elastic lamina
> 3. External elastic lamina
> 4. Intima (endothelium)
> 5. Lamina (media & smooth muscle)
> 6. Adventia

See: Underhill, chapter on "Systemic and Pulmonary Circulation." Keywords: arterial wall structures

669. **Capillaries are composed of:**
> a.   **A single layer of epithelium**
> b.   **A single layer of endothelium**
> c.   **Intima, media, and adventia**
> d.   **Intima and adventia**

ANSWER b. A single layer of endothelium or intima. They have no media or adventia. These microscopic vessels are only a single cell in thickness. They are so thin as to allow free diffusion of gases and nutrients through their cell walls. Arteries, arterioles, venules and veins are too thick to allow this. The capillary bed is the sole site of metabolic exchange between circulating blood and

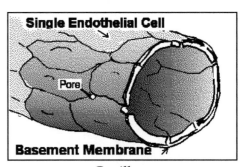

Capillary

tissues. The capillary bed connects the arterioles with the venules.

Although the cross sectional area of the capillary bed is about one square meter, the capillary - tissue interface area for diffusion is as large as a football field. See: Darovic, Chapter on "CV Anatomy and Physiology." Keywords: capillary walls - endothelium

3. Cerebral & Neck Arteries

670. **The Circle of Willis is a/an _____ located near the _____.**
    a.   **Arterial anastomosis,**   **Base of the brain**
    b.   **Arterial anastomosis,**   **Carotid sinus**
    c.   **Venous plexus,**   **Base of the brain**
    d.   **Venous plexus,**   **Carotid sinus**

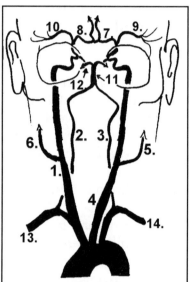

Cerebral Arteries

ANSWER a. Arterial anastomosis, base of the brain. At the base of the brain the internal carotid artery and vertebral arteries form this remarkable circular anastomosis. It encircles the hypothalamus and pituitary gland and helps protect the brain against a stroke. If any one major artery feeding the brain occludes, this circle provides an automatic collateral pathway for redirection of blood.

CORRECTLY MATCHED ANSWERS ARE:
    1. Right Common Carotid
    2. Right Vertebral
    3. Right Vertebral
    4. Left Common Carotid
    5. Left External Carotid
    6. Right External Carotid
    7. Left. Anterior Cerebral
    8. Right Anterior Cerebral
    9. Left Middle Cerebra
    10. Right Middle Cerebral
    11. Basilar
    12. Right Post Cerebral
    13. Right Subclavian
    14. Left Subclavian

Be able to match all answers above. See: Snopek, chapter on "Cerebral Angiography." Keywords: Circle of Willis

671. **Identify the artery labeled #1 in this diagram of the circle of Willis.**
   a.   Middle cerebral
   b.   Posterior communicating
   c.   Posterior cerebral
   d.   Superior cerebral
   e.   Pontine
   f.   Basilar
   g.   Vertebral arteries
   h.   Anterior spinal artery
   I.   Anterior communicating
   j.   Anterior cerebral
   k.   Internal carotid

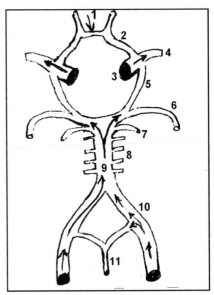
Circle of Willis

BF ABLE TO CORRECTLY MATCH ALL BELOW:
ANSWER I. The anterior communicating artery is the most anterior artery in the circle of Willis. This diagram shows as circles the two major arteries which supply the circle of Willis: Internal carotids (3) and the vertebrals (11). The three major arteries supplying the brain and arise from the circle of Willis are: the anterior cerebral (2), middle cerebral(4) and posterior cerebral (6). The circle of Willis seen in this inferior view forms the shape of a man. His hexagonal head connects these major arteries, on top by the anterior communicating artery (1) and on the sides by the posterior communicating artery (5). The eyes are the internal carotid arteries (3). The back is the basilar artery (9) and the legs are formed by the two vertebrals (10). The ribs arising from the basilar are the superior cerebral (7) and several pontine arteries to the pons(8).
CORRECTLY MATCHED ANSWERS ARE:
      1. Anterior communicating
      2. Anterior cerebral
      3. Internal carotid
      4. Middle cerebral
      5. Posterior communicating
      6. Posterior cerebral
      7. Superior cerebral
      8. Pontine
      9. Basilar
      10. Vertebral arteries
      11. Anterior spinal artery
Be able to match all answers above.
See: Snopek, chapter on "Cerebral Angiography." Keywords: ID arteries in Circle of Willis

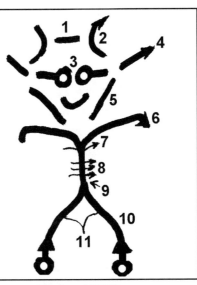
Circle of Willis

672. **The right and left vertebral arteries ascend to join in the _____ (labeled #1 in the diagram).**
a. Basilar artery
b. Common carotid artery
c. Posterior communicating artery
d. Anterior communicating artery

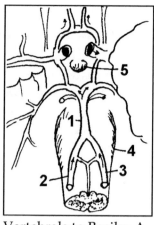

Vertebrals to Basilar A.

ANSWER a. Basilar artery. The two vertebral arteries are the first branches off each subclavian artery. They ascend through the transverse vertebral processes into the scull. They join at the brain-stem into one common basilar artery. The basilar artery then supplies the circle of Willis and posterior cerebral arteries. MATCH THE NAMES BELOW TO THE STRUCTURES SHOWN.

    1. Basilar artery
    2. Right vertebral artery
    3. Left vertebral artery
    4. Brain stem - medulla
    5. Hypophysis (pituitary gland) (*Willy's nose*)
See: Grays Anatomy. Keywords: Rt. and Lt. Vertebral A. ➔ Basilar A.

673. **Identify this artery labeled #5 in this lateral view of the internal carotid angiogram.**
a. **Ophthalmic**
b. **Anterior medial frontal**
c. **Intermediate medial frontal (collosomarginal)**
d. **Pericallosal**
e. **Middle cerebral artery group**
f. **Internal carotid**
g. **Anterior cerebral**

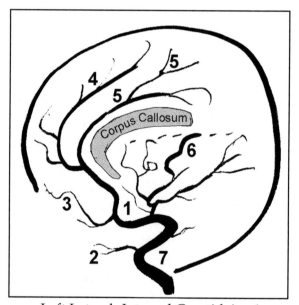

Left Lateral.-Internal Carotid Angio.

ANSWER d. The pericallosal surrounds the corpus callosum in the brain. The corpus callosum is the great white commissure connecting both cerebral hemispheres. The internal carotid (#7) makes several tortuous turns in the shape of a reverse "S" (for siphon). The ophthalmic artery originates from the internal carotid (#2) and supplies the eye. The two main branches supplying the lateral cerebral hemispheres are (#5) the pericallosal artery and (#4) the collosomarginal artery around the margins of the pericallosal. The middle cerebral (#6) supplies the lateral surface of the brain. The anterior cerebral artery runs up the midline of the brain. They appear to overlay each other in the lateral angio, but the middle cerebral is in a plane overlying the anterior cerebral artery. Note how the pericallosal moves up the midline in the comparison

picture below. Be able to match all answers below.
CORRECTLY MATCHED ANSWERS ARE:
1. Anterior cerebral
2. Ophthalmic
3. Anterior medial frontal
4. Intermediate medial frontal (collosomarginal)
5. Pericallosal
6. Middle cerebral artery group
7. Internal carotid
See: Snopek, chapter on "Cerebral Angiography." **Keywords:** cerebral arteries, lateral view, collosomarginal artery

674. **In this lateral view of the internal carotid angiogram identify the large artery labeled #1 (far left).**
  a.   **Pericallosal**
  b.   **Anterior cerebral**
  c.   **Anterior medial frontal**
  d.   **Intermediate medial frontal (collosomarginal)**
  e.   **Middle cerebral artery group**

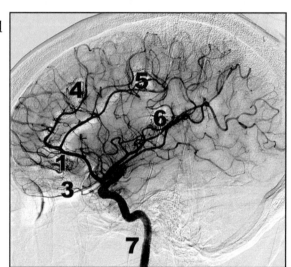
Left Lateral.-Internal Carotid Angio.

ANSWER b. Anterior cerebral artery moves anterior from the carotid siphon into (#4) intermediate medial frontal (collosomarginal) and (#5) pericallosal. The ophthalmic artery is right below it, going to the eye. Numbered same as question above.
CORRECTLY MATCHED ANSWERS ARE:
1. Anterior cerebral
3. Ophthalmic
4. Intermediate medial frontal (collosomarginal)
5. Pericallosal
6. Middle cerebral artery group
7. Left internal carotid
See: Snopek, chapter on "Cerebral Angiography." **Keywords:** cerebral arteries, lateral view, Collosomarginal artery

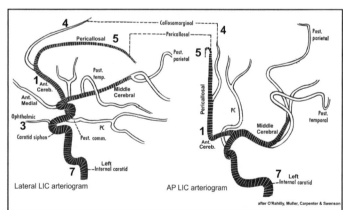
Left Lateral. & AP Carotid comparison

675. **The major artery which supplies the face is the _____.**
   a.   Internal carotid artery
   b.   External carotid artery
   c.   Internal jugular artery
   d.   External jugular artery

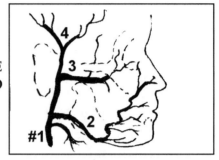
Facial arteries

ANSWER b. The external carotid artery supplies most of the face, scalp, jaw, and thyroid. This makes the ECA relatively unimportant compared to the internal carotid which is critically involved in strokes. **MATCH ALL THE LABELED BRANCHES OF THE EXTERNAL CAROTID ARTERY WITH THEIR NAMES BELOW.**
   1. External carotid
   2. External maxillary
   3. Internal maxillary
   4. Superficial temporal
There is NO "jugular" artery. Be able to match all answers above.
See: Snopek, chapter on "Cerebral angiography." **Keywords:** External carotid, facial artery

676. **In this lateral vertebral angiogram identify the artery labeled #2.**
   a.   Internal carotid artery
   b.   Vertebral artery
   c.   Basilar artery
   d.   Posterior communicating artery
   e.   Posterior cerebral artery
   f.   Superior cerebral artery
   g.   Posterior inferior cerebral artery

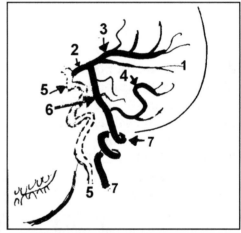
LEFT LAT. VERTEBRAL Artery

ANSWER d. This posterior communicating artery carries collateral vertebral artery blood to the circle of Willis. The internal carotid artery is shown in dotted lines to show the connection through the circle of Willis. **BE ABLE TO CORRECTLY MATCH ALL BELOW.**
   1. Superior cerebral artery
   2. Posterior communicating artery
   3. Posterior cerebral artery
   4. Posterior inferior cerebral artery
   5. Internal carotid artery
   6. Basilar artery
   7. Vertebral artery

See: Snopek, chapter on "Cerebral Angiography."

677. In this RAO view of the major neck arteries the artery labeled at #1 is the right:
   a.   Subclavian artery
   b.   Common carotid
   c.   External carotid artery
   d.   Internal carotid artery
   e.   Vertebral artery

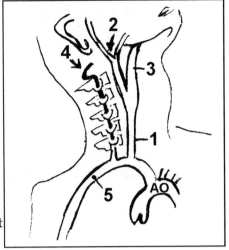
Rt. Sided neck arteries

ANSWER b. Common carotid. The internal carotid is the chief artery to the brain, while the external carotid supplies the face. This diagram shows two of the four arteries to the brain: RIC and REC (LIC and LEC are not shown). Hence the term for selective cerebral studies - **"four vessel study."**
CORRECTLY MATCHED ANSWERS ARE:
       1. Right common carotid
       2. Right external carotid artery
       3. Right internal carotid artery
       4. Right vertebral artery
       5. Right subclavian artery
See: Snopek, chapter on "Cerebral Angiography." **Keywords:** Carotid, vertebral artery

678. In this AP view of a cerebral angiogram identify the internal carotid branch labeled as #2.
   a.   Anterior cerebral artery
   b.   Sylvian artery
   c.   Middle cerebral artery
   d.   Internal carotid artery
   e.   Frontopolar artery

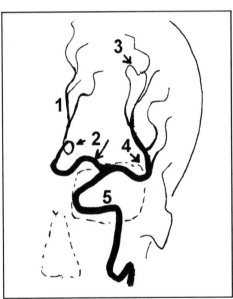
AP VIEW, Internal Carotid

ANSWER a. Anterior cerebral artery. Note the T configuration in the AP view of the internal carotid artery branches into the anterior cerebral and middle cerebral. Note how the anterior cerebral artery supplies the midbrain while the middle cerebral supplies the lateral brain. The other major cerebral artery, (the posterior cerebral) is not seen, because it usually arises from the vertebral - basilar arteries.
BE ABLE TO CORRECTLY MATCH ALL BELOW.
       1. Frontopolar artery
       2. Anterior cerebral artery
       3. Sylvian point
       4. Middle cerebral artery
       5. Internal carotid artery
See: Snopek, chapter on "Femoral Angiography."

679. In this AP - 20 degree cranial view of a vertebral angiogram, identify the artery labeled as #6.
   a.　Superior inferior cerebral artery
   b.　Basilar artery
   c.　Posterior cerebral artery
   d.　Parieto-occipital/calcarine artery
   e.　Right vertebral artery
   f.　Left vertebral artery
   g.　Posterior inferior cerebral artery

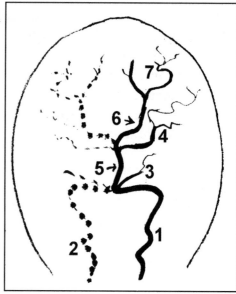

Cranial AP view of vertebral arteries

ANSWER c. Posterior cerebral artery. In this AP diagram we see a left vertebral artery angiogram. The right vertebral artery is shown in dotted lines. Note how they join at the basilar artery and branch from it into the posterior cerebral arteries.
BE ABLE TO CORRECTLY MATCH ALL BELOW.
   1. Left vertebral artery
   2. Right vertebral artery
   3. Posterior inferior cerebral artery
   4. Superior inferior cerebral artery
   5. Basilar artery
   6. Posterior cerebral artery
   7. Parieto-occipital/calcarine artery
See: Snopek, chapter on "Cerebral Arteriography." **Keywords:** AP view, vertebral arteries

4. Angiographic Anatomy: Thorax & Arch Arteries

680. The innominate artery divides into the _____ and _____ arteries.
   1. Internal thoracic (internal mammary)
   2. Right subclavian
   3. Left subclavian
   4. Left common carotid
   5. Right common carotid
       a. 1, 2
       b. 1, 4
       c. 2, 5
       d. 3, 5

ANSWER c. Right subclavian and right common carotid. The innominate artery (meaning "unnamed") is also termed the brachiocephalic artery. It normally divides into the right subclavian and right common carotid arteries. There is NO left innominate. Instead, the left common carotid and left subclavian artery arise separately from the aortic arch. The ascending cervical (vertebral) arteries each arise from their respective subclavian arteries.

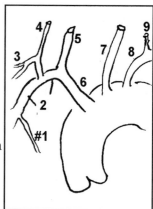

Arch vessels

BE ABLE TO CORRECTLY MATCH ALL BELOW.
  1. Right Internal Thoracic (Internal Mammary)
  2. Right Subclavian
  3. Transverse Cervical
  4. Ascending Cervical (Right Vertebral)
  5. Right Common Carotid
  6. Innominate (Brachio-cephalic)
  7. Left Common Carotid
  8. Left Subclavian
  9. Right Cervical (Right Vertebral)
See: Snopek, chapter of "Aortography." **Keywords:** AO arch vessels, innominate, branches

681. **Which vessel normally carries the most O_2 enriched blood?**
  a. **Pulmonary veins**
  b. **Pulmonary artery**
  c. **Bronchial vein**
  d. **Bronchial artery**

ANSWER a. The four pulmonary veins which empty into the LA carry red blood directly from the lungs. They are the only veins which carry O_2 rich blood. In fact, they contain the reddest blood in the body. By the time this blood gets to the LV, it has dropped 2-4% in saturation because of the bronchial and Thebesian veins which slightly reduces the O_2 saturation of the LA blood.
See: Berne and Levy, chapter on "Special Circulations." **Keywords:** Pulm. Veins, highest O_2 sat.

682. **Identify the artery labeled #2 in the thoracic angiogram shown.**
  a. **Right subclavian**
  b. **Right internal mammary**
  c. **Brachycephalic**
  d. **Right common carotid**

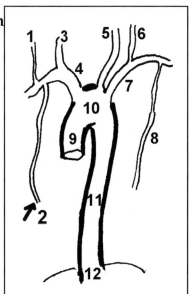
Aortic arch vessels

ANSWER b. The internal mammary (or internal thoracic artery) is commonly selectively catheterized in patients who have received internal mammary grafts to the coronary arteries.
BE ABLE TO CORRECTLY MATCH ALL BELOW.
  1. Right Vertebral
  2. Right Internal Mammary (Internal Thoracic)
  3. Right Common Carotid
  4. Innominate (Brachio-cephalic)
  5. Left Common Carotid
  6. Left Vertebral
  7. Left Subclavian
  8. Left Internal Mammary (Internal Thoracic)

9. Ascending AO
10. Aortic Arch
11. Descending AO (Thoracic AO)
12. Abdominal AO (Below diaphragm)
See: Snopek, chapter on "Aortography." **Keywords:** RIMA

683. **Identify the artery labeled #7 in the four-vessel arch angiogram shown.**

a. **Left Subclavian**
b. **Brachycephalic**
c. **Left Common Carotid**
d. **Right Common Carotid**

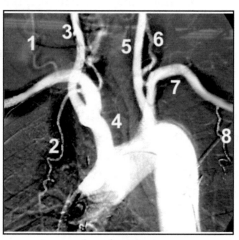

4 vessel arch arteriogram

ANSWER a. Lt. Subclavian arises directly from the aortic arch and continues to the left arm. Here it appears to originate from the Lt. Subclavian. Many variations exist.. Branches are numbered the same as in the drawing in the previous question. **BE ABLE TO CORRECTLY MATCH ALL BELOW.**

1. Right Vertebral
2. Right Internal Mammary (Internal Thoracic)
3. Right Common Carotid
4. Innominate (Brachio-cephalic)
5. Left Common Carotid
6. Left Vertebral
7. Left Subclavian
8. Left Internal Mammary (Internal Thoracic)
See: Snopek, chapter on "Aortography." **Keywords:** RIMA

684. **In this left lateral view of the left-sided neck arteries, identify the artery labeled as #4.**

a. **Common carotid artery**
b. **Internal carotid artery**
c. **External carotid artery**
d. **Vertebral artery**
e. **Thyrocervical artery**

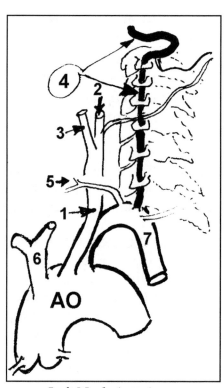

Left Neck Arteries

ANSWER d. Vertebral artery. Left vertebral arises from the left subclavian and can be seen rising through the lateral processes of the cervical spine. The vertebral artery supplies the basilar artery which feeds into the circle of Willis and the back of the brain.

BE ABLE TO CORRECTLY MATCH ALL BELOW.

1. Left common carotid artery
2. Internal carotid artery

3. External carotid artery
4. Vertebral artery
5. Thyrocervical artery
6. Innominate (brachio-cephalic) artery
7. Left subclavian artery

See: Snopek, chapter on "Cerebral Angiography."

5. Pulmonary

685. **The right lung has ____ lobes.**
   a.   2
   b.   3
   c.   4
   d.   5

ANSWER b. 3 lobes. The right lung has three lobes separated by lung fissures. The left lung has only two. Perhaps this is because of the heart takes up so much of the space of the left lung that there is no more room for another lobe. The lobes are divided from each other by fissures. **Match the lobes of the lung shown below:**
   1. Right superior (apex)
   2. Right middle lobe
   3. Right inferior lobe (base)
   4. Left superior lobe (apex)
   5. Left inferior lobe (base)

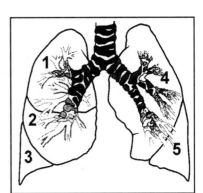
Lobes of the lung

Each lobe of the lung receives its own lobar bronchi which branches from the right or left primary bronchus as shown.
See: Tortora, chapter on "The Respiratory System." **Keywords:** Lobes of the lungs

686. **What cartilaginous structure acts like a trap door during swallowing to prevent food from entering the lungs?**
   a.   Cricoid cartilage
   b.   Carina
   c.   Epiglottis
   d.   Oropharynx

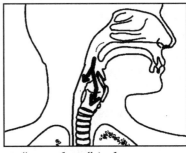
"trap door" in larynx

ANSWER c. The epiglottis is a leaf shaped structure which lies on top of the larynx. It moves freely like a trap door. During swallowing the larynx elevates causing the free edge of the epiglottis to cover and close off the trachea. This keeps food and liquid out of the trachea, which would trigger a cough reflex.
See: Tortora, chapter on "Respiratory System."

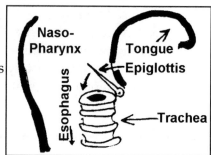
Epiglottis

687. **The space in the chest between the two lungs which contain the heart marked at #1 is called the:**
   a.   Peritoneum
   b.   Esophagus
   c.   Pleural cavity
   d.   Mediastinum
   e.   Retroperitoneal space

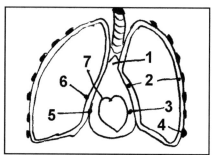
Thoracic spaces

ANSWER d. The mediastinum is the mass of tissues between the two pleural sacks (between sternum and backbone, from thoracic inlet to diaphragm). It contains the heart, pericardium, esophagus, etc. **BE ABLE TO CORRECTLY MATCH ALL BELOW.**
          1. Mediastinum
          2. Pleural space
          3. Pericardial space
          4. Rib or parietal pleura
          5. Parietal pericardium
          6. Visceral pleura
          7. Epicardium (visceral pericardium)
See: medical dictionary **Keywords:** mediastinum.

688. **In this lateral view of an RV angiogram, identify the structure labeled #4.**
   a.   RV
   b.   RPA
   c.   LPA
   d.   Main PA
   e.   Conus

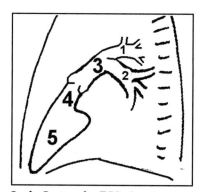
Left Lateral - RV. Angio

ANSWER e. Conus or infundibulum of the RV. The RV is a flat "U" shaped structure beneath the sternum. RV blood passes through the RV outflow tract or conus, through the pulmonary valve (most superior valve) and into the main PA. The PA divides into right and left branches going to their respective lungs. The RPA courses up through the aortic window (hole under AO arch) and into the right lung. The left PA courses down to supply the left lung.
CORRECTLY MATCHED ANSWERS ARE:

1. RPA
2. LPA
3. Main PA
4. Conus, infundibulum
5. RV

See: Braunwald, chapter on "Angiography." **Keywords:** Lt. Lat. RV gram, PA, Rt. & Lt. PA

689. Identify the structures of the lung lobule labeled at #3 on the diagram.

a. **Respiratory bronchiole**
b. **Alveolar ducts**
c. **Alveoli**
d. **Glottis**
e. **Trachea**
f. **Bronchus**

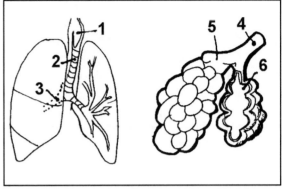

Lung and Lobule (after Anderson 16.2)

ANSWER f. Bronchus. The trachea divides into 2 main stem bronchi: the right and left bronchus. The terminal portion of the lung is the alveoli or alveolar sack (6) where the pulmonary capillary exchanges respiratory gases. This process of gas exchange is termed "internal respiration."

BE ABLE TO CORRECTLY MATCH ALL BELOW.

1. Glottis
2. Trachea
3. Right Bronchus
4. Respiratory Bronchiole
5. Alveolar Duct
6. Alveoli

Respiration Anderson, chapter on "Respiration." **Keywords:** Structures of lung and alveoli

690. In what lung structures are O_2 and CO_2 exchanged?

a. **Bronchioles**
b. **Bronchi**
c. **Alveoli**
d. **Pulmonary veins**

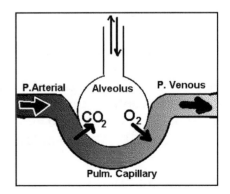

ANSWER c. Alveoli. The terminal portion of the lung is the alveoli or alveolar sack where the pulmonary capillary exchanges respiratory gases. CO_2 is very soluble, and rapidly diffuses into the alveoli. O_2 takes longer. This process of gas exchange is termed "internal respiration." Once the CO_2 and O_2 exchange across the alveolar membrane, the alveolar gas is expelled, and replaced with fresh air, low in CO_2 and high in O_2. This process of breathing is termed "external respiration."

See: Anderson, chapter on "Respiration." **Keywords:** Alveolar gas exchange

691. Which efferent (motor) nerve controls motion of the diaphragm?
- a. Vagus
- b. Phrenic
- c. Sympathetic
- d. Parasympathetic

ANSWER b. The phrenic nerve is the nerve of respiration from the respiratory center in the medulla. The vagus nerve is the afferent (from periphery to CNS) that senses stretch receptors in the lung. If the phrenic nerves are experimentally cut, respiration stops. This is a dreaded complication during AF ablation of the pulmonary veins.
See: Anderson, chapter on "Nervous System" **Keywords:** phrenic nerve

6. Angiographic Anatomy: Abdominal Arteries

692. How many pulmonary veins normally empty into the left atrium?
- a. 1
- b. 2
- c. 3
- d. 4

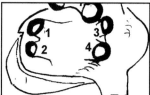
Posterior view of heart

ANSWER d. There are normally 4 pulmonary veins emptying into the posterior left atrium - 2 from each lung. This is easily seen on heart models. Get a good heart model and learn to identify every structure. These 4 veins may be misplaced in anomalous venous return - some or all emptying into the right atrium. **See:** Netter, CIBA Collection "The Heart." **Keywords:** 4 pulmonary veins

693. Where are the great vessels of the heart attached?
- a. Apex of heart
- b. Base of heart
- c. Each atrial inflow tract
- d. Each ventricular inflow tract

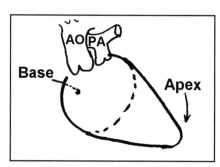
Heart as Cone (apex and base)

ANSWER b. Base of heart (basis cordis). The heart is like a cone with its apex pointing inferiorly and 60 degrees to the left. The base of this cone is where the great vessels and atria arise. Note that the apex of the lungs point up - opposite to the cardiac apex.
See: Netter, CIBA Collection "The Heart."

694. The common iliac veins unite in the pelvis to form the:
- a. Hepatic portal vein
- b. Inferior vena cava
- c. Superior vena cava
- d. Azygous vein

ANSWER b. Inferior vena cava. Iliac veins join in the abdomen to from the IVC. Memorize all major veins and arteries, especially those which are important in cardiology. Most test questions are somehow related to the field of cardiology. For example they would probably never ask about the veins in the fingers.
See: Underhill, chapter on "Cardiac Anatomy"
Keywords: Iliac veins form IVC

695. **The artery supplying the small intestine is the:**
a. Gastric
b. Celiac
c. Superior mesenteric
d. Posterior mesenteric

ANSWER c. The superior mesenteric usually arises anteriorly from the abdominal aorta, at the level of the renal arteries and just below the celiac artery. The superior mesenteric fans out to the supply all of the small intestines, while the inferior mesenteric chiefly supplies the large intestine (colon). Mesenteric venous drainage dumps into the liver for filtering and metabolic processing.
See: Gray's Anatomy. **Keywords:** Superior mesenteric a., small intestine

696. **Identify the vein in this anterior view of the portal system labeled at #1.**
a. Portal vein
b. Superior Mesenteric vein
c. Inferior Mesenteric vein
d. Hepatic vein
e. Splenic vein

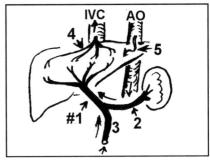
Portal circulation

ANSWER a. The portal vein collects the splenic and superficial mesenteric venous blood and funnels it into the liver. The hepatic veins drain the liver itself and feed into the IVC. the function of this system is to pass the blood from the intestines through the liver before its entering the general circulation.

The liver cleanses the blood of bacteria. It also absorbs certain nutrients from the intestinal blood such as glucose and proteins. These nutrients are stored in the liver to "buffer" their blood concentrations.

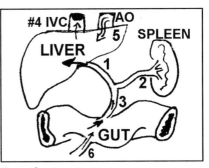
Portal system

The hepatic arteries parallel the portal veins into the liver and supply the liver itself with O_2. They are not involved in the metabolic processing of nutrients from the gut. This is a rare instance where an organ (liver) has veins feeding and draining it.

The portal vein supplies 75% of total hepatic flow. The other 25% comes from the hepatic artery which join in the "sinusoids" where macrophages clean the blood of bacteria and other impurities. This blood then empties into central hepatic veins. Note the bile ducts which run parallel but in opposite directions to the portal veins.

BE ABLE TO CORRECTLY MATCH ALL BELOW.

    1. Portal vein
    2. Splenic vein
    3. Superior mesenteric (intestinal) veins
    4. Hepatic vein
    5. Hepatic artery
    6. Mesenteric artery

See: Tortorici chapter on" Angiography of Liver and Spleen." **Keywords:** Portal veins, portal circulation

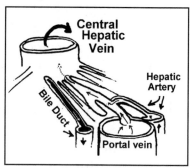

Hepatic Sinusoids

697. **The major artery arising anteriorly from the abdominal aorta labeled #3 is:**
  a.   **Celiac**
  b.   **Renals**
  c.   **Superior mesenteric**
  d.   **Testicular or ovarian**
  e.   **Inferior mesenteric**

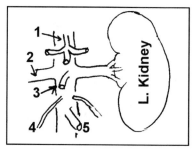

Abdominal Aorta

ANSWER c. Superior mesenteric artery. These 5 arteries all arise alphabetically from the abdominal AO, except the inferior mesenteric which is obviously the most inferior of the 5 major abdominal arteries. **BE ABLE TO CORRECTLY MATCH ALL BELOW.**

    1. Celiac
    2. Renals
    3. Superior mesenteric
    4. Testicular or ovarian
    5. Inferior mesenteric

See: "Medical dictionary," arteries. **Keywords:** superior mesenteric, abdominal arteries

698. **In the abdominal angiogram shown, identify the structure shown at #1.**
  a.   **Splenic artery**
  b.   **Common hepatic artery**
  c.   **Common celiac artery**
  d.   **Left gastric artery**

ANSWER: c. The celiac axis is a 1-2 cm. trunk from which three arteries branch in the form of a tripod feeding the gastric, splenic, and hepatic arteries.

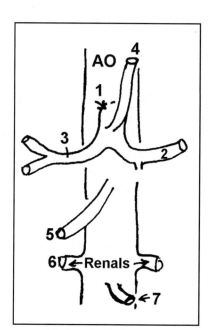

Abdominal Aorta

BE ABLE TO CORRECTLY MATCH ALL BELOW.

    1. Celiac artery
    2. Splenic artery (branches down and to the left of the spleen)
    3. Left gastric artery (branches up to the left and down to the stomach)
    4. Common hepatic artery (branches up to the liver and duodenum).
    5. Superior mesenteric artery (to small intestine)
    6. Renal artery (to kidneys)
    7. Inferior Mesenteric (to large intestine)

See: Snopek, chapter on "Abdominal Angiography." **Keywords:** Celiac axis, arteries

699. **At what vertebral level does the celiac artery normally originate?**
    a.   **T9**
    b.   **T12**
    c.   **L2**
    d.   **L4**

ANSWER b. T12. For selective celiac angiography it is helpful to know where to encounter the celiac axis. A hooked or right angle catheter is positioned at T12 and withdrawn with the point directed anteriorly. **See:** Dyer, Chapter on Celiac Arteriography.

7. Angiographic Anatomy: Arm and Leg

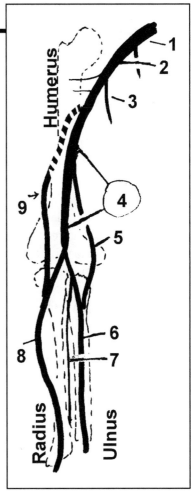

Arteries of the right arm

700. **Distal to the thorax the subclavian artery becomes the _____ artery.**
    a.   **Carotid**
    b.   **Axillary**
    c.   **Radial**
    d.   **Palmar**

ANSWER b. The axilla is the "armpit." The major subclavian arteries become axillary vessels after exiting the thorax at the shoulder. Then in the arm the axillary becomes the brachial artery, and in the forearm becomes the radial or ulnar artery. The axillary and brachial arteries are alternate arterial catheterization sites. **See:** Grays anatomy.

701. **In this right arm arteriogram identify the artery labeled at #4.**
    a.   **Subclavian artery**
    b.   **Axillary artery**
    c.   **Deep brachial**
    d.   **Radial artery**
    e.   **Brachial artery**
    f.   **Ulnar collateral**
    g.   **Ulnar artery**

h.   **Interosseous artery**
I.   **Profunda brachialis**

ANSWER e. Brachial artery arises from the axillary artery. Arteries of the arm are often used for arterial access sites in angiography. They occasionally become stenosed, although less commonly than the femoral system. **BE ABLE TO CORRECTLY MATCH ALL BELOW.**

     1. Subclavian artery
     2. Axillary artery
     3. Deep brachial
     4. Brachial artery
     5. Ulnar collateral
     6. Ulnar artery
     7. Interosseous artery
     8. Radial artery
     9. Profunda brachialis
See: "Medical Dictionary," Arteries. **Keywords:** Arm arteries, brachial

702. **The femoral artery arises from the _____ artery (labeled #2 in the diagram).**
    a.   **External iliac**
    b.   **Internal iliac**
    c.   **Popliteal**
    d.   **Profunda**

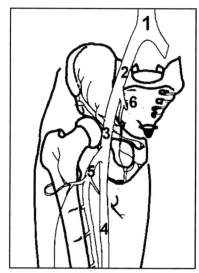

Femoral artery origin

ANSWER a. The external iliac comes from the common iliac and branches into the inferior epigastric, deep circumflex, and femoral. The internal iliac branches to pelvic organs such as the reproductive organs, buttock, and medial aspect of the thigh. Arteries shown are:

     1. Descending aorta
     2. External iliac artery
     3. Common femoral artery
     4. Femoral (superficial) artery
     5. Profunda or deep femoral artery
     6. Internal iliac artery
See: Underhill, chapter on "Cardiac Anatomy"

703. **In this AP view of the right inguinal area, identify the vessel labeled at #5.**
a. Iliac vein
b. Iliac artery
c. Deep femoral (profundus) artery
d. Superficial femoral artery
e. Femoral vein
f. Saphenous vein

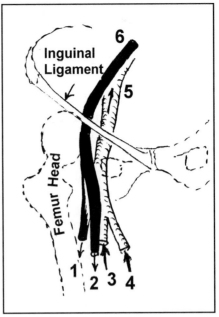

ANSWER a. Iliac vein. Note how the femoral artery and vein (#2 & #3) overlap in the lower part of the diagram. One complication of low femoral puncture is to puncture both artery and vein in one stick. This can lead to bleeding between vessels (AV fistula). Note how the femoral vein is just medial to the femoral artery.
BE ABLE TO CORRECTLY MATCH ALL BELOW.
1. Deep femoral (profundus) artery
2. Superficial femoral artery
3. Femoral vein
4. Saphenous vein
5. Iliac vein
6. Iliac artery

Pelvis, Art./veins

See: Grossman, chapter on "Percutaneous approach."

704. **What vessel is punctured with the needle shown at #3?**
a. Femoral vein
b. Iliac artery
c. Superficial femoral artery
d. Common femoral artery
e. Deep femoral (profundus) artery

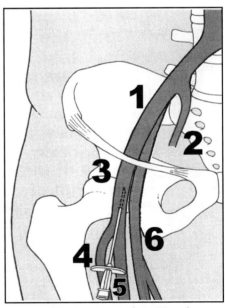

ANSWER d. Common femoral artery. This is where you are supposed to make a femoral artery puncture. Note how it is directly over the round femoral knob. Note also, how the femoral vein #6 is just medial to the femoral artery.
BE ABLE TO CORRECTLY MATCH ALL BELOW.
1. Iliac artery
2. Internal iliac artery
3. Common femoral artery
4. Deep femoral (profundus) artery
5. Superficial femoral artery
6. Femoral vein

Femoral puncture, after Kandarpa

See: Kandarpa, chapter on Peripheral arteriography." **Keywords:** Inguinal anatomy, femoral artery and vein

705. **In these views of the right calf identify the artery at #1.**

   a.   **Peroneal artery**
   b.   **Dorsal artery (anterior tibial) of foot**
   c.   **Popliteal artery**
   d.   **Anterior tibial artery**
   e.   **Lateral malleolar branch**
   f.   **Medial malleolar branch**
   g.   **Posterior tibial artery**

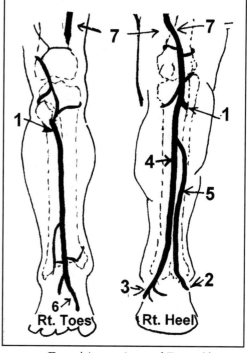

Post/Ant. view of Rt. calf

ANSWER d. The anterior tibial artery runs between the anterior aspect of the tibia and fibula and ends in the dorsalis pedis on the front of the foot. The dorsalis pedis artery is commonly palpated to check pulse quality after femoral catheterization. This shows the three trifurcation arteries arising from the popliteal artery in the right calf.
BE ABLE TO CORRECTLY MATCH ALL BELOW.
1. Anterior tibial artery
2. Lateral malleolar branch
3. Medial malleolar branch
4. Posterior tibial artery
5. Peroneal artery (last arising trifurcation branch)
6. Dorsalis pedis artery of foot
7. Popliteal artery
See: Snopek, chapter on "Femoral Angiography." **Keywords:** Arteries of calf,

706. **In this runoff arteriogram of the R & L calves, identify the artery at #5.**

   a.   **Peroneal artery**
   b.   **Dorsal artery (anterior tibial) of foot**
   c.   **Popliteal artery**
   d.   **Anterior tibial artery**
   e.   **Lateral malleolar branch**
   f.   **Medial malleolar branch**
   g.   **Posterior tibial artery**

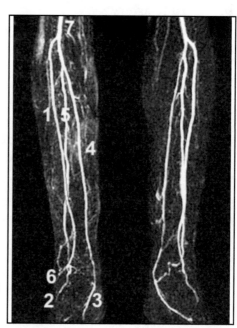

Arteriogram lower extremity

ANSWER a. Peroneal artery is the last of the 3 major arteries of the calf to branch. It appears in the middle between the other 2 major tibial branches. It continues down the posterior calf and ends in the lateral malleolar branch, which is <u>not</u> one of the ankle arteries that is easily felt. The medial malleolus is easier to feel, and is commonly checked post cath. This is an arteriogram showing the three trifurcation arteries arising from the popliteal artery in the lower extremity. Branches are numbered the same

as in the drawing in the previous question.
BE ABLE TO CORRECTLY MATCH ALL BELOW.
   1. Anterior tibial artery
   2. Lateral malleolar branch
   3. Medial malleolar branch
   4. Posterior tibial artery
   5. Peroneal artery (last trifurcation branch is between two tibial branches)
   6. Dorsalis pedis artery of foot
   7. Popliteal artery
See: Snopek, chapter on "Femoral Angiography." **Keywords:** Arteries of calf,

707. What artery supplies the anterior and posterior tibial arteries?
   a.   **Peroneal**
   b.   **Popliteal**
   c.   **Femoral**
   d.   **Iliac**

ANSWER b. Popliteal is the artery behind the knee which supplies the trifurcation arteries of the calf - the anterior tibial, posterior tibial and peroneal arteries. The dorsalis pedis artery, commonly palpated on front of the foot, is a continuation of the anterior tibial artery. See: Medical dictionary

708. Identify the 3 runoff/outflow vessels of the leg. (Select 3 below.)
   a.   **Popliteal**
   b.   **Profunda**
   c.   **Peroneal artery**
   d.   **Anterior tibial artery**
   e.   **Posterior tibial artery**

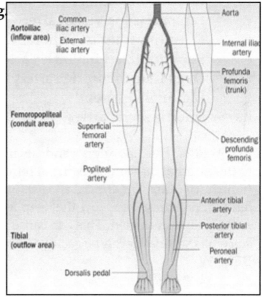

ANSWERS: c, d, & e. Peroneal, Anterior tibial, and Posterior tibial artery.

   Topol says, "The anterior tibial artery, posterior tibial artery, and the peroneal artery are considered the runoff vessels." **See:** Topo,l chapter on "Lower Extremity Interventions"

   The inflow arteries in the pelvis are iliacs. The conduit arteries of the thigh are the superficial femoral, profunda and popliteal. The calf outflow arteries are the trifurcation arteries, the 2 tibials and peroneal. The anterior tibial is usually the first to bifurcate and the most lateral. **See:** Topol, chapter on "Peripheral Vascular Interventions"

709. If a thrombus in the left common iliac <u>vein</u> becomes dislodged and embolizes, in which capillary bed will it lodge?
a.   Left leg
b.   Left arm
c.   Brain
d.   Lungs

ANSWER d. Lungs. The veins all lead back to the heart. Systemic blood then flows through the right heart and into the lungs, where clots would be filtered out. This is termed a "pulmonary embolus." The diagnosis of pulmonary embolism (PE) is commonly missed and recognized only at autopsy. It is the leading nonsurgical cause of death to hospitalized patients. Most of these thrombo-embolisms occur because of extended bed rest, immobility, clotting defects, and trauma to the vein. Therefore, you should ambulate post-op patients early to prevent "thrombo-phlebitis" and "pulmonary embolism."
See: Braunwald, chapter on "Pulmonary Embolism." **Keywords:** venous return

710. In this anterior view of the pelvic arteries (or AP abdominal angiogram of the inguinal area) identify the artery labeled #2.
a.   External iliac artery
b.   Internal iliac artery
c.   Femoral (superficial) artery
d.   Deep (profundus) femoral
e.   Superior iliac circumflex artery
f.   Deep iliac circumflex artery
g.   Inguinal ligament
h.   Middle sacral artery

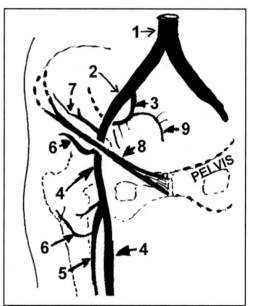

Arteries of Pelvis

ANSWER a. The iliac artery sends its main division to the external iliac and superficial femoral arteries (which we utilize for arterial access). Note that if femoral puncture is too low the deep femoral may be mistakenly cannulated. This can cause complications since it is so small it can be easily damaged. **BE ABLE TO CORRECTLY MATCH ALL BELOW**.

1. Aorta
2. External iliac artery
3. Internal iliac artery
4. Femoral (superficial) artery
5. Deep (profundus) femoral
6. Superior iliac circumflex artery
7. Deep iliac circumflex artery
8. Inguinal ligament
9. Middle sacral artery

See: "Medical Dictionary," arteries. Keywords: Pelvic arteries

8. Other Vascular Anatomy: Abdominal

711. **Which three below are functions of the spleen?**
     1. **Filtration of plasma**
     2. **Cleans blood of dead erythrocytes**
     3. **Excrete & store hormones**
     4. **Store blood**
     5. **Metabolize carbohydrates**
         a. 1, 2, 3
         b. 1, 2, 4
         c. 1, 3, 4
         d. 3, 4, 5

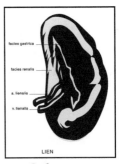

Spleen

ANSWER b. Filtration of plasma, cleans blood of dead erythrocytes, and stores blood. The spleen normally contains about 5 ml of blood, but can expand to store up to a liter. It cleanses foreign substances and erythrocytes from the blood using reticular phagocytic endothelial cells.
See: Guyton, chapter on "Special areas of the CV System." Keywords: Spleen, functions

712. **The chief function of bile is to:**
     a.   **Breakdown carbohydrates for digestion**
     b.   **Reduce surface tension of fats for digestion**
     c.   **Release the gastric enzymes-pepsin, ptyalin, & HCl**
     d.   **Digest fiber and proteins**

ANSWER b. Reduce surface tension of fats for digestion. Although bile dumps from the gallbladder into the duodenum, it is not an enzyme for digesting foods. It acts as an emulsifying detergent to lower the surface tension of fats and other water insoluble nutrients. It does this by breaking them down into smaller globules about 1 uM in diameter. This allows more efficient absorption and digestion of fats.

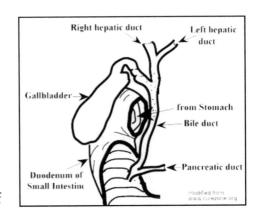

     Bile also serves to eliminate bilirubin. The principal bile pigment is "bilirubin" - a byproduct of RBC destruction in the spleen. This bilirubin eventually is broken down in the intestine and one of its byproducts gives feces its brown color. Jaundice occurs when the body cannot eliminate bilirubin from the blood.
See: Guyton, chapter on "Digestive System" Keywords: Bile, function, bilirubin

713. **This AP/PA schematic view is of the right kidney. Identify the structure labeled #4.**
  a.   **Minor calyx**
  b.   **Major calyx**
  c.   **Ureter**
  d.   **Renal artery**
  e.   **Cortex**
  f.   **Medulla**

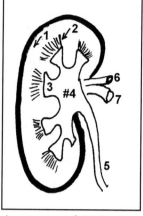

Anatomy of Kidney

ANSWER: b. Major calyx. The kidney gross structure shows the (#1) cortex (outer area), (#2) the medulla (inner area). (#3 & 4) The minor and major calyx filter and drain urine into (#5) the ureter. (#6 & 7) The renal artery and veins. Arteries are smaller in diameter and thicker walled. Be able to match all answers below. **BE ABLE TO CORRECTLY MATCH ALL BELOW.**

    1. Cortex (outer later)
    2. Medulla
    3. Minor calyx
    4. Major calyx
    5. Right ureter
    6. Right renal artery
    7. Right renal vein
See: Snopek, chapter on "Renal Arteriography."

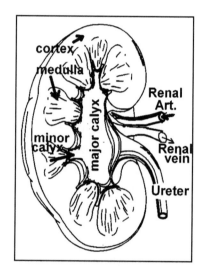

Kidney

714. **This is an anterior view of the abdominal structures that might be seen in a transhepatic cholangiogram. Identify the anatomical structure labeled at #1 (upper left).**
  a.   **Right hepatic duct**
  b.   **Light hepatic duct**
  c.   **Common hepatic duct**
  d.   **Cystic duct**
  e.   **Gall bladder**
  f.   **Common bile duct**
  g.   **Pancreatic duct**
  h.   **Duodenum**
  I.   **Right intrahepatic duct**
  j.   **Left intrahepatic duct**

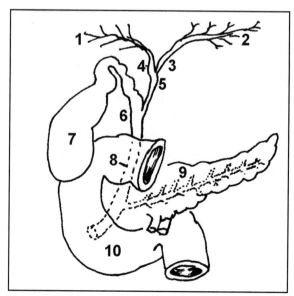

ANSWER I. The intrahepatic ducts are the

Transhepatic cholangiogram

most distal. They transport bile from the liver to the hepatic ducts. These 2 hepatic ducts combine in the common hepatic duct. The cystic duct branches from the common hepatic duct and is attached to the gallbladder. The common bile duct is the convergence of the cystic + common bile ducts. The common hepatic duct becomes the common bile duct and drains into the duodenum. The pancreatic duct continues to the pancreas. **BE ABLE TO CORRECTLY MATCH ALL BELOW.**

    1. Right intrahepatic duct
    2. Left intrahepatic duct
    3. Right hepatic duct
    4. Left hepatic duct
    5. Common hepatic duct
    6. Cystic duct
    7. Gall bladder
    8. Common bile duct
    9. Pancreatic duct
    10. Duodenum

See: Tortorici, chapter on "Transhepatic Cholangiography."

9. Other Vascular Anatomy: Lymphatic

715. **Identify the functions of the lymphatic system. (Select 4 below.)**
    a.   **Return proteins to the circulation**
    b.   **Filter and phagocytize foreign particles**
    c.   **Provide nutrition and oxygen to lymph nodes**
    d.   **Maintain low colloidal osmotic pressure in tissue spaces**
    e.   **Drain excess fluids from interstitial tissues**

ANSWERS: a, b, d, & e.
a. Return proteins to the circulation - YES
b. Filter and phagocytize foreign particles - YES
c. Provide nutrition and oxygen to lymph nodes - NO
d. Maintain low colloidal osmotic pressure in tissue spaces - YES
e. Drain excess fluids from interstitial tissues - YES

    Lymph nodes have their own arterial blood supply for nutrition. It is not supplied by the lymph itself.

    An important function of the lymphatic system is to keep the interstitial tissues "dry." It does this by removing protein from the interstitial space which has seeped out of capillaries. (See Starlings law of capillary permeability). This reduces the tissue colloidal osmotic pressure. A high osmotic pressure in tissues could pull excessive fluid out of the capillary and cause tissue edema.

    The lymphatic hydrostatic pressure is -2 mmHg due to the muscular "lymphatic pump" and lymphatic valves. In this way it is similar to the "venous pump." Both of the above properties draw fluid out of the tissue spaces until they become relatively "dry."

    Besides all these functions the lymphatic system is where lymphocytes are created and immune bodies are formed.

See: Berne and Levy, chapter on "Microcirculation and lymphatics" Keywords: lymphatic system functions

716. **Identify the major lymph node groups. (Check all that apply.)**
    a.   **Submaxillary**
    b.   **Axillary**
    c.   **Coronary**
    d.   **Inguinal**

ANSWERS: a, b, & d. Coronary is NOT correct. When you look at the lymphatic drainage areas of the body you see clusters of nodes in the neck (submaxillary), in the axilla (armpit), and in the inguinal area (crotch). Physicians often feel patients for inflammation in these lymph nodes areas.
See: Tortora, chapter on "Lymphatic System and Immunity."
Keywords: Lymph node groups

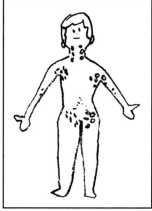

Lymph node areas

717. **The chief difference between systemic capillaries and lymphatic capillaries is that lymphatics are:**
    a.   **Open ended**
    b.   **Closed ended**
    c.   **Drain towards the heart**
    d.   **Drain away from the heart**

ANSWER b. Closed ended. Lymphatic capillaries are closed ended. They have no inlet like blood capillaries, only an outlet. This diagram shows the blind-ended plasma capillary. Plasma and other materials that accumulate in the intercellular space diffuse, may be picked by the venous capillary (shown on the bottom of diagram), or absorbed into the blind ended lymph capillary. These are conducted up through the thoracic duct and back into the bloodstream. This process helps prevent edema from occurring.

The veins and lymphatics are also similar in that they both contain valves. **See:** Anderson, Human A & P Coloring Book and Study Guide. **Keywords:** blind ended lymphatic capillaries

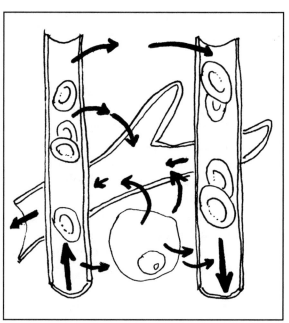

Lymphatics draining excess Intercellular fluid

718. Lymph drains from the entire lower body and left side through the _____ thoracic duct into the _____.
  a.   Right, Right subclavian artery
  b.   Right, Right subclavian vein
  c.   Left, Left subclavian artery
  d.   Left, Left subclavian vein

ANSWER d. Left, Left subclavian vein. The major lymphatic drainage from the entire lower body and the left arm and left side of head drain into the left thoracic lymphatic duct. This duct empties at the juncture of the left internal jugular and left subclavian veins. The remaining right side of the body above the waist, drains into the right side at the juncture of the right jugular and right subclavian vein.
See: Snopek, chapter on "Lymph Angiography." **Keywords:** Lymph drainage

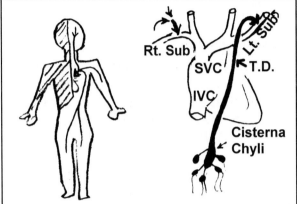

Lymph drainage from body to SVC

719. Normally the total volume of fluid transported through the lymphatics is approximately _____ ml/min.
  a.   1-2 ml/min
  b.   10-20 ml/min
  c.   50-100 ml/min
  d.   100-250 ml/min

ANSWER a. 1-2 ml/min or approximately 100 ml/hr. Compare this small flow to the normal blood flow of 5000 ml/min. The fluid and protein which escape the capillaries enter the lymphatic system. This is transported via the lymphatic system back to the blood vascular compartment via the two thoracic ducts into the right and/or left subclavian veins. The volume of fluid transported in 24 hours is about equal to an animal's total plasma volume or approximately 100 ml/hr.
See: Berne & Levy, chapter on "Microcirculation and Lymphatics." and Guyton, chapter on "Body Fluids and Lymphatics." Keywords: microcirculation, lymphatic flow

720. Lymphatic vessels originating in the villi of the small intestines which absorb fat are termed _____. They transport a type of white lymph called _____.
  a.   Cisterna, Chyle
  b.   Cisterna, Plasma
  c.   Lacteals, Chyle
  d.   Lacteals, Plasma

ANSWER c. Lacteals, Chyle. The absorbed fat forms a creamy colored lymph which drains from the lacteals of the small intestine.

BE ABLE TO CORRECTLY MATCH ALL BELOW:

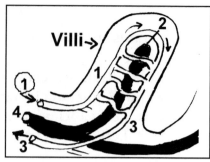

Lacteals drain Villi

1. Arteriole to villi
2. Lacteal draining chyle from villi
3. Venule from villi
4. Lymph vessels draining villi

See: Snopek, chapter on "Lymph angiography."

REFERENCES:

Anderson, P.D., *Human Anatomy and Physiology Coloring Workbook and Study Guide*, Jones and Barklett Publishers, 1990

Baim, D. S. and Grossman W., Cardiac Catheterization, Angiography, and Intervention, 7th Ed., Lea and Febiger, 2006

Pappano & Wier., Cardiovascular Physiology, 10th Ed., Mosby Year Book, 2013

Guyton & Hall, *Textbook of Medical Physiology*, WB Saunders Co., 1996

Kandarpa, K., *Handbook of Cardiovascular and Interventional Radiologic Procedures*, 3rd Ed., Little Brown and Co., 2002

Netter, *CIBA Collection of Medical Illustrations*, "The Heart", CIBA Pharmaceuticals

Snopek, A. M., *Fundamentals of Special Radiographic Procedures*, 3rd Ed., W. B. Saunders, 1992

Taylor, E. J. Ed., *Dorland's Medical Dictionary*, 27th ed., W. B. Saunders Co., 1988

Tortora, G. J., *Introduction to the HUMAN BODY*, Harper and Row Pub., 1988

Underhill, S. L., Ed., *CARDIAC NURSING*, 2nd Ed., J. B. Lippincott Co., 1989

OUTLINE: B8 - Vascular Anatomy

1. General Vascular Anatomy
   a. Anatomic positions
      i. Distal
      ii. Dorsal
      iii. Lateral
      iv. Proximal
      v. Ventral
      vi. Cephalic
      vii. Caudal
   b. Abbreviations
      i. CFA
      ii. DSA
      iii. SMA
      iv. PTA
      v. DVT
      vi. IVP
      vii. DP
      viii. V/Q
      ix. BUN
      x. PFA
      xi. NG
      xii. KUB
   c. Palpating arteries
      i. External Carotid (temporal)
      ii. Common Carotid
      iii. Subclavian
      iv. Brachial
      v. Radial
      vi. Femoral
      vii. Popliteal
   d. Grade arterial pulse 0-4
2. Vascular micro- Anatomy
   a. Capillaries = 3 billion
   b. Venous anatomy
      i. venous valves
      ii. more compliant
      iii. carry blood to heart
      iv. layers
         (1) intima (endothelium)
         (2) media (smooth muscle)
         (3) adventia
   c. Arterial anatomy
      i. carry blood away from heart
      ii. O_2 rich (except PA)
      iii. layers
         (1) intima (endothelium)

                    (a) involved with
                         atherosclerosis
                         (i) fatty lesions
                         (ii) plaque
            (2) media (smooth muscle)
                    (a) smooth muscle proliferation
                         in
                         atherosclerosis
            (3) adventia (Tunica Externa)
3. Cerebral, Neck arteries
    a. Circle of Willis
        i.   location
        ii. anastomosis
        iii. Arteries of:
            (1) Rt. Common Carotid
            (2) Lt. Anterior Cerebral
            (3) Rt. Vertebral
            (4) Rt. Anterior Cerebral
            (5) Rt. Vertebral
            (6) Lt. Middle Cerebral
            (7) Lt. Common Carotid
            (8) Rt. Middle Cerebral
            (9) Lt. External Carotid
            (10) Lt. Post Cerebral
            (11) Rt. External Carotid
            (12) Rt. Post Cerebral
        iv. Neck - Carotid Arteries
            (1) anterior communicating
            (2) anterior cerebral
            (3) Internal Carotid
            (4) middle cerebral
            (5) posterior communicating
            (6) posterior cerebral
            (7) superior cerebral
            (8) Pontine
            (9) basilar
            (10) vertebral arteries
            (11) anterior spinal artery
            (12) external carotid
            (13) vertebral
            (14) subclavian
        v.   Head arteries
            (1) ant. cerebral
            (2) sylvian
            (3) middle cerebral
            (4) internal cerebral
            (5) frontopolar
            (6) basilar
            (7) basilar
            (8) post. cerebral
            (9) parieto-occipital
            (10) post. inferior cerebral
4. Thorax,
    a. Arch arteries
        i.   Rt. Vertebral
        ii. Rt. Internal mammary
             (Internal. thoracic)
        iii. Rt. Common Carotid
        iv. Innominate (Brachio-cephalic)
        v.   Lt. Common Carotid
        vi. Lt. Vertebral
        vii. Lt. Subclavian
        viii. Lt. Internal mammary
             (Internal. thoracic)

ix.   Ascending AO
x.   Aortic Arch
xi.   Descending AO (thoracic AO)
xii. Abdominal AO. (below diaphragm)
b. PULMONARY
    i.   anatomy of
    ii. Alveoli, bronchi...
         (1) O_2 and CO_2 exchange
    iii. # lobes
    iv. carina
    v.   cricoid cartilage
    vi. epiglottis
    vii. oropharynx
    viii. mediastinum
    ix. peritoneum
    x.   pleural space
    xi. diaphragm
         (1) phrenic nerve controls
5. Abdominal arteries
    a. Branches of Aorta & IVC
        i.   gastric
        ii.   celiac
        iii. superior mesenteric
        iv.   posterior mesenteric
        v.   portal vein
        vi.   superior Mesenteric vein
        vii. inferior Mesenteric vein
        viii. hepatic vein
        ix.   splenic vein
        x.   renal arteries
        xi.   testicular or ovarian
        xii. inferior mesenteric
        xiii. common hepatic artery
    b. SPLEEN
        i.   filtration of plasma
        ii. cleans blood of dead erythrocytes
        iii. store blood
    c. Kidney
        i.   minor Calyx
        ii. major Calyx
        iii. ureter
        iv. renal artery
    d. Cholangiogram
        i.   Rt. Intrahepatic duct
        ii.   Lt. Intrahepatic duct
        iii. Rt. hepatic duct
        iv.   Lt. hepatic duct
        v.   common hepatic duct
        vi.   cystic duct
        vii. gall bladder
        viii. common bile duct
        ix.   pancreatic duct
        x.   duodenum
        xi.   Cortex
        xii. medulla
    e. function of bile
        i.   reduce surface tension of fats for
        ii. digestion
6. Arteries of the Extremities
    a. ARM
        i.   subclavian
        ii. axillary
        iii. radial

iv. palmar
v. deep brachial
vi. radial collateral a.
vii. brachial artery
viii. Ulnar collateral
ix. ulnar artery
x. interosseous artery
xi. Profunda Brachialis
b. LEG
i. anterior tibial artery
ii. lateral malleolar branch
iii. medial malleolar branch
iv. posterior tibial artery
v. peroneal artery
vi. dorsalis pedis artery of foot
vii. popliteal artery
viii. pelvic arteries
ix. aorta
x. external iliac artery
xi. internal iliac artery
xii. femoral (superficial) artery
xiii. deep (profundus) femoral
xiv. superior iliac circumflex artery
xv. deep iliac circumflex artery
xvi. inguinal ligament
xvii. middle sacral artery
xviii. pelvic arteries
xix. deep femoral (Profundus) artery

xx. superficial femoral artery
xxi. femoral vein
xxii. saphenous vein
xxiii. Iliac vein
xxiv. iliac artery
7. Lymphatic
a. function of the lymphatic system?
i. return proteins to the circulation
ii. filter and phagocytize foreign particles
iii. maintain low colloidal osmotic pressure
iv. drain excess fluids from interstitium
b. lymphatics - Closed ended
c. thoracic duct
d. drains into Lt. Subclavian vein.
e. lymph node groups
i. submaxillary
ii. axillary
iii. inguinal
f. intestinal lymphatics
i. villi
ii. lacteal draining chyle from villi
iii. venule from villi
iv. lymph vessels draining villi

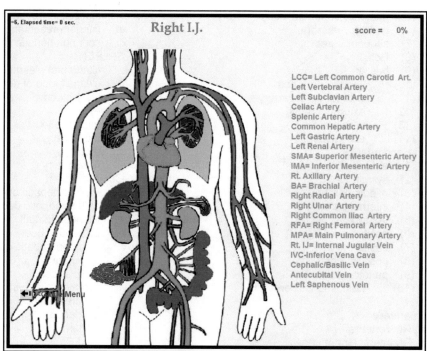

Todd CD, Vascular Anatomy Game, click on the vessel named

Vascular Physiology

INDEX: B9 - Vascular Physiology

1. Compliance

721. The elastic arteries filter and smooth out the pulsatile pressure within the aorta. This effect is termed the:

a. Pulse pressure
b. Stiffness effect
c. Peripheral resistance
d. Windkessel effect
e. Impedance

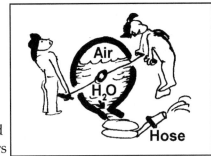

Hand operated fire hose pump

ANSWER d. A windkessel is an air ballast chamber used by the old hand pumped fire trucks. Similar air chambers are still attached to wells to smooth out pump strokes.
    The aorta stores and dampens the pulsatile pump flow by expanding the aorta in systole. This stores systolic energy and then returns that potential energy to the blood during diastole. Without this "Windkessel effect" the aortic pressure would resemble the LV pressure.
See: Berne & Levy, chapter on "Microcirculation."

722. Elderly individuals typically have _____ arterial wall compliance resulting in _____.

a. Increased, Decreased mean blood pressure
b. Increased, Increased systolic blood pressure
c. Decreased, Decreased mean blood pressure
d. Decreased, Increased systolic blood pressure

ANSWER d. Decreased, Increased systolic pressure. Old age hardens, calcifies, and reduces compliance of arteries. With this, elderly people frequently develop isolated systolic hypertension with wide pulse pressures (Eg. 180/60). The mean and diastolic BP usually don't increase as much with age. That is why many physicians consider the diastolic BP more important, because it is more indicative of the arterial resistance than systolic BP. This increasing systolic BP increases the pulse pressure as well.

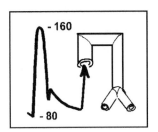

Hardening of arteries

It's like old metal plumbing, when you turn on the water, the pipes **knock** with a **water-hammer** sound.

Pulse pressure is the difference between systole and diastole:

Pulse pressure = systole - diastole

PP = S - D = 180 - 60 = 120 mmHg.

A wide pulse pressure is more easily felt (palpated) than a narrow pulse pressure.

See: Berne & Levy, chapter on "Arterial System." **Keywords**: Arterial, compliance, pulse pressure

723. **The definition of vascular COMPLIANCE is:**

(Note ∆= "change in")

a. **∆Volume /∆Pressure**
b. **∆Pressure/∆Volume**
c. **∆Volume /∆Time**
d. **∆Pressure/∆Time**

ANSWER a. ∆Volume / ∆Pressure = Compliance. Compliance is "stretchability." The more blood volume you can pump into an elastic vessel, for a given pressure the more compliant it is. Non-compliant vessels are stiff. Pumping blood into rigid vessels is like pumping up a tire - the more rigid it is the higher the pressure goes.

E.g., An aorta receives a stroke volume of 100 ml while the BP is 120/70 mmHg. The compliance is ∆V / ∆P. C = (100)/(120-70) = 100/50 = 2:1 ml/mmHg.

See: Berne & Levy, chapter on "Microcirculation." **Keywords**: Compliance, Capacitance

724. **The aorta stores blood during systole and releases it during diastole. This physical compliance is analogous to electrical:**

a. **Resistance**
b. **Capacitance**
c. **Inductance**
d. **Impedance**

ANSWER b. Capacitance is defined as C = ∆Coulombs/∆V. The number of electrons stored increases proportionately with the driving voltage. This is analogous in physiology to compliance:

C = ∆Volume / ∆Pressure.

A very compliant aorta will store more volume for the same pressure. Physiology texts use the terms compliance and capacitance synonymously.

See: Berne & Levy, chapter on "Microcirculation."
Keywords: Compliance, Capacitance

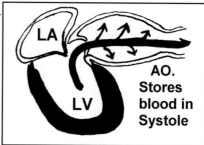

Aortic compliance

725. **Systolic arterial blood pressure normally increases with aging. What is the main factor causing this isolated systolic BP increase?**
   a.   **Increasing heart rate**
   b.   **Increased stroke volume**
   c.   **Increased arterial compliance**
   d.   **Decreased arterial compliance**

ANSWER d. Decreased arterial compliance. All these factors affect blood pressure but only a decrease in compliance (increased arterial stiffness) will increase systolic BP (while the mean BP stays the same). This compliance reduction (as in elderly stiff arteries) will raise mainly the systolic BP. However, the most compliant vessels are VEINS. They are 20 times more compliant than arteries and do not increase in pressure with aging. **See:** Berne & Levy, chapter on "The Arterial System."

726. **Hardening of the arteries in the elderly leads to:**
   a.   **Isolated diastolic hypertension**
   b.   **Isolated systolic hypertension**
   c.   **Systemic and Pulmonary hypertension**
   d.   **Systolic and diastolic hypertension**

ANSWER: b. Isolated systolic hypertension. As we age we get hardening of the arteries, which is decreased compliance (less stretchy). This tends to turn the arteries into rigid pipes, which get a water-hammer type pulse, especially higher in systole. Thus, BP tends to increase with age.
   "Isolated systolic hypertension, an elevation in systolic but not diastolic pressure, is the most prevalent type of hypertension in those aged 50 or over, occurring either de novo or as a development after a long period of systolic-diastolic hypertension with or without treatment. The increase in blood pressure with age is mostly associated with structural changes in the arteries and especially with large artery stiffness. It is known from various studies that rising blood pressure is associated with increased cardiovascular risk." **See,** Pinto, Posgraduate Medical Journal, 2007 "Blood Pressure and Aging" http://www.ncbi.nlm.nih.gov/pmc/articles/PMC2805932/
   Braunwald says, "The contour of the central aortic pressure and the pulmonary artery pressure tracing consists of a systolic wave, the incisura (indicating closure of the semilunar valves), and a gradual decline in pressure until the following systole. The pulse pressure reflects the stroke volume and compliance of the arterial system. The mean aortic pressure more accurately reflects peripheral resistance." **See:** Braunwald, chapter on "Hemodynamic Data"

727. **Venous capacitance (compliance) is normally ____ times greater than arterial capacitance.**
   a.   **5**
   b.   **20**
   c.   **30**
   d.   **40**

ANSWER b. 20. Veins can store about 20 times more blood than arteries because of their greater distensibility and vasodilation ability. This accounts for the massive venous pooling we see in some forms of shock. Nitrate drugs cause mostly veno-dilation and some arterial dilation. The veno-dilation affect probably helps angina more than the arterial dilation. It pools venous blood reducing preload.
See: Berne & Levy, chapter on "Control of CO" **Keywords:** venous capacitance, compliance, 20 times

728. In normal young individuals, when the LV pressure is compared to the femoral artery sheath pressure, the FA systolic pressure is usually _____ because _____.
a.   Slightly higher, reflected waves
b.   Significantly lower, of turbulence distal to the AO valve
c.   Slightly lower, of a slight pressure gradient across the AO valve
d.   The same, there is normally no gradient across the AO valve

ANSWER: a. Slightly higher, reflected waves. This is especially true as pressure is measured more distal to the heart. For example, pressures in the knee arteries are typically 20 mm higher in systole. Young individuals have more compliant arteries with more wave reflections and greater distal increase in systolic pressure. The arterial waveform changes distal, with more pointed and higher systolic peaks. The further the arterial pressure is measured downstream the higher the systolic peak. See diagram.

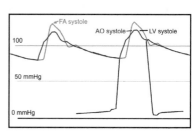

LV, AO and FA pressures

Braunwald says, "The difference in systolic pressures between the central aorta and the periphery (femoral, brachial, or radial arteries) is greatest in younger patients because of their increased vascular compliance. These potential differences between proximal aorta and peripheral artery must be considered to measure and to interpret the peak systolic pressure gradient between the left ventricle and the systemic arterial system in patients with suspected aortic stenosis. When a transvalvular gradient is present, the most accurate measure of the aortic pressure is obtained at the level of the coronary arteries." See: Braunwald chapter on Cardiac Catheterization

2. Blood Flow and Bernoulli's Equation

729. In a large vessel with fully developed laminar blood flow the velocity of the central stream is:
a.   ½ the mean velocity
b.   = to the mean velocity
c.   Twice the mean velocity
d.   Varies with viscosity

ANSWER c. Twice the mean velocity. Laminar flow is straight-line nonturbulent flow.

The velocity profile is parabolic, with the central stream being the fastest traveling blood, and the plasma next to the vessel wall not moving at all. The average or mean velocity is ½ of the central maximum velocity. **See:** Berne & Levy, chapter on "Hemodynamics." **Keywords:** Central laminar flow = 2 x mean velocity

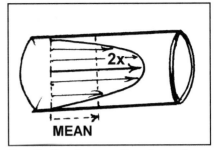

Parabolic shape - Laminar flow

730. **In normal laminar blood flow the velocity of blood at the arterial wall equals:**
a. **Zero**
b. **½ mv^2**
c. **The mean velocity**
d. **½ the peak velocity**

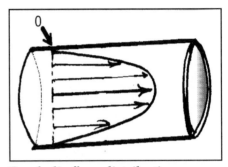

ANSWER a. Zero. The molecules of blood touching the vessel wall do not flow. Even in the most rapid forward flow phases, the velocity at the wall is always zero. Viscous drag holds it back. Remember in a river how the current at the center is fastest, flow near the shore is quiet, and the water touching the bank is not moving at all. Turbulent flow is different. **See:** Kempczinski, chapter on Instrumentation.

Parabolic flow distribution

731. **When you listen to bidirectional arterial Doppler sounds from a large high resistance peripheral artery (such as the external carotid artery) you hear 3 phases of flow in each heart cycle. What is the phase labeled #2 on the diagram (zero crossing phase)?**
a. **Zero flow**
b. **Rapid forward flow**
c. **Slow forward flow**
d. **Reversed flow**

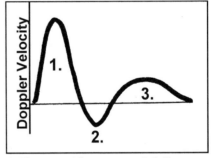

3 Phases of large arterial flow

ANSWER d. Reversed flow. Following the dicrotic notch most large arteries have a short period of reversed flow. When listening to Doppler flows in large arteries one typically hears these 3 phases; systolic forward flow (right ear), early diastolic flow reversal (also called **zero crossing** - in left ear), and end diastolic slow forward flow (in right ear). All large arteries leading to high resistance capillary beds demonstrate this 3-phase pattern. The internal carotid artery is a high flow & low resistance artery that does not show this.
CORRECTLY MATCHED ANSWERS ARE:
1. RAPID FORWARD FLOW PHASE
2. SLOW REVERSED FLOW PHASE (ZERO CROSSING): the flow reverses between systole and diastole.

3. SLOW FORWARD FLOW PHASE
See: Kempczinski, chapter on "Instrumentation." **Keywords**: Zero crossing, reverse flow

732. **Blood flow will change from laminar to turbulent at a Reynold's number:**
   a.   Under < 1.0
   b.   Under < 2000-3000
   c.   Over > 1.0
   d.   Over > 2000-3000

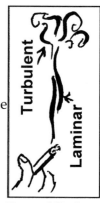

Reynold's #

ANSWER d. Over > 2000-3000. Reynold's number is a dimensionless number (no units) which represents the ratio of inertial to viscous forces. Reynold's number = N_R = pDv/n where: p is density, D is tube diameter, v is the mean velocity of flow and n is the viscosity. As Reynold's number increases with increasing blood velocity the more it is likely that turbulent flow will occur. Turbulence is generally bad in blood. It makes it more prone to clot, waste energy, and develop stenosis. The only place turbulent flow should normally occur is in the RV. Here the diameter is large, the velocity high, and the many trabeculations cause turbulence.

Flow where the Reynold's number is between 2000 and 3000 is transitional (either laminar or turbulent). A Reynold's number under 2000 indicates laminar straight line flow. A Reynold's number over 3000 always indicates turbulent flow.

A simple example is seen in rising cigarette smoke. Smoke initially rises straight up. But it eventually rises so fast that it exceeds N_R and it begins curling around in turbulence..
See: Berne & Levy, chapter on "Hemodynamics." **Keywords:** Blood Flow, Reynold's Number, turbulent flow

733. **The cerebral circulation is a:**
   a.   Low-flow,   Low resistance system
   b.   Low-flow,   High resistance system
   c.   High-flow,   Low resistance system
   d.   High-flow,   High resistance system

ANSWER c. High-flow, low resistance system Two vascular beds that are low in resistance are the cerebral vascular and pulmonary capillary beds. In the brain this leads to a unique steady and continuous blood flow. This is well known to vascular techs who scan the carotid artery flows looking for stenosis. The internal carotid artery flow does not have the zero crossing (flow reversal) that the external carotid does. This makes the Doppler phasic sound and the Doppler profile of the two arteries very different.
See: Kempczinski, chapter on "Noninvasive Testing Cerebrovascular Disease." **Keywords**: Cerebral circulation = high flow, low resistant system

734. Cerebral blood flow is normally remarkably stable and is only reduced by_____.
- a. Increased nitric oxide (NO)
- b. Hypotension (mean BP<75 mmHg)
- c. Deep REM sleep (decreased EEG activity)
- d. Significant carotid stenosis (>50% area reduction)

ANSWER b. Hypotension (mean BP<75). Cerebral perfusion only decreases in hypotension (mean BP<75 **mmHg**). Spence says: "The cerebral blood flow is relatively unaffected by changes in the systemic arterial pressure. Cerebral blood flow is remarkably constant over a very broad range of mean arterial pressures, and it does not decline significantly unless the mean arterial pressure is considerably below normal." The graph shows that as the mean BP falls below 75 mm Hg cerebral flow is forced to fall. At this point the patient may faint and if it lasts over 4 minutes brain damage may result.
See: Spencer, chapter on "Circulation"

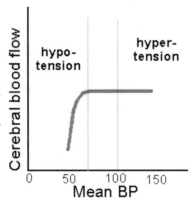

735. What happens to the metabolic rate of the brain with sleep?
- a. Brain metabolic rate increases significantly, compared to waking
- b. Brain metabolic rate decreases significantly, compared to waking
- c. Brain metabolic rate is relatively unchanged, compared to waking
- d. Brain metabolic rate increases significantly with depth of REM sleep & dreaming

ANSWER c. Brain metabolic rate is relatively unchanged. Spence says: "The overall metabolic rate of the brain varies little under widely different physiological conditions - for example, intense mental activity, muscular activity, sleep- and under most circumstances , cerebral flow does not vary greatly.... The [relative] blood flow to different local areas of the brain increases in response to increase in the activities of the areas. For example, clasping the right hand is accompanied by increased blood flow in the motor cortex on the left side of the brain. Local autoregulatory mechanisms are believed to contribute to changes that occur in local blood flow." CO_2 levels can dramatically effect blood flow. Hypothermia can reduce the metabolic rate of the brain and preserve brain function for extended periods.
See: Spencer, chapter on Circulation

736. What mechanism is PRIMARILY responsible for returning venous blood to the heart while walking?
- a. Gravity
- b. Vagal tone
- c. Skeletal muscle
- d. Arterial pressure

ANSWER c. Skeletal muscle. As the deep and superficial veins are compressed during muscular contraction, blood is propelled toward the heart. With exercise up to 30% of the total venous return is due to the pumping action of the musculature. The veins of the extremities are equipped with valves that normally prevent back-flow during skeletal muscle relaxation. This is called the muscular or calf pump. **See:** Rushmer's "CV Dynamics" chapter on effects of posture. **Keywords:** Skeletal muscle venous pump

737. When a Doppler probe is directed at an arterial stenosis the operator hears a high pitched rushing sound because of a/an:
a. Decrease in quantity of blood flow through the lesion (cc/sec)
b. Decrease in velocity of blood flow at the lesion (cm/sec)
c. Increase in quantity of blood flow through the lesion (cc/sec)
d. Increase in velocity of blood flow at the lesion (cm/sec)

ANSWER d. Increase in velocity of blood flow at the lesion (cm/sec). Blood speeds up within a restriction. Doppler ultrasound waves detect the velocity of the blood flow not quantity of blood flow. Doppler ultrasound recordings detect the high frequency jets through stenotic valves, arterial stenosis and downstream turbulence. The continuity equation is:

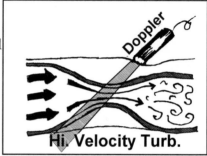

"Dopplering" arterial stenosis

Q = VA.
flow = velocity x area

When the area of a blood vessel decreases the velocity will increase to maintain flow. Q **decreases** because of small orifice area. Within a stenotic area the **velocity increases** because the pressure gradient increases across it to drive blood through. But, Doppler recordings do not evaluate quantity of flow, only velocity. Turbulence only exists after the stenosis.
See: Berne & Levy, chapter on "Hemodynamics." **Keywords:** Blood Flow, Velocity, Q=VA, Doppler jet

738. Which statements are TRUE regarding Poiseuille's law of fluid flow through tubes? Note "∝" means "directly proportional to."
1. $Q \propto$ **tube radius^4 (r^4)**
2. $Q \propto$ **tube length   (l)**
3. $Q \propto$ **pressure gradient across tube   (P_i-P_o)**
4. $Q \propto$ **fluid viscosity (η)**
    a. 1,2
    b. 1,3
    c. 2,3
    d. 2,4

ANSWER b. 1, 3. Poiseuille's Law:
Blood flow (Q in L/min) increases with driving pressure (P_{in}) and very **greatly increases** with even small charges in vessel radius(r^4). This radius to the **4th power is so significant** that almost every question dealing with Poiseuille's law emphasizes it. Double the

$$Q = \frac{\pi(P_i - P_o)r^4}{8\eta l}$$

pressure gradient and flow doubles, but double the radius and the flow increases $2^4 = 16$ times.
See: Berne & Levy, chapter on "Hemodynamics." **Keywords:** Poiseuille Law

739. **According to Poiseuille's law, which measure below will most significantly increase the flow rate through a flood catheter?**
   a.   **Reducing catheter length**
   b.   **Increasing catheter diameter**
   c.   **Increasing injection pressure**
   d.   **Adding sideholes to the catheter**

ANSWER b. Increasing catheter diameter. This is the lesson of Poiseuille's Law. Double the injection pressure and flow doubles, but double the inside radius and the flow increases $2^4 = 16$ times. **See:** Berne & Levy, chapter on "Hemodynamics." **Keywords:** Poiseuille Law

740. **Blood behaves as a _____ fluid in very small vessels.**
   a.   **Newtonian**
   b.   **Non-Newtonian**
   c.   **Viscous**
   d.   **Non-Viscous**

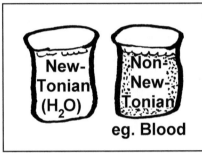
Non/Newtonian Fluids

ANSWER b. Non-Newtonian. Newtonian fluids such as water have a constant linear viscosity. But blood is **non-Newtonian** because of the suspended red blood cells. These affect the "apparent viscosity" and make blood rheology calculations difficult. Rheology is the study of the deformation and flow of blood through the circulation.

    This non-Newtonian nature of blood is especially obvious in smaller vessels were flow depends on pressing the 5-8 μm (micrometers) erythrocytes through capillaries as small as 3 μm. This is possible only because the RBCs can be compressed and deformed by the surrounding capillary walls. Miraculously, the blood appears to become less viscous (shear thinning) within the capillary.
See: Berne & Levy, chapter on "Hemodynamics." **Keywords:** Blood flow, non-Newtonian fluid, rheology

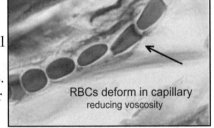
RBCs deform in capillary reducing voscosity

Non/Newtonian Fluids

741. **Poiseuille's law is not applicable in capillaries because the apparent viscosity of blood decreases as both flow rate and vessel diameter decrease. This is termed:**
   a.   **Reynold's effect**
   b.   **Zero crossing**
   c.   **Shear thinning**
   d.   **Apparent compliance**

ANSWER c. Shear thinning. Blood flow is non-Newtonian in very small vessels; i.e., Poiseuille's law is not applicable. As blood approaches the capillary both the tube diameter and the flow rate decrease. Poiseuille's law would predict that capillary blood flow is virtually impossible. Fortunately, red blood cells act as "ball bearings" to reduce the viscosity of blood in small vessels. They deform to make passage easier. Otherwise blood could not pass through capillaries.
See: Berne & Levy, chapter on "Hemodynamics." **Keywords:** Shear thinning

742. **The four tubes in the diagram are equal in length and diameter. With the inlet and outlet pressures shown, which tube will have the greatest blood flow rate (Q)?**
a.   100 mmHg ➜ 0 mmHg
b.   120 mmHg ➜ 40 mmHg
c.   140 mmHg ➜ 20 mmHg
d.   160 mmHg ➜ 90 mmHg

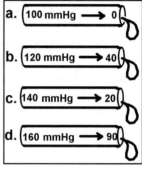

ANSWER c. 140 mmHg ➜ 20 mmHg is a 120 mm driving pressure gradient. Subtract the inlet from outlet pressure to get the driving pressure or gradient (P_i - P_o). This difference is the

Blood flow in 4 tubes

greatest driving pressure shown. The lowest tube (d) has the least flow, because its driving pressure is the lowest: 160-90=70 mmHg. Note that Poiseuille's law has pressure gradient in the numerator (P_i - P_o). Thus **pressure gradient** drives flow. That is why mean gradient is used to calculate valve area, not simple pressure.
See: Berne & Levy, chapter on " Hemodynamics." **Keywords**: Poiseuille's law

743. **Which fluid has the highest viscosity?**
a.   **Water**
b.   **Plasma**
c.   **Anemic blood**
d.   **Polycythemic blood**

ANSWER d. Polycythemic blood. "Blood is thicker than water." Especially thick blood with too many RBCs and lots of iron, is termed "polycythemic." A rise in hematocrit from 45 to 70% (as seen in polycythemia) thickens the blood so that

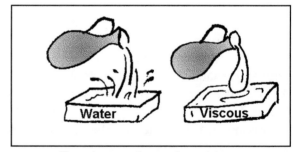

Pouring various viscosities

the viscosity doubles. This makes twice the resistance to blood flow and twice the work for the heart. Polycythemia is a natural body response to low O2 levels - as in emphysema. It produces more hemoglobin to carry more O2. But this thicker blood makes the heart work harder and makes cyanosis easier to detect. According to Poiseuille's law, blood flow is inversely proportional to fluid viscosity (η). So, the thicker the blood the slower the flow.
See: Berne & Levy, chapter on "Hemodynamics." **Keywords:** Microcirculation, blood viscosity, polycythemia

744. In aortic stenosis the systolic aortic valve flow velocity is _____, and the aortic (lateral) pressure is _____.
   a.   Increased,   Increased
   b.   Increased,   Decreased
   c.   Decreased,   Decreased
   d.   Decreased,   Increased

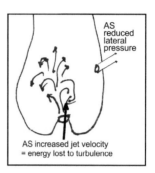

ANSWER b. Increased, decreased. Bernoulli's law explains why aortic pressure is reduced in aortic stenosis patients. The stenosis causes a rise in flow velocity through the jet and a drop in pressure between LV-AO (a gradient). However, if your catheter tip is directed directly at the aortic jet it will give incorrect readings. It acts as a pitot tube measuring increased pressure due to the inertia of the high velocity jet. Consequently gradients should be measured with side hole catheters, and not directly in the jet.

As blood flows through a stenosis, pressure gradients occur (loss of potential energy). This PE (potential energy) is transformed into velocity, turbulence, and kinetic energy. In the fluid system there exists much viscous resistance and the stenotic turbulence is so inefficient that most of the energy is lost to heat and sound energy (murmurs).

See: Berne & Levy, chapter on "Hemodynamics." **Keywords:** Bernoulli, AS, gradient

745. The hemodynamic effect of increasing a patient's peripheral vascular resistance is to: (Assume constant CO)
   a.   Increased BP
   b.   Decreased BP
   c.   Increased HR
   d.   Decreased HR

ANSWER a. increased BP.   The formula BP = CO X SVR demonstrates the direct proportionality between CO and SVR. If CO doubles so does BP. If resistance doubles so does BP. That is why administration of vasoconstrictors raises the BP.

The resistance is normally closely regulated by the baroreceptor reflex, through vasoactivity. Reflexes also regulate the CO by alerting the HR and SV. For example, the SVR lowers in exercise to allow increased blood flow with only slight elevation of the BP. Note that this is also a rearranged Ohm's Law for fluids where:

   BP = aortic mean Pressure = Voltage
   Q = Cardiac Output = Electric Current flow

See: Berne & Levy, chapter on "Hemodynamics." **Keywords:** SVR, Resistance, BP

3. Vascular Resistance & Exercise

746. Mean arterial blood pressure is approximately equal to:
   a.   CO x SVR
   b.   CO / SVR
   c.   Arterial Compliance x SVR
   d.   Arterial Compliance / SVR

ANSWER: a. CO x SVR. This formula is essential to understanding the role of vasodilators and vasoconstrictors in regulating BP. Decreasing SVR with administration of

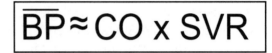

$$\overline{BP} \approx CO \times SVR$$

vasodilators decreases BP. Exercise increases CO, but since the SVR normally decreases on exercise, the mean BP may remain the same.

   The most accurate formula to calculate SVR is (AO mean - RA mean) / CO. But, since the RA pressure is relatively insignificant, an approximation can be made by eliminating the RA factor. Then SVR = AO mean / CO, or AO mean = CO x SVR. **See:** Berne & Levy, chapter on "Hemodynamics."

747. At peak exercise a normal individual's mean blood pressure may not significantly elevate, even though CO may increase up to seven times. This regulation of BP during exercise is due to _____ vascular resistance.
   a.   Increased systemic
   b.   Decreased systemic
   c.   Increased pulmonary
   d.   Decreased pulmonary

ANSWER b. Decreased systemic vascular resistance (↓SVR). With exercise, the increase in CO will raise the BP, unless peripheral vasodilation occurs. Because BP = CO X SVR, to keep a constant BP while the CO increases seven times, the SVR must decrease by a factor of seven. This peripheral vasodilation allows blood to pass the capillary bed more easily and not significantly elevate the BP. Note that the pulmonary resistance (PVR) primarily affects PA pressure, whereas systemic resistance (SVR) affects the systemic BP. **See:** Berne & Levy section on exercise.

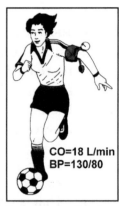

CO=18 L/min
BP=130/80

In exercise high CO and reduced SVR equalize BP

748. When a normal person exercises what happens to their BP and systemic vascular resistance (SVR) with increasing levels of exercise?
   a.   Systolic BP increases, SVR increases
   b.   Systolic BP increases, SVR decreases
   c.   Diastolic BP increases, SVR decreases
   d.   Diastolic BP increases, SVR increases

ANSWER: b. Systolic BP increases (slightly), SVR decreases (markedly). Exercise increases CO markedly, but has little effect on diastolic BP. The arterioles and capillaries dilate to reduce SVR. Braunwald says, "Physical exercise is associated with increases in heart rate, venous return, cardiac output, stroke volume, and systolic pressure. Arterial diastolic pressure remains relatively unchanged or decreases slightly... Abnormal cardiac function during maximal exercise has been based on pulmonary capillary wedge pressure or LVEDP exceeding 20 mmHg. the cardiac output failing to reach 15 liter/min, and the ejection fraction failing to rise." In the diagram below, note the dramatic drop in systemic resistance on exercise while the mean BP remains stable. **See:** Braunwald, chapter on "Pathophysiology of Heart Failure" **Keywords:** exercise > syst. BP, < SVR

749. **What factors normally rise significantly with increasing exercise? (Select 5.)**
   a. **Stroke volume**
   b. **Venous return**
   c. **O2 consumption**
   d. **Cardiac index**
   e. **Systolic BP**
   f. **Diastolic BP**
   g. **R-R interval**

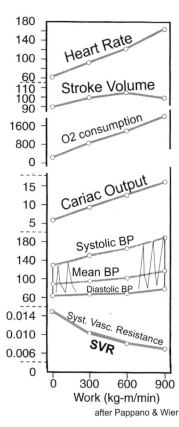

after Pappano & Wier

ANSWERS: a, b, c, d, & e all increase. Diastolic blood pressure and R-R interval decrease. Braunwald says, "Physical exercise is associated with increases in heart rate, venous return, cardiac output, stroke volume, and systolic pressure. Arterial diastolic pressure remains relatively unchanged or decreases slightly... Abnormal cardiac function during maximal exercise has been based on pulmonary capillary wedge pressure or LVEDP exceeding 20 mmHg. the cardiac output failing to reach 15 liter/min, and the ejection fraction failing to rise." Since the heart rate rises on exercise, the RR interval will shorten and decrease. **See:** Braunwald, chapter on "Pathophysiology of Heart Failure"

750. **At maximal exercise the heart rate of normal men can be estimated by the formula:**
   a. $HR^{max} = 125 \times BSA$
   b. $HR^{max} = 3.5$ mL O2/kg/min of body weight
   c. $HR^{max} = 206 - (0.88$ age$)$
   d. $HR^{max} = 220 -$ age

ANSWER: d. $HR^{max} = 220 -$ age
Braunwald says, "Cardiac output increases by four- to sixfold above basal levels during strenuous exertion in the upright position, depending on genetic endowment and level of training. The maximum heart rate and cardiac output are decreased in older persons, partly because of decreased beta-adrenergic responsivity. Maximum heart rate (HR) can be estimated from the following formula: $HR^{max} = 220 -$ age.... Thus, a 40 yom

would have a predicted maximum heart rate of 220 - 40 = 180 BPM. This formula tends to overestimate maximum heart rate in a female population. The formula HR = 206 - 0.88 (age in years) provides a more accurate estimate of maximum heart rate in women.

In current use, the term metabolic equivalent (MET) refers to a unit of oxygen uptake in a sitting, resting person; 1 MET is equivalent to 3.5 mL O2/kg/min of body weight. Measured in mL O2/kg/min divided by 3.5 mL O2/kg/min determines the number of METs associated with activity. Work activities can be calculated in multiples of METs; this measurement is useful to determine exercise prescriptions...Workloads in excess of 9 METs are compatible with heavy labor, handball, squash, and running at 6 to 7 mph"
See: Braunwald, chapter on "Exercise Stress Testing"

751. **On exercise, athletic individuals perform better compared to sedentary individuals at similar work loads because of:**
   a.   **Higher stroke volume with higher heart rates**
   b.   **Higher stroke volume with lower heart rates**
   c.   **Higher blood pressure with higher heart rates**
   d.   **Higher blood pressure with lower heart rates**

ANSWER: b. Higher stroke volume with lower heart rates.
Karve says: "The athlete has a much higher stroke volume at similar work loads. The athlete has a larger ventricular volume and slower heart rate, which allows for a greater cardiac filling during diastole (greater end-diastolic volumes); therefore the stroke volume response in the athlete is much greater compared with that of the sedentary individual." Likewise, the athletic individual's exercise BP does not rise as significantly. **See:** Integrated Cardiovascular Physiology: A Laboratory Exercise, by Patil, Karve, & DiCarlo; Advances in Physiology Education, December 1, 1993; http://advan.physiology.org/content/265/6/S20

4. Starling's & Laplace's Laws

752. **Who developed the law: T = P x R/(2 x Wall thickness)? A cardiovascular application of this law is that "When the size of a vessel or heart chamber enlarges, the wall tension must increase to hold the same fluid pressure." T= wall tension; P= pressure; R=radius**
   a.   **Charles**
   b.   **La Place**
   c.   **Bernoulli**
   d.   **Poiseuille**
   e.   **Starling**

ANSWER b. Laplace. This law relates the tension within a vessel wall to the pressure and radius of the vessel. It can be used to calculate the bursting pressure of catheters, or the tension within the ventricular wall. The term wall stress or circumferential fibers shortening all relate to this formula. Remember you can blow up a balloon until it ruptures. As its radius increases, the wall gets thinner and the wall tension increases - until it POPS! The same thing happens in aneurysms and in dilating ventricles. In CHF with volume

overload the LV dilates as it fills more. This progressive dilatation makes the myocardial wall tighter and less stable. Because it is so inefficient a dilated heart uses more O2. So it is a vicious circle of dilation - more wall tension - more inefficiency - more dilation to compensate - more wall tension...
See: Berne & Levy, chapter on "Hemodynamics."　**Keywords**: Laplace's Law

753. **Aortic aneurysms tend to grow in size and become unstable because of their:**
  a.　**Increasing blood turbulence and wall thrombus**
  b.　**Decreasing compliance and calcium content**
  c.　**Loss of elastin and smooth muscle**
  d.　**Increasing wall tension.**

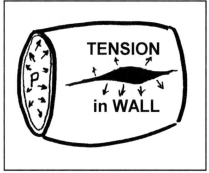
Laplace Wall Tension

ANSWER d. Increasing wall tension. Laplace's law states the wall tension = Pressure x radius. The larger aneurysms get, the thinner the wall becomes and the more tension in the wall. Like a balloon that grows too big, it will eventually rupture.

　　Dobrin says, "Aortic aneurysms encompass a vast range of aetiologies and may occur in various locations however the risk of aneurysm rupture is common to all types. This can be explained by LaPlace's Law which would follow that the pressure required to overcome the surface tension of the vessel wall is reduced with the greater the radius of the aneurysm. In practice, the greater the diameter of the aneurysm, the increased risk of rupture." **See:** Dobrin, "Mechanisms and Mechanical Properties of Aneurysms."
http://www.fdliotta.org/biblio/libro/cap5.pdf

754. **The physical principle that helps explain why dilated ventricles fail is ____ which says that____.**
  a.　**Laplace's law, LV wall tension = pressure x radius**
  b.　**Starling's, Increased hydrostatic forces cause fluid filtration and edema**
  c.　**Frank-Starling, Increased ventricular preload yields cause proximal edema**
  d.　**Poisellie's, LV wall tension = pressure / radius**

ANSWER: a. Laplace's law, LV wall tension = pressure x radius. This principle works in arteries and ventricles. The larger the LV diameter becomes the more wall tension and stress occurs in the wall. Too much stress causes thinning and weakened force of contraction, all of which can lead to a dilated failing heart.

　　Braunwald says, "in congestive heart failure, the heart dilates so that the increased radius elevates wall stress. Furthermore, because ejection of blood is inadequate, the radius stays too large throughout the contractile cycle, and both end-diastolic and end-systolic tensions are higher. . . . Overall reduction of heart size decreases wall stress and improves LV function." **See:** Braunwald, chapter on "Contractile Performance of the Intact Heart"

755. **"Thin walled capillaries can withstand high internal pressure without bursting because of their narrow lumen." Whose law explains this phenomenon?**
   a.   Ohm's law
   b.   Pascal's law
   c.   Laplace's law
   d.   Starling's law

ANSWER c. Laplace's law states that wall tension is a product of transluminal pressure and radius of the vessel:

$$T = PxR/2xWall\ thickness$$

Thus a very small capillary radius (r) times a large pressure (P) can still equal a normal wall tension. The opposite happens in aneurysmal aortas where large radii make tension excessive and cause the aneurysm to grow. This accelerated growth makes rupture inevitable. When an aortic aneurysm exceeds 6 cm in diameter surgery is recommended. **See:** Berne & Levy, chapter on "Microcirculation." **Keywords:** Microcirculation, Laplace's Law, capillary busting pressure

756. **Starling's hypothesis relating hydrostatic to oncotic pressure equilibrium across a capillary wall is:**

$$\text{Fluid Movement} = k(P_c+\Pi i) - (P_i+\Pi_p).$$

What happens to fluid movement when plasma protein oncotic pressure (Π_p) is increased significantly over hydrostatic capillary pressure (P_c)?
   a.   Filtration of fluid into tissue (edema)
   b.   Absorption of fluid into blood (hypervolemia)
   c.   Hydrostatic pressure exceeds oncotic pressure
   d.   Lateral pressure exceeds hydrostatic pressure

ANSWER b. Absorption of fluid into the vascular space (hypervolemia). A negative number will cause interstitial fluid to be drawn into the vascular space and increase the blood volume. This happens following angiography with hyper-osmolar contrast overload or increased dietary salt intake. **See**: Berne & Levy, chapter on "Microcirculation." **Keywords:** Starling's Hypothesis, Oncotic pressure, Absorption

757. **What pathologic condition is most likely to occur when the pulmonary capillary pressure is greater than plasma oncotic pressure?**
   a.   Peripheral edema
   b.   Pulmonary edema
   c.   Cor pulmonale
   d.   Dehydration of alveoli

ANSWER b. Pulmonary edema. The oncotic pressure is the plasma osmotic pressure tending to draw fluid back into the capillary. Hydrostatic pressure tends to push fluid across the capillary membrane into the tissues or alveolus causing pulmonary edema. When the capillary pressure (P_c)

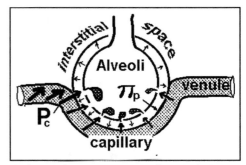

exceeds the plasma oncotic pressure (Π_p) edema occurs. As shown in the diagram when the pulmonary capillary wedge pressures are greater than about 20 mmHg acute pulmonary edema occurs. Note fluid drops seeping into the alveoli. **See**: Rushmer's "CV Dynamics" section on "Water

Pulm. Edema occurs when PAWP exceeds plasma oncotic pressure.

Balance at the Capillaries." **Keywords**: Pulmonary edema occurs when PCW pressure exceeds interstitial oncotic pressure

758. Leg stockings (sup-hose) will increase which variable of the Starling fluid movement hypothesis? Fluid Movement = $k(P_c + \Pi i) - (P_i + \Pi_p)$

a. P_c capillary hydrostatic pressure

b. P_i interstitial fluid hydrostatic pressure

c. Π_p plasma oncotic pressure

d. Π_i interstitial fluid oncotic pressure

ANSWER. b. P_i interstitial fluid hydrostatic pressure. To reduce peripheral edema surgical patients are fitted with support hose. This increases the interstitial hydrostatic pressure combating filtration into the tissues. Understand the 4 terms of Starling's equation. **Terms used in Starling's Hypothesis are:**

k =   Filtration constant

Pc=   Hydrostatic pressure of capillary (tends to force fluid out of capillary) - largest filtration force.

Pi=   Hydrostatic pressure of interstitial fluid (tends to force fluid into capillary)

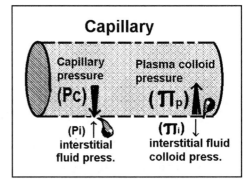

Π_p=   Plasma protein oncotic (colloidal) pressure (tends to cause osmosis of fluid into the capillary) - largest absorption force.

Forces tending to move fluid through capillary wall

Π_i=   Interstitial fluid oncotic pressure (tends to cause osmosis of fluid out through capillary walls)

Filtration (edema) occurs when the sum of these forces is positive, and absorption of fluid into the blood volume occurs when it is negative.

See: Berne & Levy, chapter on "Microcirculation." **Keywords:** Starling's hypothesis, hydrostatic pressure

759. **The key factor restraining fluid loss from a systemic capillary is:**
   a.   Osmotic pressure due to plasma proteins
   b.   Alveolar and intrathoracic pressure
   c.   Capillary hydrostatic pressure
   d.   Interstitial fluid hydrostatic pressure

ANSWER a. Osmotic pressure due to plasma proteins restrains fluid loss. Hydrostatic pressure is the main force tending to drive fluid out of the capillaries as in edema. The osmotic pressure of plasma is the main force tending to draw fluid **back into** the capillary. A good example of this is when contrast is injected. Its high osmotic pressure pulls fluid into the vascular space increasing venous pressures and blood volume. This can be fatal for severe CHF patients who already carry a fluid overload.
See: Berne & Levy, chapter on "The Microcirculation." **Keywords:** Starling's Hypothesis, Osmotic pressure

760. **When PAW pressure exceeds the plasma protein osmotic pressure ____ results.**
   a.   Pitting edema
   b.   Tissue dehydration
   c.   Interstitial pulmonary edema
   d.   Absorption and increased blood volume

ANSWER: c. Interstitial pulmonary edema occurs when the pulmonary capillary hydrostatic pressure is high enough to push plasma across the pulmonary capillary membrane into the interstitial space and alveolus. This pressure opposes the osmotic pressure in the capillary wall. When the wedge pressure exceeds around 25 mmHg, the patient increases fluid in the lungs and develops pulmonary edema . This extra fluid in the lungs impedes oxygen transport, causes coughing, and raises pulmonary vascular resistance. When this happens in the peripheral capillaries the patient gets peripheral tissue edema - usually seen as swelling in the legs. See: Berne & Levy, chapter on Microcirculation and Lymphatics

5. Vascular Autoregulation

761. **If arterial blood flow is stopped for several minutes by pumping up a BP cuff around a limb & then releasing it, the resulting flow exceeds basal flow. This is termed:**
   a.   Sympathetic discharge
   b.   Myogenic vasoconstriction
   c.   Active hyperemia
   d.   Reactive hyperemia

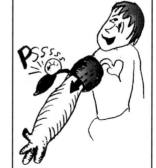
Reactive Hyperemia

ANSWER d. Reactive hyperemia. The demand for oxygen is so great that oxygen starved tissues cause the vessels to dilate. When the cuff is released, a huge blood flow results to satisfy the oxygen deficit. The resulting increased flow (hyperemia) is a reaction to the metabolic demand. This method is still used in PV labs to evaluate blood flow in people who cannot be stressed on treadmills. **See:** Berne & Levy, chapter on "Peripheral Circulation and Control." **Keywords:** Autoregulation, Reactive Hyperemia, O2 demand

762. **Local arterial vasodilation occurs after the arterial wall liberates an "endothelial-derived relaxation factor" composed of:**
- a.   **Endothelin**
- b.   **Angiotensin**
- c.   **Vasopressin**
- d.   **Nitric Oxide**

ANSWER d. Nitric Oxide. This dissolved gas dilates the arteries and arterioles upstream to the capillaries when increased flow is needed. Rapid blood flow through the arteries causes a "shear stress" on the endothelial cells because of viscous drag. This stress causes the endothelial cells to release nitric oxide which then migrates into the smooth muscle and relaxes and dilates the arterial wall. Nitric Oxide (NO) helps regulate vasomotor tone to keep blood velocity at the vessel wall within a narrow range. It prevents sluggish blood flow that might promote thrombus

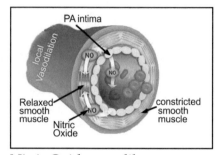

Nitric Oxide vasodilates artery

and high shear that could injure the intima. **See:** Guyton, chapter on "Local Control of Blood Flow..." **Keywords:** EDRF, Nitric Oxide

763. **Inhalation of small concentrations of nitric oxide gas is used in the cath lab to diagnose how patients with _____ will respond to _____.**
- a.   **Systemic hypertension, oxygen therapy**
- b.   **Systemic hypertension, oral vasodilators**
- c.   **Pulmonary hypertension, oxygen therapy**
- d.   **Pulmonary hypertension, oral vasodilators**

NO

ANSWER d. Pulmonary hypertension, oral vasodilators. Inchose, et al, say, "Diagnostic Use of Inhaled NO: Pulmonary Vasoreactivity Testing in the Cardiac Catheterization Laboratory Demonstration of a positive response to vasodilating agents in patients with pulmonary hypertension correlates with a favorable long-term clinical outcome. ... recent studies indicate that inhaled NO safely and effectively assesses the capacity for pulmonary vasodilation in pediatric and adult patients with pulmonary hypertension without causing systemic hypotension and predicts responsiveness to medical vasodilator therapy. For example, a >20% decrease in pulmonary artery pressure or pulmonary vascular resistance (PVR) to inhaled NO accurately predicts a subsequent response to oral vasodilators such as nifedipine....Inhaled NO is the first vasodilator to produce truly selective pulmonary vasodilation." See: (Circulation. 2004;109:3106-3111.)
http://circ.ahajournals.org/content/109/25/3106.full
Inhaled Nitric Oxide, A Selective Pulmonary Vasodilator: Current Uses and Therapeutic Potential, Fumito Ichinose, et. al. Keywords: NO test for pulmonary hypertension

764. When doing a nitric oxide right heart study on a patient with pulmonary hypertension it is important to accurately measure pulmonary resistance. One important point of technique is to:

a. Measure cardiac output on exercise.
b. Measure all pressures at end expiration.
c. Perform pulmonary flood angiography
d. Measure accurate valve pressure gradients on pullback.

ANSWER b. Measure all pressures at end expiration. Braunwald says, "In addition to confirming the diagnosis and allowing the exclusion of other causes, cardiac catheterization also establishes the severity of disease and allows an assessment of prognosis. ..,transducers must be carefully adjusted to reflect the height of the midchest on every patient. Pressures should never be determined by the digital readout from the laboratory's computer, because these measurements represent an average of several heart beats and ignore respiratory influences. In addition, the electronically integrated mean pressure can differ greatly from the actual wedge pressure. Instead, measurements of all pressures are properly made at end-expiration to avoid incorporating negative intrathoracic pressures. When a reproducible wedge pressure cannot be obtained, direct measurement of left ventricular end-diastolic pressure is advised." See: Braunwald, chapter on "Pulmonary Hypertension" Keywords: Accurate pressures on NO study

765. Brief exposure of an extremity to extreme cold temperatures results in _____ of vessels in that extremity.

a. Neural mediated vasoconstriction
b. Neural mediated vasodilation
c. Humoral mediated vasoconstriction
d. Humoral mediated vasodilation

ANSWER a. Neural mediated vasoconstriction. Moderate cooling or exposure for brief periods to extreme cold (0-15° C) results in sympathetic mediated vasoconstriction of the affected cutaneous vessels. However, prolonged exposure has a secondary vasodilator effect, thus the rosy red cheeks (vasodilation) seen in children playing in the snow. In skin, sympathetic neural control plays the most important factor in temperature regulation. Normal warm areas of the body may vasoconstrict as well, due to this neural regulation - as in the diving reflex.
See: Berne & Levy, chapter on "Special Circulations." **Keywords:** Autoregulation, temperature regulation, cold, vasoconstriction, neural mediated

766. Soldiers standing at attention for long periods often faint because:

a. Increased peripheral vascular resistance increases cardiac work
b. Arterial pooling increases BP which stimulates baro-receptor bradycardia
c. Venous pooling reduces preload and cardiac output
d. Venous reflexive vasoconstriction increases preload

ANSWER c. Venous pooling reduces preload and cardiac output. Long standing without flexing the venous pump in the large leg muscles may cause venous pooling, reduced venous return, reduced cerebral blood flow, and fainting. Another form of this pooling is "orthostatic hypotension." This is a drop in BP or even fainting due to venous pooling when someone suddenly stands up.
See: Berne & Levy, chapter on "Control of Cardiac Output."
Keywords: Autoregulation, Pooling, venous pump, orthostatic hypotension

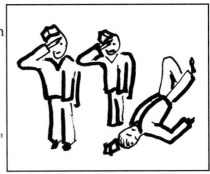

Reduced Preload, faint

6. Vascular Applications & FFR

767. **An EMBOLUS can be best described as any:**
(Remember even air can embolize.)

    a.   **Arterial fibrin clot flowing downstream**
    b.   **Venous platelet clot flowing toward the heart**
    c.   **Foreign material that travels downstream and plugs up a vessel**
    d.   **Plaque which breaks loose and is swept into the brain leading to stroke.**

ANSWER c. Foreign material that travels downstream and plugs up a vessel. An embolus is a clot or other plug brought by the blood from another vessel and forced into a smaller one. This obstructs the circulation and may lead to infarction. Even air can occlude a vessel. Because of their surface tension bubbles won't quickly dissipate, and may remain lodged in an arteriole obstructing flow.

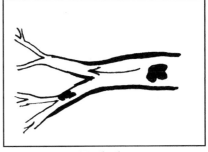

Embolus

    Other foreign body plugs include: fat embolus, tumor embolus (E.g., myxoma), and foreign body embolus such as gelfoam or spring coils intentionally inserted into the vascular system. Don't get thrombus and embolus confused. In interventional cardiology "no-reflow" after use of a Rotoblator is due to micro-emboli composed of plaque particles. **See:** Medical dictionary. **Keywords:** Terms, embolus, clot

768. **Elevated blood angiotensin II and aldosterone levels cause:**

    a.   **Capillary vasoconstriction**
    b.   **Capillary vasodilation**
    c.   **Arteriolar vasoconstriction**
    d.   **Arteriolar vasodilation**

ANSWER c. Arteriolar vasoconstriction. When the systemic arterioles constrict, blood pressure rises. These potent arterial vasoconstrictors are liberated through the renin/angiotensin system of the kidney and may actually cause systemic hypertension. Besides raising the BP they may also cause Na^+ retention which retains fluids in the body. New ACE inhibitor drugs neutralize the angiotensin through a converting enzyme (ACE inhibitors) and block this renin-angiotensin mechanism. **See:** Berne & Levy, chapter on "Special Circulations." **Keywords:** Other, angiotensin, aldosterone, vasoconstriction

769. **Angiotensin II liberates ALDOSTERONE which is a _____ causing the kidneys to _____ Na+.**
a. **Diuretic;   Retain**
b. **Diuretic;   Excrete**
c. **Corticosteroid; Retain**
d. **Corticosteroid; Excrete**

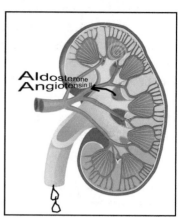

ANSWER c. Corticosteroid; Retain Na+.
 Aldosterone is a mineralocorticoid (steroid) hormone secreted by the adrenal cortex, that regulates electrolyte and water balance by promoting the renal retention of sodium. The Na$^+$ retention causes fluid retention and increased blood volume, which can be quite harmful to a failing heart. When deprived of adequate renal blood flow and perfusion pressure the kidneys produce renin which may be measured in renal veins.
 The cascade of these humors is:
  Renin → Angiotensin I → Angiotensin II → Aldosterone (also a vasoconstrictor) → Na$^+$ retention → increased BP.
 "ACE inhibitors" can break hypertension resulting from this chain of angiotensin and aldosterone.   "ACE" stands for "Angiotensin Converting Enzyme."
See: Braunwald, chapter on "Systemic Hypertension." **Keywords:** Other, Hypertension, ACE, Renin, Angiotensin

770. **The chief regulation of blood flow within the lung away from atelectatic areas is local vasoconstriction due to _____ in that atelectatic area.**
a. **Increased PA pressure**
b. **Decreased PA pressure**
c. **Increased PO$_2$ tension**
d. **Decreased PO$_2$ tension**

ANSWER d. Decreased PO$_2$ tension. Atelectatic lungs contain closed/collapsed alveoli. These are not aerated so they have a low PO$_2$. The hypoxemic blood flowing out of these alveoli causes shutdown of its capillary blood flow. This mechanism assures that only oxygenated alveoli are perfused. This is sometimes called a "physiologic shunt" because blue blood is dumping into the arterialized LA blood, and can cause cyanosis. The smooth muscles constrict in these areas shifting blood flow from poor to well-ventilated alveoli, thus nullifying the "physiologic shunt." This vasoconstriction effect is opposite to that seen in the peripheral circulation, where low O2 causes vasodilation of arterioles, better oxygenating the tissues.
See: Berne & Levy, chapter on "Special Circulations." **Keywords:** Other, Atelectasis, PO2

771. Which invasive test uses a pressure wire to evaluate the significance of a pressure gradient across a renal artery stenosis during hyperemia?
   a.   Systolic pressure gradient Ratio
   b.   Gorlin formula gradient area
   c.   Fractional Flow Reserve (FFR)
   d.   Coronary Flow Reserve (CFR)

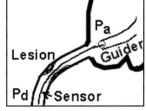

ANSWER c. Fractional Flow Reserve (FFR) is the name for the ratio of mean pressures gradients across a stenosis during adenosine induce hyperemia. Normally the coronary pressures should be the same as you move the wire down an artery. But, when you cross a lesion a gradient will occur. This is accentuated by adenosine, which increases the flow and the gradient. The ratio of distal to proximal mean pressures is the FFR. Don't confuse this with coronary flow reserve (CFR) which measures hyperemic flow using the Doppler flo-wire. More on FFR in Volume 2.
See: Braunwald, chapter on "Coronary Blood Flow and Myocardial Ischemia" Keywords: Coronary Flow Reserve (CFR)

772. What is the formula for Fractional Flow Reserve (FFR) as measured by a pressure guidewire placed distal to a stenosis during hyperemia? (Note Pa= Aortic pressure mean as measured by guiding catheter. Pd = mean Pressure distal to a stenosis)
   a.   Pa-Pd
   b.   (Pd-Pa)/Pd
   c.   (Pa-Pd)/Pa
   d.   Pd/Pa

ANSWER d. Pd/Pa = Pressure distal to stenosis / Aortic pressure measured during hyperemia. A normal FFR is 1.0. Abnormal is below 0.80. If there is a stenosis, the distal pressure will be reduced due to a gradient. This index Pd/Pa represents the maximal blood flow through an artery in the presence of a stenosis, compared to the theoretical normal maximal flow in the same artery. Just as in AS the most accurate gradients are measured at high flow (we exercise the patients), so FFR gradients should be measured at high flow (adenosine).
See: RADI Co., Coronary Pressure Measurement CD

Pressure Wire

773. When measuring FFR by pressure wire, what does the pressure waveform look like (at fast paper speeds) distal to a <u>severe</u> culprit coronary lesion?
   a.   Spike and dome pattern
   b.   Ventricularization pattern
   c.   Smoothed out and damped
   d.   Pulsus tardus with slow upstroke

ANSWER b. Ventricularization pattern with flattened low diastole and reduced systole. When a hemodynamically significant stenosis is stressed (hyperemia) it is mainly the <u>diastolic pressure that drops</u>, reflecting a ventricularized pattern. This is just like a damped main-stem left ostial lesion that shows a ventricularization pattern.

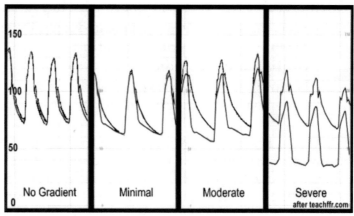

Pressure Wire

REFERENCES

Pappano & Wier, *Cardiovascular Physiology*, 10th Ed., Mosby Year Book, 2012

Braunwald, Eugene, Ed., *HEART DISEASE A Textbook of Cardiovascular Medicine*, 10th Ed., W. B. Saunders Co., 2012

Kepczinski, R. E., and Yao, J.S.T., Ed., *Practical Noninvasive Vascular Diagnosis*, 2nd Ed., Year Book Medical Publishers, Inc., 1987

Rushmer, R. F.,*CARDIOVASCULAR DYNAMICS*, W. B. Saunders Co., 1976

Spence, Alexander P., Mason, Elliott, B., Human Anatomy and Physiology, 3rd Ed, Benjamin/Cummings Publisher Co., 1987

http://circ.ahajournals.org/content/109/25/3106.full

Inhaled Nitric Oxide, A Selective Pulmonary Vasodilator: Current Uses and Therapeutic Potential, Fumito Ichinose, et. al.(Circulation. 2004;109:3106-3111.)

OUTLINE: B9 - Vascular Physiology

ARTERIAL ELASTICITY
- i. Compliance = Elasticity = dV/dP= ease of stretch
- ii. Age reduces compliance
  - (1) (hardening of arteries)
- b. Windkessel effect
  - i. Converts pulsatile to steady flow
  - ii. Systolic arterial flow stored in distensible Aorta (PE)
  - iii. Diastolic elastic recoil of artery converts PE to KE
  - iv. This elasticity reduces cardiac work
  - v. Level of mean BP depends on CO and SVR
- c. Venous elasticity - greatest
  - i. 20 x more blood stored than arteries
  - ii. Venous pooling - fainting
    - (1) Reduced preload, SV
    - (2) Venous pump = muscles

2. BLOOD PRESSURE
   - i. Mean BP = CO x SVR
   - ii. Raising SVR raises the level of mean BP
   - iii. Pulse pressure = systole - diastole
   - iv. Wider pulse pressure develop in reduce C_a
   - v. Mean Arterial estimate BP = Pd + 1/3(Ps - Pd)

3. EXERCISE
   - i. < Reduced SVR
   - ii. > SV & CI
   - iii. >Ejection Fraction
   - iv. >Venous return
   - v. > Wedge Pressure
   - vi. > Systolic BP & Pulse Pr.
   - vii. Athletes: < HR, > SV

4. BERNOULLI EQUATION
   - a. Relation between velocity and flow
   - b. Total pressure=K =Lateral pres. + KE
     - i. Total Press.=K=static pres. x ½ mv2
     - ii. Sum of PE & KE is constant K
   - c. In most arterial flow KE is negligible (except)
   - d. Aortic Stenosis: valve jet = > velocity
     - i. Turbulence
     - ii. Gradient = < lateral pressure

5. BLOOD FLOW
   - a. Velocity = distance/time
   - b. Flow = volume/time = Q/t
   - c. Q= V x A,   FLOW = Velocity x Area
     - i. Vl x Al = V2 x A2 (continuity equation)
     - ii. Used in Echocardiographic valve area calculation

6. LAMINAR FLOW = streamline flow
   - a. Parabolic flow = fully developed flow profile
     - i. Central velocity = 2 x average velocity
     - ii. Velocity at wall = 0
   - b. Concentric lamina (like layers onion)
   - c. Flow Profiles in high Res. Circuit (not brain)
     - i. Wave front blunted, flat, at entrance to tube
     - ii. Zero crossing & flow reversal @ dic. Notch
       - (1) Doppler sound Rt. - Lt.

iii. W shaped at flow reversal point
- d. Cerebral flow (brain):
  - i. Low resistance, high flow system
  - ii. Constant flow
    - (1) Cerebral flow only reduced if BP< 75 mmHg
- e. Steady state flow required
  - i. Laminar (nonturbulent) flow required
  - ii. Newtonian (homogeneous) fluid required
- f. Constant metabolic rate, even sleeping

7. TURBULENT FLOW @ jet = chaotic flow
   - a. Heart must work harder
   - b. At Stenosis = high velocity jet
     - i. Turbulence downstream
   - c. Murmurs & bruits result from turbulent flow
   - d. Thrombi more likely in turbulent areas

8. SHEAR STRESS ON VESSEL WALL
   - a. Greater flow exerts greater shear stress on intima
     - i. Greatest shear stress in AO
   - b. Tends to pull endothelium from wall
   - c. May tear intima
     - i. Resulting in DISSECTING ANEURYSM
     - ii. Most common in ascending AO

9. ARTERIAL PRESSURE CURVES
   - a. Pulse propagation wave is faster than blood flow
   - b. Propagation velocity in arterial wall
     - i. AO velocity = 50 cm/sec
     - ii. Capillary velocity =1 cm/sec
     - iii. Pressure wave velocity 500 cm/sec
       - (1) Travels down AO
       - (2) Bounces off AO bifurcation
       - (3) Reflected waves
       - (4) Antegrade and retrograde (reverberations)
   - c. Arterial Pressure wave = sum of all propagated waves
     - i. Distal peripheral vessels have elevated systole
     - ii. Knee pressures may be 20 mmHg higher

10. POISEUILLE'S LAW
    - a. Poiseuille's formula
      - i. $Q=(\pi(P_i - P_o)r^4/8\,\eta l$
      - ii. $Q \propto$ tube radius^4 (r^4)
        - (1) Main factor determining flow
      - iii. $Q \propto$ tube length (l)
      - iv. $Q \propto$ pressure gradient across tube (P_i-P_o)
      - v. $Q \propto$ fluid viscosity (η)
        - (1) Polycythemia = thick blood c RBCs
    - b. AS (LV-AO pullback) pressure gradient
      - i. Energy lost due to turbulence across tight valve
      - ii. Catheter in orifice has less lat. pres. than LV
      - iii. Sudden death risk
      - iv. ANGINA in AS
        - (1) Periodic coronary flow reversal in AS = angina
        - (2) Reduced flow & increased metabolic demand= angina

11. LAPLACE'S LAW
    - a. T = P r

    i.   T = Wall Tension = force pulling wall longitudinally
    ii.   r = radius of vessel
    iii.   Wall stress = P r / wall thickness
  b.   Aneurysms grow and rupture if > Wall Tension
  c.   Capillaries don't burst, because of Laplace Law (small r)
  d.   Critical closing pressure = vessel collapse
  e.   Hypertension - thickens AO wall = LV hypertrophy

12. STARLING'S HYPOTHESIS (not Frank-Starling law)
  a.   Balance of Hydrostatic and Osmotic Forces
    i.   Fluid movement = $(Pc-Pi) - (\pi_i - \pi_p)$
    ii.   Imbalance of Hydrostatic - Osmotic, moves fluid
  b.   Fluid leaves capillary by Filtration (hydrostatic pressure)
    i.   Tiny holes in cap. Wall
    ii.   Capillary pressure pushes fluid out
    iii.   Pulmonary edema occurs with elevated PA Wedge
  c.   Fluid enters capillary by osmotic/oncotic pressure
    i.   Absorption, can increase blood volume
    ii.   Increased salt intake
  d.   Elastic Stockings = Increase interstitial pressure
    i.   Pushes fluid back into capillary
  e.   Transcapillary Exchange
    i.   Diffusion - across capillary membrane
    ii.   Filtration - through pores in cap membrane
    iii.   Permeability due to small molecules flowing through apertures in endothelial capillary wall
  f.   Osmotic (Oncotic)Forces
    i.   Colloid osmotic pressure pulls fluid back into capillary
    ii.   Key factor restraining fluid loss from capillary
      (1) Pulls water back into capillary

    iii.   Large impermeable albumin molecules = colloid pressure

13. AUTOREGULATION
  a.   Cold causes reflexive skin vasoconstriction (sympathetic nerves)
    i.   Vagal induced bradycardia
    ii.   May be used to break SVT
  b.   Nitric Oxide (NO) - local vasodilator
    i.   Associated with adenosine release
    ii.   Pulmonary hypertension study
      (1) Evaluate PVR in Pulm. Hypertension
      (2) Measure pressure at end-expiration

14. RENAL AUTOREGULATION
  a.   Angiotensin I & II
  b.   Aldosterone
    i.   Peripheral vasoconstrictor
    ii.   Causes retention of Na
    iii.   Elevated BP
    iv.   Seen in Renal Artery Stenosis

15. THE MICROCIRCULATION AND LYMPHATIC
  a.   Capillary wall - single cell thick
  b.   Arterioles contain smooth muscle
    i.   Precapillary arteriolar sphincters
    ii.   Major resistance vessels regulate blood flow
    iii.   Chief determinant of SVR

16. VISCOSITY
    i.   Viscosity of blood varies
    ii.   Shear Thinning
    iii.   Smaller vessels have lower Hcts
      (1) RBC deform to pass capillary
      (2) Mean RBC diameter = 5-8 μm
      (3) RBCs able to pass 3 μm orifice
    iv.   Blood = non-Newtonian fluid
      (1) Polycythemia = increased Hct
      (2) Polycythemia may double viscosity

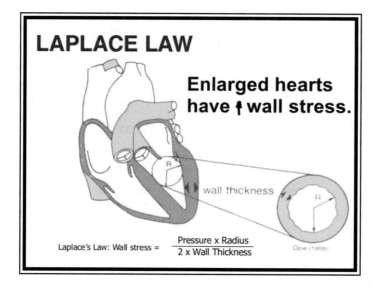

LAPLACE LAW

Enlarged hearts have ↑ wall stress.

wall thickness

R

Laplace's Law: Wall stress = $\dfrac{\text{Pressure x Radius}}{\text{2 x Wall Thickness}}$

Opie (1998)

Acquired Valvular Disease

INDEX: C1 - Acquired Valvular Disease

1. General Valve Disease

774. Other words describing a "leaky" heart valve pathology as shown at #2 are:

1. Obstructive
2. Insufficient
3. Restrictive
4. Stenotic
5. Regurgitant
6. Incompetent
   a. 1, 2, 3
   b. 1, 2, 5
   c. 2, 3, 5
   d. 2, 5, 6

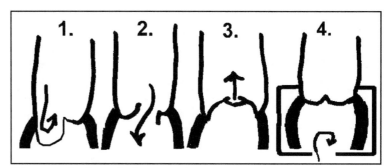

Heart pathology in heart valves

ANSWER d. 2, 5, 6. Leaky valves do not close competently. There is leakage of blood back into the proximal chamber. They may open widely during ejection, but their valve cusps don't coapt (close) properly. This diagram shows four different pathologies of the aortic valve. However, the AV valve pathologies are similarly named.

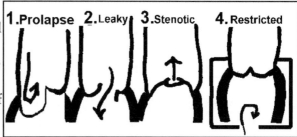

Types of valve pathology

VALVE PATHOLOGIES SHOWN ARE:

1. A prolapsing valve does not hold its position when closed. High distal pressure and an enlarged valve cause it to balloon back into the proximal chamber. The AV valves are most prone to prolapse when chordae and papillary muscles are damaged. Occasionally, a prolapsing valve may balloon or buckle so much that it leaks.

2. A **regurgitating** valve leaks. It is not "competent" to do its job of allowing flow in only one direction - it "insufficiently" coapts or closes. Leaky heart valves cause volume

overload and dilatation of the proximal chamber. They also cause loss of pressure and cardiac output to the distal chamber.

  3. A **stenosis** is a blockage or narrowing that obstructs blood flow. Stenosis restricts blood flow and pinches off the forward cardiac output. (In coronary arteries we sometimes call these obstructions "lesions.") Significant stenosis always causes a **pressure gradient** due to its high resistance to flow. It results in pressure overload and eventual hypertrophy of the proximal chamber.

  These two types of valve problems are distinctly different, with completely different physiologic consequences. However, calcified valves often exhibit both regurgitation and stenosis. Here, there is a regurgitant jet and a stenotic gradient.

  4. **Restrictive defects** form a barrier around the ventricle that limits diastolic filling and venous return. Restriction does not affect the valve leaflets. It is a "diastolic disorder." E.g., in constrictive pericarditis a tight pericardium limits (constricts) ventricular expansion in diastole. The tight pericardium allows a small initial rapid fill, then cannot expand further. Since the venous return is so restricted, the stroke volume and CO are reduced. Restriction is listed in this chapter only because it has distinct hemodynamic consequences.

SYNONYMS FOR DIFFERENT VALVE PATHOLOGIES

PROLAPSING	LEAKY	STENOTIC	RESTRICTIVE
Buckling	Insufficient	Obstructive	Encased
Billowing	Regurgitant	Narrowing	Constricted
Floppy	Incompetent	Blockage	Filling limited
Redundant	Flowing backwards	Lesion, gradient	Diastolic disorder

  See: Medical Dictionary. **Keywords:** Leaky = regurgitant = insufficient = incompetent, Stenotic = obstructive, Restrictive = constrictive

775. **Stenosis of a valve eventually causes proximal _____, and regurgitation usually causes proximal _____.**
  a. **Hypertrophy, Dilatation**
  b. **Dilatation, Hypertrophy**
  c. **Prolapse, Calcification**
  d. **Calcification, Prolapse**

ANSWER a. Hypertrophy, Dilatation. A stenosis causes a pressure overload which in turn causes hypertrophy. Stenotic valvular defects dissipate pressure energy. This causes the proximal chamber to build up more pressure to achieve the same cardiac output. Chronic pressure overload leads to hypertrophy of the chamber. Thus, as shown in the diagram, RVH results from PS.

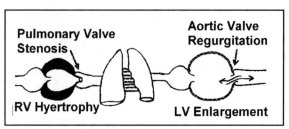

PS leads to RV hypertrophy, AR to LV dil.

  " Shunt or regurgitation leads to volume overload and chamber dilation."

Regurgitant valvular defects leak so much blood backwards that they must work harder to maintain forward cardiac output. This leads to increased filling and eventual dilatation of the upstream chamber. Thus, as shown in the diagram, LV dilatation occurs in AR. However, as dilatation stretches and thins a chamber it becomes weaker. It must increase its mass somewhat (hypertrophy) along with the dilation in order to maintain adequate pump pressure. Just as regurgitation and stenosis often occur in the same valve, volume overload is often combined with pressure overload.

See: Braunwald, chapter on "Valvular Heart Disease." **Keywords:** hypertrophy → stenosis, regurgitation → dilatation

776. **Which of the following valve diseases usually leads to an LV pressure overload?**
  a. **Ventricular septal defect**
  b. **Mitral regurgitation**
  c. **Aortic stenosis**
  d. **Aortic regurgitation**

ANSWER c. In aortic stenosis (AS) the LV pressure increases to pass the tight AO valve. The LV compensates for this pressure overload by creating parallel myofibrils. This builds LV muscle mass which is termed hypertrophy. The hypertrophy then requires more coronary flow which may be difficult to achieve, leading to ischemia especially of the sub-endocardium. Angina may develop. Myocardial cells eventually become exhausted and may be replaced with fibrous tissue and fail.

The other three answers (VSD, MR, & AR) are examples of LV "Volume Overload" where the LV fills excessively to increase forward SV.

See: Grossman, chapter on "Profiles in Valvular Heart Disease" **Keywords:** AI, LV Vol. overload

777. **Mitral stenosis pathology is classified as:**
  a. **Restrictive**
  b. **Hypertrophic**
  c. **Inflow obstructive**
  d. **Outflow obstructive**
  e. **Valvular insufficiency**

ANSWER c. Inflow obstruction refers to an inability of blood
to enter a chamber usually due to a stenosis. (E.g. Mitral Stenosis). Significant stenosis results in a pressure gradient across the stenosis, the tighter the stenosis the higher the pressure gradient. **Understand the classifications and examples below:**
  • Restrictive diseases: Constrictive Pericarditis, Tamponade
  • Hypertrophic: LV Hypertrophy, Hypertrophic Cardiomyopathy
  • Inflow obstructive: MS, TS, Cor Triatriatum, LA Myxoma
  • Outflow obstructive: AS, PS, Coarctation, IHSS/HOCM
  • Valvular insufficiency: MR, AR, varicose veins

See: Braunwald, chapter on "Valvular Heart Disease." **Keywords:** AS = Obstructive disease

778. **What condition may be associated with LV inflow obstruction?**
   a.   IHSS / HOCM
   b.   LA myxoma
   c.   Aortic stenosis
   d.   Pulmonic stenosis

ANSWER: b. LA myxoma tumors are often attached to the atrial septum by a "stalk." They may bounce around in the LA and actually "plop" down into the mitral valve to create a LV inflow obstruction. This may present signs and symptoms similar to mitral valve stenosis. MS, LA myxoma and cor triatriatum can dam up the LV inflow tract. Each can obstruct the pulmonary flow and could lead to pulmonary edema. **See:** Todd, Vol. 1, Chapter on "Acquired Valve Disease" **Keywords:** LA myxoma in LA

779. **Myxomas usually develop in the _____.**
   a.   RA
   b.   LA
   c.   RV
   d.   LV

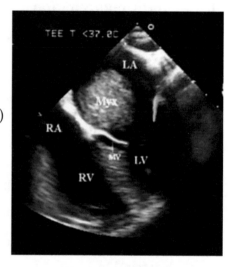

ANSWER: b. LA. "A myxoma is a primary heart (cardiac) tumor. This means that the tumor started within the heart.... Myxomas are the most common type of these rare tumors. About 75% of myxomas occur in the left atrium of the heart, usually beginning in the wall that divides the two upper chambers of the heart....The symptoms and signs of left atrial myxomas often mimic mitral stenosis... A "tumor plop" (a sound related to movement of the tumor), abnormal heart sounds, or murmur may be heard...." See: https://medlineplus.gov/ency/article/007273.htm Keywords: myxoma in LA

780. **In this RAO view of abnormal blood jets identify the valvular pathology labeled at #3 in the diagram.**
   a.   AR
   b.   AS
   c.   MR
   d.   MS

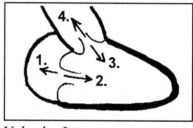
Valvular Jets

ANSWER a. AR. Note the leak regurgitating from the aorta through the aortic valve into the LV. **BE ABLE TO MATCH ALL ANSWERS.**
   1. MR = Mitral Regurgitation in systole
   2. MS = Mitral Stenosis in diastole
   3. AR = Aortic Regurgitation in diastole
   4. AS = Aortic Stenosis in systole
These jets can be imaged on angiography and Doppler color flow imaging.
See: Braunwald, chapter on, "Valvular Heart Disease." **Keywords:** AR, leak into LV

781. **Valve "doming" with distal chamber enlargement is associated with:**
   a.   Valvular regurgitation
   b.   Valvular stenosis
   c.   Supravalvular stenosis
   d.   Subvalvular stenosis

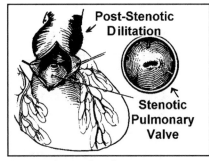

Dome shaped valve in stenosis

ANSWER b. Valvular stenosis. Stenotic valves may develop a calcified funnel shape. The valve may appear as a "dome" because of the increased pressure below it. Note in the drawing the associated post-stenotic dilatation of PA. The distal chamber below a stenosis tends to dilate, like a deep pool below a waterfall. The turbulent waterfall is analogous to the murmur. **See:** Braunwald, chapter on "Valvular Heart Disease." **Keywords:** Doming fish-mouth stenotic valve

2. Murmurs of Valvular Disease

782. **Most right sided heart murmurs are accentuated by:**
   a.   Inspiration
   b.   Expiration
   c.   Standing
   d.   Reclining

ANSWER a. Inspiration causes negative intrathoracic pressure which increases the venous return to the RA and RV. This increased flow usually increases flow through the valves and hence the right sided murmur.
See: Braunwald, chapter on "Physical Examination." **Keywords:** Right-sided murmurs increase with inspiration

783. **A patient with a decrescendo diastolic murmur and wide arterial pulse pressure probably has:**
   a.   MS
   b.   MI
   c.   AS
   d.   AI

ANSWER: d. AI = Aortic Insufficiency. Remember the hemodynamics of AI includes a wide pulse pressure with a high systolic and low diastolic reading. In severe AI, the aortic pressure may actually fall to the LVEDP. The murmur of AI decreases throughout diastole (decrescendo) just as the pressure gradient between AO and LV decreases. **See:** Todd, Vol. 1, chapter on "Acquired Valve Disease" **Keywords:** AI

BOTH QUESTIONS BELOW REFER TO THIS DIAGRAM.

784. **Describe and identify the left heart murmur labeled #1 in the diagram.**
   a.   Diastolic rumbling murmur of MS
   b.   Pansystolic murmur of MR
   c.   Systolic crescendo-decrescendo murmur of AS
   d.   Diastolic decrescendo murmur of AR

785. **The heart murmur labeled #3 in the diagram is associated with:**
   a.   AS
   b.   AR
   c.   MS
   d.   MR

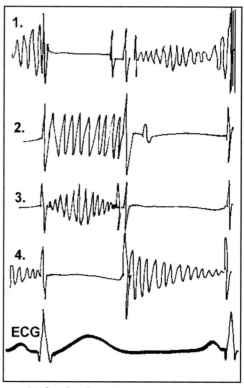

Valvular heart murmurs

BOTH ANSWERS LISTED TOGETHER BELOW

784. ANSWER a. Diastolic rumbling murmur of MS (heard best at apex).
BE ABLE TO MATCH ALL ANSWERS.
1. Diastolic rumbling murmur of MS (at apex):
   The MS jet rumbles with turbulence in the LV. In sinus rhythm this murmur gets louder (crescendos), then softer (decrescendos), and finally louder again with the atrial kick (presystolic accentuation). See LV-LA simultaneous pressure tracings in MS.
2. Pansystolic murmur of MR (at apex, spine):
   The MR murmur is pan-systolic or holo-systolic (meaning throughout all of systole). Because so much blood leaks back in systole, more blood must move into the LV during rapid diastolic filling. This rush makes the 3rd heart gallop sound

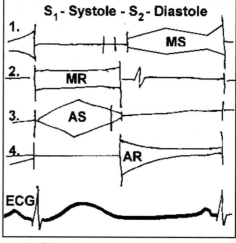

Left heart murmur envelopes

3. Systolic crescendo-decrescendo murmur of AS (at RSB):
   AS is the classic diamond shaped ejection murmur. It is harsh and high pitched because it is a high pressure jet through the tight AO valve. Its diamond shape is also termed a crescendo-decrescendo shape (louder - then softer).
4. Diastolic high frequency decrescendo murmur of AR (at LSB):
   The AR diastolic murmur is soft and high pitched diminishing in amplitude as the

gradient diminishes and may go silent by the beginning of systole. Since it decreases in intensity it is termed a decrescendo murmur - like when a symphony orchestra quiets.

The four classic left sided valve diseases have murmurs which can be reasoned out from the hemodynamics. Understanding them helps us understand the hemodynamics. Murmurs are heard at the time the turbulent jet crosses the abnormal valve. And often their shape parallels the shape of the gradient or quantity of leak.
See: Rushmer, chapter on "Valvular Heart Disease." **Keywords:** Murmurs, location

785. ANSWER a. AS is the classic diamond shaped ejection murmur (crescendo-decrescendo). This diamond shape fits the envelope of the LV-AO gradient, since the gradient causes the turbulence and the murmur. It is harsh and high pitched because it is a high pressure jet through the tight AO valve.
BE ABLE TO MATCH ALL ANSWERS.
   1. MS: Diastolic rumbling murmur
   2. MR: Pansystolic murmur
   3. AS: Systolic crescendo-decrescendo murmur
   4. AR: Diastolic high frequency decrescendo murmur
See: Rushmer, chapter on "Valvular Heart Disease." **Keywords:** Murmurs, location

786. **What type of cardiac valve sounds and murmurs would be heard best with a stethoscope at location #1 in the upper right parasternal border?**
a.   **Aortic (AS)**
b.   **Tricuspid (TS)**
c.   **Mitral - Apical (MS)**
d.   **Pulmonary (PS)**
ANSWER a. Aortic area (AS heard best).
BE ABLE TO MATCH ALL ANSWERS.
1. Aortic (AS heard best):

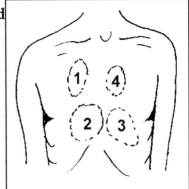

Location of murmurs

The AS murmur is heard over the aortic area 2nd RICS - RSB (2nd Right Intercostal Space - Right Sternal Border). You would think that the aortic area would be on the left side, because it is left sided. But, remember how it crosses over the top of the right PA. It also follows the right carotid blood flow and may be heard in the neck.

2. Tricuspid (TS heard best) :
Tricuspid sounds and stenotic jets travel anteriorly into the RV. Remember that the RV is the most anterior chamber. These radiate into the 4th intercostal space on both sides of the sternum.

3. Mitral, Apical (MS, AR, MR heard best):
The mitral area is at the apex and 4th LICS. Many murmurs are heard well here.   The MS jet shoots forward into the LV. It is best heard in the

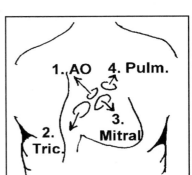

Location of murmurs

mitral area at LSB, 4-ICS just above the LV apex. The AR murmur is heard best at the apex because that is where the leaking jet is directed. The MR jet is directed back into the LA. So it may be heard at the LV apex or sometimes on the spine, trachea, or even on top the head.

4. Pulmonary (PS heard best):

The pulmonic area is where the pulmonary valve and pulmonic stenosis murmurs are heard best. Note how the PA is directed upwards and to the left - even though we consider it a right heart valve.

The location where these murmurs are loudest goes along with the direction of blood flow when the murmur is generated. Stenotic murmurs follow the stenotic jet downstream. Regurgitant murmurs radiate back upstream and are heard best near the leaking jet. So knowing where the murmur is best heard helps you tell what valve is involved.

See: Rushmer, chapter on "Valvular Heart Disease." **Keywords:** Murmurs, location

787. **A pansystolic heart murmur occurs between what heart sounds?**
   a.   S1-S2
   b.   S1-S4
   c.   S2-S3
   d.   S2-S1

ANSWER a. S1-S2. Systolic murmurs follow closure of the AV valves (S1) and end before diastole begins (S2). Pan-systolic murmurs are between S1 - S2. These murmurs are continuous throughout systole, as in mitral regurgitation. **See:** Braunwald, chapter on "Heart Sounds and Murmurs."

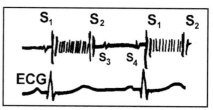

Pansystolic murmur & gallops

788. **A grade one murmur :**
   a.   **Is barely audible (faint)**
   b.   **May be heard with stethoscope barely touching chest (Very loud)**
   c.   **Is the lowest frequency murmur (<100 Hz.)**
   d.   **Is the highest frequency murmur (>1000 Hz)**

ANSWER a. Is barely audible (faint). Murmurs are graded on how loud they are, as heard through the stethoscope. This would be termed a "*grade one out of six*" murmur intensity. This intensity scale goes from 1 to 6, with 1 being so faint that it is barely audible. Grade 6 is the loudest.

Frequency or pitch varies from high to low but is not graded. The configuration or shape of a murmur is characterized as crescendo, decrescendo, crescendo-decrescendo (diamond shaped), even, or un-even. **See:** Braunwald, chapter on "Physical Exam"

789. **The most common arrhythmia associated with chronic mitral valve disease with CHF is:**
   a.   **Sinus arrhythmia**
   b.   **Atrial fibrillation**
   c.   **Heart block**
   d.   **V. tach. and/or V. fib.**

ANSWER b. Atrial fib. Atrial stretch in chronic mitral valve disease sets up reentry loops that lead to multiple ectopic foci. This may produce any of the atrial arrhythmias including atrial flutter and/or fibrillation. The danger of atrial fibrillation are:
- •Rapid ventricular response may reduce CO.
- •Loss of atrial kick reduces preload and CO.
- •Possible thrombus formation in the fibrillating atrium may lead to stroke.

See: ACLS, chapter on "Arrhythmias" Keywords: cause atrial fib. = mitral valve disease

4. Arterial Pulses

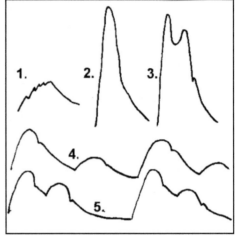

Aortic pulse tracings

BOTH OF THESE QUESTIONS REFER TO THE DIAGRAM BELOW.

790. The arterial pulse waveform labeled #1 in the diagram is termed:

a. Pulsus alternans
b. Pulsus bigeminus
c. Pulsus bisferiens
d. Pulsus tardus
e. Corrigan's pulse

791. The arterial pulse labeled #4 in the diagram may be diagnostic of:

a. Heart failure, myocardial depression
b. Alternating sinus, PVC beats (bigeminy)
c. HOCM
d. AS
e. AI

BOTH ANSWERS LISTED TOGETHER BELOW.

790. ANSWER d. Pulsus tardus.
BE ABLE TO MATCH ALL ANSWERS BELOW.
1. Pulsus tardus or parvus:
 Aortic stenosis slows the upstroke (making it tardy - "tardus"). The upstroke may have a "shudder" coincident with the ejection murmur and an anacrotic notch (notch on the upstroke wave).
2. Corrigan's pulse:
 Corrigan's pulse is seen in aortic regurgitation. It is termed "water-hammer" because it feels bounding. It shows a rapid upstroke (percussion wave) followed by a rapid collapse (regurgitation)

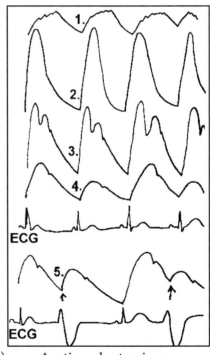

Aortic pulse tracings

early in diastole. No dicrotic notch is seen, because the aortic valve does not close completely.

3. Pulsus bisferiens:

Pulsus bisferiens is a double humped arterial pulse. Both percussion and tidal waves are distinct. It is similar to a dicrotic pulse, which has a large dicrotic notch and pulse following it, except both of the bisferiens pulses are in systole.

4. Pulsus alternans:

Pulsus alternans is an alternating systolic BP, even though the heart rate is regular. Beats alternate like this: 120/80, 115/75, 120/80, 115/75... Often seen in failing ventricles.

5. Pulsus bigeminus:

Pulsus bigeminus is caused by ventricular bigeminy. It is distinguishable from pulsus alternans only when compared to the bigeminal ECG.

Pulse contours may be palpated in the carotid artery, recorded externally with phonocardiography transducers or recorded through an intravascular catheter connected to a pressure transducer. The wave-form may be diagnostic of the pathology.

See: Braunwald, chapter on "Physical Examination." **Keywords:** Arterial pulse waves, AS=tardus, AI=Corrigan's, Alternans=CHF, Bigeminus=bigeminy

791. ANSWER a. Heart failure, myocardial depression.

BE ABLE TO MATCH ALL ANSWERS BELOW.

1. AS: In severe AS the aortic ejection is obstructed and the peak pressure reduced and delayed.

2. AI/AR:

In AI/AR the blood leaks backwards out of the AO into the LV. This loss of aortic blood rapidly drops the arterial pressure.

3. HOCM/IHSS:

Bisferiens pulse is associated with HOCM/IHSS and AR. In HOCM the LV outflow tract pinches itself off mid-systole. This makes a characteristic notch at the top of the pulse wave. The bisferiens pulse is associated with HOCM/IHSS or AR. In HOCM the LV outflow tract pinches itself off in mid-systole making a notch. This "bifid" pulse of AR is due to rapid early systolic ejection followed by a reflected wave. It may be seen in any rapid ejection - low resistance system.

4. Heart failure, myocardial depression:

In alternating pulse, the heart is so weak that it seems to rest every 2nd beat. It is an ominous sign, not specific to any disease - just a severely depressed myocardium.

5. Alternating sinus, PVC beats (bigeminy):

Bigeminal pulse is caused by a bigeminal ECG. Every other beat is a PVC followed by a compensatory pause. This pause allows more complete ventricular diastolic filling with every other beat. More preload makes for more complete contraction, and higher systolic BP with the following sinus beats.

See: Braunwald, chapter on "Physical Examination." **Keywords:** Arterial pulse waves associated pathology, AS=tardus, AI=Corrigan's, Alternans=CHF, Bigeminus=bigeminy

792. Which obstructive lesion has a <u>reduced</u> arterial pulse upstroke velocity as shown in this diagram?
a. Aortic stenosis
b. Coarctation of aorta
c. Coronary artery disease
d. Obstructive cardiomyopathy

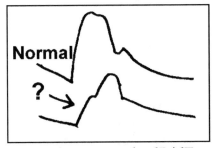

Reduced AO upstroke dP/dT

ANSWER a. AS. Note the "pulsus parvus" or "pulsus tardus" with reduced dP/dT and pulse pressure. Note the anacrotic notch seen on the arterial upstroke. These are due to the slowed ejection of blood out the tight stenotic aortic valve. Arterial pulse tracings may be recorded via invasive catheters or external transducers placed on the carotid artery.
See: Braunwald, chapter on "Physical Exam." **Keywords:** AO pulse in AS

4. Pulses and Pressures in Valvular Disease

THE NEXT 2 QUESTIONS DEAL WITH THE DIAGRAM BELOW:

793. In the simultaneous pressure tracing diagram shown, identify the chamber/vessel labeled at #3 and the valvular disease it represents.
a. AO, HOCM
b. AO, AS
c. AO, AR
d. PAW, MS
e. PAW, MR

794. Identify the valvular disease labeled at #4.
a. HOCM
b. AS
c. AR
d. MS
e. MR

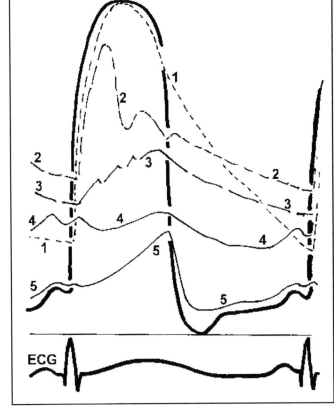

Abnormal LV, aorta and LA (PAW) pressure tracings.

ANSWERS APPEAR TOGETHER BELOW.

793. ANSWER b. AO, AS. AO tracing shows aortic stenosis pattern of pulsus tardus pattern with LV-AO gradient.
See: Braunwald, chapter on "Physical Examination." **Keywords:** valvular defects,

simultaneous pressures, HOCM, AS, AR, MS, MR

794. ANSWER d. MS. This is an LA or PAW tracing with a, c & v waves. The chief abnormality is the diastolic gradient between LA and LV indicating mitral stenosis.

BE ABLE TO MATCH ALL ANSWERS:
1. AO, AR:
> AO, AR. Note that no gradient exists (no stenosis). But the diastolic AO pressure is very low. This continues to fall as blood leaks from the AO into the LV.

2. AO, HOCM:
> AO, HOCM (previously called IHSS). Although this is not a "valvular" disease, it is similar to AS in many respects. LV-AO gradient occurs because the LV outflow tract is itself a dynamic stenosis. It obstructs flow during systole. There may be an initial (tidal wave) and then a sudden release - only to obstruct again as the LV walls come closer together. (**See:** bisferiens pulse). Pullback tracings identify two levels of pressure within the LV - one above and one below the obstruction. No gradient exists between the subvalvular LV chamber (not shown) and the AO. Gradient exists between the apical LV tracing and the AO (shown).

3. AO, AS:
> AO, AS. Note the classic pulsus tardus with slow AO upstroke. A gradient exists between the LV & AO throughout systole, but is greatest in mid-systole. The diamond shaped murmur peaks in systole just like the gradient.

4. PAW, MS:
> PAW, MS. Note the PAW-LV gradient throughout diastole.

5. PAW, MR:
> PAW, MR. Note that no gradient exists (No gradient, no stenosis). But the large v wave late in systole indicates the LA is flooded with blood from the leaky mitral valve

The LV pressure tracing is shown in dotted lines. Remember how normal simultaneous tracings overlap (See - Wiggers diagram). Normal AO-LV tracings should match in systole. Normal LV-PAW tracings should match in diastole.
See: Braunwald, chapter on "Physical Examination." **Keywords:** valvular defects, simultaneous pressures, HOCM, AS, AR, MS, MR.

795. The left heart pressures in the box, were recorded at a heart cath. What is the most likely diagnosis?

a.   AI
b.   AS
c.   MI
d.   MS

> **RECORDED PRESSURES**
> LA = 24 / 20 / 20 mmHg.
> LV = 130 / 0 / 4 mmHg.
> AO = 130 / 90 / 105 mmHg.

ANSWER d. MS. The LA pressures are considerably higher than the LV EDP indicating the end diastolic gradient or MITRAL STENOSIS. Note that the AO systole equals the LV systole indicating no gradient of AS. **See:** Kern, chapter on "Hemodynamics." **Keywords:** LA-LV gradient = MS

796. Measure & evaluate the peak to peak pressure gradient from the simultaneous AO-LV pressure tracings recorded on X200 below.
a. 75 mmHg. gradient of AS
b. 100 mmHg. gradient of AS
c. 75 mmHg. gradient of MS
d. 100 mmHg. gradient of MS

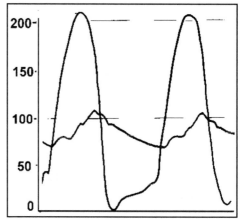
Simultaneous LV& AO X200

ANSWER b. 100 mmHg. gradient of AS. Peak LV is 210 mmHg. Peak AO is 110 mmHg, making the difference between these 2 peaks (p-p gradient) 100 mmHg. This is aortic stenosis with a characteristic pulsus parvus/tardus and anacrotic notch.
See: Kern, chapter on "Hemodynamics." **Keywords:** measure peak to peak gradient

797. The following simultaneous LV and wedge pressures were recorded on range X50 at heart cath. What abnormality is indicated?
a. Mitral stenosis
b. Mitral regurgitation
c. Constrictive pericarditis
d. Pericardial tamponade

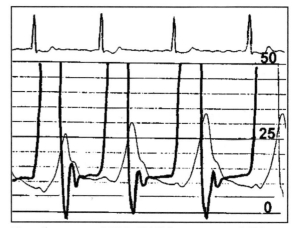
Simultaneous LV & PAW pressures X50

ANSWER b. Mitral regurgitation. The large V waves on the wedge pressure indicate mitral regurgitation - not MS - because there is no end diastolic gradient. Note the presence of atrial flutter/fib. with loss of A waves.

You might be tricked into a diagnosis of constrictive pericarditis, because of the LV diastolic dip and plateau (square root sign). But there is no elevation of the diastolic plateau (15 mmHg is not high) and this type of diastolic dip usually results from the resonant artifact of an underdamped transducer system.
See: Kern, chapter on "Hemodynamics." Keywords: ID pressures of MR - V wave

798. These simultaneous pressure tracings were recorded at cath. One catheter remains in the LV while the second is pulled back from the ascending aorta to the femoral artery. What abnormality is indicated by the pressures?

a.   Aortic aneurysm
b.   Aortic stenosis
c.   Subvalvular stenosis
d.   Coarctation of aorta

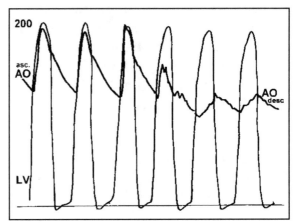

Simultaneous LV and AOa-AOd Pullback pressures x 200

ANSWER d. Coarctation of aorta. As the catheter pulls through the stenotic area, note the damping and abnormal drop in descending AO pressure. No gradient exists initially between LV and AOa (ascending AO). But in the last ½ of the tracing, as the aortic catheter pulls back - a gradient appears. This gradient occurs in the aorta, usually near the ligamentum arteriosus. Study the entire pressure tracing. All components must fit together. If you just look at the last ½ of this tracing, it mimics the gradient of AS.
See: Grossman chapter on "Congenital Heart Defects." **Keywords:** Pressure pullback in Coarctation of AO

5. Rheumatic Fever

799. What type of infection may lead to rheumatic fever?

a.   E. Coli (GI infection)
b.   Beta staphylococcus (blood infection)
c.   Alpha or hemolytic streptococcus (throat infection)
d.   Alpha or beta pseudomonas (lung infection)

ANSWER c. Streptococci throat infections cause both initial and recurrent forms of rheumatic fever. This starts as tonsillitis which is spread through the lymphatics to the heart and other organs. The acute rheumatic fever probably is an immune response to the toxins produced by the strep bacteria. This immune reaction causes inflammation of the heart, joints and skin. The valve calcification often does not appear until decades later.
See: Underhill, chapter on "Acquired Valvular Heart Disease." **Keywords:** Rheumatic fever type A. strep throat infection

800. Acute rheumatic fever is usually found in individuals between the ages of:

a.   2 and 10 years
b.   10 and 20 years
c.   30 and 45 years
d.   45 and 65 years

ANSWER: a. 2 and 10 years. Acute rheumatic fever occurs most commonly in young school age children and rarely in infancy. 40% of these strep infections occur in children 2-6 years of age. Although the strep throat is still a common illness, it is now treated with antibiotics thus preventing progression to rheumatic fever.
See: Braunwald, chapter on "Rheumatic Fever." **Keywords:** Rheumatic fever, children

801. **A child that develops a rheumatic fever usually shows what signs and symptoms? (Select 4.)**
   a.   **Chorea**
   b.   **Tiredness**
   c.   **Cyanosis**
   d.   **Diffuse joint pain**
   e.   **Fever & sore throat**

ANSWERS: a, b, d, & e. Signs of carditis and rheumatic changes are usually present. It usually starts with a strep throat infection, leading to acute rheumatic fever - an allergic reaction to the strep bacteria. Signs and symptoms include:

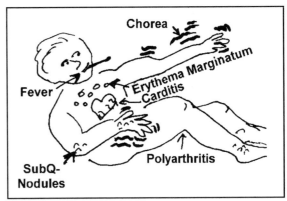
Findings in Rheumatic Fever

   1. Arthritis like joint pain - these heal with therapy to cause no residual effects.
   2. Subcutaneous nodules over body surfaces especially over fingers and toes. These tend to heal rapidly.
   3. Chorea (Sydenham's) which is a series of involuntary jerky movements (Sometimes called "St. Vitus dance")
   4. Fever may last 2-3 weeks.
   5. The heart may develop murmurs, rubs, enlarge and begin to fail.
   6. Erythema Marginatum is a round red rash which forms on the trunk.
Endocarditis is the most important manifestation of rheumatic fever. It scars the valves which continue to calcify over decades of aging and may lead to the left heart valvular defects.
See: Braunwald, chapter on "Rheumatic fever." **Keywords:** Rheumatic fever, signs, symptoms

802. **Rheumatic fever may be prevented by treating _____ infections with**

   _____.
   a.   **Viral lung, penicillin**
   b.   **Viral nasopharyngeal, steroids and antihistamines**
   c.   **Bacterial throat, penicillin**
   d.   **Bacterial throat, steroids and antihistamines**

ANSWER c. Bacterial throat, penicillin. Antibiotic therapy has almost eradicated acute rheumatic fever in the USA, though it still exists in 3rd world countries. Steroids and antihistamines should not be given, until the diagnosis is made. Penicillin is the definitive

treatment and it may be needed prophylactically to treat these patients against recurrent attacks of rheumatic fever for which they are susceptible.
See: Braunwald, chapter on "Rheumatic fever." **Keywords:** Rheumatic fever, signs, symptoms

803. Rheumatic fever most commonly damages the _____ valve.
   a.   **Tricuspid**
   b.   **Pulmonic**
   c.   **Mitral**
   d.   **Aortic**

ANSWER c. Mitral. The left sided heart valves are most affected by the endocarditis and scarring. The most common result is mitral stenosis. Some physicians say that MS is always caused by rheumatic fever, even though the rheumatic fever was decades ago. Many patients do not even remember having the rheumatic fever.

In order of frequency rheumatic valve defects are: MS, MR, AS, AR, TS, TR, PS, PR. This correlates with the hemodynamic stress placed on each valve. The closed mitral valve receives the most stress (120 mmHg) from the contracting LV. The pulmonary valve receives the least stress and seldom has acquired valve disease.
See: Underhill, chapter on "Acquired Valvular Heart Disease." **Keywords:** Rheumatic fever, most commonly causes MS

6. Mitral Valve Disease: MS and MR

804. According to Braunwald, surgery is warranted for MITRAL STENOSIS when the mitral valve area is less than _____ (critical valve area).
   a.   **0.5 square cm/M^2**
   b.   **1.0 square cm/M^2**
   c.   **2.0 square cm/M^2**
   d.   **3.5 square cm/M^2**

ANSWER b. 1.0 square cm/M^2. This is the critical number where symptoms usually begin, and valve surgery or valvuloplasty should proceed. Braunwald lists < 1.0 cm^2/M^2, or an absolute value size of 1.5-1.7 cm^2. Baim & Grossman are more conservative and list < 1.0 cm^2 as the "critical" mitral valve size (or 1.2 cm^2 for a larger individual).

The critical aortic valve area is about ½ of the mitral critical orifice size. Braunwald suggests <0.5 cm^2/M^2 to 0.8 cm^2/M^2. Baim and Grossman suggest a critical size of 0.7 cm^2. I like Braunwald's recommendation because it is easier to remember (Aortic <0.5 cm^2/M^2, or Mitral <1.0 cm^2/M^2). Valve replacement may proceed prior to these critical numbers, depending of the patient's symptoms. Better diagnostic and surgical techniques have made cardiologists and surgeons more confident about doing early surgery for valvular stenosis.
See: Grossman, chapter on "Stenotic Valve Calculations." **Keywords:** Critical MS <1.0 cm^2

805. In the simultaneous LV, AO and PAW pressures shown, which area represents the gradient used to calculate the MITRAL valve area?

a.   A
b.   B
c.   C
d.   D
e.   E

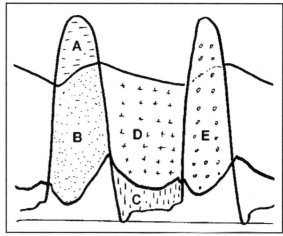

Simultaneous LV, AO, LA Pressures X200

ANSWER c. The mitral stenotic diastolic gradient is between PAW (on top) and LV pressures (on bottom). Pressure crossover points are MV opening on the left and MV closure on the right. The PAW tracing may be delayed and may need realignment. This gradient must be averaged during the diastolic filling period to evaluate the "mean" gradient for the valve area Gorlin formula.

   Note that area "A" between the LV and aortic pressures shows the gradient of aortic stenosis.

See: Grossman, chapter on "Assessment of Stenotic Valves." **Keywords:** Area to planimeter for MV area

806. The predominant cause of mitral stenosis is:

a.   Pericarditis
b.   Rheumatic fever
c.   Congenital abnormality
d.   Aging process

ANSWER b.   Rheumatic fever most commonly scars the mitral valve. In fact some physicians say it is the "only cause of MS." However, other rare causes of MS are congenital, carcinoma, lupus, and arthritis. Braunwald says that 20% of all rheumatic heart disease is MS and 40% is combined MS & MR.

See: Braunwald, chapter on "Valvular Heart Disease." **Keywords:** MS, Rheumatic Fever

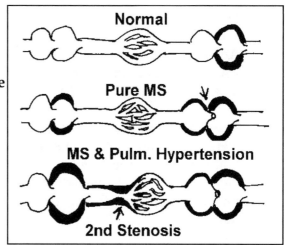

Reactive Pulm. Hypertension (after Baim)

807. Chronic mitral stenosis patients are prone to develop a "2nd stenosis" termed:

a.   Mitral valve prolapse
b.   Pulmonary valve stenosis
c.   Cor pulmonale
d.   Reactive pulmonary hypertension

ANSWER d. Reactive pulmonary hypertension. The lung capillaries are sensitive to the high LA pressures of MS. To protect the lung, the pulmonary arterioles begin to hypertrophy. This increases the pulmonary resistance so that the RV pressure must increase. This results in RV hypertrophy.

In MS the body tries to protect the lung from increasing PA pressure. In MS this "2nd stenosis" is not helpful. Symptoms of pulmonary hypertension may become worse than the MS. Other diseases which result in high LV-EDP may also develop reactive pulmonary hypertension (E.g., systemic hypertension, CHF).

In the diagram note the normal pressures, plain MS pressures, and MS with reactive pulmonary hypertension. In pulmonary hypertension PA pressures may exceed the aortic pressures. Note that pulmonary hypertension has many causes including "cor pulmonale," which involves RV hypertrophy resulting from lung diseases like COPD.

See: Braunwald, chapter on "Pulmonary Hypertension." **Keywords:** MS, reactive pulmonary hypertension, 2nd stenosis

808. **In MS with NSR (normal sinus rhythm) characteristic pressures show ___ LA "a" waves and _____ LV-EDP.**
   a.   **Elevated, Elevated**
   b.   **Elevated, Normal**
   c.   **Low, Elevated**
   d.   **Low, Normal**
   e.   **Low, Low**

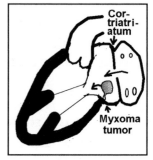
End diastolic "a" waves in MS

ANSWER b. Elevated, Normal. The "a" wave is elevated to provide better filling across the tight mitral valve. Often atrial fib. develops in which case there is no "a" wave, but the end diastolic LA pressure is still elevated above the LV-EDP. The LV diastolic is normal or low to encourage filling. This pressure is recorded on X40 - an expanded scale to better see the diastolic events (gradients). The diagram shows elevated "a" waves especially on exercise, with a normal LVEDP.

See: Braunwald, chapter on "Valvular Heart Disease." **Keywords:** MS, pressures, LA → "a wave" normal. LV-EDP

809. **Signs and symptoms of mitral stenosis may be easily confused with those of:**
   a.   **IHSS/HOCM**
   b.   **Aortic insufficiency (AR)**
   c.   **LA myxoma or cor triatriatum**
   d.   **Mitral regurgitation (MR)**

LA obstructions

ANSWER c. LA myxoma or cor triatriatum. MS, LA myxoma and cor triatriatum can dam up the LV inflow tract. Both would obstruct pulmonary flow and could lead to pulmonary edema. Cor triatriatum is three atrial chambers - a rare congenital diaphragm in the LA.

See: Braunwald, chapter on "Valvular Heart Disease." **Keywords:** LA Myxoma, Cor Triatriatum

810. **Patients with mitral valve disease in atrial fibrillation are prone to:**
  - a.   **LA clots and TIAs**
  - b.   **LA myxoma and tumor plop**
  - c.   **Subendocardial and myocardial infarction**
  - d.   **Sudden death and ventricular fibrillation**

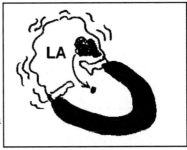

LA Thrombus, embolus

ANSWER a. LA clots and TIAs. Stagnating blood tends to clot in the LA as it dilates in advanced mitral valve disease. The large atrial size leads to atrial fibrillation. Clots can develop in the large quivering atrial appendage and break off. These emboli can lodge in the brain and cause Transient Ischemic Attacks (TIA) or stroke (CVA) the patient. That is why these patients are often anticoagulated. Atrial fibrillation reduces the cardiac output by up to 30%. It should be converted to NSR with drugs and/or electric cardio-version.
     "Stagnation clotting" happens in any chamber where blood flow slows. This also explains why reduced flow CABG veins clot off, and why apical LV clots can develop following myocardial infarction.
See: Braunwald, chapter on "Valvular Heart Disease." **Keywords:** MS, MR, atrial fibrillation, LA clots

811. **The primary complaint(s) of people with significant mitral <u>stenosis</u> is/are:**
  - a.   **Syncope and dizziness**
  - b.   **Fatigue and weakness**
  - c.   **Shortness of breath, dyspnea**
  - d.   **Signs of right heart failure, tissue edema**

ANSWER c. Shortness of breath, dyspnea. SOB is the chief symptom in both MS and MR. This is because of the increase in LA and pulmonary capillary pressure. Increased capillary pressure increases the likelihood of pulmonary edema and thus shortness of breath (SOB). Related signs and symptoms are hemoptysis (blood stained sputum), angina from RVH or coincident CAD, thromboembolism from LA, and infective endocarditis. **See:** Braunwald, chapter on "Valvular Heart Disease."

812. **What is the primary sign or symptom associated with severe mitral <u>regurgitation</u>?**
  - a.   **Syncope**
  - b.   **Chest pain**
  - c.   **Sleeplessness**
  - d.   **Shortness of breath**

ANSWER d. Shortness of breath. Individuals with acute mitral regurgitation will have the signs and symptoms of decompensated congestive heart failure (ie: shortness of breath, pulmonary edema, orthopnea, paroxysmal nocturnal dyspnea), as well as symptoms suggestive of a low cardiac output state (ie: decreased exercise tolerance). MR is the most common form of valvular heart disease. The most common cause of mitral regurgitation is mitral valve prolapse (MVP). See: https://medlineplus.gov/ency/article/000176.htm

813. **Increasing the cardiac output in mitral stenosis will_____ pressure gradient across the mitral valve.**
   a. **Increase the systolic**
   b. **Increase the diastolic**
   c. **Decrease the systolic**
   d. **Decrease the diastolic**

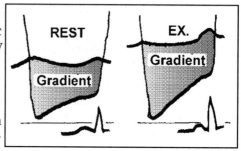

MS: LA-LV pressures, rest, Ex.

ANSWER b. Increase the diastolic. Increasing the CO or flow across a stenosis always increases the diastolic pressure gradient. This is easily seen on the PAW - LV pressures as the gradient increases with exercise, pacing, or Isuprel. Increasing the CO in patients with minimal gradients is especially important because the pressure gradient increases. This makes the valve area measurement more accurate. **See:** Braunwald, chapter on "Valvular Heart Disease." **Keywords:** MS, ↑ CO = ↑ systolic gradient

814. **A patient with mild MITRAL STENOSIS shows signs of heart failure. What could be done to increase the pressure gradient measured at cath for more accurate evaluation of his stenotic gradient? (Select 2.)**
   1. **Speed the heart rate with ventricular pacing**
   2. **Administer nitroglycerin to induce vasodilation**
   3. **Administer chronotropic drugs to increase CO (...)**
   4. **Administer negative-inotropic drugs to reduce cardiac work (beta blockers...)**
   5. **Exercise him during the cath (increase CO)**
      a. **3, 5**
      b. **4, 5**
      c. **3, 4**
      d. **4, 5**

ANSWER a. (3) Administer chronotropic drugs to increase CO (Dobutamine...), and/or (5) Exercise him during the cath (increase CO). A small gradient (under 5 mmHg) makes the Gorlin Valve area calculation inaccurate. Inaccurate valve area measurement may cause a patient to be denied surgery when he or she needs it, or prematurely push him or her into surgery. Since most stenotic valves are rigid and cannot dilate, the valve area will not change significantly with increased cardiac output. But, increasing the cardiac output will increase the gradient and make the calculation of the fixed valve area more accurate.

Grossman says that even rapid atrial pacing does not really increase the CO. Ventricular pacing would be worse without atrial synchrony. Increasing the CO increases the filling pressures and the LA-LV diastolic gradient by stressing the heart. **See:** Braunwald, chapter on "Valvular Heart Disease."

815. **Which of the following hemodynamic signs are most commonly seen in mitral stenosis pressure recordings? (Select 3.)**
a.   Diastolic isometric relaxation gradient
b.   Diastolic filling gradient
c.   End diastolic gradient
d.   Large A wave (if in sinus rhythm)
e.   Elevated systemic venous pressure

ANSWERS: b, c, & d. An isometric diastolic gradient is NOT correct. During isometric relaxation there is no flow across the valve. It occurs on the downslope of the LV pressure curve. It is brief and unrelated to the MS. MS causes elevated pulmonary venous pressures, not elevated systemic venous pressures.

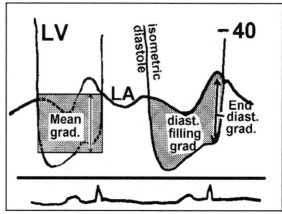
Mitral stenosis LV-LA gradients

MS pressures show: Diastolic gradient, end diastolic gradient, and large A wave (if in sinus rhythm). The characteristic MS gradient is between the LA-LV during diastole. Many physicians rely on the "end diastolic gradient" as representative of MR. This is because a small early diastolic rapid fill gradient may be normal. Also, increased atrial kick is present (increasing the "a" wave at end-diastole). This increases LV filling - to compensate for the loss of forward CO due to the leak. The mean gradient shown is the average gradient throughout diastolic filling.
See: Braunwald, chapter on "Valvular Heart Disease." **Keywords:** MS, pressure curves

816. **What is the hemodynamic effect of severe mitral stenosis?**
a.   Pulmonary artery hypotension
b.   Pulmonary artery hypertension
c.   Increased LV-end diastolic pressure
d.   Decreased LV-end diastolic pressure

ANSWER: b. Pulmonary artery hypertension. LA mean pressure increases with significant LA-LV diastolic gradient. Braunwald says, "When the mitral valve opening is reduced to 1 cm^2, which is considered to represent severe MS, ...Elevated left atrial pressure results in pulmonary artery hypertension with secondary effects on the pulmonary vasculature and right heart.... Typically the left ventricle is relatively normal, unless there is coexisting MR....Left ventricular diastolic pressure is normal in patients with isolated MS." **See:** Braunwald, chapter on "Valvular Heart Disease"

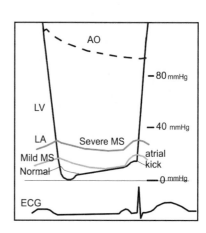

817. Which type of chamber enlargement is associated with mitral regurgitation?

   a.   LA dilatation
   b.   LA hypertrophy
   c.   LV dilatation
   d.   LV hypertrophy

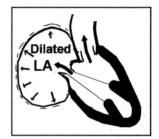
MR & enlarged LA

ANSWER a. LA dilatation. Regurgitation of a valve leads to dilation of the proximal chamber, while stenosis of a valve leads to hypertrophy of the proximal chamber. By analogy: long skinny "stretched out" muscles are seen in long distance runners, while "hypertrophied" muscles are seen in weight lifters. Note, however, that both dilatation and hypertrophy commonly exist together.
See: Braunwald, chapter on "Valvular Heart Disease" **Keywords:** LA dilatation.

818. The following asymptomatic 80 year old patient has chronic mitral regurgitation with atrial fibrillation, massive enlarged and dilated LA, normal pulmonary vascular resistance, forward cardiac output of 3.5 L/min., and regurgitation of 1.1 L/min. What wedge pressure readings would be most likely found at heart cath?

   a.   PAW = - / 12 / 10
   b.   PAW = - / 47 / 29
   c.   PAW = 15 / 12 / 10
   d.   PAW = 28 / 44 / 35

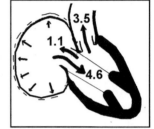
Mitral Regurg. flows

ANSWER b. PAW = - / 47 / 29. Atrial fib removes the "A" waves from the pressure tracing, so none can be read. The "-" means unreadable. Also, the second number, 47 mmHg, is the elevated "V" wave of acute MR. When the LA is chronic and dilated the "V" waves may not be as prominent as in this example. Note the regurgitant fraction here is 1.1/4.6 = 0.24 so almost one quarter of the LV flow is lost to regurgitation.
See: Kern, chapter on "Hemodynamics." **Keywords:** PAW pressure in MR with atrial fibrillation

819. Which of the following auscultatory findings is most consistent with mitral valve incompetence?

   a.   Late-diastolic crescendo murmur, best heard at the apex
   b.   Late-systolic murmur with an early diastolic component
   c.   Early-diastolic decrescendo murmur, best heard at the LLSB
   d.   Even-intensity pansystolic murmur, best heard at the apex

ANSWER d. Even-intensity pansystolic murmur, best heard at the apex. When dealing with murmurs, think of your hemodynamics and angiography. MR occurs throughout systole (pan-systolic) and is heard best in the direction of the regurgitation (apex). Understand basic murmurs, pulse tracings, and heart sounds.
See: Braunwald, chapter on "Heart sounds and Murmurs."
Keywords: MR = pansystolic murmur

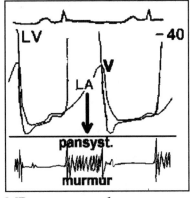

MR murmur and pressures

820. **In patients with acute mitral regurgitation the PA wedge pressures usually show a diagnostic:**
   a.   **Large V wave**
   b.   **Large A wave**
   c.   **Absent V wave**
   d.   **Absent A wave**

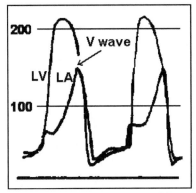

Giant V waves in VSD

ANSWER a. Large V wave. MR patients leak blood from the LV back into the LA. During ventricular systole the LA is filling both from the lungs and the LV. This overfills the LA causing the large V wave. These large V waves only develop however, if the LA has normal size and compliance. Once it dilates it becomes so compliant that regurgitant waves are damped out by the huge LA chamber.

     Grossman states that to be confident that V waves are significant they must be greater that 2-3 times the mean LA pressure. Giant V waves may also be seen in acute VSD as shown in the diagram. This is due to large pulmonary blood flow filling the LA and causing giant V waves. So, large V waves may be indicative of MR, but significant MR may be present with NO "V" waves. **See:** Kern, chapter on "Hemodynamics" and Grossman, chapter on "Profiles in Valvular Heart Disease" **Keywords:** MR, V waves

821. **In mitral regurgitation patients, which cardiac output is significantly higher than all other measures of cardiac output?**
   a.   **Increased LVMF (LV Angio CO)**
   b.   **Increased Radionuclide CO (Technetium)**
   c.   **Increased forward CO (Fick CO)**
   d.   **Increased RV cardiac output (Thermodilution CO)**

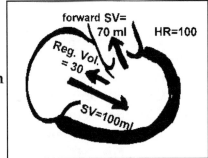

LVMF and forward C.O.

ANSWER a. Increased LVMF (LV Angio CO).
Quantitative LV cardiac output (LVMF) is measured by calculating and LV volumes at end diastole and end

systole. The difference between EDV and ESV is the SV.

EDV-ESV=SV = 250 - 150 = 100 ml.

SV x HR = LVMF = 100 x 100 = 10 L/min

LVMF = Left Ventricular Minute Flow. It is sometimes called the "angio C.O." because it is based on LV volumes for one heartbeat. But, in MR some of this LV blood leaks back into the LA. That leak is not part of the "forward C.O." Fick and Thermo are considered to be the "forward C.O." because they actually measure flow through the lungs and peripheral bed..

In the diagram note that the mitral valve diastolic inflow is large. This is the LV-angio stroke volume. It is the sum of what leaks back and what is pumped out the aorta each beat.

In MR and AR the quantitative LV cardiac output (LVMF) will be larger than either the Fick or Thermo C.O. The larger LVMF indicates that the LV is pumping more blood than is actually getting to the tissues. The difference between LVMF and Fick CO is the amount of regurgitation. Fick and Thermo. CO should theoretically be the same. LVMF-Fick CO = Regurgitation/min.

In the example shown the LV stroke volume is 100 ml while the forward SV is only 70 ml. The regurgitant volume is 100-70 = 30 ml. If the HR were 100/min, the LVMF would be 10 L/min and the Fick CO 7. L/min. **See:** Grossman, chapter on "Evaluation of Ventricular Volumes, EF,..." **Keywords:** MR, LVMF → Fick

822. **Acute severe mitral regurgitation is most often due to: (Select 2.)**

a. **Endocarditis**
b. **Chordal rupture**
c. **Mitral annulus dilatation**
d. **Papillary muscle rupture**
e. **Chest trauma**

ANSWERS: b. Chordal rupture or d. Papillary muscle rupture. Ragosta says, "Severe, acute mitral regurgitation (often due to spontaneous chordal rupture or avulsion of a papillary muscle head from acute infarction) typically occurs in the presence of a small, unadapted left atrium. The acute increase in volume rapidly raises LA and PV pressures, transmitting to the lungs and causing pulmonary edema....hypoperfusion and shock may ensue." **See:** Ragosta, chapter on "Mitral Valve Disorders" **Keywords:** acute MR = chordal or papillary muscle rupture

823. **The LA/LV size diagrams indicate the stages of development of MR. The stage labeled #3 is:**

a. **Chronic compensated MR**
b. **Chronic decompensated MR**
c. **Acute uncompensated MR**
d. **Sub-acute MR (LA**

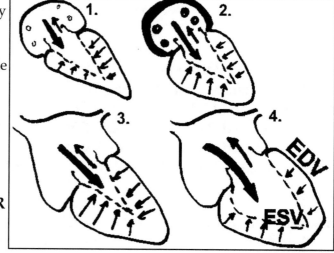

LV-EDV, LV-ESV, & LA size in stages MR

adaptation)

ANSWER a. Chronic compensated MR. **BE ABLE TO MATCH ALL ANSWERS BELOW.**

1. ACUTE UNCOMPENSATED (MR):

When severe MR appears suddenly in people with normal hearts the sudden increase in LA pressure is transmitted back into the lungs and right heart. An example of this is acute ruptured chordae tendinea with acute MI.

2. SUB-ACUTE MR (LA ADAPTATION)

Within a few weeks of this high pressure the LA begins to compensate. The LA and pulmonary vasculature begins to hypertrophy and can dramatically increase its pressure and preload. Within 6-12 months pulmonary vessels hypertrophy and pulmonary resistance increases. Also, the LV begins to adjust to this volume overload by increasing the LV EDV. LV ESV remains unchanged.

3. CHRONIC COMPENSATED MR

After a few years the LA dilates and thins to accept the increasing regurgitation. "V" waves disappear because of the compliant LA. And the LV compensates for increasing volume overload by continued dilation and hypertrophy. EDV increases ESV remains the same. SV and EF increase.

4. CHRONIC DECOMPENSATED MR

In the latter stages of MR the LV goes into failure. It dilates to the point where contraction becomes inefficient. EF and LV function both drop. ESV increases and the LV and LA both become large bags.

STAGES OF MITRAL REGURGITATION

Parameter	Normal	1.Acute MR	2. Subacute MR	3. Chronic MR	4. Decomp. MR
LA press.	10/10/8	20/40/20	30/50/30	15/25/20	20/30/25
LV edv	120 ml.	150	170	200	250
LV esv	50 ml.	30	30	30	100
LV angio SV	70 ml.	120	140	170	150
Fwd. SV	70 ml.	50	60	70	60
Reg. Vol.	0 ml.	70	80	100	110

FORMULAS: LV SV = (LV edv) - (LV esv)

fwd. SV= Fick CO / HR

Reg. Vol = LV SV - fwd. SV

EF = (LV SV) / (LV edv)

Note how there are two types of SV. The LV SV measured from the angio, and the forward SV measured from the Fick CO. The LV ANGIO CO and stroke volumes are always larger in any regurgitant situation. Note also, how the LV EDV rises consistently as the disease progresses. Also, the EF is high because the LV is volume overloaded and pumps much of its volume backwards through the leaking valve.

See: Braunwald, chapter on "Valvular Heart Disease." **Keywords:** Rx for MR

824. **Which stage of MR shows the largest "a" waves and pulmonary hypertension?**
- **a.** **Acute uncompensated MR (stage 1)**
- **b.** **Sub-acute MR with LA adaptation (stage 2)**
- **c.** **Chronic compensated MR with LV adaptation (stage 3)**
- **d.** **Chronic decompensated MR (stage 4)**

ANSWER b. Sub-acute MR with LA adaptation (stage 2). In stage #2 (see previous diagram) the LA and pulmonary vasculature hypertrophy in response to the high LA pressure. The hypertrophied LA contraction ("a" waves) can better preload the LV. As the LA dilates, LA pressure declines. The LA has not yet dilated to the point where atrial fibrillation is likely. As the pulmonary arterioles hypertrophy due to the increased pulmonary capillary pressure the pulmonary resistance (PVR) increases which in turn increases the RV and PA pressures. The LV continues to take in more blood (EDV) in response to the need for larger stroke volumes. **See:** Braunwald, chapter on "Valvular Heart Disease." **Keywords:** MR, Stage with largest PVR

825. **At which stage of MR progression will large "v" waves disappear from PA wedge pressure tracings?**
- **a.** **Acute uncompensated MR (stage 1)**
- **b.** **Sub-acute MR with LA adaptation (stage 2)**
- **c.** **Chronic compensated MR with LV adaptation (stage 3)**
- **d.** **Chronic decompensated MR (stage 4)**

ANSWER c. Chronic compensated MR with LV adaptation (stage 3). When the LA dilates and thins to the point where it can absorb the LV regurgitation without reflecting it back into the lungs, "v" waves will decrease in size. The increased LA compliance dramatically affects the LA and wedge pressures. These later stages of MR usually show NO significant "v" waves unless the regurgitation volume is tremendous.
See: Braunwald, chapter on "Valvular Heart Disease." **Keywords:** MR, Stage where "v" waves disappear

826. **When mitral regurgitation occurs as the mitral valve "billows" into the LA, as shown, it is termed:**
- **a.** **Flail mitral valve**
- **b.** **Mitral valve prolapse**
- **c.** **Left atrial myxoma**
- **d.** **Myxomatous mitral valve**

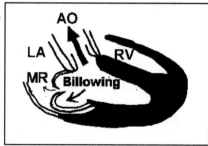
Mitral Valve Prolapse

ANSWER b. Mitral valve prolapse. MVP is called by many names: Barlow's syndrome, floppy valve syndrome, ballooning mitral cusp syndrome, systolic click syndrome, hooded valve...
Here the mitral leaflets become so enlarged that they flop back into the LA in systole. The

middle collagen layer of the valve tissue is overabundant or myxomatous (tumorous). This enlarges the valve and it becomes floppy (redundant). MVP is diagnosed on 2D echocardiography or LV angiography when the mitral leaflet coaptation point is behind/superior to the mitral annulus. If the MR is due to ruptured chordae tendinea it is termed a "Flail leaflet."
See: Underhill chapter on "Acquired Valvular Heart Disease." Keywords: MVP, post. mitral leaflet, diastole

827. **Which type of angiogram would best define a "flail" posterior mitral valve leaflet or ruptured chordae tendinea?**
    a. **Aortic root, LAO angiogram**
    b. **Aortic root, RAO aortogram**
    c. **Left ventriculogram, LAO view**
    d. **Left ventriculogram, RAO view**

ANSWER d. Left ventriculogram, RAO view. LV gram for leaky mitral valves. The RAO views the mitral valve on edge. It best lays out the LA and LV chambers so they do not overlap. Note the RAO view in the previous question. Both prolapse and flail leaflet may result in MR. Braunwald says that the RAO view best defines posterior mitral leaflet prolapse, while the LAO view best defines anterior leaflet prolapse.
See: Kern, chapter on "Angiography." **Keywords:** RAO LV gram injection to Dx MR flail leaflet

828. **A patient recovering from acute MI in the CCU becomes cold and clammy, dyspneic, drops his BP, and develops a holosystolic murmur. What condition is probable?**
    a. **Aortic stenosis**
    b. **Septal rupture - VSD**
    c. **Acute aortic dissection**
    d. **Ruptured chordae Tendinea**

ANSWER: d. Ruptured chordae tendinea can result from MI affecting the papillary muscles. This may lead to mitral regurgitation, increased pulmonary wedge pressures, and dyspnea. Remember that MR results in a holosystolic murmur. See: Braunwald chapter on "Valve Disease" **Keywords:** MI complication = ruptured chordae tendinea

829. **Therapy for mitral regurgitation includes: (Select 2.)**
    1. **Vasodilators (nitrates, ACE inhibitors)**
    2. **Vasoconstrictors (aramine, neosynephrine)**
    3. **Stimulants (dobutamine, epinephrine)**
    4. **Mechanical counterpulsation (IABP)**
        a. 1, 2
        b. 1, 4
        c. 2, 3
        d. 2, 4

ANSWER b. (1) Vasodilators (nitrates, ACE inhibitors), and (4) Mechanical counterpulsation (IABP). In MR forward LV stoke volume is reduced due to the mitral leak (similar to a VSD). Anything which will make it easier to eject blood out the AO will increase SV and reduce regurgitant volume. Afterload reduction therapy includes:

1. YES: Vasodilator drugs (nitrates & ACE inhibitors) may be life saving by making it easier to eject blood forward than to leak backward.

2. NO: Vasocostrictors increased the afterload/resistance and thus reduce the CO and EF. They raise the BP at the expense of maintaining blood flow.

3. NO: Stimulants increase the force of contraction, which may make regurgitation worse.

4. YES: Mechanical counterpulsation (IABP) reduces the afterload during deflation. It helps "pull" blood out of the LV away from the leaking valve.

See: Braunwald, chapter on "Valvular Heart Disease." **Keywords:** Rx for MR

830. **The hallmark hemodynamic sign of acute mitral regurgitation is:**
a. **Large "V" waves in wedge pressure**
b. **Large "A" waves in wedge pressure**
c. **Diastolic dip and plateau in wedge pressure**
d. **Spike and dome arterial pressure**
e. **Pulsus paradoxus arterial pressure**

ANSWER: a. Large "V" waves in wedge or LA pressure. This is true in acute MR when the LA is normal in size. Blood regurgitating back through the mitral valve quickly fills the LA and increases its V wave pressure. However, as the LA dilates and becomes more compliant, the regurgitant wedge V wave is damped out and may not appear large. Besides, there are many other diseases that also present with large V waves. Remember, atrial V waves are seen after the T wave on the ECG.

See: Kern chapter on "Hemodynamic Data" **Keywords:** acute MR = V waves

831. **This simultaneous LV - wedge pressure tracing demonstrates:**
a. **Chronic MS with atrial fibrillation**
b. **Acute MS with sinus rhythm**
c. **Chronic MR with atrial fibrillation**
d. **Acute MR with sinus rhythm**

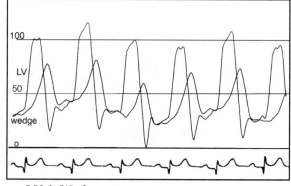

LV & Wedge   after Ragosta Cardiac Catheterization Text

ANSWER: d. Acute MR with sinus rhythm. Note large V waves of 4+ mitral regurgitation. The wedge is delayed in transmission through the lungs, so the V wave peak does not line up with the LV downslope as it would in a transseptal LA tracing. There is no end diastolic gradient, thus no mitral stenosis. P waves of sinus rhythm are evident.

Ragosta says, "A prominent "V" wave on the pulmonary capillary wedge pressure

waveform represents the classic hemodynamic finding of acute, severe mitral valve regurgitation....The presence of a "V" wave depends on the size, pressure, and compliance of the left atrium. Patients with chronic, well compensated, severe mitral regurgitation often have normal, physiologic "V" waves on the pulmonary capillary wedge pressure tracing."
See: Ragosta, chapter on "Classic Hemodynamic Waveforms" **Keywords:** MR= V waves

832. **The "MitraClip" device reduces _____ by creating a _____.**
  a. **MR, single orifice mitral valve**
  b. **MR, double orifice mitral valve**
  c. **MS, more complaint mitral valve**
  d. **MS, larger mitral valve ring**

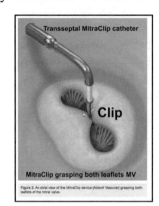

ANSWER: b. MR, double orifice mitral valve - with a figure 8 shape.
The single MitraClip basically staples the center of the 2 mitral leaflets together forming 2 smaller orifices, one on each side of the clip. This is most helpful when regurgitation is from the center of the valve with a torn chordae tendinea.

   The MitraClip is made of chromium and cobalt and is covered in polyester to promote the growth of tissue around the clip. **See:** https://www.vascular.abbott/us/products/structural-heart/mitraclip-mitral-valve-repair.html.

   EchoNavigator software can merge the images from echocardiography and fluoroscopy making it easier to navigate the catheter and position the clip to best reduce regurgitation. **See:** https://www.youtube.com/watch?v=40iHkbPTcb0
See: https://www.usa.philips.com/healthcare/product/HCOPT08/echonavigator

7. Aortic Valve Disease: AS, AR & IHSS

833. **Which of the following murmurs is most consistent with aortic stenosis (AS)?**
  a. **Diastolic blowing murmur heard at apex**
  b. **Diamond-shaped ejection murmur radiating toward the neck**
  c. **Holosystolic murmur radiating toward shoulder**
  d. **Pansystolic murmur radiating toward sternum**

ANSWER b. Diamond-shaped ejection murmur radiating toward the neck. This is a classic phono cardiographic description of AS. Note that the shape of the murmur parallels the gradient, which is also "diamond" shaped. Know the murmurs.
See: Braunwald, chapter on "Heart Sounds and Murmurs." **Keywords:** MR = pansystolic murmur

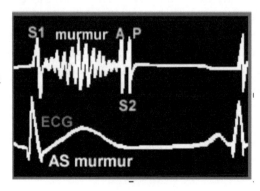

834. **In the USA the most common form of aortic valve stenosis in younger patients under 70 years old is:**
   a. **Calcific AS**
   b. **Rheumatic AS**
   c. **Congenital bicuspid AS**
   d. **Congenital tricuspid AS**

ANSWER c. Congenital bicuspid AS. With the decrease in rheumatic fever in the USA most AS is now found in younger patients with congenital aortic valve defects. More than half of all younger valve replacement patients (< 70 years) have such congenital valve defects. The congenital "bicuspid" valve goes unnoticed for years until calcification develops from the turbulence around the misshaped valve. Although commonly called "congenital bicuspid" they may be either uni, bi, or tricuspid malformed valves.
See: Braunwald, chapter on, "Valvular Heart Disease." **Keywords:** Congenital AS, bicuspid

835. **Aortic stenosis patients may develop angina type pain in the absence of coronary disease because the LV work is _____, and the coronary driving pressure is _____.**
   a. **Increased,   Increased**
   b. **Increased,   Decreased**
   c. **Decreased,   Decreased**
   d. **Decreased,   Increased**

ANSWER b. Increased, Decreased. We tend to think all angina is associated with CAD. But severe AS can manifest with angina. Angina results when the myocardial demand for O2 exceeds the supply. In AS the myocardium becomes hypertrophied to generate the high LV systolic pressures required to push blood through the tight valve. This requires lots of work and O2. Note increased LV work area in diagram (LVs-LA). The coronary arteries are usually normal or even enlarged, but the AO has reduced pressure with which to push it through the coronaries. Note, reduced coronary driving pressure in diagram (AOd - RA). In AS diastolic coronary flow is vital, because the high

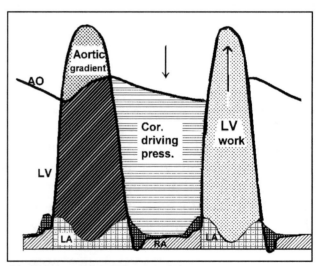

Aortic stenosis with simultaneous AO, LV, & RA pressures

LV wall tension constricts the myocardial capillaries even more than normal - so no coronary systolic flow occurs.
See: Braunwald, chapter on "Valvular Heart Disease." **Keywords:** AS with angina

836. In aortic stenosis, the pressure gradient occurs between the _____ chambers and during the _____ phase of the heart cycle.
a. LA-LV, Systolic
b. LA-LV, Diastolic
c. LV-AO, Systolic
d. LV-AO, Diastolic

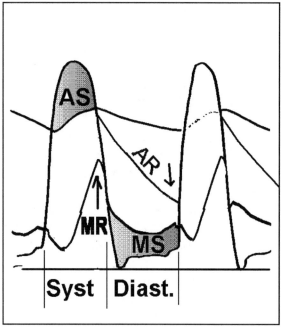

ANSWER c. LV-AO, Systolic. In AS the aortic valve closes but won' open enough. The aortic valve is between LV-AO and opens in systole. **EACH OF THE ABOVE ANSWERS IS ASSOCIATED WITH ONE VALVULAR DISEASE.**

1. LA-LV (mitral regurgitation): leaks in systole
2. LA-LV (mitral stenosis): obstructed in diastole
3. LV-AO (aortic stenosis): obstructed in systole
4. LV-AO (aortic regurgitation): leaks in diastole

Systolic/diastolic valve disease

Note that the time when these abnormal obstructions or leaks occur is the same time that the murmur is loudest.
See: Braunwald, ch.r on "Rheumatic Fever."

THE NEXT 2 QUESTIONS DEAL WITH THE DIAGRAM BELOW.

837. Identify the obstruction seen at #2 in this LV-AO pullback tracing.
a. Valvular AS
b. HOCM/IHSS
c. Coarctation of AO
d. Combined HOCM & AS

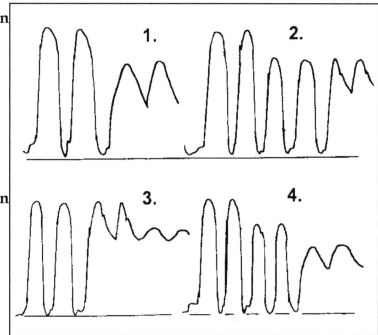

838. Identify the obstruction seen at #4 in this LV-AO pullback tracing.
a. Valvular AS
b. HOCM/IHSS
c. Coarctation of AO
d. Combined HOCM & AS

Left heart catheter pullback pressures

ANSWERS APPEAR TOGETHER BELOW. MATCH ALL.

837. ANSWER b. HOCM/IHSS. The classic valvular aortic stenosis tracing shows a drop in systolic pressure as the catheter tip crosses the AO valve. The valve is crossed between the two distinctive pressure tracings of the LV and then the AO.
These three gradients would not normally be seen together in one patient.
MATCH THE CHAMBERS AND PRESSURES SHOWN IN THIS DIAGRAM WITH PATHOLOGY BELOW.
      1. Valvular AS
      2. HOCM/IHSS = Subvalvular Stenosis
      3. Coarctation AO = Supravalvular
      4. Combined HOCM & AS
Note how the systolic pressure drops suddenly across each stenosis. HOCM is a subvalvular stenosis within the outflow tract of the LV. Valvular AS is in the valve itself. Coarctation of the AO is above the valve (just beyond the aortic arch).
See: Kern, chapter on "Hemodynamics." **Keywords:** AS

838. ANSWER d. Combined HOCM & AS. Gradients will occur within the LV outflow tract and at the aortic valve. As the catheter is pulled out of the apex into the LV outflow track the systolic pressure drops across the obstruction. Then as the catheter is pulled across the AO valve, the LV AO systolic is lower than the LV outflow systolic pressure.
See: Kern, chapter on "Hemodynamics." **Keywords:** Pullback, combined HOCM & AS

839. **Identity the type of aortic stenosis labeled at #2 in the diagram? (NOTE: Small circles indicate calcium deposits on valve.)**
  a.   **Congenital bicuspid**
  b.   **Rheumatic AS**
  c.   **Normal AO valve**
  d.   **Atherosclerotic calcific**

ANSWER b. Rheumatic thick calcified fused cusps. Calcium deposits occur in characteristic places on AS valves.

BE ABLE TO MATCH ALL ANSWERS BELOW.
      1. Normal thin pliable leaflets open completely in systole and no show gradient. Note the coronary artery orifices in the images.

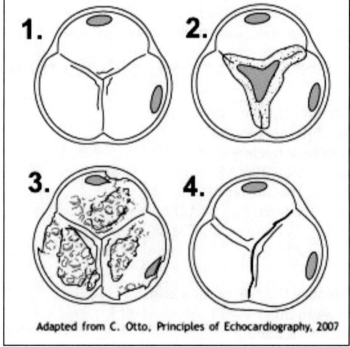

Adapted from C. Otto, Principles of Echocardiography, 2007

Aortic cusp pathologies in AS

      2. Rheumatic AS shows calcium deposits along commissure. It results from rheumatic fever which is now rare in the USA. A streptococcal throat infection results in cartitis and cusp thinkening.

3. Calcific/Atherosclerotic AS shows generalized calcium throughout valve.and may be seen in patients with severe hyper-cholesterolemia and some bone diseases. Degenerative (senile) calcification is the most common type of AS in older patients. The cusps are immobile due to calcium deposits near the wall of the AO where they flex.

4. Congenital bicuspid valve shows thickening and fusion of the commissures leading to stiff valve borders. The orifice may be a rounded triangle or even circular. These valves are often so stiff they may be leaky as well as stenotic. This may not be noticed at birth. But in later years the turbulence causes calcium to deposit on the lips of the cusps **See:** Braunwald, chapter on, "Valvular Heart Disease."

840. **A patient has severe aortic stenosis, LVH, and is in sinus rhythm. The PA wedge pressure tracing will likely show:**
a.   **Large "V" waves**
b.   **Large "A" waves**
c.   **No "A" waves**
d.   **No "V" waves**

ANSWER b.   Large "A" waves. Left ventricular hypertrophy (LVH) increases the stiffness of the LV so it is difficult to fill in diastole. The LA comes to the rescue by increasing the atrial kick and thus the LV-EDP. Note how loss of P wave on ECG beat#3 decreases the systolic LV and AO pressure. **See:** Braunwald, chapter on "Valvular Heart Disease."

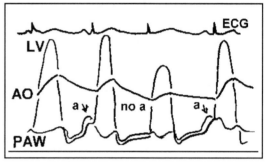

PAW/LA "a" wave in AS

841. **What is the natural history of untreated aortic stenosis patients that begin to develop symptoms such as angina or syncope?**
a.   **It is too late to operate (pulmonary hypertension likely)**
b.   **Cardiac transplantation should be considered**
c.   **Sudden death is likely within 3 years**
d.   **Stroke is likely within 5 years**

ANSWER c. Sudden death is likely within 3 years. When significant symptoms do develop it's time to aggressively evaluate the patient for valve aortic replacement surgery - which is the definitive therapy. Most AS patients live for decades without symptoms. But, watch out when symptoms do develop. The risk of sudden death dramatically increases.

The natural history of these patients indicates that most die of sudden death (ventricular fibrillation) within 3 years of developing these symptoms. Note the sudden drop in the survival curve at the point of symptom development. Thus, it is essential to quickly treat AS patients with symptoms of syncope, angina, or CHF.

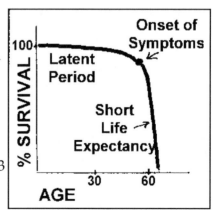

Natural history of AS after symptoms develop

See: Braunwald, chapter on "Valvular Heart Disease."

842. **Arterial pressure showing pulsus parvus/tardus with low aortic dp/dt suggests:**
a. **Aortic stenosis**
b. **Aortic regurgitation**
c. **Aortic valve prolapse**
d. **Aortic mechanical valve dehiscence**

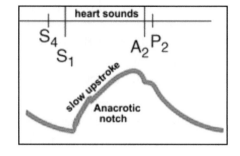

ANSWER: a. Aortic stenosis. The tight aortic valve restricts flow into the AO, so the arterial upstroke is slowed. Because of this reduced outflow, the AO systolic pressure does not rise as fast or as high as the LV systolic pressure. dp/dt is the maximum pressure up-slope. Low slope is tardy, thus pulsus parvus or pulsus tardus.
See: Braunwald, chapter on "Evaluation of the Patient" **Keywords:** pulsus parvus = AS

843. **Current candidates (2018) for transcatheter semilunar valve replacement are severely symptomatic patients that are not candidates for valve replacement surgery with: (Check all 3 that qualify for transcatheter replacement below.)**
a. **MS and MR**
b. **Hypertrophic Obstructive Cardiomyopathy**
c. **AR**
d. **AS**
e. **Pulmonary regurgitation in children over 5 years of age**
f. **Stenosis of PA valve prosthesis conduit in children over 5 years of age**

ANSWERS: d. AS, e. PR, & f. PA conduit stenosis. TAVR in adults is for AS patients that are not candidates for valve surgery. In children, the Melody transcatheter valve has multiple uses.

Topol says: "In the United States, no indications for TAVI have been established, as the devices are still under investigation. Inclusion in the PARTNER trial required patients to have severe symptomatic AS, be considered high risk for surgical complications (STS risk score >10%), have a greater than 1 year survival with regard to their comorbidities, and might benefit from valve replacement.... Transcatheter mitral valve implantation has not yet been applied clinically. In large part, this is because radial force, which is used to secure aortic prostheses in a calcified aortic root, cannot be applied in the mitral position."

Topol says, "[transcatheter] valve replacement is also considered reasonable if severe pulmonary regurgitation is accompanied by moderate to severe right ventricular dysfunction or enlargement, symptomatic or sustained atrial and/or ventricular arrhythmias, or moderate to severe tricuspid regurgitation.... In conduit dysfunction, percutaneous intervention may be useful where the diameter narrowing of the prosthesis is >50%.... TPVI is a transcatheter approach that can treat both pulmonary regurgitation and stenosis in patients with suitable RVOT anatomy" Pulmonary valve replacement is done with the *Melody Transcatheter Pulmonary Valve* system of Medtronic. See: Topol, chapter on Pulmonary and Tricuspid Valve interventions

844. **During TAVR, when the Sapien balloon is inflated in the aortic valve:**
    a.   **Pace the RV at 180 bpm**
    b.   **Remove the ventricular guide wire**
    c.   **Inflate as quickly, and deflate as quickly as possible**
    d.   **Administer adenosine to increase AV block and reduce HR**

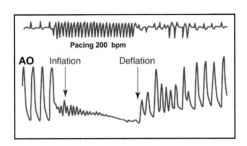

ANSWER: a. Pace the RV at 180 bpm. (TAVR = Transcatheter Aortic Valve Replacement).
    Kern says, "Following the angiography, a temporary transvenous pacemaker is positioned.... The pacer was to be used for the rapid ventricular pacing needed to reduce left ventricular ejection force, permitting more stable balloon inflation across the aortic valve. After crossing the aortic valve with a stiff guide wire, aortic balloon dilation was performed. The 4cm x 20mm balloon catheter was then exchanged for the Sapien Edwards stent 26mm valve system and during rapid ventricular pacing (180bpm), the stent valve is deployed, and the catheter is removed." **See:** Kern, TAVR – A Personal Experience, Cath lab Digest, 2013

845. **What access route is preferred for balloon inflated TAVR in patients with tortuous aortic arch and femoral artery?**
    a.   **Radial**
    b.   **Transseptal**
    c.   **Transapical**
    d.   **Subclavian**

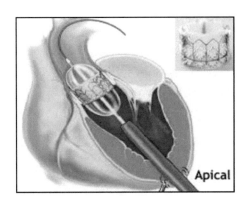

ANSWER: c. Transapical through the cardiac apex. Cheung & Lichtenstein say, "Transfemoral (TF-TAVR) retrograde and transapical (TA-TAVR) antegrade approaches are the most widely practiced. TA-TAVR is the preferred procedure where the peripheral access is limited due to size, calcification and tortuosity. TA-TAVR provides a more stable platform for TAVR, due to the more direct and shorter distance to the native aortic valve. Access via the subclavian artery and ascending aorta are emerging to be viable alternatives." Currently only the Sapien valve is balloon expandable and can be placed apically. **See:** Cheung & Lichtenstein, Illustrated Techniques for Transapical Aortic Valve Implantation, Annals of Cardiothoracic Surgery, 2012

IHSS/HOCM - Coarctation AO

(Although not strictly a valve pathology - IHSS and Coarctation fit here because they both obstruct the LV Outflow.)

846. This hypertrophied LV which pinches off its own outflow tract in systole has what pathology?
   a.   (RC) Restrictive cardiomyopathy
   b.   (HOCM) Hypertrophic obstructive cardiomyopathy
   c.   (CP) Constrictive pericarditis
   d.   (MVP) Mitral valve prolapse
   e.   Coarctation of aorta

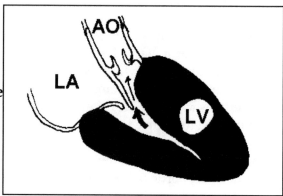
LV Outflow obstruction

ANSWER b. HOCM (Hypertrophic Obstructive Cardio-Myopathy), HCM (Hypertrophic Cardio-Myopathy) or IHSS (Idiopathic Hypertrophic Subaortic Stenosis) are different names for this myopathy. It is a genetically transmitted myopathy characterized by myocardial muscle cell disarray. The myocardial cells are not lined up parallel to each other. The LV wall is so hypertrophied that there is almost no end-systolic volume (rat-tail ventricle). This tends to trap blood in the apex during systole. The location of the obstruction is between the anterior leaflet of the mitral valve and the hypertrophied LV septum. Usually the hypertrophy is greater on the septal side of the LV, thus the echocardiographic term "asymmetrical septal hypertrophy (ASH)." The muscle itself is the obstruction, and it is dynamic. It comes and goes. Obstruction is accentuated with increased contractility (E.g. exercise, post-PVC beats...) Although some Hypertrophic Cardiomyopathy (HCM) patients show minimal gradients, HOCM/IHSS patients usually show an intra-LV gradient is seen as the LV catheter is pulled out of the LV apex. Pressures may read: apex = 200/10, LV outflow = 150/10, AO = 150/90 mmHg. **See:** Grossman, chapter on "Profiles in Dilated and Hypertrophic Cardiomyopathies."

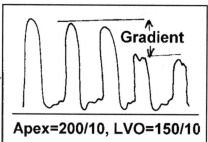
LV apex - LV outflow gradient

Gradient

Apex=200/10, LVO=150/10

847. While monitoring the arterial pressure you notice that post PVC beats show reduced systolic BP and increased gradient. This abnormal hemodynamic phenomenon is termed _____ sign and is associated with _____.
a.   Kussmaul's, AS
b.   Kussmaul's, HOCM
c.   Brockenbrough's, AS
d.   Brockenbrough's, HOCM

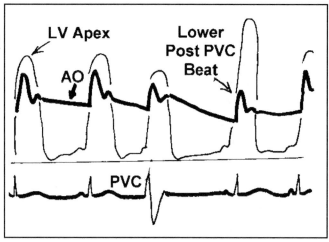

Post PVC drop in systolic BP

ANSWER d. Brockenbrough's, HOCM. PVCs are usually followed by a compensatory pause. This increases the preload and makes the post PVC beat harder. So this post PVC beat should normally have higher systolic pressure. But in HOCM the opposite happens as shown. In HOCM when the LV beats harder it pinches off.

The apical LV pressure is high, but the LV outflow tract and AO are lower. Make yourself a hero by diagnosing HOCM just by noting the post PVC drop in arterial pressure.

In AS the relationship between LV systole and AO systole is constant. It is not dynamic. The AO systolic will be a constant % of the peak LV. Post PVC beats in AS will increase the AO pressure just like in normal physiology.
See: Braunwald, chapter on "Valvular Heart Disease." **Keywords:** IHSS, HOCM, Brockenbrough's sign

848. A patient has coarctation of the AO near the ligamentum arteriosus. When compared to the right carotid pulse wave the _____ pressure wave is reduced in pressure and delayed in time.
a.   Right radial
b.   Right brachial
c.   Left brachial
d.   Right femoral

ANSWER d. Right femoral. In coarctation of the aorta the aortic pressures below the coarctation (stenosis) will be reduced and delayed. The ligamentum arteriosus is over the top of the arch, after the 3 arch vessels. Aortic vessels below the left subclavian will show reduced systolic pressures. Both femoral arteries will be reduced.
See: Braunwald, chapter on "Physical Examination."

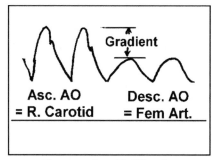

Coarctation Pullback

849. **Medical therapy for HOCM/IHSS includes:**
      1. Beta blockers
      2. Calcium channel blockers
      3. Digitalis
      4. Vasodilator
            a. 1, 2
            b. 1, 3
            c. 2, 3
            d. 3, 4

ANSWER a. (1) Beta blockers and (2) Calcium channel blockers. Since the muscle itself is the obstruction the harder the LV contracts the more it obstructs. So therapy involves reducing the LV contractility.
    1. YES: Beta blockers
    2. YES: Calcium channel blockers
    3. NO: Digitalis
    4. NO: Vasodilator

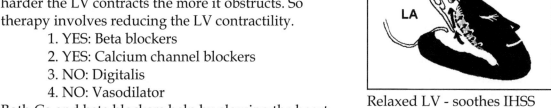
Relaxed LV - soothes IHSS

Both Ca and beta blockers help by slowing the heart rate and reducing contractility. Digitalis and vasodilators are contraindicated, since digitalis makes the heart beat harder, and dilators reduce the afterload. Reducing the afterload and resistance lets the LV eject blood so forcefully that the LV may obstruct. Surgery can be done to excise the obstructing LV septum, but has limited success. AV sequential pacemaker implantation may help IHSS (HOCM) patients. The increased atrial kick increases preload and may keep the LV-edv volume large enough to prevent LV muscular obstruction in systole.
See: Underhill, chapter on "Cardiomyopathies." **Keywords:** HOCM, IHSS, medical therapy, Ca blockers, beta blockers

Aortic Insufficiency - Regurgitation

850. **In severe AR the presystolic apical rumble (sounding like an MS murmur) commonly heard is termed a/an:**
a.   **Austin Flint murmur**
b.   **Diamond shaped ejection murmur**
c.   **Graham Steel murmur**
d.   **Bruit murmur**

ANSWER a. Austin Flint murmur. The AR jet impinges on the anterior leaflet of the mitral valve making it vibrate in systole. This vibration is also seen on the anterior valve leaflet in this M-mode echocardiogram. Note the "f" (flutter) waves seen on this mitral valve M-mode echocardiogram in AR.
See: Braunwald, chapter on "Valvular Heart Disease."

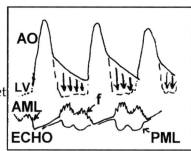
Austin Flint on Echo

Keywords: Austin Flint, AI

851. This diagram shows the LV-EDV and LV-ESV seen in various stages of the natural history of aortic regurgitation. The LV labeled at #4 (↑EDV & ↑ESV) best represents what stage?
a. Normal LV
b. Severe acute AR
c. Chronic compensated AR
d. Chronic decompensated AR

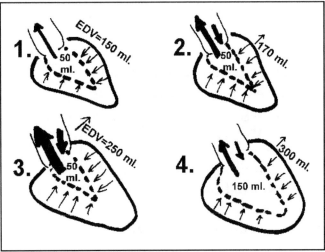

LV contraction in stages of AR

ANSWER d. Chronic decompensated AR. Since so much leaks back as AR progresses from acute to chronic the LV progressively dilates and hypertrophies in an attempt to pump an adequate stroke volume. Note how as AI progresses the EDV increases but the ESV stays about the same. Then when it "goes" the LV can no longer maintain the small ESV and the EF goes to "pot" (decompensated LV failure). Chronic AR has the largest LV volumes found in any heart disease. **BE ABLE TO MATCH ALL ANSWERS BELOW.**

　　1. Normal LV (here EF = 66%)
　　2. Severe acute AR - begins to fill more - inadequate SV - barely pumps out all the blood that leaks back (here EF = 71%)
　　3. Chronic compensated AR - fills (dilates) even more in diastole - maintaining adequate SV (here EF = 80%)
　　4. Chronic decompensated AR - dilated even at end systole - dilates so much that heart failure develops - reduced BP (here EF = 50%)

Sample LV measurements in AR are:	EDV	ESV	SV	EF
1. Normal LV	150	50	100	.67
2. Severe acute AR	170	50	120	.71
3. Chronic compensated AR	250	50	200	.80
4. Chronic decompensated AR	00	150	150	.50

Acute AR may be caused by aortic dissection, trauma, or infective endocarditis.
See: Braunwald, chapter on "Valvular Heart Disease." **Keywords:** stages of LV dilation secondary to rheumatic AR

852. Which type of AR has the greatest EF and LV-stroke volume as measured by quantitative LV angiography.
a. Normal LV
b. Severe acute AR
c. Chronic compensated AR
d. Chronic decompensated AR

ANSWER c. Chronic compensated AR. The LV attempts to compensate for the increasing diastolic regurgitation volume. It compensates by increasing its end diastolic volume. It fills to the max, because so much of its SV leaks back.

Essential formulas are: SV = EDV - ESV and EF = SV/EDV

See: Braunwald, chapter on "Valvular Heart Disease." **Keywords:** AR stages of LV dilation

853. This diagram shows simultaneous LV and AO pressures seen in the various stages of AR. The pressure tracings shown at #2 indicate:

a. Chronic decompensated AR
b. Normal LV
c. Severe acute AR
d. Chronic compensated AR

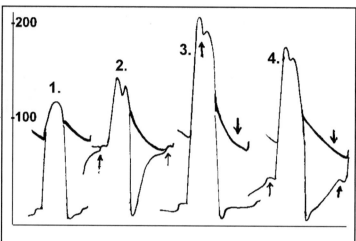

LV-AO pressures seen in stages of AR

ANSWER c. Severe acute AR. The most devastating pressures are seen in the acute phase where so much blood leaks back into the ventricle that pressures equalize early in diastole. The LV-EDP may equal the aortic diastolic pressure.

CORRECTLY MATCHED STAGES OF AORTIC REGURGITATION ARE:
Pressures measured in mmHg are:

Type of Ao. Regurgitation..	Aortic BP in mmHg.	LV edp in mmHg
1. Normal LV	120 /80	10
2. Severe acute AR	130 /70	↑↑ 50
3. Chronic compensated AR	↑ 190 /↓ 60	12
4. Chronic decompensated AR	↑ 170 /↓ 60	↑ 25

See: Braunwald, chapter on "Valvular Heart Disease." each

854. Which type of AR has the highest LV-edp?

a. Normal LV
b. Severe acute AR
c. Chronic compensated AR
d. Chronic decompensated AR

ANSWER b. Severe acute AR. In severe acute AR the AO and LV end-diastolic pressures equalize. For example the stages of AR shown below are:

STAGES OF AR	Sample LV-EDP in mmHg.
1. Normal LV	10
2. Severe acute AR	↑↑ 50
3. Chronic compensated AR	12

4. Chronic decompensated AR   ↑   25
See: Braunwald, chapter on "Valvular Heart Disease." **Keywords:** AR stages of LV dilation

855. What valve disease is most likely to complicate manual hemostasis, by increasing the likelihood of femoral hematoma post cath?
- a.   AS
- b.   MS
- c.   AR
- d.   MR

ANSWER c. AR. Aortic regurgitation has a wide pulse pressure. Hematomas are more common because of the bounding pulse. **See:** Braunwald, chapter on "Valvular Heart Disease."

856. Some AI and MVP patients suffer from an autosomal connective tissue syndrome which includes: long spindly limbs and digits, scoliosis, joint hyper-mobility, and myopia. What syndrome is this?
- a.   Kawasaki syndrome
- b.   Cushing's syndrome
- c.   Dressler's syndrome
- d.   Marfan's syndrome

ANSWER d. Marfan's syndrome. This is the syndrome "Abraham Lincoln" may have had. It is a genetic syndrome affecting all connective tissue. Diagnosis is made by clinical findings in the eye, skeleton (pectis excavatum), aorta, and other signs. It effects the heart by dilating the aorta (increased risk of AR and AO dissection). It also is associated with mitral valve prolapse. Related diseases which dilate the aorta are: Ehlers-Danlos syndrome, syphilis, ankylosing spondylitis, arthritis, and systemic hypertension.

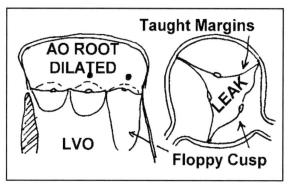
Dilation of Aorta in Marfan

See: Braunwald, chapter on "Genetics and Cardiovascular Disease."

857. What type of LV work is associated with chronic aortic regurgitation?
- a.   ↓ Diastolic filling (decreased LV preload)
- b.   ↑ LV pressure work (increased aortic obstruction)
- c.   ↓ Volume work (decreased LV stroke volume)
- d.   ↑ Volume work (increased LV stroke volume)

ANSWER d. ↑ Volume work (increased LV stroke volume). The continued dilation of the LV in AR results from the need to increase stroke volume, just to keep ahead of the amount of the regurgitation. The LV stroke volume may exceed 300 ml in an effort to maintain an average forward stroke volume of 100 ml (200 ml of regurgitation). This increase in volume

work causes dilation (enlargement) of the LV. But dilated LVs are inefficient according to Laplace's Law and so hypertrophy develops because of the increased wall tension and increasing blood pressure.
See: Braunwald, chapter on "Valvular Heart Disease." **Keywords:** AI, ↑ SV

858. **Appropriate definitive therapy for acute symptomatic aortic insufficiency (AR) is:**
   a. **Afterload reducing agents (Nitrates)**
   b. **Aortic balloon valvuloplasty (Cath)**
   c. **Valve replacement (Surgery)**
   d. **Balloon pump (IABP)**

ANSWER c. Valve replacement (Surgery). Immediate surgery is usually required, because cardiac output is severely reduced. In chronic AI surgery is called for once symptoms develop. If the AI is due to infective endocarditis it is best to "sterilize" the patient with antibiotics before the surgery. IABP is contraindicated since it would inflate during diastole and increase the regurgitation.
See: Underhill, chapter on "Acquired Valvular Heart Disease." **Keywords:** AI, surgery

859. **Appropriate MEDICAL THERAPY for acute symptomatic aortic insufficiency (AR) is:**
   a. **Afterload reducing agents (nitrates)**
   b. **Afterload increasing agents (pressors)**
   c. **Preload reducing agents (diuretics)**
   d. **Preload increasing agents (IV fluid)**

ANSWER a. Afterload reducing agents (Nitrates: E.g., nitroprusside)
Vasodilators may be used to stabilize acute AR patients. Nitrates reduce the afterload and make it easier to eject blood into the aorta. Reduced BP reduces the amount of regurgitation because there is less diastolic pressure to drive leaking blood retrograde through the valve. This improves forward flow and reduces the amount of regurgitation. What you do NOT want to do is increase the diastolic pressure with IABP (contraindicated in AR). **See:** Underhill, chapter on "Acquired Valvular Heart Disease." **Keywords:** Acute symptomatic RX for AI = Nitrates

860. **A 7 year old with a mechanical heart valve was taken to your cath lab with loud diastolic and systolic murmurs. You record this simultaneous LV - AO pressure tracing which demonstrates:**
   a. **Pure aortic stenosis**
   b. **Aortic stenosis with pulmonary hypertension**
   c. **Pure aortic regurgitation**
   d. **Combined aortic regurgitation and stenosis**

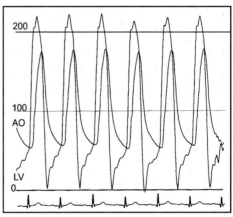

LV-AO   After Ragosta Cardiac Catheterization Text

ANSWER: d. Combined aortic regurgitation and stenosis, because of the low diastole and systolic gradient. The arterial pulse pressure is wide (170/55 mmHg) and diastole falls dramatically to the level of the LV-edp. There is also a 40 mmHg systolic gradient. The artificial aortic valve may be stuck in a open position, so that it both leaks and is stenotic. The LV-edp is 50 mmHg, which means the PA pressure must be elevated. There will be signs of right heart failure along with the loud murmurs. Time for a new valve. **See:** Ragosta, chapter on "Classic Hemodynamic Waveforms" **Keywords:** Combined AR & AS

9. Other Acquired Valve Disease

861. **An example of congenital RV pressure overload is:**

    a.   **PR**
    b.   **PS**
    c.   **ASD**
    d.   **TS**
    e.   **TR**

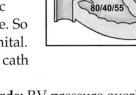

ANSWER b. Pulmonic Valve Stenosis (PS). The tight pulmonic valve forces the RV to build up pressure. This takes RV muscle. So the RV hypertrophies. The most common form of PS is congenital. Congenital PS can often be repaired with valvuloplasty in the cath lab. This diagram shows RV pressure overload due to PS.
See: Braunwald, chapter on "Valvular Heart Disease." **Keywords:** RV pressure overload, congenital PS

862. **Elevated central venous pressure and large right atrial systolic "V" waves, as shown at #1 on the diagram, indicate:**

    a.   **Mild TR**
    b.   **Severe TR**
    c.   **Over-compliant RV**
    d.   **Non-compliant RV**

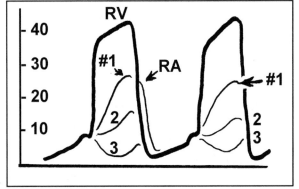

Elevated "V" waves

ANSWER b. Severe Tricuspid Regurgitation (TR). RA and RV-EDP are elevated. The RA tracing shows absence of "x" descent and prominent "v" wave in systole. When the atrial "v" wave is so large that it resembles the RV tracing it is termed "ventricularization." Pressures in the RV of 40/5/10 mmHg. **BE ABLE TO MATCH ALL ANSWERS.**

        1. Severe TR - ventricularization - large "v wave" to 30 mmHg
        2. Mild TR - small "v wave" to 18 mmHg.
        3. Normal RA pressure - "v wave" to 8 mmHg.

The most common cause of TR is dilation of the tricuspid annulus as complication of RV failure. The valve ring is stretched so much that the leaflets fail to coapt correctly. Compensatory dilation of the RV develops. TR usually requires no surgical treatment unless pulmonary hypertension develops.

See: Braunwald, chapter on "Valvular Heart Disease." **Keywords:** RA "v" wave, severe TR pressures

863. **This diagram shows right heart pullback pressure tracings on four patients. What abnormality is labeled at #1?**
   a. **Pulmonary arteriolar gradient**
   b. **Pulmonary valvular gradient (PS)**
   c. **Intra RV gradient (infundibular stenosis)**
   d. **Tricuspid valvular gradient (TS)**

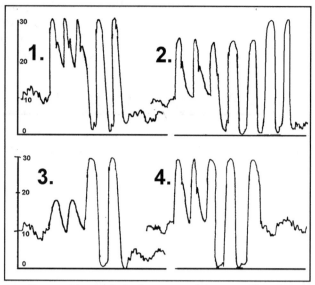

Swan-Ganz right heart catheter pullbacks

ANSWER a. Pulmonary arteriolar gradient usually indicates pulmonary disease.

BE ABLE TO MATCH ALL ANSWERS BELOW.
1. Pulmonary Arteriolar Stenosis:
   Compare the initial PAW to the PA pressure that follows. The PAW mean should equal the PA end-diastolic pressure or not be more than 6 mmHg higher. Here there is a 10 mmHg. gradient between the PA and the LA in the pulmonary arterioles indicating possible stenosis. This can happen in pulmonary hypertension and various lung diseases. However, increased CO can accentuate this gradient in normal individuals.
2. Infundibular Stenosis:
   Compare the RV outflow with RV inflow. They should be the same. An intra-cavity systolic gradient due to infundibular stenosis exists (analogous to HOCM/IHSS.)
3. Pulmonary Valve Stenosis:
   Compare the PA systolic to the RV systolic. They should be equal. A systolic gradient exists due to a tight pulmonic valve (analogous to AS.)
4. Tricuspid Valve Stenosis:
   Compare RV diastolic with RA mean pressure. They should be the same. A tricuspid valve gradient exists (comparable to MS.)
NORMAL RIGHT HEART PULLBACK should look like this.
Chambers recorded here are:
   1. PAW
   2. PA
   3. RV outflow
   4. RV inflow
   5. RA
Note normal pressure equalization at the arrows. Normally PAW ≈ PA-edp,

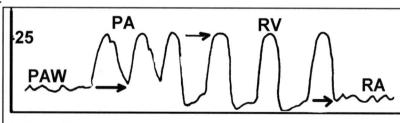

Normal Rt. Heart pullback: PAW-PA-RVO-RV-RA

PA syst. = RV syst., and RV-edp = RA mean.
See: Grossman, chapter on "Profiles in Valvular Heart Disease." Keywords: Rt. Heart
Pullback, arteriolar stenosis, PS, Infundibular. St., TS

864. **What valvular heart disease is indicated by these**
pressures taken during right heart catheterization?
    a.   **Pulmonic valve stenosis (PS)**
    b.   **Pulmonary valve insufficiency (PI)**
    c.   **Tricuspid valve stenosis (TS)**
    d.   **Tricuspid valve insufficiency (TI)**

Right Heart Pressures
PAW = 12 / 10 / 7 mmHg.
PA = 25 / 10 /15 mmHg.
RV = 25 / 4 / 5 mmHg.
RA = 5 / 15 / 6 mmHg.

ANSWER d. Tricuspid Insufficiency (TI) or Tricuspid Regurgitation. Note the elevated "V"
wave (15 mmHg) in the RA, indicating possible tricuspid insufficiency (regurgitation).
Understand hemodynamic changes for all valvular, vascular, and constrictive lesions.
Know how to read and interpret pressures for all cardiac chambers. Readings are taken and
noted as follows:
        PAW = "a" / "v" / mean
        PA = systolic / diastolic / mean
        RV = systolic / begin diastolic / end diastolic
        RA = "a" / "v" / mean
See: Kern, chapter on "Hemodynamics."

865. **This is a simultaneous PAW and LV**
pressure tracing run on X50. Pathology
indicated is:
    a.   **Pure PS**
    b.   **Mixed PS - MR**
    c.   **Pure MR**
    d.   **Mixed MR - MS**

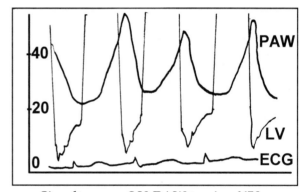

ANSWER d. Mixed MR - MS. Here we see   Simultaneous LV-PAW tracing X50
large "v" waves indicating probable MR, and a diastolic LA-LV gradient indicative of MS.
Mixture of stenosis and insufficiency in the same valve is common when leaflets are
calcified. They neither open nor close adequately.
See: Kern, chapter on "Hemodynamics."

866. **This is a simultaneous LA and**
LV pressure tracing. The wave
at the ? is a ____ suggesting __.
    a.   **C wave, MS**
    b.   **V wave, MS**
    c.   **C wave, MR**
    d.   **V wave, MR**

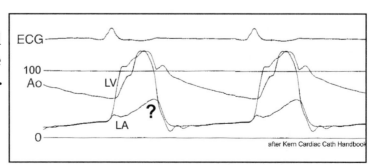

Simultaneous LV-PAW tracing X40

ANSWER: d. V wave, MR = mitral regurgitation. This giant V wave is due to build up of regurgitating blood backwards through the mitral valve filling the LV in systole. The arterial pressure falls from 130 to 60 mmHg (wide pulse pressure) while the LA pressure builds from 20 up to 60 mmHg (large V wave). All are features of AR. There is a slight intrinsic LV-AO gradient in early systole probably due to the large LV stroke volume required - not AS. Note, the fast paper speed that makes it hard to appreciate these striking hemodynamic features. **See:** Kern, chapter on "Hemodynamic Data."

REFERENCES:

Baim, D. S and Grossman W.., Cardiac Catheterization, Angiography, and Intervention, 7th Ed., Lea and Febiger, 2006

Braunwald, Eugene, Ed., HEART DISEASE A Textbook of Cardiovascular Medicine, 9th Ed., W. B. Saunders Co., 2012

Criley J. M., and Ross, R. S., CARDIOVASCULAR PHYSIOLOGY, Tampa Tracings, 1971

Kern, M. J., Ed., The Cardiac Catheterization Handbook, 6th Ed., Mosby-Year Book, Inc., 2016

Netter, CIBA Collection of Medical Illustrations, "The Heart", CIBA Pharmaceuticals

Ragosta, Textbook of Clinical Hemodynamics, Saunders Elsevier, 2008

Rushmer, R. F.,CARDIOVASCULAR DYNAMICS, W. B. Saunders Co., 1976

Textbook of ADVANCED CARDIAC LIFE SUPPORT, American Heart Association, 2010

Underhill, S. L., Ed., CARDIAC NURSING, 2nd Ed., J. B. Lippincott Co., 1989

OUTLINE: C1 - Acquired Valvular Heart Disease

General Acquired Heart Disease
- a. Definitions
    - i. regurgitation = insufficiency = leak
    - ii. stenosis = obstruction = blockage
    - iii. restrictive = encased = constricted
    - iv. hypertrophy
        - (1) caused by pressure overload
        - (2) LV hypertrophy in AS
        - (3) Atrial hypertrophy is MS
    - v. dilation = enlargement
        - (1) caused by volume overload
        - (2) LV dilation in AR
- b. Echo Doppler in valvular disease
    - i. M-mode patterns normal
    - ii. M-mode in valve disease
    - iii. CW Doppler patterns nml. & dis.
    - iv. simultaneous presentation
- c. Murmurs in valvular disease
    - i. AS = diamond systolic ejection
    - ii. AR = decrescendo diastolic
    - iii. MS = diastolic rumble
    - iv. MR = pansystolic
    - v. Locations of murmurs
    - vi. Splitting S2
        - (1) normal is A2 - P2
        - (2) paradoxic split is P2 - A2 in AS
    - vii. S3 = rapid ventricular filling (MR)
    - viii. S4 = atrial contraction
    - ix. breathing effects on murmurs
- d. Hemodynamics - pressures
    - i. simultaneous pressures in AS, AR, MS, MR
    - ii. Gradients, V waves
- e. Pulses
    - i. Pulsus tardus
    - ii. Corrigan's pulse
    - iii. Pulsus alternans
    - iv. Pulsus Bisferiens
    - v. Pulsus bigeminus

2. Rheumatic Fever
- a. etiology
    - i. strep throat
    - ii. valves affected
        - (1) chiefly Mitral
- b. clinical manifestations
    - i. use of Echocardiography
    - ii. ages of children (2-10 yrs old)
- c. physical assessment
    - i. chorea
    - ii. nodules
- d. Therapy
    - i. antibiotics
    - ii. Rheumatic fever still prevalent in underdeveloped countries

3. Mitral Stenosis (MS)
- a. etiology

        i.   rheumatic
- b. clinical manifestations
    - i. LA myxoma
    - ii. Cor tri atratus
    - iii. clots in LA, stroke
    - iv. Chief complaint = SOB
    - v. second stenosis in pulm. arterioles
    - vi. stages
        - (1) chronic = enlarged/hypert. LA
- c. physical assessment
    - i. murmur
- d. Cath. findings
    - i. hemodynamics
        - (1) diastolic PAW - LV gradient
        - (2) elevated a wave
        - (3) elevated LAedp
        - (4) gradient accentuated with exercise or inotropic agents
        - (5) angiography
- e. Therapy
    - i. Mitral valvulo-plasty
    - ii. Mitral valve replacement surgery

4. Mitral regurgitation (MR)
    - a. etiology
        - i. Mitral valve prolapse
        - ii. ruptured chordae tendinea
        - iii. Ruptured chordae or pap. Muscle
    - b. clinical manifestations
        - i. SOB, pulmonary edema
        - ii. Stages
            - (1) acute
                - (a) elevated V wave
            - (2) chronic compensated
                - (a) elevated PAW pressure
                - (b) LA dilates
                - (c) pulmonary vessels hypertrophy
            - (3) decompensated
                - (a) increased regurg.
                - (b) reduced SV
    - c. physical assessment
        - i. murmur
    - d. Cath. findings
        - i. V wave
        - ii. regurgitant fraction
        - iii. LV angiography
    - e. Therapy
        - i. valve repair or replacement surgery

5. Aortic Stenosis (AS)
    - a. etiology
        - i. rheumatic
        - ii. bicuspid congenital valve

       iii. Prosthetic valve
          (1) valve area meaningless
- b. clinical manifestations
    - i. valvular AS
    - ii. IHSS, HOCM, Subvalvular stenosis
    - iii. coarctation
    - iv. combined
    - v. turbulent jet on echo
    - vi. calcification vs. congenital valve appearance
    - vii. angina with AS
    - viii. Sudden death often occurs when symptoms develop
- c. physical assessment
    - i. murmur
- d. Cath. findings
    - i. LV - AO systolic gradient
    - ii. pullback pressures
    - iii. elevated a wave
    - iv. gradient to planimeter for valve area
    - v. LV angiography
- e. Therapy
    - i. Valvuloplasty
    - ii. Valve replacement surgery
    - iii. TAVR

6. Aortic Insufficiency (AI)
    - a. etiology
        - i. Marfans syndrome
    - b. clinical manifestations
        - i. stages
            - (1) acute
            - (2) chronic compensated
            - (3) decompensated
    - c. physical assessment
        - i. murmur
        - ii. pulse (bounding)
    - d. Cath. findings
        - i. wide pulse pressure
        - ii. regurgitant fraction
        - iii. Aortic angiography
    - e. Therapy
        - i. valve replacement surgery

7. Other valvular Heart Disease
    - a. Pulmonary valve stenosis - gradient
    - b. Infundibular stenosis - gradient
    - c. Pulmonic Regurgitation
    - d. Pulmonary arteriolar stenosis
    - e. Tricuspid stenosis
    - f. Tricuspid regurgitation
    - g. mixed stenotic - regurg. lesions

Types of Structural Heart Disease

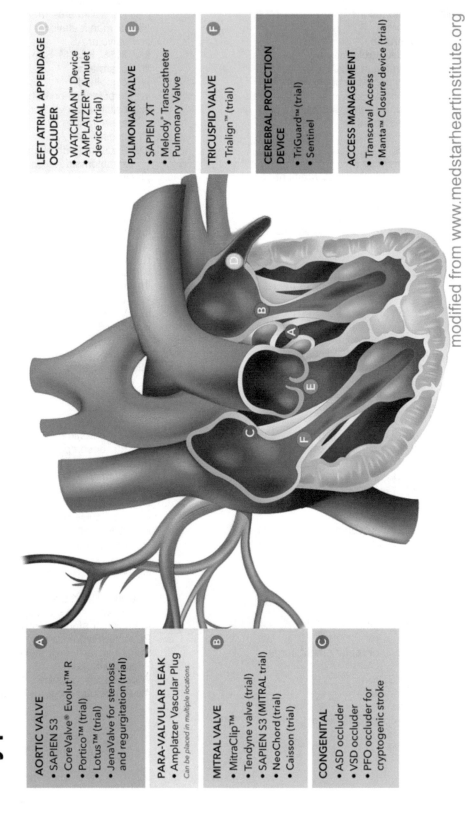

A AORTIC VALVE
- SAPIEN S3
- CoreValve® Evolut™ R
- Portico™ (trial)
- Lotus™ (trial)
- JenaValve for stenosis and regurgitation (trial)

PARA-VALVULAR LEAK
- Amplatzer Vascular Plug

Can be placed in multiple locations

B MITRAL VALVE
- MitraClip™
- Tendyne valve (trial)
- SAPIEN S3 (MITRAL trial)
- NeoChord (trial)
- Caisson (trial)

C CONGENITAL
- ASD occluder
- VSD occluder
- PFO occluder for cryptogenic stroke

D LEFT ATRIAL APPENDAGE OCCLUDER
- WATCHMAN™ Device
- AMPLATZER™ Amulet device (trial)

E PULMONARY VALVE
- SAPIEN XT
- Melody® Transcatheter Pulmonary Valve

F TRICUSPID VALVE
- Trialign™ (trial)

CEREBRAL PROTECTION DEVICE
- TriGuard™ (trial)
- Sentinel

ACCESS MANAGEMENT
- Transcaval Access
- Manta™ Closure device (trial)

modified from www.medstarheartinstitute.org

Pericardial and Myocardial

INDEX: C2 - Pericardial and Myocardial

1. General Myo/Pericardial Pathology

BOTH QUESTIONS BELOW REFER TO THIS DIAGRAM.

867. These are diagrams of hearts showing types of RESTRICTIVE or CONSTRICTIVE CARDIAC pathology. Identify the pathology seen at #3 on the diagram.

a.   Cardiac tamponade (effusive)
b.   Cardiac tamponade (hemorrhagic)
c.   Constrictive pericarditis
d.   Restrictive cardiomyopathy

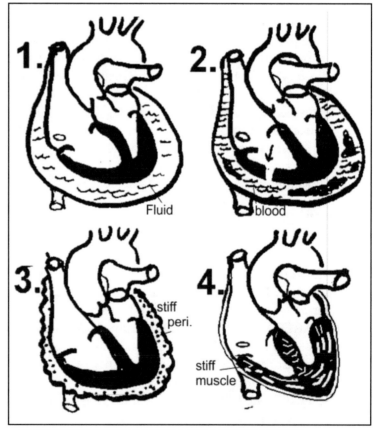

CONSTRICTIVE CARDIAC PATHOLOGIES

868. The most likely etiology (cause) associated with the cardiomyopathy pathology shown at #4 is:

a.   Amyloidosis
b.   Cancer, radiation therapy, or uremia
c.   Recent trauma or MI
d.   History of pericarditis

ANSWERS LISTED CONSECUTIVELY BELOW.

867. ANSWER c. Constrictive pericarditis is shown in diagram #3.
BE ABLE TO CORRECTLY MATCH ALL ANSWERS BELOW.
1. CARDIAC TAMPONADE - EFFUSIVE:
> When irritated the pericardium secretes a straw colored serous fluid into the pericardial cavity, rather like a burn develops a boil. Irritants include neoplasm (cancer), radiation therapy, uremia, or infection. When this begins to constrict filling of the heart it is termed effusive tamponade.

2. CARDIAC TAMPONADE - HEMORRHAGIC:
> The pericardium is filled with blood and clots. But once blood in the pericardial space often does not clot because of the nature of the pericardial fluid (sero-sanguinous fluid). Still, clots may develop. Blood may enter the pericardium through a ruptured transmural myocardial infarction (shown). Or it may enter because of a catheter puncture through the myocardium. Pericardial-centesis can be lifesaving in tamponade. The heart cannot fill properly because the effusion compresses it. If it cannot fill - it has nothing to pump.

3. CONSTRICTIVE PERICARDITIS:
> The pericardium becomes stiffened and encases the heart in a shell. The surgeons compare doing a CP pericardiectomy to peeling off an "orange rind." This rind limits the diastolic filling of the heart and elevates the filling pressures.

4. RESTRICTIVE CARDIOMYOPATHY:
> This heart is so stiff that it impedes diastolic filling. Hemodynamics of CP and RC are similar and often confused with constrictive pericarditis. Biopsy may be needed to differentiate the two pathologies.

See: Braunwald, chapters on "Pericardial Diseases." **Keywords:** Pericardial tamponade, pericardiocentesis

868. ANSWER a. Amyloidosis is a common etiology of diagram #4 (restrictive cardiomyopathy.)
BE ABLE TO CORRECTLY MATCH ALL ANSWERS BELOW.
l. **PERICARDIAL EFFUSION:** Since PE is often chronic, the pericardium has a chance to expand. These signs of tamponade do not appear until compression of the heart impedes venous return and reduces SV.

2. **PERICARDIAL TAMPONADE:** Tamponade means "compression." When pericardial pressure rises, RV collapse can suddenly reduce SV and CO Since hemorrhagic pericardium usually occurs suddenly (as from trauma or cath) the pericardium does not have time to expand.

3. **CONSTRICTIVE PERICARDITIS:** CP is associated with patients who have a history of pericarditis. The thick scarred pericardium often can be heard as a sandpaper-like rubbing sound "friction rub." The thick pericardium limits filling in diastole. The ventricles fill until they "hit" the pericardial shell. The moment they "hit" - a systolic "pericardial knock" may be heard. Etiology includes tuberculosis and pericarditis.

4. **RESTRICTIVE CARDIOMYOPATHY:** Amyloidosis is a common cause of RC. This thickened ventricle is too stiff and hard to fill adequately. Hemodynamics are similar to those of constrictive pericarditis. Restrictive cardiomyopathy may be idiopathic, due to MI scars, or associated with "Amyloidosis." Amyloidosis is a disease in which sheets of protein are deposited in the muscle, stiffening it and

impairing diastolic filling. Etiology includes myocardial fibrosis, infiltrative diseases (amyloid & sarcoid), Hemochromatosis, and endomyocardial scarring (common in Africa).

See: Braunwald, chapter on "Pericardial Diseases." **Keywords:** Obstructive pathology: PE, CP, RC

869. **This diagram shows the effect of inspiration on the pressure curves from four patients. Identify the hemodynamic pattern shown in the diagram labeled #2.**
   a.   **Normal physiology**
   b.   **Normal underdamped tracing**
   c.   **Constrictive pericarditis**
   d.   **Pericardial tamponade**

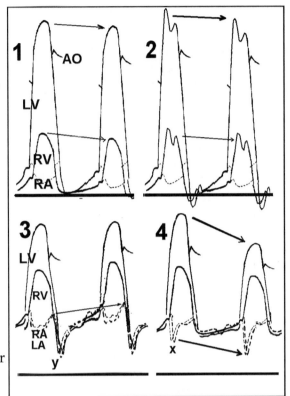

Constrictive pressures patterns
Simultaneous LV, RA, RV X 100

ANSWER b. Normal underdamped tracing.
BE ABLE TO CORRECTLY MATCH ALL ANSWERS BELOW.
1. NORMAL PHYSIOLOGY:
   Normal pressure levels, with a slight drop in all systolic and diastolic pressures with inspiration.
2. NORMAL UNDERDAMPED TRACING:
   This tracing is normal as above except for a resonant artifact in the ventricular pressure tracings. Note the systolic overshoot, diastolic undershoot, and ringing at the systems resonant frequency.
3. CONSTRICTIVE PERICARDITIS:
   Elevated venous pressure with prominent "y" descent is seen on the diastolic portion of the RA, RV and LV pressures. This is usually seen in the LA also. There is an elevated diastolic plateau on these pressures. Right and left-sided diastolic pressures equilibrate so that RA-Edp = RV-Edp = LV-Edp and usually = LA-Edp. This pattern of dip and plateau is termed a "square root sign" ($\sqrt{\ }$). Inspiration does not change the systolic pressure, since the rigid case around the heart prevents transmission of the negative intrathoracic pressure. Inspiration results in no change in venous pressures or an actual increase, termed *Kussmaul's sign*.
4. PERICARDIAL TAMPONADE:
   This shows elevated venous pressures with a prominent "x" descent. NO "y" descent or square root sign $\sqrt{\ }$ is usually seen on atrial pressures. Inspiration dramatically reduces the systolic pressure. Brachial pulses may disappear or reduce with inspiration termed pulsus paradoxus. Tamponade can be either effusive or hemorrhagic. The term tamponade means that the heart is compressed enough to restrain diastolic filling. On echocardiography the RV and RA chamber may actually collapse during diastole due to this pericardial compression.
See: Braunwald, chapter on "Pericardial Disease." **Keywords:** Four constrictive diseases:

Hemorrhagic tamponade, effusive tamponade, restrictive cardiomyopathy, constrictive pericarditis

870. **Identify the hemodynamic signs associated with advanced pericardial tamponade. (Select 4.)**
   a.   Arterial pulsus paradoxus
   b.   Prominent venous "x" descent wave
   c.   Prominent "y" descent
   d.   Elevated venous pressures
   e.   Equalized diastolic pressures

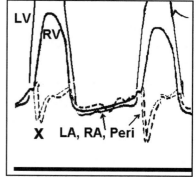
Diastolic pressures in PT x 40

ANSWERS: a, b, d, & e. Prominent "y" descent is NOT associated with tamponade. It occurs during rapid filling in early diastole. This is the first portion of the square root sign. It is associated with constrictive pericarditis and restrictive cardiomyopathy. Square root sign is **not** characteristic of tamponade. In tamponade, as the pericardial pressure rises with increasing effusion, it pushes up the RA, RV diastolic, and eventually the LA and LV diastolic pressures with it. In the end there is pressure equalization of all venous pressure levels as shown.
See: Braunwald, chapter on "Pericardial Diseases." **Keywords:** Pericardial tamponade, Pulsus paradoxus, definition

871. **Which hemodynamic signs are associated with advanced constrictive pericarditis? (Select 4.)**
   a.   Pulsus paradoxus
   b.   Kussmaul's sign
   c.   Square root sign
   d.   Elevated venous pressures
   e.   Equalized diastolic pressures

ANSWERS: b, c, d, & e. Pulsus paradoxus is NOT associated with advanced constrictive pericarditis. Inspiration does not change the systolic pressure, since the rigid case around the heart prevents transmission of intrathoracic pressures. Inspiration usually results in no change in venous pressures or occasionally an actual increase, termed *Kussmaul's sign*.

Constrictive pericarditis shows classic square root sign (rapid filling "y" wave). There may occasionally be an "x" wave following atrial contraction. Together these X and Y waves make an M or W configuration. But, there is never a prominent "x" wave alone as in tamponade.

RV, LV, and RA pressures are identical in diastole, (At least within 5 mmHg of each other). Usually LA = the other diastolic pressures. These pressures equilibrate in

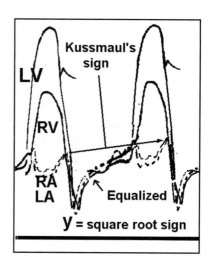
Pressures in CP x 100

diastole because the heart is surrounded by a rigid shell which transmits these overfilled pressures equally to all four heart chambers like balloons filled in a tin can. See tin can analogy later.
See: Braunwald, chapter on "Pericardial Diseases." **Keywords**: Constrictive pericarditis

872. **At catheterization this patient had an RA and LA mean pressure of 15 mmHg. Ventricular pressures in the box show this characteristic pattern of:**
a.   **Constrictive pericarditis**
b.   **Pericardial tamponade**
c.   **Mitral stenosis with secondary pulmonary hypertension**
d.   **CHF with underdamping**

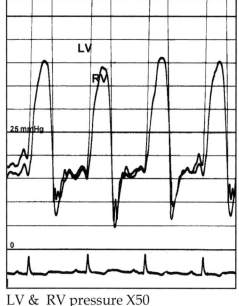

ANSWER a. Constrictive pericarditis or Restrictive cardiomyopathy. These ventricular pressures show the square root pattern seen in these two constrictive diseases.
PRESSURE MEASUREMENTS ARE:
    LV EDP is 17 - high.
    RV systolic is 40 - high.
    RV EDP is 17 - high and = LV EDP

LV & RV pressure X50
(after Peterson fig 22-13)

Noting the square wave pattern, you should wonder if this diastolic dip is "resonance" caused by a resonant pressure line. These resonant lines are very commonly due to long large bore pressure tubes and catheters. Filling them with contrast will reduce this resonance.

This diastolic "dip and plateau" or "Square root sign (√) pattern" is characteristic of constrictive pericarditis or restrictive cardiomyopathy, but not tamponade. In constrictive pericarditis the diastolic plateau is at the same pressure level in all heart chambers (LV, LA, RA, & RV). Since these pressures show similar EDP levels, it is most likely constrictive pericarditis. This plateau may be obscured in rapid heart rates. If this occurs and you suspect CP, induce a PVC to observe the long compensatory pause. Shabeteai says, "in tamponade, the y descent is absent from the vena caval and right atrial pressure curves, and no early diastolic dip appears in the right ventricular pressure tracing....Pulsus paradoxus is almost invariably present. " **See:** Peterson, chapter on "Catheterization and Angio. in Restrictive and Constrictive Disorders of the Heart." **See:** Shabctai, http://www.sciencedirect.com/science/article/pii/000291497090706X **Keywords**: constrictive pattern

873. **An inflammation in the area of the heart labeled at #2 on the diagram is termed:**

a. **Myocarditis**
b. **Endocarditis**
c. **Pericarditis**
d. **Pericardial effusion**

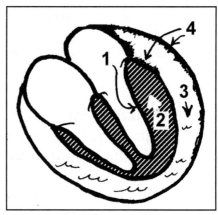
Types of -carditis

ANSWER **a.** Myocardial inflammation = myocarditis. Be able to match all answers below.
CORRECTLY MATCHED ANSWERS ARE:
1. **ACUTE BACTERIAL ENDOCARDITIS** inflames the inner membrane lining of the heart and the external lining of a valve. It is usually caused by a bacteremia which attaches to the valves or endocardial layer.
2. **MYOCARDITIS:** When the middle muscle layer (myocardium) becomes inflamed it is termed "myocarditis." In the USA this is usually caused by viral infection. In South America it is associated with Chagas' disease: a protozoan infection transmitted by an insect bite.
3. **PERICARDIAL EFFUSION:** When the pericardium is irritated it begins to secrete a fluid termed "pericardial effusion." This can occur chronically with no symptoms, when the pericardium stretches slowly (over months). If it accumulates rapidly, it may begin to compress the heart. This is termed "pericardial tamponade" or "PT."
4. **PERICARDITIS:** When the pericardium or epicardium becomes inflamed it is termed "pericarditis." Both layers become infected, scar over, and grow together.
See: Braunwald, chapter on either "Infective Endocarditis" or "Pericarditis." **Keywords:** types of carditis

2. Pericardial Pathology

874. **A patient's cardiac pressure readings are shown in the box. The tracings all show deep "y" waves and a diastolic plateau (square root sign) usually associated with:**

a. **Restrictive cardiomyopathy**
b. **Constrictive pericarditis**
c. **Pericardial tamponade**
d. **IHSS/HOCM**

HEMODYNAMIC FINDINGS
RV = 36/15/25 mmHg
RA = 26/28/20
LV = 95/10/25
LA = 27/22/20

ANSWER b. Constrictive pericarditis. Constrictive disease pressures all show elevation of the diastolic plateau, but only constrictive pericarditis causes the equalization of diastolic pressures and square root sign (√) as described by deep "Y" wave. Distinguish between the hemodynamics of the 3 major constrictive diseases. **See:** Grossman, chapter on "Profiles in Constrictive Disease." **Keywords:** ID pressures of constrictive pericarditis

875. Which of these hemodynamic signs is commonly associated with cardiac tamponade?
   a.   Arterial pulsus paradoxus
   b.   Wide arterial pulse pressure
   c.   Venous square root sign
   d.   Venous rapid "y" descent

ANSWER a. Arterial pulsus paradoxus. Note the dramatic BP drop with inspiration. This is not really "paradoxical" because it normally drops a few mmHg with inspiration. But pulsus paradoxus seen here is an exaggeration of this normal phenomenon. Note how the RV pressure increases with inspiration, while the aortic pressure falls. The pulse pressure also drops. Pulsus paradoxus is a drop of more than 10 mmHg in the aortic systolic pressure with inspiration. **See:** Braunwald, chapter on "Pericardial Diseases." **Keywords:** Pericardial tamponade, pulsus paradoxus, definition

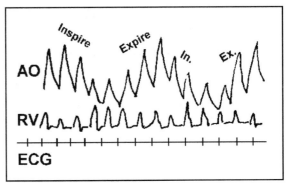

Pulsus paradoxus/tamponade

876. The mechanism of pulsus paradoxus, shown above, is due to bulging of the interventricular septum into the:
   a.   RV in diastole.
   b.   LV in diastole.
   c.   RV in systole.
   d.   LV in systole.

ANSWER b. LV in diastole. The mechanism of this drop is due to the normal increase in venae cava flow as the thoracic pressure drops with inspiration. (This alone causes a 2-4 mmHg drop in all thoracic pressures.) But the critical thing is that the RV septum bulges into and compresses the LV during part of its diastolic filling phase. Because of the tamponade LV output and pressures fall. **See:** Braunwald, chapter on "Pericardial Diseases." **Keywords:** Pericardial tamponade, pulsus paradoxus, definition

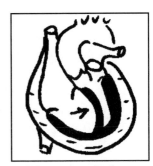

IV septum bulges

877. **Functions of the pericardium include: (Select 4)**
  a.   **Prevent shifting of the heart with position**
  b.   **Reduce friction between heart and other organs**
  c.   **Prevent chronic cardiac dilation**
  d.   **Prevention of acute cardiac dilation**
  e.   **Assist in diastolic filling of the heart**
  f.   **Assist in systolic emptying of the heart**

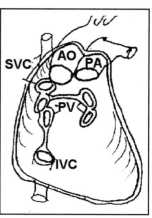
Pericardium

    ANSWERS: a, b, d, & e. Functions of the pericardium include:
      a. TRUE: Prevent shifting of the heart with position
      b. TRUE: Reduce friction between heart and other
            organs
      c. FALSE: Prevent chronic cardiac dilation
      d. TRUE: Prevent acute cardiac dilation
      e. TRUE: Assist in diastolic filling of the heart
      f. FALSE: Assist in systolic emptying of the heart

FURTHER INFORMATION on functions of pericardium:
    1. **ATTACHMENTS:** The pericardium is attached to the
origins of the great vessels, sternum, vertebral column, and
diaphragm. It fixes the position of the heart in the mediastinum.
Shifting of the heart can choke off venous return as we see in
surgery when a surgeon pulls the heart up to work on the
circumflex coronary artery.
    2. **FRICTION REDUCED:** The fluid between the visceral
pericardium (this inner layer is also called the epicardium) and
the parietal pericardium acts as a lubricant. It allows the heart to
twist and turn without seriously disturbing nearby organs. Like
the oil in your car it lubricates moving parts and increases
efficiency.

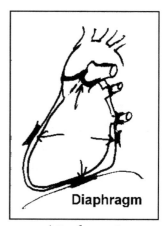
Attachments

    3. **THE PERICARDIUM ALLOWS SLOW DILATION:**
The heart can dilate and hypertrophy as can the pericardium.
When excessive pericardial fluid is produced slowly the pericardium stretches and the
accumulation may not be noticed. This slow pericardial stretching happens in all
cardiomegaly.
    4. **RESTRICTS SUDDEN DILATION:** Sudden dilation of the heart can damage the
sarcomere by pulling apart. In open heart surgery, bypass pump suckers are placed in the
heart to prevent this acute distension. When fluids accumulate rapidly in the pericardium,
it cannot stretch. The accumulation increases pericardial pressure. When this exceeds
cardiac filling pressure, it will compress that chamber, reduce venous return, and cardiac
output. Hemorrhagic pericardial tamponade is an example of this acute tamponade.
    5. **AIDS FILLING:** The normal negative pressure within the pericardium acts as a
suction cup to help distend the heart during filling. When the pericardial pressure
increases with pericardial effusion instead of aiding, it may impair filling and collapse the
RA and RV during their filling phases.

6. **SYSTOLIC EMPTYING:** In systole the AV ring and valves are "pulled down." Since the apex and base of the heart are fixed by pericardial attachments, as the LV contracts, it pulls down the AV ring. This sucks more blood into the atria in ventricular systole. This results in the drop in atrial pressure labeled the "x" wave. This drawing down of the AV ring creates a potential space in the atrium and aids in atrial filling. This "pull down" is easily seen in RAO nuclear gated blood pool studies where the heart appears to stays the same size throughout systole and diastole. The only thing that appears to move is the AV valve and ring. This gives the impression that the AV ring is a diaphragm pumping blood. Note: the drawing shows motion of the AV ring (solid arrows) and blood flow (dotted arrows).

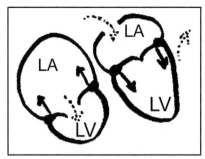
DIASTOLE - SYSTOLE

See: Braunwald, chapter on "Pericardial Diseases." **Keywords:** Functions of pericardium

878. **Constrictive cardiac pathology seen in acute cardiac tamponade shows REDUCED:**
   a.   **Systolic ejection (EF)**
   b.   **RV diastolic filling**
   c.   **Heart rate**
   d.   **LV contractility**

ANSWER b. RV diastolic filling. Filling of the LV is also impaired because the RV is compressed and pushed into the LV. This septal bulging impairs all ventricular filling. In addition the RV collapses in diastole from the increased pressure of the pericardial fluid. Because the RV is not feeding adequate blood to the lungs, the LV filling will be further decreased. Systole is OK. Diastole is the problem. Heart rate and contractility increase to compensate for the reduced stroke volume.

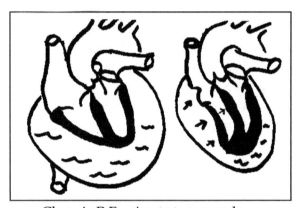
Chronic P.E. - Acute tamponade

     In a chronic pericardial effusion the pericardium has time to stretch. It can hold more than 2 liters of fluid if given time to stretch. The problems arise only when it cannot stretch as fast as the production of pericardial fluid. A chronic pericardial effusion may accumulate huge volumes of fluid without hemodynamic compression. But, this can only occur if the pericardium stretches slowly. The diagram on the right shows tamponade where the pericardial fluid accumulates so fast it cannot stretch - pericardial pressure increases. **See:** Braunwald, chapter on "Pericardial Diseases." **Keywords:** Pericardial tamponade, pericardiocentesis

879. **Electrocardiographic changes associated with pericarditis consist of: (Circle 3)**
   a.   **Lowered PR segment**
   b.   **Enlarged R-waves**
   c.   **Elevated S-T segment**
   d.   **Prolonged Q-T intervals**
   e.   **T-wave inversion**

ANSWERS: a, c, & e.
       a. **TRUE**: Lowered PR segment
       b. FALSE: Enlarged R-waves
       c. **TRUE**: Elevated S-T segment
       d. FALSE: Prolonged Q-T intervals
       e. **TRUE**: T-wave inversion.

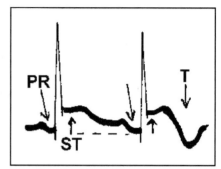

ECG of pericarditis

Pericarditis patients show characteristic ECG changes which set in shortly after sharp chest pain. The inflamed pericardium touches the epicardium which then shows signs of electrical injury (ST ↑). Most of the ECG leads are affected in pericarditis, as opposed to MI where specific leads near the injury are most affected.

        Most leads in pericarditis show "ST" elevation (injury current) which is concave upward. The "PR" segment is also depressed, possibly because of atrial injury. The "T" waves are inverted later in pericarditis showing ischemia. The diastolic ECG waves seem to coast "downhill" toward the "PR" segment baseline.
See: Braunwald, chapter on "Pericardial Diseases." **Keywords:** Pericarditis, ECG

880. **When does pericardial effusion become pericardial tamponade?**
   a.   **When blood enters pericardium (hemorrhagic)**
   b.   **When the effusion is acute**
   c.   **When cardiac compression begins.**
   d.   **When it becomes constrictive pericarditis**

ANSWER c. When cardiac compression begins. Effusion continues until pericardial pressure equals the RA and RV diastolic filling pressures. At this point RA and RV collapse begins; RV preload falls, and hence LV preload and SV fall. BP drops and death is imminent as long as the rate of pericardial pressure increase is greater than the rate of filling pressure increases.

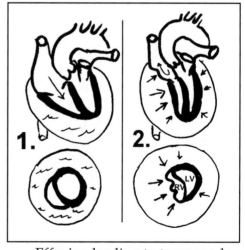

        The left diagram (#1) shows the chronic effusive pericardium filling. However, in the right diagram (#2), the RA and RV collapse, because the effusion occurs faster than the pericardium can stretch. **See:** Braunwald, chapter on "Pericardial Diseases." **Keywords:** Pericardial effusion becomes tamponade when cardiac compression begins

Effusion leading to tamponade

881. **As pericardial effusion progresses to tamponade what happens to the CVP (RA) and systemic blood pressure (BP)?**
  a.   Increased CVP,   Increased BP
  b.   Increased CVP,   Decreased BP
  c.   Decreased CVP,   Increased BP
  d.   Decreased CVP,   Decreased BP

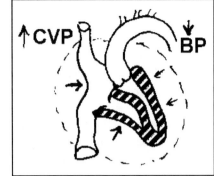
Tamponade Hemodynamics

ANSWER b. Increased CVP, Decreased BP. As pericardial pressure increases the heart becomes increasingly compressed as shown in the diagram. Venous return is pinched off as the RA and RV collapse. This reduces SV, BP, and CO. The heart rate and venous pressure increase to compensate for these reductions. **See:** Braunwald, chapter on "Pericardial Diseases." **Keywords:** Constrictive compensation, →CVP, →BP

882. **In pericardial tamponade the heart rate will be _____ and the right and left sided diastolic filling pressures will be _____.**
  a.   Decreased,   Equal but both decreased
  b.   Decreased,   Unequal but both increased
  c.   Increased,   Unequal but both decreased
  d.   Increased,   Equal but both increased

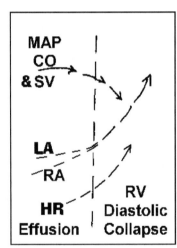
Pericardial tamponade

ANSWER d. Increased, Equal but both increased. As intra-pericardial pressure increases (IPP) the heart becomes increasingly compressed. Venous return is pinched off as the RA and RV collapse. This reduces SV, BP, and CO. The heart rate and venous pressures increase to compensate for these reductions. The ventricles try to fill more by increasing their filling volume, but they cannot because the pericardial pressure exceeds ventricular filling pressures.

    Both RV and LV filling pressures eventually equalize as the pericardial fluid transmits it evenly to both atria and ventricles in diastole. The diagram graphs parameters which fall: CO, SV, and MAP (Mean Arterial Pressure.) It also graphs parameters which rise: HR, RA pressure and IPP (Intra Pericardial Pressure.) These all get most severe when RV diastolic collapse begins at the dotted vertical line. **See:** Braunwald, chapter on "Pericardial Diseases."

883. Diastolic pressures usually equalize in which of the following diseases? (Select 3)

a. Hypertrophic cardiomyopathy
b. Constrictive pericarditis
c. Pericardial tamponade
d. Restrictive cardiomyopathy
e. Mitral Regurgitation

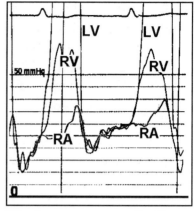
Diast. pressure equalization

ANSWERS: b, c, & d. Hypertrophic cardiomyopathy (HOCM/IHSS) **DOES NOT** display pressure equalization. The two classic pathologies with equalization of diastolic pressures are constrictive pericarditis (shown in the figure) and advanced pericardial tamponade. Restrictive cardiomyopathy is very similar to constrictive pericarditis (with square root sign √) and may be indistinguishable from it. Although with exercise, a restricted heart usually increases its left sided venous pressures more than its right sided pressures. The restriction is usually localized in the thick layers of calcified LV myocardium.

In all the restricted, constricted, and tamponade pathologies the heart's diastolic filling is restricted. In CP it is a rigid pericardium, in PT it is an overfilled pericardium, and in RC it is a rigid calcified muscle. After a certain point is reached, the elevated diastolic pressure flattens out. This point is termed the "plateau." It ends in the atrial "a" wave. Here is why:

TIN CAN ANALOGY: Imagine the 4 chambers of the heart as 4 water balloons. Imagine trying to fill these balloons in a closed tin can. They would fill only to the limit of the can size. Also, all 4 balloons would be at the same pressure when filling because fluid transmits pressure perfectly and in all directions. **See:** Grossman, chapter on "Profiles in Constrictive... Restrictive... Tamponade."

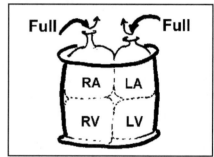
Tin Can compression analogy

884. Which of the following typically have a "square root sign" (√‾) pattern in the LV and RV pressure tracings? (Circle 3.)

a. Restrictive cardiomyopathy
b. Constrictive pericarditis
c. Pericardial tamponade
d. Underdamped CHF

ANSWERS: a, b, & d.
THE DISEASES WITH SQUARE ROOT SIGN ARE:

a. **TRUE:** Restrictive cardiomyopathy (√‾)
b. **TRUE:** Constrictive peri-carditis (may show M or W diastolic pattern with √‾ and =)
c. FALSE: Pericardial tamponade (= diast. pressures and prominent "x"wave but no √‾)

d. **TRUE**: Underdamped CHF (false $\sqrt{}$)
Square root sign begins with the atrial "y" wave and the "beginning diastolic" ventricular wave. It is the sudden drop in pressure when the AV valve opens and the ventricles fill by the "suction cup effect." In CP this is the only filling the ventricle gets. The rapid diastolic dip ("y wave") is followed by a plateau in which it can't fill further because of its tight "tin can" "constrictive" pericardium. **See :** Grossman, chapter on "Profiles in Constrictive ... Restrictive ... Tamponade." **Keywords:** square root sign seen in RC & CP

885. **Medical treatment with anti-inflammatory agents (NSAIDS) is used for:**
a. **Pericarditis with friction rub**
b. **Endocarditis of tricuspid valve**
c. **Myocarditis in heart transplant patients**
d. **Idiopathic hypertrophic cardiomyopathy**

ANSWER: a. Pericarditis with friction rub. "Acute idiopathic pericarditis [with friction rub], is a self-limited disease without significant complications . . . If laboratory data supports the clinical diagnosis, symptomatic treatment with nonsteroidal anti-inflammatory drugs (NSNAIDS) should be initiated....Constrictive pericarditis is a progressive disease...." Nonsteroidal anti-inflammatory drugs, usually abbreviated to NSAIDs or NSAIDs, are drugs with analgesic, antipyretic (fever-reducing) and anti-inflammatory effects (reducing inflammation). The term "nonsteroidal" is used to distinguish these drugs from steroids, which have a similar anti-inflammatory action. As analgesics, NSAIDs are unusual in that they are non-narcotic. Common NSAIDS drugs include aspirin, ibuprofen, and naproxen. **See:** Braunwald chapter on "Pericardial Disease"

886. **What pathology shows pressure equalization of LVEDP and RVEDP and square root pattern?**
a. **Underdamped CHF**
b. **Pericardial tamponade**
c. **Constrictive pericarditis**
d. **Restrictive cardiomyopathy**

ANSWER: c. Constrictive pericarditis. Elevated venous pressures, with M or W pattern. Square root sign on the diastolic RA, RV and LV pressures. This is the "tin can effect" with a rigid and tight pericardium. Because all chambers are constricted equally, all 4 chambers may have the same diastolic pressure and pattern.

3. Myocardial Pathology

887. **Chronic excessive consumption of alcohol may lead to:**
a. **Dilated cardiomyopathy**
b. **Restrictive cardiomyopathy**
c. **Hypertrophic cardiomyopathy**
d. **Idiopathic cardiomyopathy**

ANSWER a. Dilated cardiomyopathy. Alcoholism is the major cause of dilated cardiomyopathy in the Western world. This is believed due to the toxic effects of alcohol on tissues. Thiamine and other nutritional deficiencies are also found in chronic alcohol abusers. Dilated cardiomyopathy has also been found in AIDS patients.
See: Braunwald, chapter on "Cardiomyopathy" **Keywords:** Dilated cardiomyopathy, alcoholic cardiomyopathy

888. **What myocardial disease is associated with sudden death of athletes? Children going out for athletics should all be screened for this inherited cardiac condition.**
   a.   Ideopathic cardiomyopathy
   b.   Restrictive cardiomyopathy
   c.   Dilated cardiomyopathy
   d.   Hypertrophic cardiomyopathy

ANSWER d. Hypertrophic cardiomyopathy. "Hypertrophic Cardiomyopathy (HCM) causes disability and death in patients of all ages, with the most devastating component of its natural history being sudden death in youth. For example in American athletes under the age of 30, HCM is the first cause of sudden death (36% of total). Thus, there is general agreement that preparticipation screening in all athletes will increase the number of suspected cases of HCM and allow more definitive diagnoses." **See:** e-journal of the ESC Council for Cardiology Practice, Piro, 2015

889. **Septal muscle fiber "disarray" is a common pathologic tissue finding in:**
   a.   Dilated cardiomyopathy
   b.   Restrictive cardiomyopathy
   c.   Hypertrophic cardiomyopathy
   d.   Idiopathic cardiomyopathy

ANSWER c. Hypertrophic cardiomyopathy. Disarrayed hypertrophy is usually found in the LV septum of hypertrophic cardiomyopathy patients. The muscle cells are not aligned parallel to each other. A myocardial biopsy is used to obtain tissue samples for microscopic diagnosis of this muscle disarray.
See: Braunwald, chapter on "Cardiomyopathy."
Keywords: HCM, muscle fiber disarray

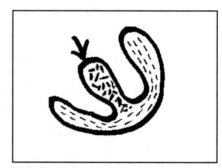
HOCM Muscle Disarray

890. **The DYNAMIC systolic ejection murmur and bisferiens pulse shown is most common in _____ cardiomyopathy?**
   a.   Dilated cardiomyopathy
   b.   Restrictive cardiomyopathy
   c.   Hypertrophic cardiomyopathy
   d.   Alcoholic cardiomyopathy

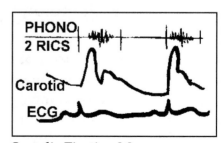
Systolic Ejection Murmur

ANSWER c. Hypertrophic cardiomyopathy. The murmur of HCM (HOCM/IHSS) is similar to an AS murmur - systolic and diamond shaped. It increases with Valsalva maneuvers, upon standing and with Amyl Nitrate (vasodilator). It may disappear upon squatting or other maneuvers that increase afterload. Associated findings are: SAM= Systolic Anterior Motion (of Mitral Valve), ASH= Asymmetric Septal Hypertrophy (of LV), and midsystolic closure of the aortic valve.

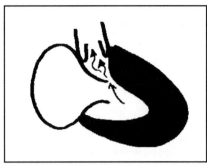

HOCM, ASH, SAM

See: Braunwald, chapter on "Cardiomyopathy."
Keywords: HCM, systolic ejection murmur

891. **Hypertrophic obstructive cardiomyopathy (HOCM) differs from aortic stenosis (AS) in that:**
   a.   **HOCM is treated with large balloon valvuloplasty**
   b.   **HOCM is associated with a bicuspid semilunar valve**
   c.   **HOCM arterial pressure is slow rising (pulsus parvus/ tardis)**
   d.   **HOCM pulse pressure decreases following a PVC beat**

ANSWER d. HOCM pulse pressure decreases following a PVC beat. This is the Brockenbrough effect brought on by the hypercontractile LV that obstructs more the harder it contracts. With HOCM the arterial pulse has a rapidly rising spike and dome pattern with smaller pulse pressure. The Post PVC beat in AS will have a slow rising arterial pulse with larger pulse pressure. Only AS often has a bicuspid semilunar valve and may be treated with valvuloplasty.

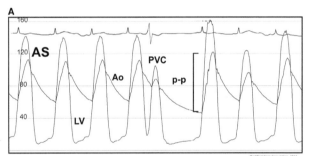

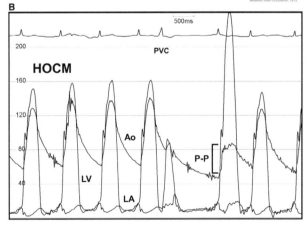

Nishimura &. Carabello say, "Response of the aortic pressure after a long pause is useful in differentiating between the fixed obstruction of valvular aortic (Ao) stenosis and the dynamic obstruction of hypertrophic cardiomyopathy. A, In this patient with valvular aortic stenosis, the beat after the premature ventricular contraction (PVC) has an increase in pulse pressure (P-P). B, In this patient with hypertrophic cardiomyopathy, there is a reduction in the pulse pressure on the beat after the premature ventricular contraction. LV indicates left ventricle; LA, left atrium." **See:** Hemodynamics in the Cardiac Catheterization Laboratory of the 21st Century, Nishimura &. Carabello, Circulation May, 2012

892. Alcohol septal ablation is used to treat:
   a.   Acute infectious septal pericarditis
   b.   Reciprocating bundle branch tachycardia
   c.   Acute endocarditis of the ventricular septum
   d.   Hypertrophic obstructive cardiomyopathy

ANSWER d. Hypertrophic obstructive cardiomyopathy.
Braunwald says, "Some patients with hypertrophic obstructive cardiomyopathy (HOCM) have refractory symptoms resulting from outflow obstruction produced by hyperdynamic LV contraction with a hypertrophied septum. A controlled septal infarction can be produced with a new method of nonsurgical septal mass reduction that uses alcohol. In brief, a small balloon catheter is inserted into the septal artery with angioplasty technique and alcohol is instilled. This causes the septal muscle to infarct, become noncontractile, and scar, which eliminates the LV outflow tract gradient." **See:** Braunwald chapter on "Transluminal Alcohol Septal Ablation for HOCM"

893. The arterial pressure pattern associated with hypertrophic obstructive cardiomyopathy is_____.
   a.   Spike and dome
   b.   Pulsus paradoxus
   c.   Square root sign
   d.   Pulsus alternans

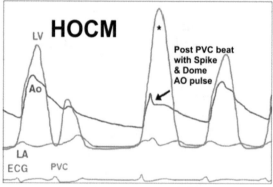

ANSWER a. Spike and dome This spike and dome arterial pattern has a rapid upstroke and second arterial rounded tidal wave. It is also termed as jerky, bifid or a bisferiens pulse. This is due to systolic anterior motion (SAM) of the mitral valve, as it is pulled into the hypertrophic IV septum in early systole causing an interventricular obstruction and gradient. It then momentarily relaxes and is followed by a second rise in the pulse pressure (dome). Pulsus paradoxus is a drop in BP on inspiration with tamponade. Square root sign is a diastolic pattern seen in constrictive pericarditis. Pulsus alternans is alternating arterial systolic pressure seen in heart failure.

894. Which type of ventricular myopathy is shown in the diagram at #2?
   a.   Normal ventricle
   b.   Hypertrophic cardiomyopathy
   c.   Restrictive cardiomyopathy
   d.   Dilated cardiomyopathy

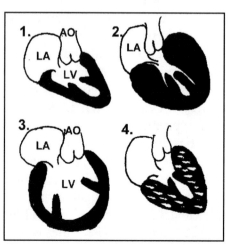

Types of Cardiac Myopathy

ANSWER b. Hypertrophic cardiomyopathy. Hypertrophy involves thickening of the muscle wall. This increased muscle bulk may be in response to pressure overload or due to some primary pathologic condition - as in cardiomyopathy. The outer LV diameter increases, but the internal dimensions may not change. Be able to match all answers below.

CORRECTLY MATCHED ANSWERS ARE:
1. Normal ventricle
2. Hypertrophic cardiomyopathy
3. Dilated cardiomyopathy
4. Restrictive cardiomyopathy

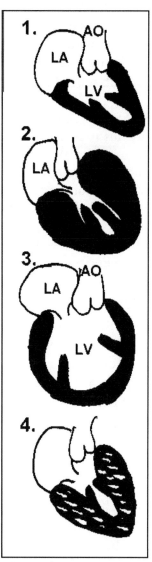

All of the cardiomyopathies show heart muscle dysfunction. Many of these cardiomyopathies are of unknown cause (idiopathic). Most are progressive with poor prognosis. Cardiac transplantation may be considered. RV myocardial biopsy may help make the diagnosis. Constrictive pathologies shown are:

1. **NORMAL**

2. **HYPERTROPHIC CARDIOMYOPATHY:** Here the LV septum is usually inappropriately and asymmetrically hypertrophied (ASH). Muscle fibers in the septum may be disarrayed. The anterior leaflet of the mitral valve is so close to the LV outflow tract that it may get trapped or sucked anteriorly during systole with a Venturi effect (SAM=Systolic Anterior Motion of MV). The LV hypertrophy makes the heart contract vigorously - too vigorously. It may pinch itself off causing a systolic intra LV gradient. When the SAM causes obstruction of the outflow tract it is termed HOCM or IHSS. Both hypertrophic obstructive cardiomyopathy (HOCM/IHSS) and idiopathic obstructive cardiomyopathy tend to be an inherited defects.

3. **DILATED CARDIOMYOPATHY:** This was formerly called congestive cardiomyopathy. The LV is dilated and shows signs of CHF. The dilation stretches the valve rings and AV valve regurgitation is common. It is also associated with contractile or systolic dysfunction.

Myopathies

4. **RESTRICTIVE CARDIOMYOPATHY:** Various types of proteins may be deposited in the muscle making a granular or "sparkling" appearance on 2D echo. The most common "deposition" disease is amyloidosis. This stiff ventricle makes diastolic filling so difficult that the venous filling pressures are all elevated - but not equally on both sides. (LV-EDP > RV-EDP).
See: Grossman, chapter on "Profiles in Constrictive... Restrictive... Tamponade." **Keywords:** Types of cardiomyopathies

4. Endocarditis

895. **The condition where bacteria from the blood stream grow on normal cardiac valves is known as:**
  a.   Septicemia/bacteremia
  b.   Valvulitis/atrial myxoma
  c.   Acute bacterial/infective endocarditis
  d.   Subacute bacterial/infective endocarditis (SBE)

ANSWER c. In acute infective endocarditis extremely virulent bacterial organisms can rapidly destroy a **NORMAL** cardiac valve. Bacterial growths called vegetations may grow on the valve, break off and embolize. Death occurs in less than six weeks without vigorous antimicrobial therapy. A normal endothelium surface does not grow vegetations.

Sub-acute endocarditis is an infection of an "abnormal" valve. Damaged valves may have a denuded area where platelets and bacteria can lodge and grow. The course of the "subacute" infection is years in duration. Currently most of the valvulitis occurs in patients with artificial valves, mitral valve prolapse or IV drug abusers. **See:** Braunwald, chapter on "Infective Endocarditis or Pericarditis." **Keywords:** Infective Endocarditis

896. **A patient with infective endocarditis also has MVP and MR. If vegetations are present, they would most likely be attached to the:**
  a.   Atrial appendage
  b.   Ventricular apex
  c.   Mitral valve atrial surface (underside)
  d.   Mitral valve ventricular surface (flow surface)

ANSWER c.   Mitral valve atrial surface (underside). Vegetations are clumps of bacterial and thrombin which grow on the endocardium or valves. They tend to accumulate just beyond any narrowing which causes a high velocity jet of blood like the underside of a leaky mitral valve. They also grow where the jet stream strikes a wall. "MVP" = Mitral Valve Prolapse.

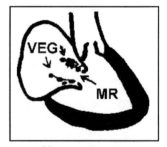
Vegetations

This jet turbulence may denude an area of the endocardium. These injured areas attract platelets and bacteria. Germs find this a good growing medium. These vegetations can embolize and form hemorrhages on the skin called "petechiae."
See: Braunwald, chapter on "Infective Endocarditis." **Keywords:** Endocarditis, vegetation location

897. An older patient with severe MR and acute endocarditis is being considered for valve replacement. Is a heart cath indicated prior to surgery?
    a.   NO: risk of secondary infection is too great
    b.   NO: risk of embolizing a vegetation is too great
    c.   YES: risk of embolizing a vegetation is small, coronary angio is essential
    d.   YES: but only after the patient is sterilized and all vegetations have disappeared, LV angio is essential

ANSWER c. YES: risk of embolizing a vegetation is small, Coronary angio is essential. Grossman states that the risk of a catheter breaking off vegetations is negligible and a heart cath may be done safely. Certainly the patient will be on intensive antibiotic therapy to reduce the infection. Valve surgery may be lifesaving and CABG surgery may need to be done during the same operation. **See:** Grossman, chapter on "Indications for Heart Cath." **Keywords:** Infective endocarditis, heart cath OK = yes.

898. Bacterial endocarditis is commonly associated with a patient history of:
    a.   **Infectious hepatitis**
    b.   **IV drug abuse**
    c.   **Alcohol abuse**
    d.   **Cocaine abuse**

ANSWER b. IV drug abuse spreads many diseases. Bacteremia is common and often affects the tricuspid valve of drug abusers. The bacteria also find their way into the left side of the heart as well and infect the mitral and aortic valves. Other pathologies commonly associated with infective endocarditis are patients with an artificial valve or mitral valve prolapse. Braunwald says, "Endocarditis occurring in intravenous drug abusers has a unique propensity to infect right heart valves. . . . In clinical series the typical distribution of valve involvement is tricuspid in 78%, mitral in 24% and aortic in 8%." **See:** Braunwald, chapter on "Infective Endocarditis or Pericarditis." **Keywords:** Infective Endocarditis, IV drug abuse

5. Other Myocardial / Pericardial Pathology

899. What is the most appropriate treatment for symptomatic cardiac tamponade?
    a.   **Pericardiectomy**
    b.   **Administration of IV fluids**
    c.   **Pericardiocentesis**
    d.   **IABP**

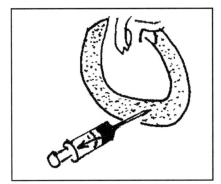

Pericardiocentesis

ANSWER c. Pericardiocentesis can be lifesaving in tamponade. The accumulating fluid compresses the heart so much that it cannot fill properly. If it cannot fill, it has nothing to **pump. See:** Braunwald, chapter on "Pericardial Diseases." **Keywords:** Pericardial tamponade, pericardiocentesis

900. Check the 3 classic hemodynamic features of constrictive pericarditis below.
a. Brockenbraugh sign with a PVC
b. Increased atrial pressures
c. Square root sign in ventricular diastole
d. Equalization of end-diastolic pressures
e. Pulsus paradoxus

ANSWERS: a, b & d, Brockenbraugh sign, increased atrial pressures and pressure equalization in diastole.

Mayo Clinic Proceedings say, "Increased atrial pressures, equalization of end-diastolic pressures, and dip-and-plateau or square-root sign of the ventricular diastolic pressure recording have traditionally been considered hemodynamic features typical of constrictive pericarditis." Brockenbraugh sign is seen in HOCM, and pulsus paradoxus is seen in tamponade.

901. The distinctive heart sound associated with pathology seen in diagram #2 (constrictive pericarditis) is/are:
a. Friction rub
b. Pericardial "knock"
c. Systolic ejection murmur
d. Distant, quiet heart sounds

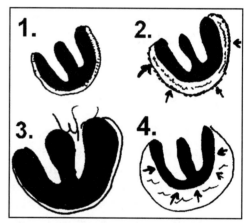

Myocardial, pericardial sounds

ANSWER b. Pericardial "knock." Be able to match all answers below.
CORRECTLY MATCHED ANSWERS ARE:
1. **PERICARDITIS:** friction rub
2. **CP:** systolic "pericardial knock" (See diagram ➡)
3. **HOCM:** systolic ejection murmur
4. **Cardiac Tamponade or Effusion:** distant, quiet heart sounds

This diagram explains the square root sign and the pericardial "knock" sound heard in constrictive pericarditis.

In early diastole the LV fills rapidly ("y" wave) until it "knocks" against the rigid pericardium (PK = pericardial knock). Pressure then plateaus because filling stops between PK and S1. Following atrial contraction (note "a" wave on CVP) the QRS fires and S1 signals the beginning of contraction. Systole pulls down the atria causing the "x" descent wave.
See: Braunwald, chapter on "Infective Endocarditis, Myopathies or on Pericardial Diseases." **Keywords:** auscultation CP, PT, HOCM

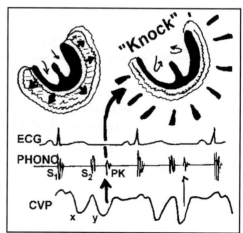

Constrictive pericarditis

BOTH QUESTIONS BELOW REFER TO THIS M-MODE ECHO SCAN.

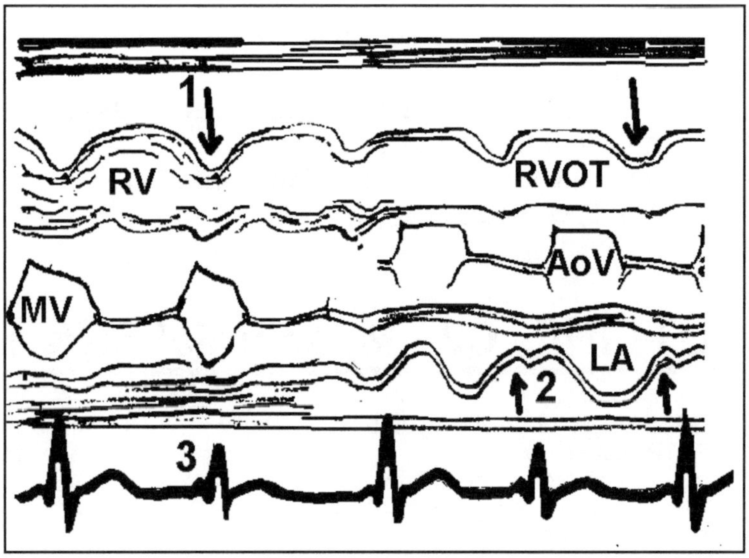

902. The ECG of electrical alternans shown at #3 in this echo is usually diagnostic of:
  a. Constrictive pericarditis
  b. Cardiac tamponade
  c. Endocarditis
  d. Bigeminy

903. The arrows at #1 and #2 indicate:
  a. Rapid filling waves(√)
  b. IHSS/HOCM
  c. Systolic heart compression
  d. Diastolic heart compression

M-mode parasternal echocardiographic scan from LV-AO
(after Braunwald fig. 43-9)

ANSWERS LISTED CONSECUTIVELY BELOW:

902. ANSWER b. Cardiac or pericardial tamponade. Braunwald says, "Total electrical alternans, involving P, QRS, and T complexes, is almost diagnostic of cardiac tamponade." The heart swings within the distended pericardial sack (swinging heart). In the anterior leads, the ECG voltages increase as the heart moves closer to the chest wall. The pattern may cycle at 2:1 (as shown here) or even 3:1. Partial electrical alternans of only one part of the ECG complex, may be seen in pericarditis (without tamponade), SVT, VT, and CAD. **See**: Braunwald, chapter on "Pericardial Diseases." **Keywords:** Pericardial tamponade, electrical alternans

903. ANSWER d. Diastolic heart compression. As the pericardial pressure rises it begins to collapse the RV in diastole and occasionally the atria in late diastole. Note that the compression occurs while the mitral valve is open in diastole. The unlabeled spaces containing the arrows are the enlarged pericardial spaces containing the pericardial effusion fluid around the heart. The pericardial effusion is also well seen surrounding the heart on 2D echo. This makes echocardiography a primary diagnostic tool for pericardial tamponade.
See: Braunwald, chapter on "Pericardial Diseases." **Keywords:** Pericardial tamponade, cardiac compression on echo

REFERENCES

Baim, D. S and Grossman W.., Cardiac Catheterization, Angiography, and Intervention, 7th Ed., Lea and Febiger, 2006

Kern, M. J., Ed., The Cardiac Catheterization Handbook, 4th Ed., Mosby-Year Book, Inc., 2016

Braunwald, Eugene, Ed., HEART DISEASE A Textbook of Cardiovascular Medicine, 7th Ed., W. B. Saunders Co., 2012

Peterson K. and Nicod P., Cardiac Catheterization Methods, Diagnosis, and Therapy, 1st Ed., W.B. Saunders Co., 1997

OUTLINE: C2 - Myocardial & Pericardial Pathology

1. GENERAL MYO / PERICARDIAL PATHOLOGY
   a. Cardiac tamponade (effusive)
   b. Cardiac tamponade (hemorrhagic)
   c. Constrictive pericarditis
   d. Restrictive cardiomyopathy
   e. Myocarditis
   f. Endocarditis
   g. Pressure waveforms in each

2. PERICARDIAL
   a. Functions of pericardium
   b. attachments
   c. etiology
   d. clinical manifestations
      i. Pericardial effusion
         (1) becomes tamponade when RV and RA collapse occurs
      ii. Pericardial tamponade
         (1) acute diastolic dysfunction
         (2) increased CVP & HR
         (3) decreased BP
         (4) no square root sign
      iii. Constrictive pericarditis
         (1) Equalization of diastolic pressures
         (2) elevated diastolic pressures
         (3) square root sign
         (4) ECG changes - ST elevation
   e. physical assessment
      i. pulsus paradoxus
      ii. mechanism of pulsus paradoxus
   f. Cath findings
   g. Therapy
      i. pericardial-centesis

3. MYOCARDIAL
   a. etiology
      i. alcoholism - dilated cardiomyopathy
   b. clinical manifestations
      i. Restrictive cardiomyopathy (RC)
      ii. Hypertrophic cardiomyopathy (HOCM
         = IHSS)
         (1) muscle fiber disarray
         (2) Systolic Ejection murmur
      iii. Dilated cardiomyopathy
      iv. Restrictive cardiomyopathy
   c. physical assessment
   d. Cath findings
      i. characteristic hemodynamics in diastole
   e. Therapy

4. ENDOCARDIAL
   a. etiology
      i. bacterial / infective endocarditis
   b. clinical manifestations
      i. vegetation embolization
      ii. history of IV drug abuse
   c. physical assessment
   d. Cath findings
      i. hemodynamics
      ii. cath recommended in older patients
   e. Therapy
      i. antibiotics
      ii. surgery if life threatening

5. OTHER
   a. Heart sounds in each form of restrictive / constrictive disease
      i. pericardial knock
      ii. friction rub
      iii. murmur

Coronary Artery Disease & M.I.

1. General Ischemic Heart Disease

904. A patient has signs and symptoms of myocardial infarction. Myocardium may be preserved from necrosis if _____ is administered within _____ hours of the symptom onset.
   a.   A heparin drip, 3-4 hours
   b.   A heparin drip, 24-48 hours
   c.   A thrombolytic drug, 3-4 hours
   d.   A thrombolytic drug, 24-48 hours

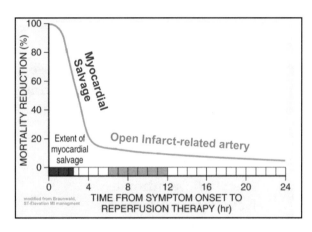

ANSWER c. Thrombolytic drug, **3-4** hours. Thrombolytic drugs can dissolve clots that cause the infarction. The sooner blood flow is reestablished, the better. The window of opportunity to salvage myocardium is generally considered to be within the first 4-6 hours after the initial symptoms of MI. Time is critical. It has led to rapid response STEMI cath teams.

Thrombolysis is effective at restoring blood flow, but cannot revive dead myocardial cells. Acute PCI for MI may have important advantages over thrombolytic drugs, but this requires urgent coronary arteriography, which may not be available in outlying areas of the country. This diagram shows the window for myocardial salvage and successful intervention.
See: Braunwald, chapter on "MI."

905. What coronary vein drains the inferior LV and usually runs alongside the PDCA?
   a.   Small
   b.   Middle
   c.   Great
   d.   Crux

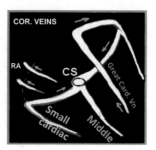

ANSWER: b. Middle coronary vein.

Medscape says, "The middle cardiac vein is seen to run in the posterior interventricular groove [often alongside the posterior descending artery (PDA) branch which usually arises from the right coronary artery] and drains directly into the coronary sinus."

906. Atherosclerosis is best defined as:
   a.   **Thickening of the arterial walls**
   b.   **Hardening of the arterial walls**
   c.   **Deposits of fatty plaques within arterial lumen**
   d.   **Thrombus formation in the lumen of the arteries**

ANSWER c. Deposits of fatty plaques within arterial lumen. The Greek roots of atherosclerosis are: "atheroma" from "porridge" and "sclerosis" from "hardening." In atherosclerosis yellow plaques (atheromas) develop just below the intima of arteries and arterioles. These plaques contain cholesterol and other lipoproteins. They become the instigator in most myocardial infarctions and ischemic heart disease.

Atherosclerotic heart disease (ASHD) begins silently, and fatty streaks are found in very young individuals. The fatty plaques eventually become complex lesions overgrown with smooth muscle and intimal cells and mixed with lymphocytes and lipoproteins. Arteriosclerosis is "hardening" of arteries from any cause: age, arteritis, or most commonly atherosclerosis.
See: Medical dictionary. **Keywords:** Atherosclerosis, arteriosclerosis, plaque

907. What is the name of the syndrome associated with central obesity, elevated lipids, elevated BP, and elevated fasting glucose levels. It increases a patient's risk of developing cardiovascular disease and diabetes? It is_____.
   a.   **Hyperlipidemia syndrome**
   b.   **Diabetic heart syndrome**
   c.   **Belly fat syndrome**
   d   **Metabolic syndrome**
   e.   **Kawasaki syndrome**

ANSWER: d. Metabolic syndrome is a common condition that increase the risk of developing cardiovascular disease and diabetes. It affects one in five people, and its prevalence increases with age. Metabolic syndrome is also known as syndrome X or insulin resistance syndrome. The US National Cholesterol Education Program Adult Treatment Panel III (2001) definition of metabolic syndrome requires at least three of the following:
   -Central obesity: waist circumference > 40 inches (male), > 36 inches(female)
   -Dyslipidemia: TG >150 mg/dl and/ or HDL-C < 40 mg/dL (male), < 50 mg/dL (female)
   -Blood pressure > 130/85 mmHg
   -Fasting plasma glucose > 6.1 mmol/L (110 mg/dl)
See: http://www.webmd.com/heart/metabolic-syndrome/

908. **Which of the following is NOT a form of acute coronary syndrome (ACS) and is usually treated medically?**
a.   Stable angina
b.   Unstable angina
c.   ST elevation MI
d.   Non-ST elevation MI

ANSWER: a.   Stable angina is not an acute coronary syndrome. It should first be treated medically. Only if that fails should PCI be considered, and then only for improving the quality of life.

The sub-types of acute coronary syndrome include unstable angina and two forms of myocardial infarction in which heart muscle is damaged - NSTEMI and STEMI. Unstable angina is similar to NSTEMI in that there is no ST elevation. **See:**
http://www.heart.org/HEARTORG/Conditions/HeartAttack/AboutHeartAttacks/Acute-Coronary-Syndrome_UCM_428752_Article.jsp
Keywords: acute coronary syndrome

909. Death **of heart tissue due to occlusion of a coronary artery is called:**
a.   **Myocarditis**
b.   **Myocardial infarction**
c.   **Myocardial insufficiency**
d.   **Myocardial ischemia**

ANSWER b. Myocardial infarction. Infarcted tissue is dead tissue (necrotic) due to local ischemia resulting from obstruction to blood flow. Any tissue deprived of O2 and nutrients will eventually infarct and die. The brain tissue begins to die after four minutes. Heart tissue takes longer, usually 1-4 hrs to die. This is the narrow window of time to salvage myocardium following acute MI.

Infarction is followed by progressive degradation of the dead tissue and release of cardiac enzymes: CK, LDH, and SGOT.
See: Medical dictionary. **Keywords:** Infarction, necrotic, dead tissue

910. **Select the three major histologic changes characteristic of the** fully developed **atherosclerotic fibrous plaque.**
           1. Smooth muscle proliferation
           2. Intimal proliferation
           3. Medial destruction and atrophy
           4. Accumulation of collagen
           5. Fatty streaks on the wall of intima
           6. Cholesterol accumulating in adventia
           7. Accumulation of fat inside the wall of intima
                   a. 1, 4, 7
                   b. 1, 2, 6
                   c. 2, 5, 7
                   d. 2, 6, 7

ANSWER a. 1, 4, 7

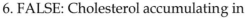

1. **TRUE:** Smooth muscle proliferation (Smooth muscle cells migrate into the plaque and may build it up so much that it occludes the lumen.)

2. FALSE: Intimal proliferation (This occurs in response to injury such as PCI.)

3. FALSE: Medial destruction and atrophy

4. **TRUE:** Accumulation of collagen (Fibrous tissue accumulates with the smooth muscle cells.)

5. FALSE: Fatty streaks on the wall of intima. This occurs in the first stages of ASHD that leads to this "plaque stage."

6. FALSE: Cholesterol accumulating in Adventia (Adventia is the outer layer - the buildup is inside the lumen.)

Morphology of fibrous plaque

7. **TRUE:** Accumulation of fat inside the intimal wall (THE cholesterol seems to build up inside the plaque along with the collagen and smooth muscle.)

The three stages of lesion development are: (1) Fatty streaks, (2) Raised fibrous plaque, and (3) Complicated lesions. This latter stage includes calcification, rupture under the plaque, with hemorrhage, and probable thrombus on the plaque.

See: Underhill, chapter on "Pathogenesis of Atherosclerosis." **Keywords:** Plaque formation

911. **Which type of coronary artery lesion is most likely to lead to clot formation and STEMI?**
a.   **Stenotic, with no vessel enlargement (no remodeling)**
b.   **Stenotic, with compensatory vessel enlargement (remodeling)**
c.   **Nonstenotic with no vessel enlargement (no remodeling)**
d.   **Nonstenotic with compensatory vessel enlargement (remodeling)**

ANSWER: d. Nonstenotic with compensatory vessel enlargement (remodeling). The stenoses we usually see on angio are not usually the ones that lead to STEMI.

Libby says "This schematic depicts 2 morphological extremes of coronary atherosclerotic plaques. Stenotic lesions tend to have smaller lipid cores, more fibrosis, and calcification; thick fibrous caps; and less compensatory enlargement (positive remodeling). They typically produce ischemia appropriately managed by combined medical therapy and often revascularization for symptom relief. Nonstenotic lesions generally outnumber stenotic plaques and tend to have large lipid cores and thin, fibrous caps susceptible to rupture and thrombosis. They often undergo substantial compensatory enlargement that leads to underestimation of lesion size by angiography. Nonstenotic plaques may cause no symptoms for many years but when disrupted can provoke episode of unstable angina or MI. ...Many coronary atherosclerotic lesions may lie between these 2 extremes, produce mixed clinical manifestations, and require multipronged management. Because both types of

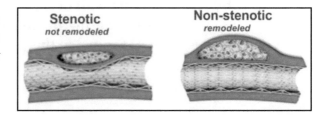

lesions usually coexist in given high-risk individual, optimum management often requires both revascularization and systemic therapy." **See:** http://circ.ahajournals.org/content/111/25/3481.full Peter Libby, "Pathophysiology of Coronary Artery Disease", Basic Science for Clinicians, 2005

912. **In the coronary artery atherosclerotic process, when do macrophages become "foam cells?"**
   a.   **When nitric oxide reduces endothelial function**
   b.   **When nitric oxide gas builds up in macrophages**
   c.   **When they become necrotic through apoptosis**
   d.   **When they ingest excess lipoprotiens**

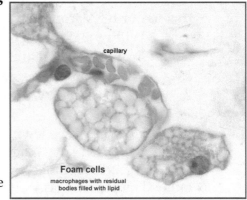

ANSWER: d. When they ingest excess lipoproteins.
   The white blood cell monocytes entering the intimal wall become macrophages that ingest the stored fat molecules. As you can see from the image, they appear to contain large fat bubbles.
   Yu, et. al, say,"Atherosclerosis is a chronic disease characterized by the deposition of excessive cholesterol in the arterial intima. Macrophage foam cells play a critical role in the occurrence and development of atherosclerosis. The generation of these cells is associated with imbalance of cholesterol influx, esterification and efflux. ..When inflow and esterification of cholesterol increase and/or its outflow decrease, the macrophages are ultimately transformed into lipid-laden foam cells, the prototypical cells in the atherosclerotic plaque." **See:** Yu, et al., Foam Cells in Atherosclerosis, 2013, at http://www.sciencedirect.com/science/article/pii/S0009898113002477

913. **The most common cause of death in the U.S. is:**
   a.   **Cancer**
   b.   **Stroke**
   c.   **Trauma and suicide**
   d.   **Coronary artery disease**

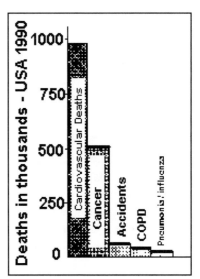

ANSWER d. Coronary artery disease is the most common cause of death in the western world. Approximately one million Americans died of cardiovascular disease in 1990. As shown on the diagram, the cardiovascular death rate was twice as frequent as the next leading cause of death - cancer.
   Approximately 1,500,000 MI's occur in the USA each year and approximately one fourth of ALL American deaths occur from Acute Myocardial Infarction (AMI). Of this year's 1 ½ million acute MI's, 60% will within one hour of the onset, most of sudden death (SD) due to ventricular fibrillation (VF).
   These numbers are impressive but the mortality (death rate) for AMI has declined dramatically in recent

Leading Causes of death in USA

years due to a general decline in ASHD and better in hospital care. In 20 years the MI in-hospital mortality has fallen from 30% to 5%. This dramatic reduction in hospital mortality for AMI is believed due to the better in-hospital care and interventional cardiology. Also, risk factor modification has reduced the general incidence of ASHD in the USA by 25%. Of course the general population is growing so fast that the total number of AMI patients each year continues to escalate.
See: Braunwald, chapter on "Acute MI." **Keywords:** The incidence of AMI,

914. **It is safest to do a left main coronary PCI when there is a functioning bypass graft to a major left coronary artery (LAD/Circ). What is this termed?**
a. **Widowmaker rescue**
b. **Protected left main PCI**
c. **CABG Impella rescue**
d. **High risk PCI with Impella**

ANSWER: b. Protected left main PCI.
Vekatesan says, "The term protected left main, was not coined by cardiovascular physiologists but by interventional cardiologists. Hence it connotes an anatomical meaning rather than physiological. Protected LMD meant there must be at least one graft to either LAD or circumflex. And this graft should be functional. The presence of this graft is supposed to increase the comfort levels of the interventionist as well as the patient." This is because there is a second source of blood supply available retrograde from the grafted vessel. **See:** Dr. Vekatesan, MD, "What is protected left main disease?", 2011 https://drsvenkatesan.com/2009/09/15/what-is-protected-left-main-coronary-artery-how-good-is-the-protection-if-good-why-should-it-need-another-protection/
Abiomed has coined the term "Protected PCI" to describe high-risk PCI with an Impella. They say, "Protected PCI™ involves a minimally-invasive procedure plus support of your blood pressure, like that from the Impella 2.5 heart pump."
See: http://www.protectedpci.com

915. **What is the average mortality rate for untreated LEFT MAIN coronary artery occlusion?**
a. **35%**
b. **50%**
c. **75%**
d. **90%**

ANSWER d. 90%. This vessel supplies approximately 3/4 of the blood to the heart and feeds the LAD and circumflex coronary arteries. This is the hypercritical "widow-maker" lesion which puts most of the LV at risk. Total occlusion is near fatal. When a "widow-maker" lesion is seen, GET THE PATIENT TO SURGERY STAT. PCI is generally contraindicated for "widow-maker" lesions.
See: Braunwald, chapter on "Coronary Arteriography." **Keywords:** Cor. physiology, widow-maker, main-stem lesion, mortality 90%

916. A 70 year old man had a severe bout of coronary ischemia and was admitted to the ER. His echo shows severe LV dysfunction. But, then he gradually improved over a period of hours and was discharged. This suggests he had:
a.   Infarcted myocardium
b.   Injured myocardium
c.   Stunned myocardium
d.   Hibernating myocardium

ANSWER c. Stunned myocardium recovers function after a transient period of ischemia. If the recovery occurs within hours, it is said to have been "stunned." If its depression was more persistent and it recovers within days or months it is said to have been "hibernating." The ischemic dysfunction usually involves LV wall segment abnormalities where the most severely ischemic areas bulge (are dyskinetic) and the mildly ischemic areas fail to contract vigorously (become hypokinetic). The permanence and recovery

(hours)	*(days)*	*(dead)*
Stunned →	**hibernating →**	**infarcted**

from cardiac damage progresses like this: Stunned (hours) - hibernating (days) - infarcted (dead).

     Although once infarcted (dead) the tissue cannot recover, ischemic tissue gets just enough flow to remain alive (viable). This is the basis for "myocardial salvage" and recent "interventional" techniques such as acute PCI and thrombolysis. Often these salvaged hearts do not recover immediately but gradually after these interventions. Hibernating myocardium is often seen after bypass surgery where patients need to be supported on IABP to get them off the pump. But with time the "hibernating myocardium" may recover its function. **See:** Braunwald, chapter on "Coronary Blood Flow and Myocardial Ischemia."
Keywords: Stunned, hibernating myocardium

917. A "critical coronary stenosis" significantly impairs maximal EXERCISE coronary blood flow. A "critical coronary stenosis" occurs when the stenosis exceeds _____%.
a.   >50 % reduction in diameter
b.   >75 % reduction in diameter
c.   >90 % reduction in diameter
d.   >99 % reduction in diameter

ANSWER a. >50 % reduction in diameter. Mild stenoses are not usually significant. They only reduce coronary flow at high flow rates. That is why exercise stress tests are most sensitive in detecting CAD. To be significant on exercise a stenosis must be at least 50% in diameter (75% area reduction). Only when they reach this level is intervention or surgery considered. Below 50% flow is not impaired and even on exercise does not cause symptoms. Remember a 50% diameter stenosis is the same as a 75% area reduction stenosis. See next question.
     Disease must be quite severe to cause resting

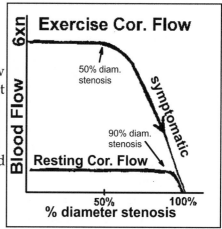

% coronary stenosis

angina. **Resting** coronary flow is only impaired when the stenosis exceeds 90% diameter reduction (99% area reduction). See the graph. **See:** Braunwald, chapter on "Coronary Angiography." **Keywords:** Significant reduced coronary flow at < 50% diameter stenosis.

918. **A blood vessel 2-mm in diameter becomes stenosed, down to 0.8 mm diameter as shown. Calculate the percentage reduction in this stenosis diameter?**
   a.   20%
   b.   40%
   c.   60%
   d.   75%

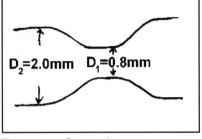
Diameter Stenosis

ANSWER c. 60%. Instead of the % orifice <u>area</u> reduction, we can calculate the % of <u>diameter</u> reduction or blockage.
       If we represent the original vessel diameter as D_2 and the reduced vessel diameter as D_1 the formula for % stenosis becomes:
       % Diameter Stenosis = $(D_2 - D_1) / D_2$ or $\{1 - (D_1/D_2)\}$
Substituting 2.0 and 0.8 mm. diameters from the problem:
       % Diameter Stenosis = $1 - (.8/2) = 1 - .4 = .6 = 60\%$
Since a 50% diameter reduction = a 75% area reduction, this example will have an area reduction of more than a 75%. In the next question we will calculate the % area reduction. **See:** Braunwald, chapter on "Coronary Blood Flow and Myocardial Ischemia." **Keywords:** % diameter stenosis calculation

919. **A 50% DIAMETER stenosis equals a _____ % AREA stenosis.**
   a.   50%
   b.   75%
   c.   85%
   d.   95%

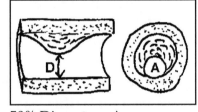
50% Diameter - Area

ANSWER b. 75%. Area stenoses always have higher numbers then diameter stenoses. (Perhaps that's why Dr's usually quote the area stenosis # to patients - to make it sound more severe.)
Area stenosis is based on the formula for area of a circle and thus varies as the square of the radius or diameter. $A = \pi r^2$ or $A = \pi (D/2)^2$

       To make it sound even worse we speak of these stenoses as "percentage of reduction." So instead of the % orifice, we calculate the % of blockage. Thus a stenotic area which is 40% of the original vessel area is termed a 60% stenosis (see previous question).
       If we represent the original vessel diameter as D_2 and the reduced vessel diameter as D_1, and using the formula above:
       % Diameter Stenosis = $\{1 - (D_1/D_2)\}$
       To change the Diameter into Area we use the formula for area of a circle: $A = \pi r^2$ or $A = \pi (D/2)^2$.

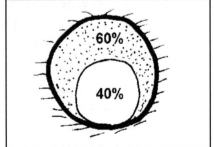
60% Area Reduction

After substituting and dividing out common elements in the numerator and denominator the formula becomes:

% Areas Stenosis - $\{1 - (D_1/D_2)^2\}$

Thus we see that the % area stenosis varies as 1 minus the square of the diameter ratios. Now let's substitute the numbers given in the question. E.g., Original = 2 mm. Diameter, reduced to 1 mm = 50% diam. reduction. This becomes a 75% Area reduction as shown:

% Area Stenosis = $\{1 - ((2-1)/2)^2\} = 1 - .5^2 = 1 - .25$

% Area Stenosis = $.75 = 75\%$

These are two easy numbers to remember (50% Diam. = 75% Area reduction), and they also happen to be the critical stenosis numbers from the question above. Remember the area stenosis reduction varies as the square of the diameter subtracted from one. Thus NOT $(50\%)^2$. but $1 - (50\%)^2 = 1 - 25\% = 75\%$

See: Braunwald, chapter on "Coronary Blood Flow and Myocardial Ischemia." **Keywords:** % Convert % diameter stenosis to % area stenosis calculation

920. **Some endocardial micro-veins do not drain into the coronary sinus. What is the name of coronary veins that bypass the CS and drain directly into the ventricle?**

a. **Small cardiac veins**

b. **Thebesian veins**

c. **Arterio-sinusoid veins**

d. **Anterior RV veins**

ANSWER: b. Thebesian veins. Note in the diagram vein #1 drains directly into a cardiac chamber. Others drain into sinusoids in the chamber.

Ajay, et. al., say: "Early vertebrates (e.g., hagfish and lampreys) nourished the myocardium simply by absorbing blood from the lumen of their single-chambered ventricles. Simple diffusion is the classic method of nutrition and waste disposal for lower organisms lacking vascular systems.... Thebesian veins. These veins form a "lesser" venous system of the heart. Careful anatomical analysis has identified three distinct forms of these Thebesian vessels. The first type of Thebesian veins drain blood from the capillary bed into the ventricular cavity. The second type, arterioluminal vessels, drain blood directly from the arteries into the ventricles without traversing capillary beds and thus have a larger diameter. The third type, the venoluminal vessels, form direct communications with the coronary veins, shunting blood from these vessels into the ventricular cavities. Most of the Thebesian veins in the

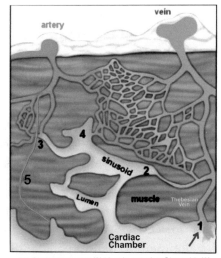

(1) Thebesian vein; (2) Venule entering Sinusoid; (3) Arteriosinusoidal vessel entering Sinusoid; (4) Capillary entering Sinusoid; (5) Arterioluminal vessel

ventricles appear to be venoluminal in nature. The presence of an extensive Thebesian venous network, which in the healthy state carries 5-10% of the venous return, does allow for an alternative route of venous drainage of the myocardium. It has been established that the Thebesian veins are capable of carrying the bulk of venous return in situations where the epicardial coronary veins are compromised." **See:** Ajay, et.al., The Coronary Venous System: An Alternative Route of Access to the Myocardium, The Journal of Invasive

2. Coronary Angiographic Pathology

921. **What coronary artery normally feeds the inferior interventricular septum?**
   a. **LAD**
   b. **Diagonal**
   c. **Circumflex**
   d. **PDCA**

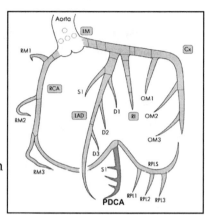

ANSWER: d. PDCA. The PDCA runs in the posterior interventricular groove at the bottom of the heart and sends up septal perforators into the inferior IV septum. In a normal right dominant coronary system, the PDCA arises from the RCA at the crux. One of these branches usually supplies the His bundle and AV node. The LAD also has septal perforators but, they dive down into the IV septum from above. Note that this diagram shows a Ramus Intermedius artery between the LAD & Circumflex.

922. **Compensatory coronary circulation that comes to ischemic tissue by an alternative route is called:**
   a. **Collateral circulation**
   b. **Vein bypass circulation**
   c. **Thebesian circulation**
   d. **Greater circulation**

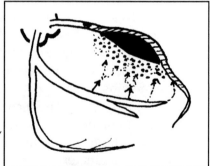

Collateral circulation

ANSWER a. Collateral circulation. Latin root of "collateral" comes from "lateral" meaning "beside." This is a circulation through secondary channels occurring after obstruction to the principal vessel supplying an area. It is also called "compensatory" circulation because it develops to compensate an ischemia area.

    Little is known about how collaterals develop. They may have been there all along and simply recruited, or they may "grow" into ischemic areas. Exercise encourages their development, but most collaterals develop slowly in response to chronic ischemia. Ischemic areas may be injured and yet recover if the heart has time to develop collateral vessels to the injured area.

    Note in the diagram how the RCA RV branches have developed collateral vessels (dotted lines) to the LAD. The LAD is blocked so this is the only blood flow the anterior part of this heart receives.

See: medical dictionary. **Keywords:** "collateral" definition

923. What abnormality is seen in this RAO coronary angiogram at #5 & #6?

    a.   **Subtotal LAD stenosis**

    b.   **Vein bypass graft to RCA**

    c.   **PDCA to LAD collateral**

    d.   **LAD to PDCA collateral**

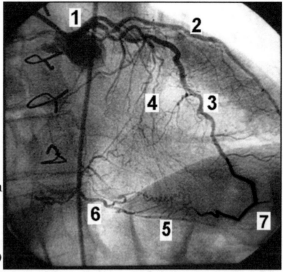

RAO cranial view, LCA injection

ANSWER d. LAD (7) to PDCA collateral (5 & 6). The PDCA branch of the RCA is filling retrograde by collateral channels in the septum and at the apex. An RCA stenosis must exist which makes the inferior wall ischemic. Fortunately, the inferior wall is now collateralized by the LAD. Note the distal LAD wrapping around the apex (7) and continuing on to small branches of the distal PDCA. Additional collateral channels provide fresh blood through the septal branches (4) of the LAD to the septal branches of the PDCA. Identify all anatomy shown.

LABELED VESSELS ARE:

    1. Main left coronary

    2. Diagonal branch

    3. LAD

    4. Septal perforators - with collateral to septal branches of PDCA

    5. Distal PDCA showing collateral from LAD entering from the apex

    6. Distal RCA, PDCA and posterior lateral branches.

    7. Distal LAD wraps around LV apex and sends collateral to PDCA

See: Grossman, chapter on "Coronary Arteriography." **Keywords:** collateral

924. The CONUS coronary artery frequently collateralizes to the:

    a.   **LAD**

    b.   **Circumflex**

    c.   **PDCA**

    d.   **AV node**

ANSWER a. LAD. Remember the conus is the first branch off the RCA, and normally feeds the RV outflow tract (infundibulum). If the conus continues past the RV into the LV, these branches may be feeding the adjacent ischemic LAD branches. Grossman demonstrates dozens of possible collateral locations where branches of one coronary circulation contact the branches of another coronary circulation. The conus to LAD is a common collateral pattern.

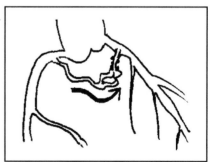

Collateral - Conus to LAD

See: Grossman, chapter on "Coronary Arteriography."

Keywords: RCA, Collateral, Conus

925. **The bypass graft shown in the drawing is a/an:**
a. **IMA graft to LAD**
b. **IMA skip graft to circumflex and LAD**
c. **CABG skip graft to diagonal and circumflex**
d. **CABG skip graft to LAD and RCA**

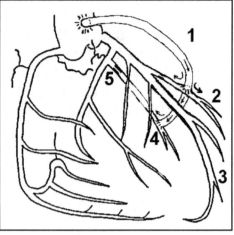

? Graft ➡ to coronary

ANSWER c. CABG skip graft to diagonal and circumflex (obtuse marginal) coronary artery. This is a standard RAO view of both coronary arteries. Surgeons commonly draw these diagrams to explain where the bypass grafts were placed on a patient. #1 is a CABG bypass from the aorta to the 1st diagonal (2). Then it skips over to the obtuse marginal branch of the circumflex (4). The fresh blood from the aorta travels through the vein bypass distal to the stenosis in each vessel. Note the stenosis drawn in each bypassed vessel (5).
See: Braunwald, chapter on "Coronary Arteriography." **Keywords:** CABG to Diag. & LAD

926. **The coronary lesion shown on the diagram at #1 is:**
a. **Acute marginal stenosis**
b. **PDCA stenosis**
c. **Posterior lateral stenosis**
d. **Conus ➡ LAD collateral**
e. **Acute marginal ➡ circ. collateral**

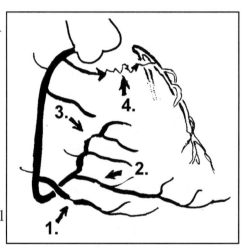

Coronary arteriogram

ANSWER a. Acute marginal stenosis. This is a standard RAO right coronary arteriogram. Be able to match all answers shown below. Be able to identify all lesions shown on this diagram.
BE ABLE TO MATCH ALL ANSWERS.
1. Acute marginal stenosis
2. PDCA stenosis
3. Posterior lateral stenosis
4. Conus ➡ LAD collateral
    The conus coronary frequently collateralizes to the LAD across the RV outflow track. It is termed "Vieussen's Ring." Collateral vessels that develop usually grow in from another system supplying an adjacent area. The LAD is probably totally obstructed at the origin.
See: Braunwald, chapter on "Coronary Arteriography." **Keywords:** Coronary lesions: RAO, RCA

927. **The coronary lesion on the diagram at #3 is:**
   a.   **LAD → RCA (PDCA) collateral**
   b.   **Circumflex → posterior lateral (RCA) collateral**
   c.   **Main stem stenosis**
   d.   **Circumflex stenosis**
   e.   **Diagonal stenosis**
   f.   **LAD stenosis**

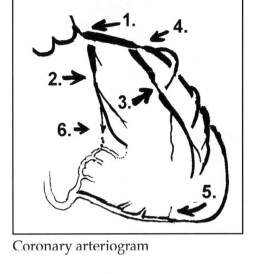
Coronary arteriogram

ANSWER e. Diagonal stenosis. This is a standard RAO left coronary angiogram. Identify all lesions on this diagram. **BE ABLE TO MATCH ALL ANSWERS.**

   1.   **Main stem LCA stenosis**
   2.   **Circumflex LCA stenosis**
   3.   **Diagonal stenosis**
   4.   **LAD stenosis**
   5.   **LAD → RCA (PDCA) collateral**
       The LAD can wrap around the apex like this to provide collateral to the PDCA (or vice versa). This LAD is thus supplying the entire ventricular septum. Since the LAD and main-stem LCA both have stenosis it would be very unusual to find the LAD helping the RCA like this. The RCA would be more likely to provide collateral to the LAD.
   6.   **Circumflex → posterior lateral (RCA) collateral:**
       The circumflex can grow collateral to the posterior lateral branches of the RCA (or vice versa).

See: Braunwald, chapter on "Coronary Arteriography." **Keywords:** Coronary lesions: RAO, RCA

928. **The coronary lesion shown on the diagram at #3 is:**
   a.   **Circumflex stenosis**
   b.   **LAD stenosis**
   c.   **LAD → PDCA division of RCA**
   d.   **Circumflex → posterior lateral branch of RCA collateral**
   e.   **LAD → PDCA branch of RCA collateral**

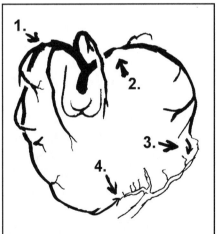
Coronary arteriogram

ANSWER d. Circumflex → posterior lateral branch of RCA collateral. This is a caudal LAO left coronary arteriogram (spider view). Identify all lesions shown on this diagram. **BE ABLE TO MATCH ALL ANSWERS.**

   1. **LAD stenosis**
   2. **Circumflex stenosis**
   3. **Circumflex → posterior lateral branch of RCA collateral**
       The circumflex travels toward the crux in the left AV groove. The posterior lateral branches of the RCA also travel in the AV groove. Where both end is a natural place to exchange collateral circulations.

4. LAD ➜ PDCA division of RCA collateral.
The LAD goes to the apex in the anterior IV groove. The PDCA goes to the apex in the inferior IV groove. Where they both end, the LAD may grow collaterals over to help the starving RCA. We would expect to find a severely stenosed or obstructed RCA on that coronary arteriogram.
See: Braunwald, chapter on "Coronary Arteriography." **Keywords:** lesions RAO, RCA

929. The coronary lesion shown on the diagram at #5 on the diagram is:
a. LAD lesion
b. 2nd diagonal lesion
c. 2nd septal lesion
d. Circumflex lesion (2nd OM)

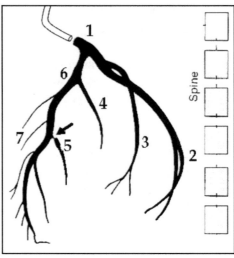
LAO coronary arteriogram

ANSWER b. 2nd diagonal lesion. Note how nicely this 55° LAO view lays out the diagonal branches. The circumflex branches on the right side overlap. Match all answers below. LCA arteries shown are:
1. Main left coronary
2. Obtuse marginal branch of circ.
3. Distal circumflex artery
4. 1st diagonal branch of LAD
5. 2nd diagonal branch of LAD - 80% proximal lesion
6. Proximal LAD
7. Septal branches of LAD
See: Kern, chapter on "Angiographic Data" **Keywords:** lesion in 2nd diagonal coronary

930. The coronary artery lesion shown on the diagram at #2 is a:
a. Diagonal stenosis
b. Obtuse marginal stenosis
c. PDCA stenosis
d. Posterior circumflex stenosis

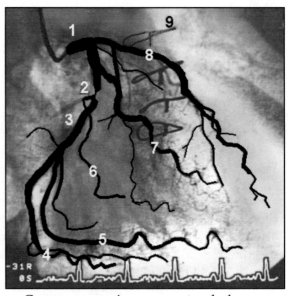
Coronary arteriogram - *retouched*

ANSWER d. Posterior circumflex stenosis. Identify all vessels shown on this diagram. **BE ABLE TO MATCH ALL ANSWERS.**
1. Main left coronary artery
2. Lesion in proximal circumflex
3. Circumflex
4. PDCA in posterior IV groove
5. Obtuse marginal #2
6. Obtuse marginal #1
7. Acute marginal
8. Small LAD or diagonal branch (probable graft to LAD system)
This left coronary artery shown in the RAO view is dominant. **See:** Braunwald, chapter on "Coronary Arteriography." **Keywords:** AV node artery from Circ.

931. **What coronary artery lesion is shown on the diagram at #4?**
   a.   **Diagonal branch occlusion**
   b.   **PDCA occlusion**
   c.   **Subtotal LAD stenosis**
   d.   **Subtotal main-stem LCA stenosis**

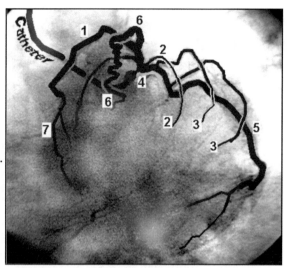

40 deg LAO, 20 deg caudal
Spider view left coronary

ANSWER d. Subtotal main-stem LCA stenosis. The main-stem left coronary is shown well in this LAO caudal view (spider). The lesion shown at #4 is nearly occluded (subtotal). Because of the high risk of these "widowmakers", this patient should go immediately to CABG surgery. Be able to identify all vessels shown on this diagram.
CORRECTLY MATCHED VESSELS ARE:
   1. LAD
   2. Ramus medianus
   3. Obtuse marginal
   4. Left main
   5. Circumflex
   6. Diagonal
   7. Distal LAD
See: Braunwald, chapter on "Coronary Arteriography." **Keywords:** Main stem left lesion

932. **What coronary artery lesion is shown on the diagram?**
   a.   **Subtotal main-stem left**
   b.   **Obtuse marginal**
   c.   **Proximal circumflex**
   d.   **LAD**

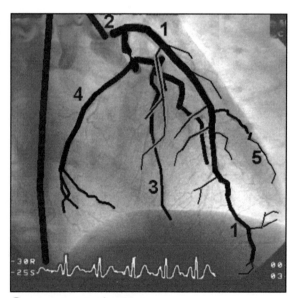

Coronary arteriogram

ANSWER c. Proximal circumflex. ID all
BE ABLE TO MATCH ALL ANSWERS.
   1. LAD
   2. Main-stem left
   3. Obtuse marginal branch of Cx.
   4. AV groove branch of Cx.
   5. Diagonal branch of LAD
See: Braunwald, chapter on "Coronary Arteriography." **Keywords:** lesion in prox. circ.

933. What coronary artery lesion is shown on the diagram?

    a.   SA node
    b.   Proximal RCA
    c.   Distal RCA
    d.   PDCA

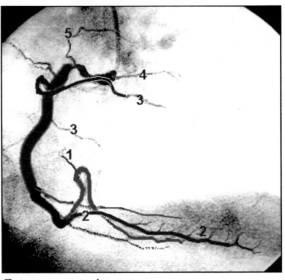

Coronary arteriogram

ANSWER b. Proximal RCA. ID all -
CORRECTLY MATCHED VESSELS ARE:
    1. AV node branch of RCA
    2. PDCA
    3. RV branch (Acute marginal)
    4. Conus branch of RCA
    5. SA node branch of RCA
See: Braunwald, chapter on "Coronary Arteriography." **Keywords:** lesion in prox. RCA

BOTH QUESTIONS BELOW REFER TO THIS ANGIOGRAM.

934. What coronary angiographic view is shown in this diagram?

    a.   Shallow RAO
    b.   Steep RAO
    c.   Shallow LAO
    d.   Steep LAO

935. What coronary artery is labeled #1?

    a.   Obtuse marginal
    b.   Acute marginal
    c.   PDCA branch of RCA
    d.   Diagonal branch of LCA

BOTH ANSWERS LISTED TOGETHER BELOW.

Coronary arteriogram

934. ANSWER b. Steep RAO. The apex points to the right making it an RAO view. Up to 45 degrees RAO the RCA is C shaped. Then at about 45 degrees it looks L shaped. In steeper RAO views, past about 60 degrees, it takes on this reverse C shape. It's like looking at the base of the RA from the patient's right shoulder - steep RAO.
See: Braunwald, chapter on "Coronary Arteriography." **Keywords:** RCA, steep RAO view

935. ANSWER c. PDCA branch of RCA. ID all -
CORRECTLY MATCHED ARTERIES ARE:
    1. PDCA branch of RCA
    2. Acute marginal branch of RCA
    3. RV branch of RCA
    4. Conus branch of RCA
    5. Mid RCA (note small eccentric lesion)

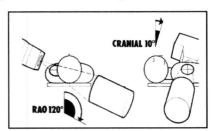

Steep RAO cran.- After Kern

The diagram shows how this view (almost lateral) nicely lays out the main segments of the right coronary artery.

See: Kern chapter on "Angiographic Data" Keywords: ID coronary arteries

BOTH QUESTIONS BELOW REFER TO THIS ANGIOGRAM.

936. On this coronary angiogram identify the wire labeled #2?

a.   ECG lead wire
b.   Defib. pad wire
c.   RV pacing wire
d.   RA pacing wire

937. Which coronary artery is labeled # 3?

a.   AV node artery
b.   SA node artery
c.   Conus artery
d.   Obtuse marginal

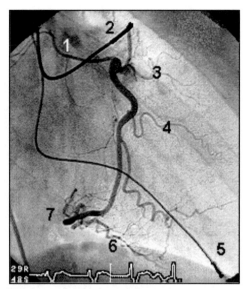

Right coronary arteriogram

BOTH ANSWERS LISTED TOGETHER BELOW.

936. ANSWER d. RA pacing wire. This patient has a permanent dual chamber dual chamber or AV sequential pacemaker. The atrial lead is in the right atrial appendage just above the RCA. The ventricular lead is in the RV. These two leads provide stimulus for synchronized atrial and ventricular contraction. Dual chamber pacemaker leads such as these are usually connected to a DDD pacemaker.
See: Braunwald, chapter on "Coronary Arteriography." Keywords: pacer leads on angio.

937. ANSWER c. Conus artery. This artery is usually the first branch of the RCA. It supplies the outflow track of the RV. It is to the right of the main RCA, as opposed to the SA node artery which is to the left of the RCA in this view. Be able to identify all vessels shown in this RAO view.
CORRECTLY MATCHED ARTERIES ARE:
    1. SA node artery of RCA
    2. RA pacing wire
    3. Conus branch of RCA
    4. RV or marginal branch of RCA
    5. RV pacing wire
    6. PDCA branch of RCA
    7. Posterior lateral LV branch of RCA
See: Braunwald, chapter on "Coronary Arteriography." Keywords: Right coronary arteries ID, conus branch of RCA

938. A 50 year old man has a 95% left main coronary lesion, a 90 % LAD lesion, and a 75% circumflex lesion as shown. This is termed _____ and is best treated with _____.

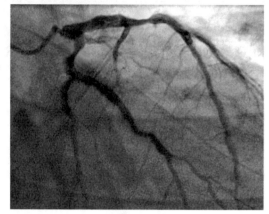

a. Protected left main disease, CABG
b. Protected left main disease, DES
c. Unprotected left main disease, CABG
d. Triple vessel coronary disease, DES

ANSWER: c. Unprotected left main disease, CABG. Grossman says, "For many years coronary artery bypass graft surgery has been considered the therapy of choice for the left main coronary artery disease....surgery still must be considered the standard of care for good operative candidates with left main disease." Triple vessel disease refers to disease in all 3 major coronary vessels: LAD, CX and RCA. The left main may be protected by receiving significant collateral circulation. **See:** Grossman, chapter on "Coronary Stenting"

3. Physiology & Mechanisms of CAD/MI

939. Some acute MI's affect only the inner layers of the myocardium. This type of heart attack is called:
a. Epicardial infarction
b. Transmural infarction
c. Subendocardial infarction
d. Subdural infarction

ANSWER c. Subendocardial infarction. These MI's are more common than transmural infarcts, that affect all three walls of the LV. The endocardial layer is most vulnerable to ischemia because the blood has to travel through the contracting myocardium to get there. **See:** Braunwald, chapter on "Coronary Blood Flow and Myocardial Ischemia." **Keywords:** Acute thrombosis most common in transmural total blockage

940. Which of the following mechanisms is thought to close the coronary artery in acute myocardial infarction?
a. Coronary spasm without a plaque lesion
b. Coronary spasm on top of a plaque lesion
c. Thrombus formation without a plaque lesion
d. Thrombus formation on top of a plaque lesion

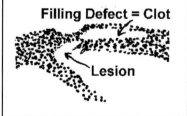

Coronary Thrombosis

ANSWER d. Thrombus formation on top of a plaque lesion. Spokane is proud to have aided in recognizing the importance of "thrombus" in acute transmural MI's. Prior to this time, the medical community was unsure about the role of thrombosis in MI. In the

1970's we did heart caths on acute MI patients and found a preponderance of **filling defects** due to clot in the effected coronary vessel. We used to call them "cigars" because of their rounded appearance. This observation was published in 1980 by Dr. DeWood. Because of this Spokane has been a pioneer in interventional procedures, especially emergency CABG surgery for acute MI.

See: DeWood, Spores, Notske, et al, "Prevalence of total coronary occlusion during the early hours of transmural myocardial infarction" N. Engl J Med 303:897, 1980. **Keywords:** Acute thrombosis most common in transmural MI

941. **Acute coronary thrombosis (clots) are most commonly found in:**
   a.   Acute transmural MI due to a partially occluded coronary artery
   b.   Acute transmural MI due to a totally occluded coronary artery
   c.   Subendocardial MI due to spasm of a major coronary artery
   d.   Subendocardial MI due to sub-total stenosis of a major coronary artery

ANSWER b. Acute transmural MI due to a totally occluded coronary artery. An incomplete blockage of a vessel is more often associated with subendocardial MI - where the necrosis does not extend through all three layers of the heart.
See: Braunwald, chapter on "Coronary Blood Flow and Myocardial Ischemia." **Keywords:** Acute thrombosis most common in transmural total blockage

942. **The diagram shows angiographic classification of coronary artery dissections from mildest to most severe types (NHLBI classification). Match each dissection type with its description below.**
   a.   New persistent filling defect
   b.   Extraluminal cap. Contrast persists after dye clears from lumen
   c.   Minor radiolucency in lumen
   d.   Parallel tracts or double lumen separated by a radiolucent area
   e.   Spiral luminal filling defect
   f.   Impaired flow or occlusion

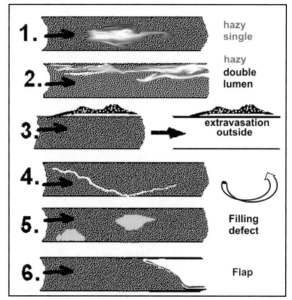

Coronary Angios of dissection types

BE ABLE TO MATCH ALL ANSWERS:
1 or type A. = c. Minor radiolucency in lumen
2 or type B. = d. Parallel tracts or double lumen separated by a radiolucent area
3 or type C. = b. Extraluminal cap. Contrast persists after dye clears from lumen as perivascular extravasation through coronary wall.
4 or type D. = e. Spiral luminal filling defect
5 or type E. = a. New persistent filling defect
6 or type F. = f. Other types that lead to impaired flow or occlusion
   Freed says: "Coronary artery dissection is usually defined angiographically; of

various classification schemes, the NHLBI classification is the most popular. Types A and B are considered "minor" dissections since they do not appear to adversely impact procedural outcome. In contrast, Types C-F are considered "major" dissections and are associated with a 5-fold risk of myocardial infarction, emergency CABG, or death."
See: Freed, chapter on "Dissection and Acute Closure"

943. On this coronary angiogram identify the tiny defect at #2.
   a. Type F, Flap dissection in mid circumflex
   b. Type F, Flap dissection in mid LAD
   c. Type E, Thrombus in circumflex
   d. Type E, Thrombus in LAD

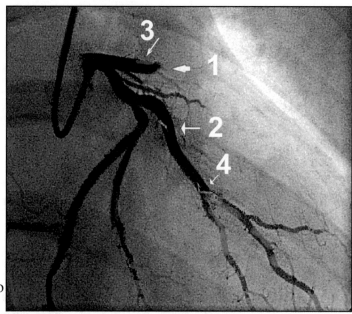

Multiple Coronary Lesions

ANSWER. a. Type F, flap dissection in mid circumflex. Flaps are very prone to clot formation or may act as a valve to shut off flow. Just remember "F" is for FLAP, E is for a Embolus or clot. Such flaps of intima can usually be plastered down with a balloon and the vessel held open by a stent. Be able to identify all defects shown in this RAO view of the LCA. This is an RAO view of the left coronary artery. Note ribs descending toward the sternum. Be able to identify all lesions described below.
CORRECTLY CLASSIFIED LESIONS SHOWN IN THE DIAGRAM ARE:
   1. Total LAD occlusion, Due to acute thrombus.
   2. Type F, Flap dissection in mid circumflex.
   3. Type E, Thrombus in proximal LAD. Cigar shaped filling defect at #3 arrow.
   4. Type D, Spiral luminal filling defect/dissection

944. On this coronary angiogram identify the defect seen in the angio and IVUS images?
- a.   Calcified plaque in LAD
- b.   Calcified plaque in CX
- c.   Thrombus filling defect in LAD
- d.   Thrombus filling defect in CX

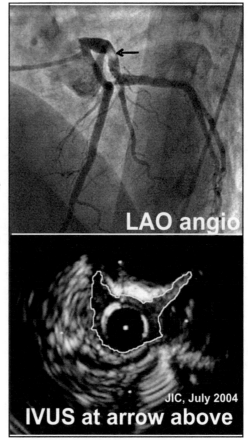

ANSWER. b. Calcified plaque in CX. This filling defect appears in the origin of the circumflex. The IVUS shows reflective calcium on the surface of the plaque, which causes shadowing (absent echos) behind the calcium. Note the catheter going up the AO near the spine. Remember the CX is nearest the spine. It was felt this plaque extended into the left main coronary artery, so the patient was sent to surgery.

IVUS, filling defect from JIC 2004

945. Acute ST Elevation Myocardial Infarction (STEMI) usually occurs when a coronary lesion has a/an:
- a.   Total thrombotic occlusion
- b.   Severe obstruction (>75% narrowing)
- c.   Large heavy calcified (>75%) plaque burden
- d.   Inadequate coronary flow to sustain the myocardium

ANSWER: a. Total thrombotic coronary occlusion. Braunwald says, "Acute total occlusion of a coronary artery usually causes STEMI, whereas UA/NSTEMI usually results from severe obstruction, but not total occlusion, of the culprit coronary artery.... The acute event, which usually involves thrombus formation at the site of a ruptured or eroded atherosclerotic plaque, is currently referred to as 'atherothrombosis' a term that is replacing 'atherosclerosis' because it more fully describes the pathophysiology of the disease that involves both progression and disruption of the atheroma and superimposed thrombus."
See: Braunwald, chapter on "Unstable Angina and Non-ST Elevation MI"
Thrombus is essentially the final common pathway for ACS. Plaque disruption/rupture with consequent exposure of the highly prothrombotic lipid core to the bloodstream generally results in complete thrombotic occlusion (Q-wave myocardial infarction) or high-grade, intermittent obstruction (non-Q wave myocardial infarction, unstable angina, sudden cardiac death). **See:**
http://www.invasivecardiology.com/articles/myocardial-infarction-and-culprit-plaque-myths-data-and-statistics

946. **When considering a lesion for PCI, which <u>type of lesion</u> below is most likely to receive successful PCI and have the least associated complications?**
   a.   Irregular contour (as opposed to smooth)
   b.   Tubular (as opposed to discrete)
   c.   Concentric (as opposed to eccentric)
   d.   Thrombus present (as opposed to no thrombus)
   e.   Calcium present (as opposed to no calcium)

ANSWER c. Concentric lesions are easier to dilate than eccentric lesions. Concentric lesions occur equally around the lumen, whereas eccentric lesions occur on just one side of the vessel. Eccentric lesion PCI tend to dilate the uninvolved wall which springs back with elastic recoil. Other factors increasing difficulty are long diffuse lesions, tortuosity, increasing angulation, total occlusion, vein grafts, ostial location, irregular contour and involved side branches.

The ACC/AHA Task Force on Assessment of Diagnostic and Therapeutic Cardiovascular Procedures developed a classification of type A, B and C lesions. Each type of lesion has progressively worse PCI outcomes. Type A is low risk with >85% success. Type B is moderate risk, with 60-85% success. Type C is high risk, with < 60% success. **See:** Braunwald, chapter on "Cardiac Catheterization" **Keywords:** Lesion morphology concentric

947. **The earliest appearance of atherosclerosis is:**
   a.   Calcification on intima wall
   b.   Elevated plasma HDL cholesterol
   c.   Foam cells and fatty streaks on intima
   d.   Smooth muscle cells proliferate and accumulate in the intima

ANSWER: c. Foam cells and fatty streaks in arteries. Fatty streaks are the earliest lesions seen with atherosclerosis in arteries. Increased total cholesterol and decreased HDL cholesterol contribute to this process. "The precursors (of atherosclerotic lesions) are arranged in a temporal sequence of three characteristic lesion types. Types I and II are generally the only lesion types found in children, although they may also occur in adults. Type I lesions represent the very initial changes and are recognized as an increase in the number of intimal macrophages and the appearance of macrophages filled with lipid droplets (foam cells). Type II lesions include the fatty streak lesion, the first grossly visible lesion, and are characterized by layers of macrophage foam cells and lipid droplets within intimal smooth muscle cells and minimal coarse-grained particles and heterogeneous droplets of extracellular lipid. Type III (intermediate) lesions are the morphological and chemical bridge between type II and advanced lesions. Type III lesions appear in some adaptive intimal thickenings (progression-prone locations) in young adults and are characterized by pools of extracellular lipid in addition to all the components of type II lesions." **See**: Arteriosclerosis and Thrombosis, Vol 14, 840-856, 1994 by American Heart Association, "A Definition of Initial, Fatty Streak, and Intermediate Lesions of Atherosclerosis." **Keywords:** Foam cells and fatty streaks

4. Coronary Disease Effects on LV

948. If an embolus were to lodge in the origin of the posterior descending coronary artery (PDCA) at the crux, which heart segment would suffer damage?
   a.   Right ventricle
   b.   Inferior LV wall
   c.   Anterior LV wall
   d.   Lateral LV wall

ANSWER b. Inferior LV wall infarctions result from RCA infarction. The RCA's posterior descending artery feeds the lower 1/3 of the IV septum and descends in the inferior interventricular groove. The crux is the anatomic area in the back of the heart where all 4 chambers intersect and the RCA makes a sudden dip, then it turns 90 degrees and descends to the PDCA. Usually there are also posterior-lateral branches from the RCA at the crux that supply the posterior-lateral LV wall. Understand the coronary distribution to various areas of the LV that may "infarct" when thrombosed. Besides inferior MI, the AV node may become ischemic resulting in some form of heart block on ECG .
See: Grossman, chapter on "Coronary Arteriography."

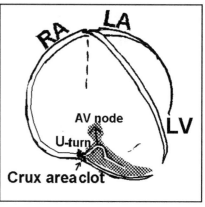

Clot at crux

949. Obstruction of a dominant right coronary artery usually causes myocardial infarction of the _____ region of the LV.
   a.   Apical
   b.   Lateral
   c.   Anterior-septal
   d.   Infer-posterior

ANSWER d. Infer-posterior. In a dominant RCA the PDCA feeds the inferior IV groove, and the posterior lateral branches (LV branches of RCA) feed the inferior posterior LV wall. Inferior MI is seen on ECG leads II, III and aVF. **See:** Braunwald, chapter on "Coronary Arteriography."

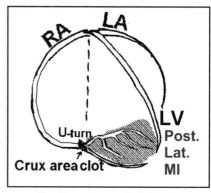

Rt. Dominant RCA MI

950. When evaluating the rate of coronary blood flow in an artery, what is the TIMI grade indicating <u>normal</u> runoff (full opacification within 3 cardiac cycles)?
   a.   0
   b.   3
   c.   4
   d.   10

ANSWER: b. grade 3 TIMI. The TIMI grade is also termed the TIMI myocardial perfusion grade (TMPG).

Kern says,"The Thrombolysis In Myocardial Infarction (TIMI) study group developed a grading scale for coronary blood flow based on visual assessment of the rate of contrast opacification of the infarct artery. The TIMI flow grade has become the standard for semiquantitative evaluation of myocardial perfusion before and after coronary reperfusion therapies. Determination of TIMI flow grade after coronary reperfusion yields important prognostic information in patients with acute myocardial infarction."

This is related to "myocardial blush grade" which is the stained glass appearance as contrast fills the capillary bed beyond a stenosis. TIMI 0 represents minimal or no blush, while TIMI 3 represents a normal myocardial blush. This becomes important if there is collateral circulation around a stenosis.

This TIMI classification was developed by the TIMI (Thrombolysis In Myocardial Infarction) study group to semiquantitatively assess coronary artery perfusion beyond point of occlusion on coronary angiography.

TIMI Grade	Description
TIMI 0 - no perfusion	no antegrade flow beyond the point of occlusion
TIMI 1 - penetration without perfusion	faint antegrade coronary flow beyond the occlusion with incomplete filling of the distal coronary bed
TIMI 2 - partial perfusion	delayed or sluggish antegrade flow with complete filling of the distal territory
TIMI 3 - complete perfusion	normal flow with complete filling of the distal territory

PAMI (Primary Angioplasty in Myocardial Infarction) investigators precised the description of TIMI 3 as "opacification of the vessel within three cardiac cycles).

See: Determination of Angiographic (TIMI Grade) Blood Flow by Intracoronary Doppler Flow Velocity During Acute Myocardial Infarction, Kern, et. al., Circulation, 1996

951. These diagrams show the various patterns of LV regional wall motion in systole. The outer line is the EDV outline. The inner line is the ESV. What type of LV wall motion is shown at #3 on the diagram?

a. Normal
b. Akinetic
c. Dyskinetic
d. Local hypokinetic
e. Global hypokinetic
f. Asynchronous

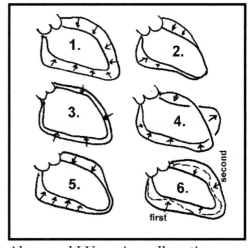

Abnormal LV angio wall motion

ANSWER e. Global hypokinesis.
BE ABLE TO MATCH ALL ANSWERS.
   1. **Normal**
   2. **Akinetic**
   3. **Global hypokinetic**
   4. **Dyskinetic**
   5. **Local hypokinetic**
   6. **Asynchronous**

Further explanations of each type of asynergy:
1. Normal: The normal EF is greater than 50%. Ejection fraction (EF) is the ratio between
   how much blood is pumped each beat to its EDV. **EF = 100% x (SV/EDV)**
A large ejection fraction usually shows a healthy vigorous myocardium. The contraction
should be concentric with all points moving toward the center. This is called synergy.
Myocardial ischemia and infarction produce asymmetrical contractions. This is also termed
asynergy. All the abnormal patterns below show asynergy.
2. Akinetic: No contraction is part of the LV.
3. Global hypokinetic: A diminished but visible motion of the entire LV. Often seen in
   dilated failing hearts.
4. Dyskinetic: A bulging or aneurysmal segment of the LV. This is also termed paradoxical
motion.
5. Local hypokinetic: A diminished but visible motion of part of the LV.
6. Asynchronous: The LV wall does not beat synchronously. Part of the wall beats first -
another part follows.
   A hyperkinetic LV wall is commonly seen on the wall opposite an acute MI in order
to compensate for the akinetic infarcted wall. **See:** Kern, chapter on "Angiography."
Keywords: LV wall motion abnormalities, akinesis, dyskinesis, global hypokinesis...

BOTH QUESTIONS BELOW REFER TO THIS DIAGRAM.

952. **This LV gram of superimposed EDV and ESV**
   frames shows:
   a.   **Inferior wall akinesis**
   b.   **Inferior wall dyskinesis**
   c.   **Septal wall akinesis**
   d.   **Septal wall dyskinesis**

953. **What coronary artery obstruction could cause the**
   LV wall abnormality seen in the abnormal LV
   gram shown?
   a.   **LAD**
   b.   **Circumflex**
   c.   **Diagonal**
   d.   **RV branch of RCA**

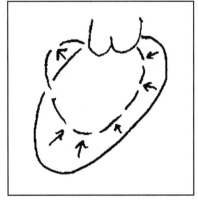
Abnormal LAO LV gram

BOTH ANSWERS LISTED TOGETHER BELOW.

952. ANSWER d. Septal wall dyskinesis. This is an LAO LV gram (apex on the lower left). The septal wall is on the left side in this view. It is bulging or dyskinetic - perhaps from a septal MI. Rupture of the dyskinetic septal wall could lead to a VSD. Actually it is rare to see a septal wall bulging like this, because of the opposing RV pressure.
See: Kern, chapter on "Angiography." **Keywords:** LAO LV angio, septal wall dyskinesis

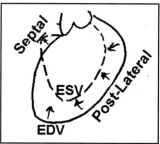
LAO LV Walls

953. ANSWER a. LAD. Normally the LAD supplies the superior 2/3 of the LV septum. But the RCA feeds the inferior 1/3 of the LV septum.
See: Kern, chapter on "Angiography."
Keywords: LAO LV angio, septal wall dyskinesis

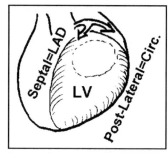
LAO Cor. Supply

954. Acute myocardial infarction of the posterior-lateral wall of the left ventricle is associated with obstruction of what coronary artery?
a. Circumflex
b. Anterior descending
c. Posterior descending
d. Main-stem left

ANSWER a. The circumflex normally feeds the posterior lateral LV wall. In a dominant RCA system the right coronary may also supply part of the posterior lateral wall.
See: Kern, chapter on "Angiography." **Keywords:** LAO LV angio, septal wall dyskinesis

955. LAD coronary artery occlusion may lead to which 3 complications? (Select 3.)
a. Cardiac rupture with tamponade
b. Cardiac rupture with VSD
c. Papillary muscle rupture with MR
d. Sinus of Valsalva AV fistula
e. Sinus node block on ECG

ANSWERS: a, b, & c. Sinus of Valsalva AV fistula is NOT correct. The LAD feeds the LV not the aorta or aortic valve. Coronary A-V fistula is a congenital deformity where one coronary artery empties directly into a cardiac chamber - without passing though a capillary bed. SA node is high in the RA, and not supplied by the LAD.
See: Braunwald, chapter on "Myocardial Infarction."

5. Complications CAD/MI

956. **What is the most common location for a left ventricular aneurysm following acute myocardial infarction?**
a. RV free wall
b. Inferior wall
c. Anterior/apical wall
d. Anterolateral wall

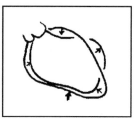

ANSWER c. Anterior/apical wall. An LV aneurysm is a thin walled noncontractile out-pouching which bulges with each systole. It "steals" stroke volume from the LV wasting the LV's contraction on the "dyskinetic" aneurysm. The soft wall of an infarcted ventricle can bulge and even rupture. Most MI aneurysms eventually fibrose and as it becomes firmer can improve the SV.

Ant. wall bulge

  The infarcted artery is usually the LAD coronary artery. Thus these aneurysms usually occur at the apex (thinnest part of LV) or on the anterior LV wall.
See: Braunwald, chapter on "Acute MI." **Keywords:** LV aneurysm, location=apex=LAD

957. **Cardiac rupture only occurs with:**
a. Subendocardial infarction
b. Transmural infarction
c. Diaphragmatic infarction
d. RV infarction

ANSWER b. Transmural infarction. All three walls of the LV must be weakened to allow rupture of the heart. Most ruptures are through the LV free wall into the pericardium and are fatal. **See:** Braunwald, chapter on "Acute MI." **Keywords:** Transmural MI > cardiac rupture

958. **What type of ventricular aneurysm is shown on the diagram at #2.**
a. Wide neck, true anatomic aneurysm
b. Wide neck, true functional aneurysm
c. Narrow neck, false anatomic aneurysm
d. Narrow neck, false functional aneurysm

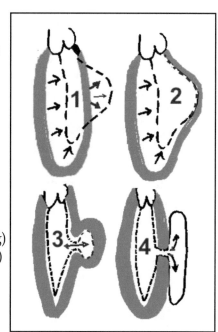

ANSWER a. Wide neck, true anatomic aneurysm.
BE ABLE TO MATCH ALL ANSWERS:
 1. Wide neck, true functional aneurysm (soft - bulging)
 2. Wide neck, true anatomic aneurysm (akinetic - scar)
 3. Narrow neck, true aneurysm
 4. Narrow neck, false aneurysm

TYPES OF LV ANEURYSMS
Dotted line = end systole

All aneurysms are bulges in the outline of the heart or vessel. Anatomic aneurysms are scar tissue and relatively fixed (akinetic). They protrude in both systole and diastole. Whereas, functional aneurysms protrude only in systole (dyskinetic). True aneurysms are composed of scar tissue from all three walls of the heart or artery; whereas, false aneurysms have one or two layers of the heart or artery ruptured. The remaining layers hold the blood in. Besides the anatomic-functional and true-false classifications, aneurysms can be classified by the size of their neck - narrow or wide neck.

1. **WIDE NECK TRUE FUNCTIONAL ANEURYSMS** occur with scarred over MI which contain elements of all three wall layers (endo, myo, and epicardium). Being a "functional" aneurysm it is "dyskinetic" and bulges out in systole and returns in diastole. This bulging action "steals" stroke volume from the LV. These seldom rupture.

2. **WIDE NECK TRUE ANATOMIC ANEURYSMS** occur with a scarred over MI which weakens a large area of myocardium. True aneurysms contain elements of all three wall layers (endo, myo, and epicardium). Anatomic aneurysms are scarred over and NON-FUNCTIONAL or AKINETIC. These seldom rupture.

3. **NARROW NECK TRUE ANEURYSMS** occur with MI's which do not rupture through all three walls of the LV. This soft wall bulges through a narrow neck in systole making a dyskinetic diverticulum of thinned LV wall. These seldom rupture.

4. **NARROW NECK FALSE ANEURYSMS** occur with a rupture of the ventricle which communicates through a narrow neck with a pouch (usually of pericardium). It looks like a blister bulging with each systole. The walls of a false aneurysm contain clot and hematoma and are at a **high risk of rupture. Be able to identify all aneurysm types.**

See: Braunwald, chapter on "Chronic Coronary Artery disease." **Keywords:** Types of aneurysms, fusiform, mycotic, narrow - wide neck, anatomic - anatomic, true - false

959. **A false LV ventricular aneurysm is composed of bulging:**
a. RV which appears to be an LV aneurysm
b. Pericardium and clotted hematoma
c. All three layers of myocardium
d. Only one layer of myocardium

ANSWER b. Pericardium and clotted hematoma. These narrow necked thin aneurysms usually result from rupture of a transmural MI. The aneurysm is composed of pericardium, hematoma, and clot. All this debris helps prevent LV rupture and cardiac tamponade. Some false aneurysms bulge in systole. Others seal completely. If the narrow neck remains open, the aneurysm bulges and enlarges - it may rupture.
See: Braunwald, chapter on "Acute MI." **Keywords:** False LV aneurysm

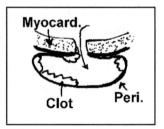

False Aneurysm

960. Identify the abnormality in this ventriculogram.

a. Mycotic LV false aneurysm
b. Fusiform anterior LV aneurysm
c. True functional apical aneurysm
d. Anatomic scarred LV aneurysm

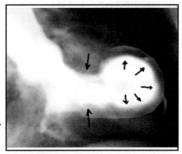
RAO LV gram

ANSWER c. True functional apical aneurysms are dyskinetic. They are "true" in that they contain all three wall layers (endo, myo, and epicardium) and are "functional" because they bulge out in systole and return in diastole, as shown. This bulging action "steals" stroke volume from the LV. Here you can see the LV apical wall is bulging, and appears to still have intact LV wall around it, although somewhat thinned because the bulge causes wall thinning. **See:** Braunwald, chapter on "Acute MI." **Keywords:** True functional aneurysm

6. Signs and Symptoms CAD/MI

961. Which cardiac enzyme peaks earliest, usually within a few hours after myocardial infarction, and declines most rapidly?

a. Troponin (TnT)
b. CK-MB
c. Myoglobin
d. LD (Lactate dehydrogenase)

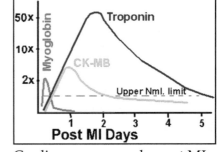
Cardiac enzyme peaks post MI

ANSWER c. Myoglobin is released into the circulation from injured myocardial cells and can be detected within 1-4 hours after the onset of infarction or reperfusion. It is usually below normal within one day post MI. However, myoglobin is not completely cardiac specific and should be supplemented by more specific enzymes such as troponin (cTnT). It rises and declines rapidly as shown. Creatine Kinase - Muscle/Brain (CK-MB) peaks at 24 hours.

Braunwald says, "elevated levels of CK-MB isoenzyme may be considered, for practical purposes, to be the result fo AMI (except in cases of trauma or surgery...)."

Post MI troponin rise may be tremendous, up to 50 times normal upper limit. Its peak and decline show a delayed time course making it useful for the late diagnosing of MI.

LDH reaches a peak at 3-6 days after initial MI and may take 2 weeks to decline to normal. The timing of the peaks of these curves help time an MI. Understand all cardiac enzymes. **See:** Braunwald chapter on "Acute MI" **Keywords:** Myoglobin cTnT enzyme peaks earliest

962. **The most specific and commonly used biomarker to detect myocardial necrosis is:**
   a.   Myoglobin
   b.   CK-MB
   c.   Troponin
   d.   Creatine kinase-MB

ANSWER: c. Troponin.
   Patient.Info says, "Cardiac troponin I and T have displaced myoglobin and creatine kinase-MB as the preferred markers of myocardial injury.... Troponin is a protein released from myocytes when irreversible myocardial damage occurs. It is highly specific to cardiac tissue and accurately diagnoses myocardial infarction with a history of ischemic pain or ECG changes reflecting ischaemia. Cardiac troponin level is dependent on infarct size, thus providing an indicator for the prognosis following an infarction." **See:**
http://patient.info/doctor/cardiac-enzymes-and-markers-for-myocardial-infarction

963. **In acute MI what is the pattern of troponin rise following successful revascularization (PCI or thrombolysis) compared to an untreated MI?**
   a.   Rises to higher peak, then falls early with less area under the curve
   b.   Rises to higher peak, then falls late with more area under the curve
   c.   Lower peak, then falls early with less area under the curve
   d.   Lower peak, then falls late with more area under the curve

ANSWER: a. Rises to higher peak, then falls early. The area under the troponin-time curve is smaller following successful revascularization, indicating myocardial salvage. Following successful revascularization the peak circulating enzyme levels tend to occur earlier and are often higher following successful thrombolytic therapy because accumulated metabolites are flushed out of the newly opened artery.

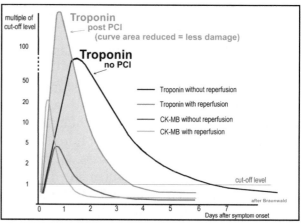

964. **What are the 3 serum markers for cardiac damage in acute MI? (Select 3.)**
   a.   Troponin (cTnI)
   b.   Lactic Dehydrogenase (LDH)
   c.   Glucose -6-phosphatese (G6P)
   d.   Creatine Kinase - (CK-MB isoenzyme)
   e.   BNP (Brain Natriuretic Hormone)

ANSWERS: a, b, & d. Glucose -6-phosphatese (G6P) is NOT a cardiac enzyme. BNP is an indicator of heart failure.
   Babuin says, "Troponin is the biomarker of choice for the detection of cardiac injury. .... Cardiac isoforms of troponin are specific for the heart. Elevated troponin levels indicate cardiac injury but do not define the mechanism. In patients with acute coronary ischemia

and elevated troponin levels, myocardial infarction should be diagnosed; treatment should be guided by the elevated troponin levels." **See:** Babuin & Jaffe,"Troponin: the biomarker of choice for the detection of cardiac injury", 2005, online at http://www.ncbi.nlm.nih.gov/pmc/articles/PMC1277047/

   McCord says, "Acute myocardial infarction can be excluded rapidly in the emergency department by use of point-of-care measurements of myoglobin and troponin I during the first 90 minutes after presentation." **See:** McCord, et. Al., "Ninety-Minute Exclusion of Acute Myocardial Infarction By Use of Quantitative Point-of-Care Testing of Myoglobin and Troponin I." Circulation, 2001

965. **The most common arrhythmia found in patients recovering from MI is:**
 a. V. Fib.
 b. V. Tach.
 c. PACs (APCs)
 d. PVCs (VPCs)

ANSWER d. PVCs are most common, especially in the setting of myocardial ischemia. Ischemic tissue may set up a reentry loop which cause unifocal PVCs or multifocal PVCs. Runs of 3 or more PVCs are called ventricular tachycardia. Runs are more serious than single PVCs. Treatment for MI includes: O2, pain relief, and alteration of hemodynamics with nitroglycerine and beta blockers. Routine lidocaine is no longer routinely recommended for patients with frequent PVCs post MI. ***Treat the patient not the monitor.***
See: ACLS, chapter on "Evaluation and treatment of arrhythmias associated with MI."

966. **Identify the 3 warning symptoms of a heart attack. (Select 3)**
 a. **Resembling indigestion**
 b. **Pressure in the center of the chest**
 c. **Intermittent sharp stabbing pains in the chest**
 d. **Pain in chest that move to shoulders, neck, arms.**
 e. **Acute intense headache**

ANSWERS: a, b, & d.
 a. Resembling indigestion - YES
 b. Pressure in the center of the chest - YES
 c. Intermittent sharp stabbing pains in the chest - NO
 d. Pain in the chest that moves to the shoulders, neck, and arms - YES
 e. Headache more commonly associated with stroke - NO
Stabbing pains termed "pleuritic" are NOT commonly associated with heart attack. Angina pain is more commonly described as choking, dull, or a pressure sensation.
See: AHA manual BLS **Keywords:** sharp stabbing pains not angina

967. Referred angina pain from myocardial ischemia is most commonly located in the patient's precordium and :
a.   Along the ulnar aspect of the left arm
b.   Along the radial aspect of the right arm
c.   Between the shoulder blades
d.   Between backbone and sternum

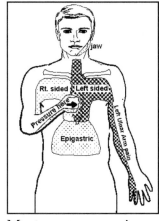

ANSWER a. Along the inner or ulnar aspect of the left arm. Referred angina pain most often occurs in the center of the sternum, inner aspect of the left arm and up the left neck and jaw. This is usually described not as "pain" but as pressure, squeezing or a gasping tightness. It may be described as the patient clenches his fist on his chest.

   With severe ischemia other areas may become involved such as the: right arm, jaw, epigastrium, and back. Much related useful knowledge can be acquired by taking a CPR instructors class, available through the American Heart Association.
See: Underhill, chapter on "Myocardial Ischemia." **Keywords:** location of angina

Most common angina locations

968. Which of the following is termed STABLE angina?
a.   New onset of angina, brought on by mild exertion
b.   Severe angina relieved with rest or beta blockers
c.   Angina at rest not relieved by rest or nitroglycerine
d.   Angina brought on by exertion, relieved by rest or nitroglycerine

ANSWER d. Angina brought on by exertion, relieved by rest or nitroglycerine. Stable angina comes on with exertion and is relieved by rest or nitroglycerine. The other answers are types of UNSTABLE angina usually associated with a complicated plaque lesion in a coronary artery. These types of lesions usually need intervention such as PCI to prevent an platelet aggregation, thrombosis, and impending heart attack. Stable angina is usually treated with rest and medications.
See: Braunwald, chapter on "Chronic Coronary Artery Disease." **Keywords:** Stable angina

969. What type of angina is this: "An attack of chest pain at rest during which the electrocardiogram shows changes identical with those of the early stage of myocardial infarction, but returns to the previous pattern after the attack."
a.   Chronic stable angina
b.   Variant or Prinzmetal angina
c.   Syncopal angina
d.   Preinfarction or unstable angina

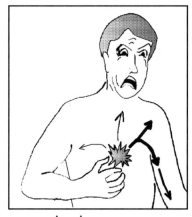

ANSWER b. Variant or Prinzmetal angina is a dynamic

Angina

angina. Dynamic because it appears without warning, even while the patient is at rest. Variant angina is due to coronary spasm and is quickly relieved with nitroglycerine and Ca blocker medications. This is not the type of lesion you would angioplasty. The smooth muscle spasm will just return. (Understand how this differs from a fixed atheromatous lesion.) **See:** Braunwald, chapter on "Examination of the Patient." **Keywords:** variant or Prinzmetal angina

970. **A special type of angina at rest caused by SPASM of a coronary artery is termed:**
   a.   **Silent or ischemic angina**
   b.   **Unstable or pre-infarction angina**
   c.   **Stable or classic angina pectoris**
   d.   **Prinzmetal or variant angina**

ANSWER d. Prinzmetal or variant angina. This angina pain feels like classic angina except it usually occurs at rest and is seldom induced by exertion or stress as classic angina is. ST segments elevate as in acute MI injury pattern and may spontaneously resolve. It may cause MI, arrhythmia or sudden death. It may be induced with ergonovine. Nitroglycerine usually reduces the spasm.
See: Braunwald, chapter on "Acute MI." **Keywords:** Prinzmetal or variant angina

971. **Angina pectoris is an unpleasant chest sensation which is most often described by patients as: (Select 3)**
   1. **"Dull ache"**
   2. **"Sharp stabbing pain"**
   3. **"Band across my chest"**
   4. **"Sharp pain" aggravated by breathing**
   5. **"Squeezing or strangling sensation"**
   6. **"Jabbing pain" which lessens upon sitting**
   7. **Pressure sensation like a "weight on my chest"**
      a. 1, 3, 6
      b. 2, 4, 6
      c. 3, 5, 7
      d. 4, 6, 7

ANSWER c. 3, 5, 7
   1. NO: Dull ache
   2. NO: Sharp stabbing pain
   3. **YES:** Band across my chest
   4. NO: Pinching pain aggravated by breathing
   5. **YES:** Squeezing or strangling sensation
   6. NO: Jabbing pain which lessens upon sitting
   7. **YES:** Pressure sensation like a weight on my chest

The feelings associated with angina pectoris are due to myocardial ischemia. These feelings may be mild (sometimes as indigestion) or very intense and are usually relieved with nitroglycerine. It is sensed not so much as a pain but as pressure or strangulation. A classic sign is the patient clenching his fist and pressing to his/her sternum as he/she describes it.

In contrast **ANSWER B. 2, 4, 6** is how patients most commonly describe the pain of acute pericarditis - sharp and jabbing exaggerated by position or breathing.
See: Braunwald, chapter on "Physical Examination." **Keywords:** Angina pectoris sensations = pressure, strangling

972. **A patient with angina is brought for coronary arteriography. His coronary arteries all appear normal even when stressed. This is termed:**
a.   **Syndrome Y**
b.   **Syndrome X**
c.   **Variant Angina**
d.   **Stable Angina**

ANSWER b. Syndrome X. This is a syndrome of angina like chest pain with a normal coronary arteriogram. Even coronary stressors such as hand-grip exercises or ergonovine challenge do no usually reveal any coronary defects. These patients may constitute 10-20% of the patients brought to cath. Although the cause of syndrome-X is unclear, many of these patients may have microvascular dysfunction due to small resistance vessels not visible on angiography. Although many of these patients have ischemic defects on ECG or Thallium abnormalities during exercise, their prognosis is usually excellent. Nitroglycerine is usually ineffective at relieving this angina, so calcium blockers may be used.
See: Braunwald, chapter on "Chronic Coronary Artery Disease." **Keywords:** Syndrome X

973. **The three <u>major</u> risk factors associated with heart attacks are:**
1. **Diabetes**
2. **Cigarette smoking**
3. **Stress/ Type "A" behavior**
4. **High blood cholesterol**
5. **Hypertension**
        a. 1, 2, 4
        b. 1, 4, 5
        c. 2, 3, 4
        d. 2, 4, 5

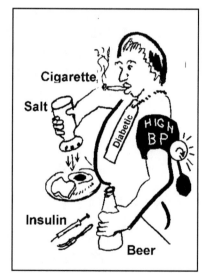

ANSWER d. 2, 4, & 5. The American Heart Association teaches these three major risk factors. They happen to be the three factors which can be changed. As medical professionals we need to encourage all our patients to reduce these risk factors.
        1. NO: Diabetes
        2. YES: Cigarette smoking
        3. NO: Stress/ Type "A" behavior
        4. YES: High blood cholesterol
        5. **YES:** Hypertension

Cardiovascular Risk Factors

See: American Heart Association, ACLS manual, chapter on "Risk Factors." **Keywords:** Risk factors, 3 main

974. **Persons experiencing early signs & symptoms of a heart attack most commonly:**

a.   Begin exercising to "work it off"
b.   Deny they are having a heart attack
c.   Drive themselves to the Dr.
d.   Go to sleep to relieve the pain

ANSWER b. Denial is a common sign of heart attack. MI victims often say "it's just indigestion." or "It will go away." The fear of having an MI is too great. "Macho Men" especially tend to deny the pain, even when it is excruciating. The American Heart Association teaches family members to override the protests of a symptomatic individual and call 911 immediately.
See: American Heart Association, ACLS manual, chapter on "Risk Factors."

975. **A person with an acute RCA myocardial infarction may develop a condition known as "Stokes-Adams Syndrome." The physical signs of this syndrome are:**
a.   Cyanosis and dyspnea
b.   Cold clammy skin with a pallid coloration
c.   Pain in the chest radiating to the arms and neck
d.   Vertigo, fainting, and convulsions

ANSWER d. Vertigo, fainting, and convulsions. Stokes-Adams attack or syndrome involves fainting due to insufficient cerebral blood flow. It is usually preceded by the eyes rolling up and labored breathing (tongue swallowing). It is often associated with complete heart block, due to AV node ischemia from the RCA insufficiency. Repeating Adam-Stokes attacks and bradycardia are classic indications for pacemaker implantation.
See: Medical Dictionary **Keywords**: Adams-Stokes syndrome

7. ECG Changes CAD/MI

976. **The ECG change most associated with transmural myocardial infarction is:**
a.   Pathologic Q-wave
b.   Inverted T wave
c.   Prolonged QT interval
d.   Depressed ST segment

ANSWER a. Pathologic Q waves appear in the first day of an MI. Although they may resolve with time, they usually remain on the ECG throughout the patient's life as telltale markers of the dead myocardium. Q waves are pathologic when they are SIGNIFICANTLY LARGE - both deep and wide. Significant Q waves are seen in any of the first 3 V leads or if they are over >.04 sec. (1 box) in duration (or over ⅓ the height of the R wave) in leads 1, 2, aVL, aVF, V4, V5, or V6.

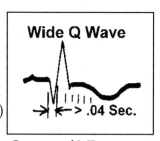
Q wave of MI

Q wave being a negative wave means that the depolarization forces are "away" from the electrode. It's like the "infarcted" dead tissue beneath the electrode is a "window" looking into the LV and watching the remaining viable LV depolarize "away" from it. Q wave vectors point "away" from the area of infarction.

The term "Q wave infarct" describes a significant transmural infarct with pathologic Q waves where the ECG "looks through" this window of dead tissue.

See: Braunwald, chapter on "Electrocardiography..." **Keywords:** MI = pathologic "Q" wave

977. **An OLD myocardial infarct is seen on the ECG as a significant:**
- a.   **Q wave**
- b.   **Inverted "T" wave**
- c.   **Elevated ST segment**
- d.   **Depressed ST segment**

ANSWER a. Q waves never go away. Since dead myocardial tissue does not conduct, it makes an electrically silent area. The Q wave looks through this window at the remaining myocardium depolarizing away from it. Note how the infarction enlarges the Q wave, and drags down the QRS complex. To be significant the Q wave must be wide (>1 box) and deeper than 1/3 of the QRS complex.
See: Braunwald, chapter on "Myocardial Infarction." **Keywords:** Q wave = old MI

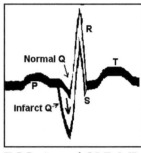
ECG sign of OLD MI

978. **Which of the following ECG changes results from acute myocardial INJURY?**
- a.   **Pathologic Q-wave**
- b.   **T wave inversion**
- c.   **ST segment elevation**
- d.   **ST segment depression**

ANSWER c. Elevated ST segments signal an acute INJURY to the heart. They are seen in the first hours after MI, also during PCI inflation. Injury is a reversible process that may lead to infarction if allowed to progress. If this diagram were from lead II, it would signify acute inferior wall injury.
See: Braunwald, chapter on "Electrocardiography..."

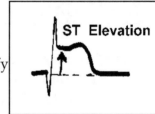
ST - Injury

979. **Which of the following ECG changes results from myocardial ischemia?**
- 1. **Pathologic Q-wave**
- 2. **T wave inversion**
- 3. **ST segment elevation**
- 4. **ST segment depression**
    - a. 1, 2
    - b. 2, 3
    - c. 2, 4
    - d. 3, 4

ANSWER c. 2 & 4 (T wave inversion, & ST segment depression.) Ischemia is the lack of sufficient oxygenated blood to the LV. It shows on the ECG as symmetrically inverted T waves or ST depression.

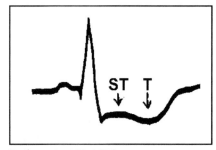

Ischemic ↓T, ↓ST waves

Normally the T waves should be upright in all leads (except III, aVR, and V1). When T waves are present in several leads it means that an infarction has occurred some time ago - how long is uncertain. It is neither an "acute" infarction or an "old" infarction but somewhere in between. These are termed "age indeterminate" inverted or ischemic T waves.

ST depression is a common symptom of ischemia on exercise. Treadmill testing relies heavily on ST depression markers. They may also be seen as reciprocal ST changes of an acute MI. Remember the leads OVER an acute infarction show ST elevation. This forces the leads beneath an infarction to be depressed. It's like looking at a vector from the opposite direction. It appears to be going the other way. An acute inferior MI will show ST elevation in lead III, but inversion in lead aVL (which is an almost opposite lead direction).
See: Davis, chapter on Ischemia, Injury, and Infarction.

980. **In ACS (acute coronary syndrome) N-STEMI cases are associated with:**
a. **Transmural infarction, ST elevation on ECG**
b. **Transmural infarction, ST & T wave depression**
c. **Subendocardial infarction, ST elevation on ECG**
d. **Subendocardial infarction, ST & T wave depression**

ANSWER: d. Subendocardial infarction, ST & T wave depression.

Dr. Svenkatesan says: "The pain of UA [Unstable Angina] is due to subtotal occlusion and endocardial ischemia, while STEMI is sudden total occlusion and the resultant transmural ischemia. In STEMI epicardial surface is always involved (Which lifts the ST segment in ECG.)" **See:**
https://drsvenkatesan.com/tag/how-is-chest-pain-different-between-nstemi-and-stemi/

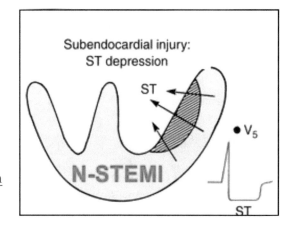

ACLS.net says: "High-risk unstable angina (UA) or NSTEMI (non-ST-segment elevation myocardial infarction). Definition: Ischemic ST-segment depression of 0.5 mm (0.5 mV) or greater -OR- Dynamic T wave inversion with pain or discomfort." **See:**
https://www.acls.net/acute-coronary-syndromes-algorithm.htm

981. This is a diagram of the rings of cell damage during acute inferior MI. What ECG finding is usually associated with the middle "injured" area labeled #2 on the diagram?

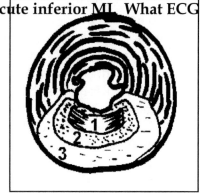

Area of Acute MI

a. ST segment elevation
b. T wave depression
c. Pathologic Q wave

ANSWER a. ST segment elevation.
BE ABLE TO MATCH ALL ANSWERS.
    1. **INFARCTION:** pathologic Q wave
    2. **INJURY:** ST segment elevation
    3. **ISCHEMIA:** symmetric inverted "T" wave depression

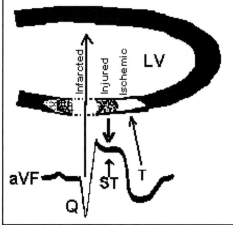

MI's Three I's

This is the classic triad of acute MI. They are used to tell how old the MI is. Normally only 1 or 2 of these will be present at one time. The diagram shows the inferior wall of the LV undergoing a myocardial infarction. The middle stage of an acute MI may show all 3 of these signs at the same time.

    ● The inferior ECG leads closest to the MI (aVF, I & II) will show pathologic Q waves, that see through the dead tissue (due to infarcted area #1).
    ● ST elevation waves (vectors) point toward the acute injury (area #2)
    ● T wave inversion (vectors) point away from ischemic area (#3)

See: Dubin, chapter on "MI." **Keywords:** Injury = ST elevation

REFERENCES:

Baim, D. S and Grossman W.., Cardiac Catheterization, Angiography, and Intervention, 7th Ed., Lea and Febiger, 2006

Braunwald, Eugene, Ed., HEART DISEASE A Textbook of Cardiovascular Medicine, 9th Ed., W. B. Saunders Co., 2012

DeWood, Spores, Notske, et al, "Prevalence of total coronary occlusion during the early hours of transmural myocardial infarction" N. Engl J Med 303:897, 1980.

Kern, M. J., Ed., The Cardiac Catheterization Handbook, 6th Ed., Mosby-Year Book, Inc., 2016

Underhill, S. L., Ed., CARDIAC NURSING, 2nd Ed., J. B. Lippincott Co., 1989

Textbook of ADVANCED CARDIAC LIFE SUPPORT, American Heart Asn., 2017

Dubin, Dale, RAPID INTERPRETATION of EKG's, 3rd Ed., Cover Publishing Co., 1982

Davis, Dale, How to Quickly and Accurately Master ECG Interpretation, 2ND Ed., J. B. Lippincott Co., 1985

Teo, et.al. "Utility of Intravascular Ultrasound in the Diagnosis of Ambiguous Calcific Left Main Stenoses" JIC, Jul 03 2004

OUTLINE: C3 - Coronary Artery Disease and MI

1. Coronary Anatomy
   a. Review normal Cor. Art. anatomy
      i. Left Main
      ii. LAD
      iii. Circumflex
      iv. RCA
         (1) PDCA
   b. Micro-anatomy
      i. Epicardial arteries & veins
      ii. Endocardial arteries & veins
         (1) Compressed in systole
         (2) Thebesian veins / plexus
         (3) TMR - Laser surgery
   c. Coronary Regions
      i. Right Coronary LV region
         (1) AV block
      ii. LAD Coronary LV region
         (1) Ant. Apical MI
            (a) (most common)
      iii. Cx. Coronary LV region
      iv. Left Main = widowmaker
         (1) 90% mortality
   d. MI effect on LV contraction
      i. Akinetic
      ii. Global hypokinetic
      iii. Dyskinetic
      iv. Local hypokinetic
      v. Asynchronous
   e. Review Cor. Vein Anatomy
      i. CRT (Lat. LV vein)
      ii. Coronary Sinus
      iii. Same grooves as arteries
         (1) LAD - Great Card. Vn.
         (2) PDCA - Middle Vn.
         (3) RCA - small Vn.
      iv. Collateral circulation
         (1) Bridge severe stenosis
         (2) Natural bypasses
         (3) Minimize effect of MI
         (4) Large epicardial collaterals
         (5) Capillary size usually subendocardial
         (6) Recruitment
         (7) Building collaterals = Exercise
   f. Critical stenosis >50% diam.
      i. Critical area >75%
   g. Calculation of % stenosis

2. General Ischemic Ht. Disease
   a. Atherosclerosis & CAD
      i. Ischemia = O2 starved = T
      ii. Injury = damage = ST
      iii. Infarction = necrosis, death
         (1) Q waves
   b. Acute Coronary Syndrome
      i. STEMI =
         (1) ST elevation MI

      ii. N-STEMI
         (1) NonST elevation MI
      iii. Stunned / hibernating myocardium
   c. Etiology CAD
      i. Histologic changes in CAD
         (1) Fatty streaks
         (2) Plaque
         (3) Ruptured plaque
         (4) Thrombosis
      ii. Kawasaki CAD
      iii. Syndrome X
   d. Most common cause of death

3. Coronary Flow
   a. Diastole
   b. Systolic endocardial compression
   c. HR effect of flow
   d. CFR

4. Pathophysiology of CAD
   a. Transmural infarction
      i. STEMI, CAD thrombosis
      ii. ST elevation - tombstones
      iii. Braunwald's theorem: time is muscle
   b. Subendocardial Infarction
      i. Raised Plaque
      ii. N-STEMI
         (1) ST & T depression
         (2) Loss endo. Fn. (NO)
   c. Plaque
      i. 3 contents
         (1) Lipid
         (2) Smooth muscle
         (3) Collagen
   d. Spasm
      i. Prinzmetal angina
      ii. Provocation c methylergonovine
   e. Thrombus - MI
   f. Classes of lesions (4)
      i. Type I
      ii. Type II
      iii. Type III
      iv. Type IV
      v. Concentric/eccentric
   g. Coronary Dissections (6)
      i. D = Spiral
      ii. F = total occlusion

5. Complication CAD/MI
   a. Anterior MI most common
   b. Transmural MI with rupture
   c. LV Aneurysms
      i. true
      ii. functional
      iii. false
      iv. wide - narrow neck
      v. fusiform

vi. mycotic

6. Signs and symptoms CAD/MI
   a. Stable angina
   b. Unstable angina
   c. Prinzmetal angina
   d. PAIN: Type & location
   e. Risk factors
      i. Denial
      ii. 3 major (AHA)
         (1) hypertension
         (2) smoking
         (3) cholesterol
      iii. Unchangeable - changeable
   f. Adam-Stokes attack

7. Biomarkers
   a. Myoglobin
   b. Troponin

c. CK-MB

8. CAD Therapy
   a. Thrombolytics
   b. Other medications
      i. Nitro, Aspirin, Plavix, heparin, Morphine
      ii. Beta blockers, Ace inhibitors
   c. CABG
      i. Grafts
         (1) IMA
         (2) Radial Artery
         (3) Saphenous
         (4) Skip
   d. PCI
      i. Angioplasty (balloon)
      ii. Stent (BMS, DES, bioabsorbable)
   e. Gene therapy

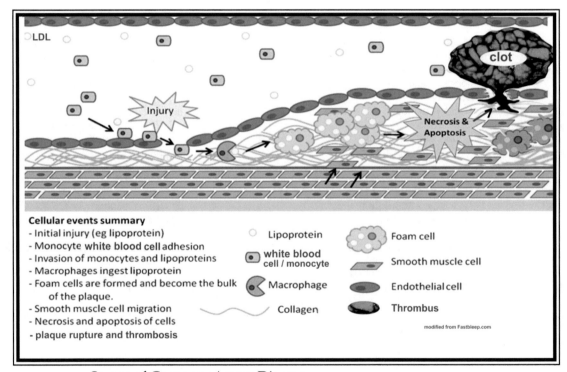

Stages of Coronary Artery Disease

Heart Failure and Shock

1. General CHF Pathology

982. Heart failure is an abnormal state of cardiac function which fails to meet the needs of metabolizing tissues or can only meet them with:
a. Increased coronary flow
b. Increased cholinergic stimulation
c. Increased blood pressure
d. Increased venous pressure

ANSWER d. Increased venous pressure. Heart failure is a pathologic state where poor cardiac function fails to pump enough blood to meet the requirements of metabolizing tissues, or it can only do so with an elevated filling pressure.

CHF is caused by either a weakening of myocardial contraction (as from acute MI) or an inability of the heart to meet some acute volume or pressure load (such as acute AI or AS); or the diastolic function is impaired (as in pericardial tamponade). CHF has many causes. But THE COMMON DENOMINATOR IS COMPENSATORY **ELEVATION OF THE VENOUS PRESSURES. This means increased CVP in right heart failure, and/or increased Wedge, PAedp, and LVEDP in left heart failure.**
See: Braunwald, chapter on "Clinical Aspect of Heart Failure." **Keywords:** CHF ➜ failure to meet metabolic needs, elevated venous pressures

983. Identify 3 compensatory mechanisms used to maintain cardiac output in CHF.
a. Increased preload
b. Reduced afterload
c. Myocardial hypertrophy
d. Increased catecholamines

ANSWERS: a, c, & d. Reduced afterload is NOT correct. The afterload (resistance) increases in CHF. This results from the increased sympathetic and catecholamine levels. Here is a list of the short term compensatory effects on failing hearts. Note how the long term effect is usually bad and in the end stages of CHF leads to cardiac exhaustion.

RESPONSE TO IMPAIRED CARDIAC PERFORMANCE

Compensatory mechanism	Short term effect	Long term effect
Na & H20 retention	↑ Preload	Congestion (PE)
Vasoconstriction	Maintains BP	↑ Cardiac work
↑ Sympathetic tone	↑ Heart rate	↑ Cardiac work
↑ hypertrophy	Unloads individual myocardial fibers	Cell deterioration & cardiomyopathy
Collagen deposition		Impairs relaxation

See: Braunwald, chapter on "Pathology of Heart Failure." **Keywords:** CHF, compensatory mechanism, NOT reduced afterload

984. **In CHF, elevation of Ventricular End Diastolic Pressure (LV-EDP) increases ventricular performance but in the long term leads to deleterious:**
a. Myocardial atrophy
b. Decreased work load on the heart
c. Vasoconstriction in periphery
d. Venous congestion

ANSWER d. Venous congestion. The increased venous pressures increase diastolic filling which increases the force of contraction according to Starling's law. But the price patients pay for this is venous congestion and pulmonary edema. This reduces arterial O2 saturation and increases the work of breathing. It eventually dilates the heart, weakens it, and backs up into the right heart.
See: Underhill, chapter on "Heart Failure." **Keywords:** CHF, increased preload

985. **Congestive heart failure patients retain excessive amounts of:**
a. Bicarbonate
b. Acid
c. Sodium
d. Potassium

ANSWER c. Sodium. The reduced CO in CHF makes the kidneys retain Na+. This results in fluid retention and increased blood volume, which leads to increased preload. This is accomplished by increased renin-aldosterone levels through the kidneys and adrenal gland. ACE inhibitors break this renin-aldosterone cycle and prevent sodium retention.
See: Braunwald, chapter on "Clinical Aspect of Heart Failure." **Keywords:** CHF, NA retention

986. **In response to an acute MI the LVs first hemodynamic compensatory mechanism is to _____ LV end diastolic PRESSURE and _____ LV end diastolic VOLUME.**
    a.   ↑LV-edp, ↑LV-edv
    b.   ↓LV-edp, ↓LV-edv
    c.   ↓LV-edp, ↑LV-edv
    d.   ↑LV-edp, ↓LV-edv

ANSWER a. ↑LV-edp, ↑LV-edv. The failing heart tries to compensate for acute injury which overtaxes its ability to pump. The sequence of events is:

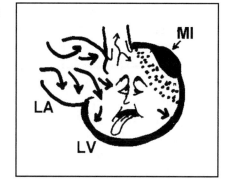

   1. ↑Ventricular EDV & EDP
   2. Increasing LA pressure and atrial kick
   3. Increasing pulmonary capillary and venous pressure
   4. Transudation of fluid into the pulmonary capillary bed, leading to pulmonary edema.

These are important compensatory mechanisms in response to pump failure, but they cause their own problems. The high preload leads to pulmonary congestion and a vicious cycle of increasing cardiac work, increasing wall tension, and myocardial cell deterioration.

Hemodynamic compensation in acute MI

See: Braunwald, chapter on "Pathology of Heart Failure." **Keywords:** CHF, compensation, ↑LV-edp, ↑LV-edv

987. **Chronic left heart failure, if allowed to progress, usually leads to:**
    a.   **Atherosclerotic heart disease (ASHD)**
    b.   **Dilated aortic root and AR**
    c.   **Hypertension (systemic)**
    d.   **Right heart failure**

ANSWER d. Right heart failure. As the failing LV "fails" to pump out all the blood brought to it, it in effect "dams up" the venous blood. Blood backs up through the LA, pulmonary capillaries, pulmonary arteries, RV, and eventually the RA. Just like a dam backs liquid upstream. Thus the term "backward failure."

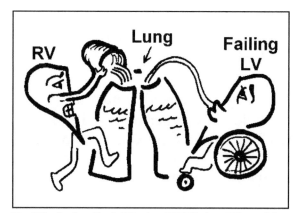

   With time the pulmonary congestion backs up of into the right side of the heart. Then the right heart must increase its pressure and work to support the ailing left heart. So left sided failure leads to right sided failure.

Rt. Ht. helps Left Ht. in CHF(after Tipp 64)

See: Braunwald, chapter on "Clinical Aspect of Heart Failure." **Keywords:** Lt. sided CHF ➔ Rt. sided CHF ➔ backward failure

988. **Right sided CHF eventually leads to:**
a.   SOB and DOE
b.   Left sided CHF
c.   LVH with strain
d.   RVH, RAD, and atrial hypertrophy

ANSWER d. RVH, RAD, and atrial hypertrophy. Right sided CHF dilates and hypertrophies the RV (RVH), leading to right axis deviation on the ECG and pulmonary hypertension. This also leads to Jugular Venous Distension (JVD), hepatomegaly, and edematous ankles. The pressure in the systemic tissues (RA pressure) is not great enough to back up into the systemic arterial circulation (AO pressure).
    NO: SOB = Shortness of Breath: DOE = Dyspnea On Exertion - all signs of LEFT sided heart failure.
    NO: Left sided CHF = Congestive Heart Failure
    NO: LVH with strain = Left Ventricular Hypertrophy associated with hypertension and left sided heart failure
    YES: RVH = Right Ventricular Hypertrophy, RAD = Right Axis Deviation.
See: Braunwald, chapter on "Clinical Aspect of Heart Failure." **Keywords:** Lt. sided CHF
➡ Rt. sided CHF

989. **Which of the following is considered the primary cause of LV hypertrophy without dilatation?**
a.   Increased volume load
b.   Decreased volume load
c.   Increased pressure load
d.   Decreased pressure load

ANSWER c. Increased LV pressure leads to a thick muscular LV. Pressure overload as seen in AS or hypertension develops hypertrophied LV muscle mass and strength. It's like the weight lifter pumping iron - his muscles thicken. More sarcomeres are added in parallel to thicken and strengthen the muscle, not dilate it.
See: Braunwald, chapter on "Pathology of Heart Failure." **Keywords:** CHF, pressure overload ➡ hypertrophy

990. **This diagram shows LV myocardial dilatation and hypertrophy patterns seen in CHF. The pattern seen at #3 in the diagram is _____ and is usually a compensation for _____.**

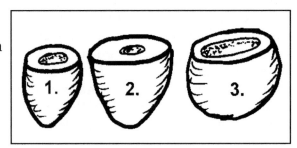
LV Dilation - hypertrophy patterns

a.   Dilation, Volume overload
b.   Dilation, Pressure overload,
c.   Hypertrophy, Volume overload
d.   Hypertrophy, Pressure overload

ANSWER a. Dilation, Volume overload.
CORRECTLY MATCHED ANSWERS ARE:
1. Normal
2. **Hypertrophy** which is a parallel replication of myofibrils, **(pressure overload.)** Increased LV pressure, as seen in AS, leads to a thick muscular LV - like pumping iron. The LV wall is disproportionally thickened. This thickening is due to parallel (side by side) building of sarcomeres.
3. **Dilation** which is a "series" replication of myofibrils **(volume overload.)** As increasing volume stretches the LV it adds myofibrils onto the ends of others (in series) and thus lengthening them. However, an LV that is dilated too thin could rupture - according to Laplace's law. So, some hypertrophy must thicken the wall to keep the ratio of wall

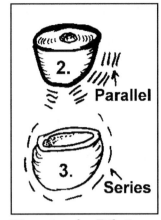

Hypertrophy Dilation

thickness to LV radius normal. For this reason, we seldom see pure dilatation.
See: Braunwald, chapter on "Pathology of Heart Failure." **Keywords:** CHF, pressure & volume overload, dilatation

991. **Your patient comes to the cath lab with a diagnosis of left heart failure with diastolic dysfunction. You would expect his hemodynamics to show:**
a. EF > 40% and LVEDP > 18 mmHg
b. EF > 40% and LVEDP < 18 mmHg
c. EF < 40% and LVEDP > 18 mmHg
d. EF < 40% and LVEDP < 18 mmHg

ANSWER a. EF > 40% and LVEDP > 18 mmHg. Most CHF is systolic dysfunction with a low EF usually associated with by CAD, but some CHF is termed diastolic dysfunction because the EF is almost normal. "The symptoms of left ventricular dysfunction and the physical signs are all due to increased left arterial pressure, capillary pressure, and pulmonary congestion. If the EF is less than 40%, it is labeled systolic heart failure. If it is greater than 40%, it is labeled diastolic heart failure. In diastolic dysfunction, a lower total volume of blood is ejected even though the EF may be normal." In all heart failure patients filling pressures are higher than normal because of poor ventricular compliance (LVEDP> 18).

2. Forms of CHF

992. **The "backward" theory of heart failure states that when a ventricle fails to adequately discharge its contents it causes a/an:**
a. Reduced cardiac output and BP
b. Insufficient blood supply to the myocardium
c. Damming up of blood behind it
d. The kidneys to retain sodium

ANSWER c. Damming up of blood behind it. This is analogous to closing a dam. The water behind it backs up and floods the upstream areas. Thus when a ventricle fails, it backs up blood into the upstream veins and organs. In right heart failure blood backs up into the systemic veins. In left heart failure it backs up into the lungs. Thus, the term "backward failure"

See: Braunwald, chapter on "Pathology of Heart Failure." **Keywords:** CHF, backward theory of

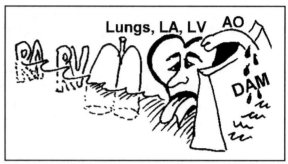

Backward CHF

993. The "forward" theory of heart failure states that an insufficient cardiac output tends to cause:
  a.   A dilated ventricle and reduced EF%
  b.   A "damming up" of venous blood
  c.   Insufficient coronary blood supply
  d.   The kidneys to retain sodium

ANSWER d. The kidneys to retain sodium. This theory relates to the aspects of heart failure relating to the inadequate "forward" delivery of arterial blood. Here reduced cardiac output diminishes perfusion to vital organs, especially the kidneys.

   Reduced kidney flow leads to the retention of $Na+$, $H2O$, and vasoconstriction. This happens through the renin - aldosterone mechanism. Like the "backward theory" the "forward theory" also leads to increased fluid retention, congestion, and edema behind the failing ventricle.

See: Braunwald, chapter on "Pathology of Heart Failure." **Keywords:** CHF, forward theory of CHF

994. At low cardiac output states activation of the "renin-angiotensin-aldosterone" system results in:
  1. Vasoconstriction
  2. CA++ inhibition
  3. NA+ retention
  4. Autonomic cholinergic stimulation
  5. Release of acetylcholine
      a. 1, 4, 5
      b. 1, 3
      c. 2, 3, 5
      d. 4, 5

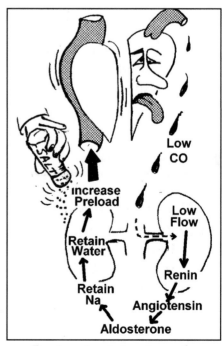

ANSWER b. 1, 3
  1. **YES:** Vasoconstriction
  2. NO: CA++ inhibition
  3. **YES:** NA+ retention

Renin - Angiotensin cycle

4. NO: Autonomic cholinergic stimulation

5. NO: Release of acetylcholine

The low CO triggers the baroreceptors in the kidneys to release renin. This is the triggering hormone which stimulates angiotensin I, angiotensin II, and aldosterone release.

• Angiotensin II is a potent vasoconstrictor.

• It also stimulates the adrenergic nerves to liberate norepinephrine - another potent vasoconstrictor

• Aldosterone causes the kidneys to retain NA+

• These act as a vicious cycle in CHF to increase venous distension and exaggerate the CHF.

See: Braunwald, chapter on "Pathology of Heart Failure." **Keywords:** CHF, Renin, Angiotensin, Aldosterone

995. **A common cause of isolated right heart failure (cor pulmonale) is:**
  a. **Diabetes**
  b. **Emphysema**
  c. **Increased salt intake**
  d. **Left heart failure**

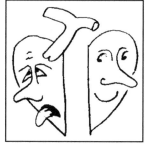

Right Heart Failure

ANSWER b. Emphysema. Chronic Obstructive Pulmonary Disease (COPD) destroys pulmonary alveoli and capillaries. This increases the pulmonary vascular resistance to the point where the right heart may begin to fail. It increases the RV and PA pressure, hypertrophies, and backs up, congesting the RA and peripheral veins. Since it fails to supply the left heart with adequate filling, the LV cardiac output declines as well.

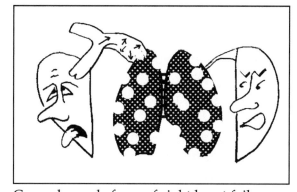

Cor pulmonale form of right heart failure

See: Braunwald, chapter on "Pathology of Heart Failure." **Keywords:** CHF, Cor Pulmonale, Rt. Ht. Failure

996. **Which condition below is associated with elevated venous pressure, edema, ascites, and renal failure?**
  a. **Hypotonicity**
  b. **Hypertonicity**
  c. **Hypovolemia**
  d. **Hypervolemia**

ANSWER d. Hypervolemia. Hyper = increased, vol = volume, emia = blood: thus too much blood increases the preload on the ventricles which makes them pump harder according to Starling's law. Hypervolemia is a common result of congestive heart failure - the backward damming up of blood. It may be treated with diuretics and a low salt diet. **See:** Braunwald, chapter on "Pathophysiology of Heart Failure." **Keywords:** signs and symptoms of hypervolemia

997. **Patients with <u>diastolic</u> left heart failure, or HfpEF, have pulmonary congestion and:**
a.   EF >50%, LV hypertrophy (concentric)
b.   EF >50%, LV dilation (eccentric)
c.   EF <40%, LV hypertrophy (concentric)
d.   EF <40%, LV dilation (eccentric)

ANSWER: a. EF >50%, LV hypertrophy (concentric) is parallel sarcomere addition causing hypertrophy of the LV wall similar to pressure overload. Some consider diastolic failure the precursor to systolic heart failure. Remember a normal EF is >50%. Diastolic heart failure is also termed HFnEF (normal EF) or HfpEF (preserved EF).

   Diastolic failure is characterized by an elevated diastolic pressure in the left ventricle, despite an essentially normal physiologic end diastolic volume (EDV) and stroke volume (SV). Diastolic failure appears when the ventricle can't be filled properly because it can't relax or because its wall is thick or rigid. This situation presents as a concentric thickened hypertrophic heart. In contrast systolic heart failure presents with an eccentric hypertrophied heart [enlarged, baggy thin heart wall, asymmetrical in shape.]

998. **Common signs of isolated right heart failure in patients include:**
   1. Swollen and puffy legs
   2. Orthopnea
   3. Claudication
   4. Enlarged liver
   5. Distended neck veins
   6. Pulmonary rales
      a. 1, 2, 6
      b. 1, 4, 5
      c. 2, 3, 5
      d. 3, 5, 6

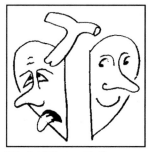
Right Heart Failure

ANSWER b. 1, 4, 5
   1. **YES: SWOLLEN AND PUFFY LEGS** (tissue edema)
   2. NO: ORTHOPNEA (dyspnea upon reclining due to pulmonary edema)
   3. NO: CLAUDICATION (leg pain on exercise = femoral artery stenosis)
   4. **YES: ENLARGED LIVER** (increased systemic venous pressures congest the liver, enlarge it, and causes "hepato-jugular reflux."
   5. **YES: DISTENDED NECK VEINS** (Increased RA -

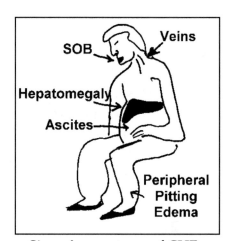
Signs & symptoms of CHF

CVP pressures will distend neck veins even upon sitting up.)
    6. NO: PULMONARY RALES (this is a pulmonary edema problem)
Other signs and symptoms of right heart failure resulting from the high CVP are: tissue edema, ascites, tiredness, SOB, PND, and congestive hepatomegaly.
See: Braunwald, chapter on "Clinical Aspects of Heart Failure." **Keywords:** CHF, signs right sided CHF

999. Hypertrophic obstructive cardiomyopathy (HOCM) is a:
    a.   **Atherosclerotic disease with a dilated and hypokinetic LV**
    b.   **Atherosclerotic disease with a hypertrophied and hypercontractile LV**
    c.   **Genetic disorder with a dilated and hypokinetic LV**
    d.   **Genetic disorder with a hypertrophied and hypercontractile LV**

ANSWER: d. Genetic disorder with a hypertrophied and hypercontractile LV. Grossman says, "Hypertrophic cardiomyopathy is a common autosomal dominant genetic disorder....The most common dramatic hemodynamic feature of HCM is the dynamic intraventricular pressure gradient. Ventriculography typically demonstrates a hypercontractile state, ventricular hypertrophy, and a small ventricular cavity. Dynamic outflow obstruction may even be visible..." **See:** Grossman chapter on "Cardiomyopathy and CHF" **Keywords:** HOCM = genetic LV defect

3. Hemodynamics of CHF

1000. Match each cause of CHF with a diseased heart in that category.
    A. Loss of cardiac muscle
    B. Restricted filling
    C. Volume overload
    D. Pressure overload

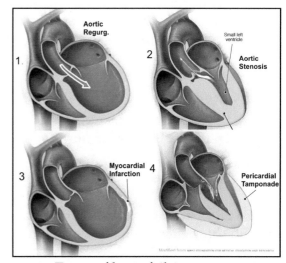

ANSWERS:
A-3. Loss of cardiac muscle E.g., MI makes for dilated asynchronous heart beat.
B-4. Restricted filling, E.g., Tamponade. Pressure around heart won't allow heart to fill completely.
C-1. Volume overload, E.g., AR. Aortic Regurgitation into LV. Heart must pump large stroke volume because of leakage back into atrium.

Types of heart failure

D-2. Pressure overload, E.g., AS. Aortic Stenosis prevents full ejection of blood and increases pressure in LV, causing LV hypertrophy.
See: http://slideplayer.com/slide/3721431/ - "Cardiac Pathophysiology: A Short Overview"

1001. Acute pulmonary edema occurs when there is inadequate emptying of the:
   a. Right ventricle
   b. Left ventricle
   c. Pulmonary artery
   d. Aorta

ANSWER b. Left ventricle. If the LV becomes inefficient and it cannot adequately pump out the LA's volume then it backs up in the lungs causing pulmonary edema. It is a "damming up" effect which floods everything upstream. The pulmonary edema causes the chief CHF symptoms - shortness of breath (SOB) and dyspnea. **See:** Braunwald, chapter on "Clinical Aspect of Heart Failure." **Keywords:** CHF, inadequate emptying LA

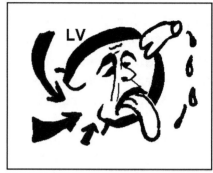
Flooded exhausted LV

1002. What is the usual hemodynamic finding in left heart failure?
   a. Elevated systolic arterial pressure
   b. Reduced systolic arterial pressure
   c. Elevated pulmonary capillary pressure
   d. Reduced pulmonary capillary pressure

ANSWER c. Elevated pulmonary capillary pressures reflect the increased "back-up" of blood in the LA. This elevates the PA wedge pressure. Since PA diastolic pressure is only 2-6 mmHg higher than the LA, PA pressures elevate in CHF also. Since PA pressure is elevated the RV systolic pressure is also elevated, and if it continues the RV diastolic will become elevated. Thus, left heart failure leads to right heart failure.
See: Braunwald, chapter on "Pathology of Heart Failure."

1003. Advanced left heart failure is most associated with:
   a. Systolic heart murmurs
   b. Diastolic heart murmurs
   c. Interstitial pulmonary edema
   d. Non-cardiogenic pulmonary edema

ANSWER: c. Interstitial pulmonary edema. It is due to failure of the heart to remove fluid from the lung circulation ("cardiogenic pulmonary edema"). Cardiogenic edema results in increased interstitial fluid, as determined by the balance of fluid homeostasis, and increased secretion of fluid into the interstitium or impaired removal of this fluid. Generation of interstitial fluid is regulated by the forces of the Starling equation. Whereas, a direct injury to the lung parenchyma is termed "noncardiogenic pulmonary edema" which may be due to inhalation of toxic gases, pulmonary contusion, aspiration, etc. **See:** Todd, Vol. 1, chapter on "Vascular Physiology"

1004. **What level of pulmonary capillary wedge pressure leads to pulmonary edema? (Assume normal plasma colloid pressure and normal lymphatic flow.)**
a.   Wedge < 15 mmHg
b.   Wedge < 28 mmHg
c.   Wedge > 15 mmHg
d.   Wedge > 28 mmHg

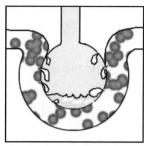
Pulmonary Edema

ANSWER d. Wedge > 28 mmHg. Capillary wedge pressures greater than 28 mmHg lead to pulmonary edema, if everything else remains normal. Besides the wedge pressure there are many other variables affecting edema:
   1) Oncotic pressure can increase plasma Na^+ and draw additional fluid into the vascular space.
   2) Lymphatic flow can elevate - removing more edematous fluid
   3) The significant time it takes to build up enough fluid to become a significant edema.
Nevertheless, it is well recognized that elevated pulmonary hydrostatic pressure is the chief imbalance of Starling forces leading to edema (see "Starling's Law" of capillary permeability). Normal wedge pressures average = 8 mmHg.
See: Braunwald, chapter on "Pulmonary Edema" **Keywords:** CHF > wedge > 28 mmHg.

1005. **Pitting and/or peripheral edema usually begins when:**
a.   Wedge pressure > 10 mmHg
b.   Wedge pressure > 28 mmHg
c.   CVP > 10 mmHg
d.   CVP > 28 mmHg

ANSWER: c. CVP > 10mmhg.
CVP pressure monitoring evaluates caval and RA pressure. Peripheral edema starts when CVP or RA pressure exceeds 10 mmHg. Remember normal RA is 1-5 mmHg. Normal Wedge mean pressure is 5-13 mmHg and pulmonary edema starts around 20 mmHg. So, edema normally begins at about twice the normal value.

1006. **What serum biomarker is elevated in all forms of CHF?**
a.   BNP
b.   Troponin
c.   Myoglobin
d.   CK-MB

ANSWER: a. BNP. Brain natriuretic peptide is a hormone secreted from the ventricles in response to elevated filling pressures that occur when heart failure develops. Its level increases proportionally to the level of CHF: 100 is normal, 300 is mild CHF, 900 is severe CHF, and decreases with effective therapy.
   NIH says, "Heart failure (HF) biomarkers have dramatically impacted the way HF patients are evaluated and managed. B-type natriuretic peptide (BNP) and N-terminal proBNP (NT-proBNP) are the gold standard biomarkers in determining the diagnosis and

prognosis of HF, and studies on natriuretic peptide-guided HF management look promising." **See:** http://www.ncbi.nlm.nih.gov/pubmed/23313577

1007. **Hemodynamics diagnosis of cardiogenic shock includes a systolic BP ___ mmHg, CI___ L/min/M² and wedge__ mmHg:**
   a.   BP <90, CI < 1.5, Wedge over 15
   b.   BP <90, CI < 2.2, Wedge over 15
   c.   BP <120, CI < 2.2, Wedge over 25
   d.   BP <100, CI < 1.5, Wedge under 6

ANSWER: b. BP <90, CI < 2.2, Wedge over 15
BP < 90 mmHg for over 30 minutes, CI < 2.2 L/min/M², and Wedge >15 mmHg.

1008. **These pressure tracings are show the various stages of <u>diastolic</u> heart failure or HFpEF. This type of heart failure is associated with:**
   a.   **Increased LV stiffness and increasing LVEDP**
   b.   **Increased LV stiffness and decreased LVEDP**
   c.   **Reduced Ejection fraction and increasing LVEDP**
   d.   **Reduced Ejection fraction and decreased LVEDP**

ANSWER: a. Increased LV stiffness and increasing LVEDP. Heart failure with preserved ejection fraction (HFpEF) is a form of heart failure in which the LV ejection fraction - is normal, defined as greater than 50% EF. But, what is abnormal is diastolic filling.

  We think of heart failure as a reduction in ejection fraction, But, approximately half of people with heart failure have preserved ejection fraction (HFpEF), also termed diastolic heart failure.

  Diastolic heart failure is characterized by an increase in LV stiffness, which decreases the suction cup effect during the early diastolic rapid filling phase. This results in elevated the wedge and LVEDP filling pressures as shown. It is most common in older people with hypertension, diabetes and/or hardening of the arteries.

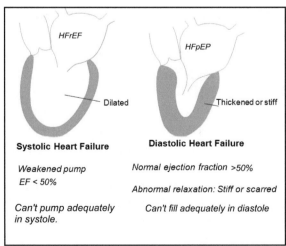

1009. **Increasing the stiffness (decreasing compliance) of the left ventricle has the greatest effect on _____ properties of the LV.**
a. **Diastolic filling**
b. **Diastolic ejection**
c. **Systolic ejection**
d. **Systolic filling**

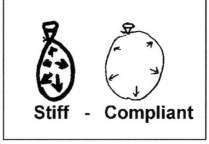

BALLOON Compliance

      ANSWER a. Diastolic filling. Diastole is the period of LV filling. In the initial rapid filling phase the LV sucks in blood like a suction cup. In the remainder of diastole the atria push blood into the ventricle - especially during the atrial "kick."
   It's like filling a balloon. The stiffer the balloon the less air you can blow into it. The more compliant the LV the easier it fills. In CHF the LV shows impaired ability to accept blood. CHF is an example of how "**DIASTOLIC DYSFUNCTION**" can be as big a problem as "**SYSTOLIC DYSFUNCTION." The heart acts as both a diastolic suction pump and a forward systolic pump.**
See: Braunwald, chapter on "Pathology of Heart Failure." **Keywords:** CHF, pressure & volume overload, hypertrophy and dilatation

1010. **Congestive dilatation of the left ventricle may also dilate the mitral valve annulus, resulting in: (Note MR = Mitral Regurgitation, MVP = Mitral Valve Prolapse)**
a. **MR and a diastolic murmur**
b. **MR and a systolic murmur**
c. **MVP and a diastolic murmur**
d. **MVP and a systolic murmur**

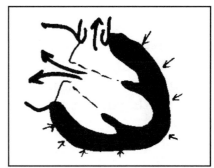

CHF ➡ MR ➡ Murmur

ANSWER b. MR and a systolic murmur. Stretching of the annulus can separate the mitral leaflets so much that they leak. This is mitral regurgitation (MR) which is a systolic event, and leads to the holo-systolic blowing murmur of MR.
See: Braunwald, chapter on "Pathology of Heart Failure." **Keywords:** CHF, stretched annulus > MR > systolic murmur

4. Signs & Symptoms of CHF

1011. **A common sign of right sided congestive heart failure is:**
a. Dyspnea
b. Pulmonary congestion
c. Pulmonary hypertension
d. Neck vein distension

ANSWER d. Neck vein distension occurs when the right heart fails and the RA and systemic veins become engorged with blood. Pulmonary hypertension is only a compensation to left-sided failure (understand how in left-sided failure the pulmonary veins become engorged, increasing PAW pressure.) **See:** Braunwald, chapter on "Physical Examination." **Keywords:** Right sided CHF causes neck vein distension

1012. **Moist or crackling rales in CHF are auscultatory sounds heard best at the:**
a. Apex of the lung indicating interstitial edema
b. Apex of the heart indicating volume overload of LV
c. Base of the lung indicating fluid in bronchi & alveoli
d. Base of the heart indicating pressure overload of LV

ANSWER c. Base of the lung indicating fluid in bronchi & alveoli. Moist rales are the bubbling or gurgling lung sounds due to transudation of fluid into the alveoli. This fluid then moves into the airways and gurgles on inspiration. These sounds are often accompanied by expectoration of frothy, blood-tinged sputum. This fluid in the lungs settles to the bottom or base of the lung and is heard best there. Pulmonary pressure is highest there due to gravity effects.
See: Braunwald, chapter on "Clinical Aspect of Heart Failure." **Keywords:** CHF, inadequate emptying LA

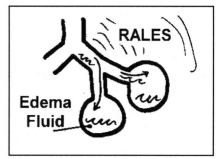
Pulmonary RALES

1013. **The "New York Heart Association Functional Classification" is used to classify patients in heart failure. How would you rate the patient in the box?**

Symptoms of SOB occur with LESS THAN ORDINARY activities, Comfortable at rest, Marked limitation of physical activity.

a. I
b. II
c. III
d. IV

ANSWER c. III. The first class is no limitation due to CHF. The worst class IV is unable to do ANY physical activity. They have symptoms of CHF even at rest. Match all below.

NYHA CLASS	LIMITATIONS	SYMPTOMS
I	No limitation	No undue symptoms with ordinary activities
II	Slight limitation of physical activity	Comfortable at rest. Ordinary activity causes dyspnea, fatigue, Palpitations
III	Marked limitation of physical activity	Comfortable at rest. Symptoms with less than usual activity.
IV	Inability to carry on any physical activity	Symptoms CHF at rest. Discomfort with any physical activity.

See: Braunwald, chapter on "Physical Examination." **Keywords:** New York Heart Association Functional Classification

1014. A rare form of heart failure in which the patient is warm and pink, with good pulse pressure and stroke volume is:
a. Low output heart failure
b. High output heart failure
c. Acute heart failure
d. Chronic heart failure

ANSWER b. High output heart failure. In most forms of CHF the patients have a low CO are vasoconstricted, cold, pale, and sometimes cyanotic. But in high cardiac output syndromes the patient is warm, pink, with a good pulse pressure and stroke volume. These diseases overwork the heart so much it may fail. Diseases which may lead to high output CHF are: AV fistula, thyrotoxicosis, beriberi, anemia and pregnancy. Similarly, in septic shock the CO is elevated and the patient is pink. **See:** Braunwald, chapter on "Clinical Aspects of Heart Failure." **Keywords:** CHF, signs left sided CHF

1015. The most common symptom found in patients with congestive left heart failure is:
a. Shortness of breath
b. Abdominal pain of ascites
c. Chest pain
d. Claudication

ANSWER a. Shortness of breath. Most signs and symptoms in pure left sided CHF result from pulmonary edema. These shortness of breath (SOB) signs and symptoms include :
    1. Exertional - Dyspnea On Exertion (DOE)

2. Orthopnea - Dyspnea in a recumbent position (CHF patients breath better sitting up)
3. Paroxysmal Nocturnal Dyspnea (PND) - Awaking at night gasping for breath. This is due to bronchospasm precipitated by the pulmonary edema. Alternately called cardiac asthma. **See:** Braunwald, chapter on "Clinical Aspects of Heart Failure." **Keywords:** CHF, signs left sided CHF

1016. **A CHF patient must sit up to get his breath. This is termed:**
a.   **Hypopnea**
b.   **Orthopnea**
c.   **Pulmonary dysplasia**
d.   **Orthostatic hypotension**

ANSWER b. Orthopnea is discomfort in breathing in any but the erect or standing position. This is often associated with pulmonary congestion due to heart failure. The partial upright position or several pillows help lower the pulmonary capillary pressure that often promotes the pulmonary edema. **See:** Medical Dictionary.

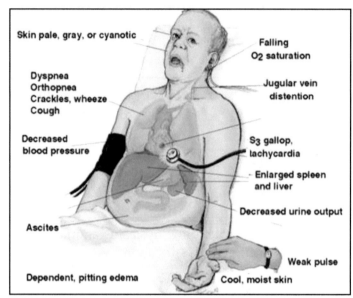

Skin pale, gray, or cyanotic

Falling O2 saturation

Dyspnea Orthopnea Crackles, wheeze Cough

Jugular vein distention

Decreased blood pressure

S3 gallop, tachycardia

Enlarged spleen and liver

Decreased urine output

Ascites

Dependent, pitting edema

Weak pulse

Cool, moist skin

Left Heart Failure - orthopnea

1017. **Post MI your patient develops orthopnea, tachypnea, and bilateral lung crackles. He has most likely developed:**
a.   **Right heart failure**
b.   **Left heart failure**
c.   **Right to left VSD shunt**
d.   **Left to right VSD shunt**
e.   **Pulmonary embolus**

ANSWER: b. Left heart failure. Common respiratory signs of left heart failure are tachypnea (increased rate of breathing) and increased work of breathing (non-specific signs of respiratory distress). Rales or crackles, heard initially in the lung bases, and when severe, throughout the lung fields suggest the development of pulmonary edema (fluid in the alveoli). Common causes of heart failure include myocardial infarction and other forms of ischemic heart disease, hypertension, valvular heart disease and cardiomyopathy. Left heart failure can cause a large variety of symptoms such as shortness of breath (typically worse when lying flat, which is called orthopnea), coughing and exercise intolerance. Right heart failure (which, may result from left heart failure) is seen in the periphery and associated with increased jugular pulses, ankle swelling, and peripheral edema. Shunts may also result in pulmonary edema and CHF.
See: http://emedicine.medscape.com/article/163062-clinical

1018. What results when PAW pressure significantly exceeds the plasma protein osmotic pressure?
a. Cardiac asthma
b. Pulmonary stenosis
c. Interstitial pulmonary edema
d. Paroxysmal nocturnal dyspnea

ANSWER: c. Interstitial pulmonary edema occurs when the pulmonary capillary hydrostatic pressure is high enough to push plasma across the pulmonary capillary membrane into the interstitial space and alveolus. This pressure opposes the osmotic pressure in the capillary wall. When the wedge pressure exceeds around 25 mmHg, the patient gets fluid in the lungs and pulmonary edema. This extra fluid in the lungs impedes oxygen transport, causes coughing, and raises pulmonary vascular resistance. When this happens in the peripheral capillaries you get peripheral tissue edema - usually seen as swelling in the legs. **See:** Braunwald, chapter on CHF **Keywords:** PE when wedge > 25

5. Management of CHF

1019. When a congestive heart failure patient exhibits dyspnea, orthopnea, and basilar "rales" the most effective relief is brought by:
a. Reducing RA pressure
b. Reducing pulmonary capillary pressure
c. Increasing cardiac output
d. Increasing blood pressure

ANSWER b. Reducing pulmonary capillary pressure. The congestive symptoms of left heart failure are best relieved by reducing the high pulmonary capillary pressures which cause them. A Swan Ganz catheter is the best diagnostic tool here. Diuretics, digitalis, O2, and positive end expiratory pressure breathing (PEEP) are among the best therapeutic tools. **See:** Daily, "Techniques in Bedside Hemodynamic Monitoring"

1020. The use of diuretics in the treatment of congestive heart failure is intended to:
a. Increase CO
b. Decrease preload
c. Increase afterload
d Decrease contractility

ANSWER b. Decrease preload. Diuretics make you "diurese" or "pee." Eliminating water from the system reduces the elevated blood volume and brings less blood back into the veins. This is reflected in lower venous pressures and lower preload. Diuretics can help with the "edema" problem, but by reducing preload they may make the heartbeat weaker. Diuretics are often given with digitalis to strengthen the weakened contractility. **See:** Braunwald, chapter on "Pathology of Heart Failure." **Keywords:** CHF, diuretics, < preload

1021. Medical treatment for acute CHF (congestion with hypoperfusion syndrome) includes: (Select 3 below.)

1. Diuretics
2. IV fluid therapy
3. Vasoconstrictors
4. Vasodilators
5. ACE inhibitors
6. Beta blockers

    a. 1, 3, 6
    b. 1, 4, 5
    c. 2, 3, 4
    d. 2, 4, 5
    e. 1, 4, 6

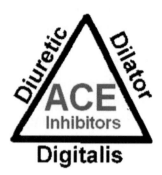

CHF Rx - 3D's

ANSWER b. 1, 4, 5

1. **YES:** DIURETICS - (Furosemide)"Dry out" the wet lungs
2. NO: IV FLUID THERAPY - Would further fluid-overload the flooded lungs
3. NO: VASOCONSTRICTORS - Already too vasoconstricted.
4. **YES:** VASODILATORS (Hydralazine and nitroglycerine) "open up" shut down peripheral capillaries
5. **YES:** ACE inhibitors (Angiotensin Converting Enzyme inhibitor). Renin, aldosterone, angiotensin II are natural hormones released by the kidney in hypoperfusion states. Their release causes sodium and water retention, and makes CHF worse. The increase in fluid leads to volume overload and ventricular remodeling. ACE inhibitors can prevent this.
6. NO: BETA BLOCKERS. May be deleterious in CHF.

Congestion is usually treated with diuretics to eliminate the excess fluid (E.g., Furosemide). In chronic CHF a Na+ restricted diet also helps reduce the fluid levels.

The low CO is often caused by the sympathetic stimulation, catecholamines, and vasoconstriction. This may be corrected with vasodilator therapy such as ACE-inhibitors, nitroglycerine or sodium nitroprusside. If these excessively drop the BP then inotropic agents should be added to the regimen like digitalis or dopamine. The classic "3D" drugs for CHF are Diuretic, Dilator, Digitalis, but ACE inhibitors are now added. ACE inhibitors are now the cornerstone of treatment for heart failure, because they break the bad renin - angiotensin cycle.

See: Braunwald, chapter on "The Management of Heart Failure." **Keywords:** Rx for acute CHF

1022. A class of drug specifically used to interrupt the "renin-angiotensin-aldosterone" system in CHF is:

a.   Beta blockers
b.   Ca channel blockers
c.   ACE inhibitors
d.   Digitalis

ANSWER c. ACE-inhibitor is an Angiotensin Converting Enzyme inhibitor. Know the

other drugs listed:
a.   BETA BLOCKERS (E.g., Inderol) block the beta adrenergic receptors.
b.   CA CHANNEL BLOCKERS (E.g., Nifedipine) block the Ca+ fast channels. Slow HR and vasodilate smooth muscle.
c.   ACE INHIBITORS (E.g., Captopril) block conversion of angiotensin I to angiotensin II. These reduce renin, angiotensin II, and aldosterone blood levels and thus the Na+ retention and vasoconstriction problems.
d.   DIGITALIS, cardiotonic or inotropic drug.
See: Braunwald, chapter on "The Management of Heart Failure."

1023. These Starling curves are from a patient in CHF. He is at point A and is experiencing symptoms of mild dyspnea. Which management regimen below would move him to point #4 on the curve?
a.   **VOLUME EXPANSION:** or increased salt intake
b.   **DECOMPENSATION:** continued deterioration
c.   **DIURETIC:** or Na restricted diet
d.   **DIGITALIS:** or other inotropic drug

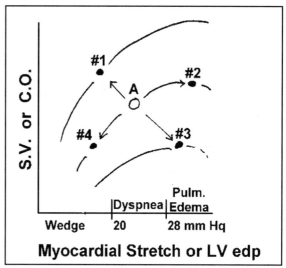

Starling curves in CHF

ANSWER c. DIURETIC: or Na restricted diet. These curves can be divided into 4 quadrants called the Forrester Subsets. Be able to describe each subset below.
CORRECTLY MATCHED ANSWERS ARE:
   1. DIGITALIS: or other inotropic drug such as a catecholamine. This will move him to a higher contractile state - a whole higher "supercharged" curve. Digitalis will move up the CO and down the wedge pressure which will help the dyspnea.
   2. VOLUME EXPANSION: or increased salt intake, veno-constriction, continued IV infusions. These do not move him to a new contractile state - only moves up the preload along the same curve to point #2. May increase CO slightly but also moves up the wedge pressure above the acute pulmonary edema point.
   3. DECOMPENSATION: continued deterioration - no therapy.
   4. DIURETIC: or Na restricted diet or veno-dilator to pool venous blood away from the main circulating volume. Moving down the same contractility curve will reduce wedge pressure and CO. The patient will breath better, but may feel more tired.
Note how the best therapy would be to combine #1 (Digitalis) with #4 (Diuretic). This would move the patient to the higher curve and move him down that curve to a new point not shown on the diagram, but on the far left of the upper curve.
See: Todd, chapter B7 on Frank-Starling Law and Underhill, chapter on "Heart Failure."

1024. Your 54-year old patient has had several untreated heart attacks and a 25% EF. He enters the ER with severe angina unrelieved with nitrates. In the cath lab, your cardiologist sees 3 vessel disease and decides to send him to acute CABG surgery. Before taking him to surgery you will probably:
a. Put in an IABP or Impella
b. Put in an RVAD or Tandem Heart device
c. Put in a Swan-Ganz catheter
d. Start him on a GP IIb/IIIa inhibitor & heparin drip

ANSWER: a. Put in an IABP or Impella. This is a high risk patient for CABG surgery. High risk surgical candidates benefit from preoperative IABP with improved survival, reduced hospital stay, and decreased cost. High risk surgical patients that need preoperative IABP are those with any 2 of the following: poor LVEF, prior CABG, unstable angina, left main disease (>75% stenosis). Impella may be used instead of balloon pump.
See: e-learning modules at https://getinge.training/DesktopShell.aspx?tabId=1135

1025. A 62-year-old female with significant ST elevation, severe angina, RBBB and shortness of breath, comes for emergency catheterization. She is pale with dilated neck veins, has a BP of 90/55 mmHg, HR 95 bpm, with runs of ventricular tachycardia. Which of the following should be available at the time of catheterization?
a. IABP or Impella
b. A cutting balloon
c. A permanent pacemaker
d. A transcutaneous pacemaker

ANSWER a. IABP or Impella. This STEMI patient appears to be in cardiogenic shock, in which case a lifesaving balloon pump or Impella may be inserted before or during PCI. These will unload the LV and improve coronary supply.
See: Braunwald, chapter on "Percutaneous Coronary Intervention"

6. General Pathology of Shock

1026. Shock is an acute inability of the heart to maintain adequate perfusion to:
a. Maintain an average BP > 80 mmHg.
b. Maintain an average BP > 100 mmHg.
c. Sustain function of the vital organs at rest
d. Sustain metabolism of all organ systems at rest

ANSWER c. Sustain function of the vital organs at rest.
Braunwald states that "Shock encompasses the syndromes associated with an acute reduction in effective blood flow with failure to maintain the transfer and delivery of essential substrates to sustain the function of vital organ systems." In shock, blood is

shunted to vital organs (such as the brain), and away from less essential tissues (like skin) and BP < 90 systolic. **See:** Braunwald, chapter on "Acute Circulatory Failure (Shock)."

1027. **In severe shock vasoconstriction redistributes blood flow to vital organs. To protect them from ischemia, arterial blood is redirected to the:**
1. Kidneys
2. Lungs
3. Heart
4. Brain
     a. 1, 4
     b. 2, 3
     c. 2, 4
     d. 3, 4

ANSWER d. 3 & 4
  1. NO: KIDNEYS. The kidneys do receive less flow in shock. Urine output diminishes or ceases in severe shock.
  2. NO: LUNGS. All the blood must pass through the lungs anyway

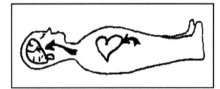
Vital Core Organs - spared

  3. **YES:** HEART. Coronary flow is preserved.
  4. **YES:** BRAIN. The brain is the most vital organ sensitive to ischemia (4 minutes). The brain and heart are the core organs whose circulation is preserved. Evidence of the vasoconstriction and redistribution of blood away from non-vital organs is seen in the signs and symptoms of pale cool skin, oliguria, and respiratory muscle fatigue. **See:** Braunwald, chapter on "Acute Circulatory Failure (Shock)." **Keywords:** Shock, selective vasoconstriction

1028. **Failure of compensatory mechanisms in shock leads to:**
a.   **Anaerobic metabolism in tissues**
b.   **Aerobic metabolism in tissues**
c.   **Right heart CHF**
d.   **Left heart CHF**

ANSWER a. Anaerobic metabolism in tissues. The fundamental defect in shock is the failure to maintain O2 delivery to the essential organs of the body. When inadequate O2 is available O2 consumption is reduced and the tissues switch to anaerobic metabolism. Glycolysis byproducts are pyruvate and lactate - classical markers for anaerobic metabolism. This anaerobic energy pathway produces less than 10% of the ATP which would normally be available through the Kreb's cycle. Lactic acid/lactate is the best blood test to quantitate O2 deficit and severity of shock. It also produces the metabolic acidosis characteristic of shock.

  Shock victims with lactate levels over 4 mM/L have less than a 50% survival rate. Severe shock is associated with severe oxygen deficit and ushers in terminal perfusion failure. When this occurs it is called the "irreversible stage of shock." **See:** Braunwald, chapter on "Acute Circulatory Failure (Shock)." **Keywords:** Shock, anaerobic metabolism

1029. A serious consequence of the low CO found in shock is "sludging" of blood cells which commonly leads to:
a. Disseminated Intravascular Coagulation (DIC)
b. Hypertrophic Obstructive Cardiomyopathy
c. Transient Ischemic Attack (TIA)
d. Myocardial Infarction

ANSWER a. Disseminated Intravascular Coagulation (DIC) is spontaneous micro-embolism within the vessels. It may lead to pulmonary embolism, pulmonary edema, and purpura fulminans (purple skin lesions due to micro-emboli). DIC is treated with heparin to prevent further clotting. **See:** Braunwald, chapter on "Acute Circulatory Failure (Shock)."

1030. The acute pulmonary edema pattern of "shock lung" or "ARDS" often found in the "non-cardiac" forms of shock is associated with:
a. Reduced peripheral resistance
b. Elevated wedge pressure
c. Increased capillary permeability
d. Increased surfactant production

ANSWER c. Increased capillary permeability. **The rationale for each answer is:**
a. NO: Peripheral resistance INCREASES due to the reduced CO found in most shock states.
b. NO: Elevated wedge pressure is found only in cardiogenic shock. Right heart pressures decrease because of sudden loss of circulating volume.
c. **YES:** Increased capillary permeability allows plasma to leave the circulation and move across the capillary membrane. Tissue edema occurs (including skin rash and airway edema) because of massive hypersensitivity reaction.
d. NO: DECREASED surfactant production may be a contributing factor in Adult Respiratory Distress Syndrome (ARDS) just as it is in Infant Respiratory Distress Syndrome (IRDS). The surface tension within the alveoli must be low enough to easily inflate.
See: Braunwald, chapter on "Acute Circulatory Failure (Shock)." **Keywords:** Shock, pulmonary edema, shock lung, increased capillary permeability

7. Types and Classification of Shock

1031. What type of shock is described by an immediate allergic reaction to a drug or dye which results in life-threatening respiratory distress, with skin rash and wheals, followed by vascular collapse?

SHOCK

a. Vaso-vagal reaction
b. Gram-negative sepsis
c. Congestive heart failure
d. Anaphylaxis

ANSWER d. Anaphylaxis. Respiratory distress often begins within minutes of the allergic antigen-antibody reaction. Mucosal edema of the airway causes strider, and bronchiolar constriction resembling asthma. Circulatory shock follows the respiratory distress. Cardiac output and BP both decrease. Anaphylactic shock may be treated with large volume IV infusions or epinephrine administration. Don't waste time in an emergency like this with Benadryl, hydrocortisone, etc. **See:** medical dictionary. **Keyword:** anaphylaxis

1032. **The hemodynamic cause of ANAPHYLACTIC SHOCK is:**
a. **Mechanical pump failure and loss of CO**
b. **Vasoconstriction and loss of BP**
c. **Pooling of circulating blood volume**
d. **Obstruction to blood flow**

ANSWER c. Pooling of circulating blood volume. Anaphylaxis (allergic reaction) = Loss of circulating blood volume. Anaphylactic shock is a form of hypovolemic shock where plasma water is lost to the tissues due to increased capillary permeability. This allows the large molecule blood proteins to pass through the now permeable membrane. The Starling osmotic forces then allow more water to escape from the capillary into the interstitial spaces as shown. The skin and other tissues become edematous, reddened and develop wheals and a rash. The bronchial mucosa inflames and may cause "cardiac asthma."

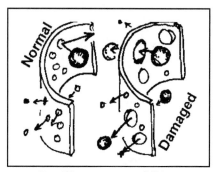

Capillary permeability

Respiratory distress often begins within minutes of the antigen-antibody reaction. Mucosal edema of the airway causes strider, and bronchiolar constriction resembling asthma. Circulatory shock follows the respiratory distress. Cardiac output and BP both decrease. Anaphylactic shock may be treated with large volume IV infusions and/or epinephrine administration.

Anaphylaxis is also associated with histamine, serotonin, and bradykinin release, which cause direct vasodilation and increased capillary permeability. **See:** Braunwald, chapter on "Acute Circulatory Failure (Shock)." **Keywords:** Anaphylactic shock = hypovolemia

1033. **Anaphylactic shock is a form of:**
a. **Hemorrhagic shock**
b. **Obstructive shock**
c. **Hypovolemic shock**
d. **Low resistance septic shock**

ANSWER c. Hypovolemic shock. Significant quantities of plasma can be lost during anaphylactic reactions. It crosses the damaged capillary membranes and causes edema. Part of the edema is manifested as skin rash, inflammation, wheals, and mucosal edema and bronchiolar constriction (cardiac asthma). The altered permeability of the tissue membranes is due to histamine, kinins, serotonin and platelet activating factor. **See:** Braunwald, chapter on "Acute Circulatory Failure (Shock)." **Keywords:** Anaphylaxis ➡ a form of hypovolemic shock

1034. Bacterial hyperdynamic septic shock leads to fever, _____, and _____.
- a. Vasodilation; ↑CO
- b. Vasodilation; ↓CO
- c. Vasoconstriction; ↑CO
- d. Vasoconstriction; ↓CO

ANSWER a. Vasodilation; ↑CO (or normal). Gram-negative enteric bacilli are the most common cause of this type of SEPTIC shock. It is most commonly acquired during invasive or surgical procedures. This type of bacteremia, common to IV drug abusers, is the only form of shock with vasodilation of the periphery and normal or increased CO. Many patients succumb in this hyperdynamic state. Some patients with septic shock continue into a lethal "hypo-dynamic" shock state.
See: Braunwald, chapter on "Acute Circulatory Failure (Shock)."

1035. Within minutes after LV angiography the patient starts wheezing and becomes short of breath. The BP falls to 90/50 mmHg. The PA wedge pressure falls to 3 mmHg and the RA pressure falls to 1 mmHg. The pulse rises to 120. Frequent PVCs are seen. He becomes pale and diaphoretic. How should the patient be positioned?
- a. Supine, elevate the legs 6 - 12 inches
- b. Sit the patient up 30-45 degrees
- c. Turn in left lateral position - legs flexed
- d. Reverse Trendelenburg position

ANSWER a. Supine, elevate the legs 6 - 12 inches. These are classic signs and symptoms of anaphylactic shock. It is due to loss of plasma volume with an increase in hematocrit. These are the same characteristics of hypovolemic shock. Both are treated by administration of IV fluid. Raising the patient's legs provides an immediate "transfusion" of lower limb blood into the thorax. This is the Trendelenburg position.
See: Braunwald, chapter on "Acute Circulatory Failure (Shock)."

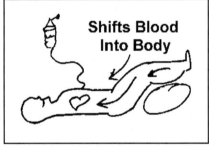

Raising legs in shock

1036. Mortality in untreated cardiogenic shock with pump failure is approximately:
- a. 20%
- b. 40%
- c. 60%
- d. 80%
- e. 100%

ANSWER e. 100%. Prognosis of severe cardiogenic shock is POOR. If these patients do not respond to a simple fluid challenge, the death rate approaches 100%. If less rigorous criterions for pump failure are used, the

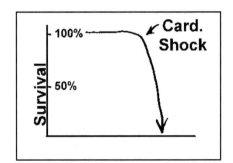

Card. Shock Mortality

mortality is between 85-95% - still very poor. The high mortality has not improved much through the years. The trick is to keep patients OUT of cardiogenic shock. We now have powerful interventional therapies like thrombolysis, PCI, IABP, Impella, ECMO and CABG surgery which if used early may salvage myocardium.
See: Braunwald, chapter on "Acute Circulatory Failure (Shock)."

8. Signs and Symptoms of Shock

1037. **Identify 3 clinical manifestations of shock. (Select 3 answers)**
   a.   **Pallor**
   b.   **Metabolic acidosis**
   c.   **Slow bounding pulse**
   d.   **Falling blood pressure**
   e.   **Increased diuresis**

ANSWERS: a, b, & d. Tachycardia usually results to compensate for decreased tissue perfusion. Falling BP and metabolic acidosis are common signs of shock states. The kidneys shut down in shock. Understand the vicious circle of shock. **See:** Braunwald, chapter on "Acute Circulatory Failure - Shock." **Keywords:** tachycardia in shock

1038. **During periods of shock which major blood reservoir veno-constricts and causes <u>pallor</u>?**
   a.   **Skin bed**
   b.   **Liver bed**
   c.   **Lung bed**
   d.   **Coronary bed**

ANSWER a. Skin bed. In shock blood flow is redirected to core organs and away from the skin. The skin feels cool and looks pale (pallor) - both signs of poor blood flow.
See: Braunwald, chapter on "Acute Circulatory Failure (Shock)." **Keywords:** Shock

1039. **Identify 4 causes of hypovolemic shock. (Select 4 answers.)**
   a.   **Anaphylaxis**
   b.   **Hemorrhage**
   c.   **Excessive diarrhea or vomiting**
   d.   **Extravasation (e.g., hematoma)**
   e.   **Congestive heart failure**

ANSWERS: a, b, c, & d. All of the above reduce the circulating fluid volume EXCEPT heart failure. CHF patients have an increased blood volume. The chief difference between shock and CHF is in the venous distension of CHF compared to the venous collapse of most shock patients. In low preload shock states (hypovolemia & blood pooling) the pump works OK,

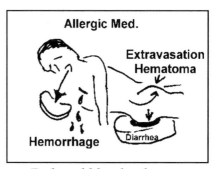

Reduced blood volume

but there is not enough blood to pump. **See:** Braunwald, chapter on "Acute Circulatory Failure (Shock)."

1040. **What are the signs of circulatory shock? (Exclude septic shock.)**
   1. Cold and clammy skin
   2. Decreased heart rate
   3. Collapsed neck veins
   4. Decreased urine output
   5. Dilated unresponsive pupils
   6. Hypotension
      a. 1, 2, 3, 4
      b. 1, 3, 4, 6
      c. 2, 3, 4, 6
      d. 3, 4, 5, 6

ANSWER b. 1, 3, 4, 6

1. **YES**: COLD AND CLAMMY SKIN results from adrenergic vasoconstriction in the periphery.

2. NO: DECREASED HEART RATE Tachycardia is an important compensation mechanism for the decreased SV and CO.

3. **YES:** COLLAPSED NECK VEINS. Preload is reduced in most forms of shock. In cardiogenic shock CVP is usually normal. The exceptions are right heart infarction, pulmonary hypertension, and right heart failure. LV-EDP and wedge pressures are elevated due to the "backward failure" pattern of CHF.

4. **YES:** DECREASED URINE OUTPUT. This is a classic tool to evaluate the severity of shock. Urine output ceases in severe shock.

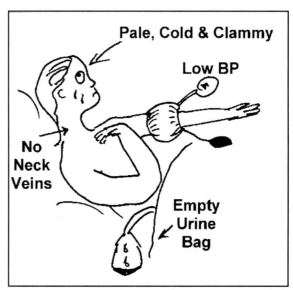

Signs and Symptoms of Shock

5. NO: DILATED UNRESPONSIVE PUPILS. They are a sign of brain death or narcotic overdose.

6. **YES**: HYPOTENSION. Blood pressure is commonly below 90 mmHg. systolic.
Other clinical signs of shock are: prostration, pallor, mental confusion. **See:** Braunwald, chapter on "Acute Circulatory Failure (Shock)." **Keywords:** Shock, signs and symptoms

1041. A patient with acute total occlusion of the LAD coronary artery has the hemodynamic findings shown in the box. This patient shows the clinical signs of:
a. Hypovolemic shock
b. Hypervolemic shock
c. Pump failure
d. Right heart failure

Wedge pressure	= 20 mmHg.
CVP	= 8 mmHg.
CI	= 1.8 L/min/M²,
BP (by doppler)	= 60 mmHg.

ANSWER c. Pump failure is cardiogenic shock. These limits (CI < 2.2, wedge > 18, and BP < 60) define a failing LV. CVP is normal, so the right side of the heart is normal unless pulmonary factors elevate the CVP.

CHF may lead to acute cardiogenic shock. It looks like severe CHF but is acute, and tissue viability is in jeopardy. Most pump failure is caused by infarction of major coronary arteries. **See:** Braunwald, chapter on "Acute Circulatory Failure (Shock)." **Keywords:** Cardiogenic shock, signs, < CO, > wedge, < BP

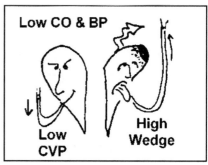
Cardiogenic shock

1042. The clinical picture of cardiogenic shock includes abnormal hemodynamic values. Match each borderline value for cardiogenic shock to its hemodynamic measure.
1. Systolic BP < _____ mmHg for more than 1 hour
2. Cardiac index < _____ L/min/M²
3. Urine output < _____ mL/hr
4. PCWP > _____ mmHg

a.90.
b.30.
c.18.
d.2.2

ANSWERS:
1. a. Systolic BP < 90 mmHg for more than 1 hour
2. d. Cardiac index < 2.2 L/min/M²
3. b. Urine output < 30 mL/hr.
4. c. PCWP > 18 mmHg
See: E-learning modules at https://getinge.training/d/

9. Management and Therapy of Shock

1043. **In the acutely dyspneic anaphylactic shock patient, what two medical therapies are indicated? (Select 2 answers.)**
- a. **IV fluid administration (200-500 ml IV)**
- b. **IV lidocaine (100 mg IV)**
- c. **IV epinephrine (.5 mg IV)**
- d. **Atropine (.5 mg IV)**
- e. **Double dose of beta blockers**

ANSWERS a & c (IV fluid administration and epinephrine)

　a. **YES:** IV fluid administration (200-500 ml IV). This will replace the fluid lost due to the altered capillary permeability.
　b. NO: IV lidocaine (100 mg IV). Although the patient has some PVCs, this is not the life threatening problem. Anaphylactic shock is.
　c. **YES:** IV epinephrine (.5 mg IV)
　d. NO: Atropine (.5 mg IV). This would further speed the heart rate. The increased HR is a necessary compensation for the low CO.

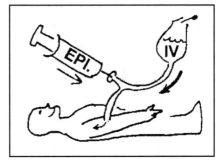

IV infusion & epinephrine

　e. Beta blockers slow and relax the heart. The CO is already too low.
In the early stages "anaphylactic shock" is reversible with administration of large volumes of fluid and/or immediate administration of epinephrine 0.5-1.0 mg IV.
See: Braunwald, chapter on "Acute Circulatory Failure (Shock)."

1044. **Because of the low vascular flow rates in severe shock the most reliable type of BP monitoring is:**
- a. **Swan-Ganz catheter**
- b. **Intra-arterial catheter**
- c. **Auscultatory BP cuff method**
- d. **Doppler BP cuff method**

ANSWER b. Intra-arterial catheter
- a. NO: Swan-Ganz catheter is used to monitor right heart pressures, not arterial blood pressure.
- b. **YES:** Intra-arterial catheter. Usually radial artery lines are used to accurately assess current BP.
- c. NO: Auscultatory BP cuff method. With low flow rates found in shock there may be no Karotkoff sounds or there may be considerable error in hearing the distorted Karotkoff sounds.
- d. NO: Doppler BP cuff method, is better than auscultatory BP, but it too often errs in measuring the diminished flow through the vasoconstricted arteries of shock patients. Even in normal patients only systolic BP can be accurately measured with

Doppler.
See: Braunwald, chapter on "Acute Circulatory Failure (Shock)."

1045. **In cardiogenic shock due to an acute MI, what therapy best provides rapid hemodynamic stabilization?**
a.   IV digitalis and diuretics
b.   IABP or Impella
c.   CABG
d.   PCI

ANSWER b. IABP. Intra-Aortic Balloon Pump or Impella
a.   NO: Digitalis and diuretics are used for CHF with chronic volume overload. Many forms of shock are volume under loaded.
b.   YES: IABP. Intra-Aortic Balloon Pump was originally designed for cardiogenic shock. It is a temporary measure that rapidly increases CO by reducing the systolic afterload and improving diastolic coronary flow. Impella is even better for shock.
c.   NO: CABG. Coronary Artery Bypass Graft surgery
d.   NO: PTCA. Percutaneous Transluminal Coronary Angioplasty
Intra-Aortic Balloon Pump is also termed counterpulsation because the balloon inflates counter to systole. IABP has the advantage of gaining time for definitive invasive or surgical therapy. It will not cure the problem. **See:** Braunwald, chapter on "Acute Circulatory Failure (Shock)." **Keywords:** Shock, Rx, IABP

1046. **For cath lab personnel the first priority toward a patient who develops signs of any acute shock is to:**
a.   Prepare to administer epinephrine IV
b.   Prepare the defibrillator
c.   Give chest compressions when BP can no longer be measured
d.   Administer O2 by nasal cannula

ANSWER d. Administer O2 by nasal cannula. The priorities in shock therapy use the acronym - VIP.
  V = Ventilation. All shock patients need O2. Severe hypoxemia patients may need intubation and ventilator support. But to start with - give them O2.
  I = Infusion. All shock patients need an IV line for fluid and drug infusion. All shock patients (except severe cardiogenic) need volume infusion.
  P = Pump. After ventilation and infusion are taken care of then proceed to improve pump performance and BP. The auscultatory BP may not be measurable in low flow shock states.

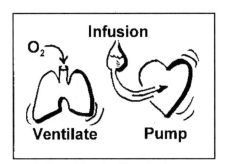

V.I.P - R$_x$ - in Shock

Like the ABCs of CPR, get the airway and ventilation taken care of before proceeding. Administer fluid, elevate legs, and then treat the MI with inotropic agents.
See: Braunwald, chapter on "Acute Circulatory Failure (Shock)." **Keywords:** Shock, priorities of therapy - VIP, Ventilation & O2

1047. This is the aortic pressure tracing from a patient in cardiogenic shock. What therapy is demonstrated at #B?

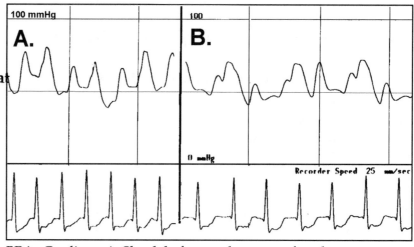

BP in Cardiogenic Shock before and   -   after therapy

a. Large dose dopamine IV
b. Medium dose beta blocker
c. IABP (1:1)
d. IABP (2:1)

ANSWER d. IABP (2:1). Balloon counterpulsation is commonly used in cardiogenic shock. Note the low BP in panel A (70 mmHg). When the balloon pump is turned on, in panel B, it is set on 2:1 ratio to time the inflations. Note the two QRS complexes between each balloon inflation. The high peaks seen every other beat are due to balloon inflation during diastole. The beat following inflation is lower and reduces the work of the LV. In this example the heart rate drops showing the heart is working less. In IABP the diastolic inflation sends additional blood flow into the coronary tree. **See:** Underhill, chapter on "Circulatory Assist Devices." **Keywords:** IABP in cardiogenic shock

1048. What approved hemodynamic support device is most effective in urgent high-risk PCI for STEMI patients with shock?

a. ECMO
b. Tandem Heart
c. Impella
d. HeartMate 3

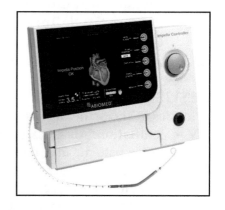

Answer: c. Impella.

ProtectedPCI.com says, "FDA APPROVES IMPELLA ® FOR HIGH-RISK PCI. Impella is the only hemodynamic support device proven safe and effective in elective and urgent High-Risk PCI patients. Impella is designed to protect the patient hemodynamically during a high-risk procedure." See: protectedPCI.com

Current standards say, "The most recent guidelines relating to percutaneous coronary intervention and management of acute coronary syndromes recommend consideration of hemodynamic support devices in the settings of HR-PCI [High Risk PCI] and STEMI with cardiogenic shock and for use in unstable patients being transported from one hospital center to another." Expert Consensus Statement on the Use of Percutaneous Mechanical Circulatory Support Devices in Cardiovascular Care says, **JACC 2013**

1049. The Impella 2.5 device pumps blood from _____ into _____.
- a. FV to FA
- b. LV to ascending AO
- c. LV apex to descending AO
- d. LA via Transseptal catheter to FA

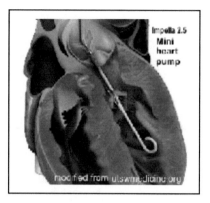

ANSWER: b. LV to ascending AO across the aortic valve. It is placed percutaneously and passed retrograde up the femoral artery into the LV. The inlet area pulls blood from the LV and expels it into the aorta to unload the LV and increase cardiac output up to 2.5 L/min. There are no oxygenators or filters, only direct increase in CO. This unloads the LV reducing it's work level and ischemia.

REFERENCES:

Baim, D. S and Grossman W.., Cardiac Catheterization, Angiography, and Intervention,   7th Ed., Lea and Febiger, 2006

Kern, M. J., Ed., The Cardiac Catheterization Handbook, 4th Ed., Mosby-Year Book, Inc.,   2016

Braunwald, Eugene, Ed., HEART DISEASE A Textbook of Cardiovascular Medicine, 9th   Ed., W. B. Saunders Co., 2012

Tipp, Alice, Basic Pathophysiological Mechanisms of Congestive Heart Failure,
        McGraw-Hill, 1979

Underhill, S. L., Ed., CARDIAC NURSING, 2nd Ed., J. B. Lippincott Co., 1989

Daily, E. K., and Schroeder, J. S., Techniques in Bedside Hemodynamic Monitoring, 4th   Ed., C. V. Mosby Company, 1989

Taylor, E. J. Ed., Dorland's Medical Dictionary, 27th ed., W. B. Saunders Co.,1988

OUTLINE: C4 - Heart Failure and Shock

1. General CHF Pathology
   a. Definitions
      i. CHF = Congestive Ht. Failure
      ii. RHF = Rt. Ht. Failure
      iii. LHF = Left Ht. Failure
      iv. PE = Pulm Edema
   b. Etiology
      i. Abnormal Relaxation - asynchronous fill
      ii. pericardial restraint - compression
      iii. intrinsic myocardial disease
         (1) stiff ventricle
         (2) Amyloidosis
      iv. Volume Overload
         (1) Hypervolemia
      v. Pressure Overload
         (1) hypertension
      vi. Dilation of ventricle
         (1) usually volume overload
      vii. Hypertrophy of ventricle
         (1) usually pressure overload
      viii. Coronary artery disease
         (1) Myocardial Infarction
      ix. myopathy
   c. Compensatory mechanisms in CHF
      i. Na & H2O retention (kidneys)
         (1) Renin-Angiotensin-Aldosterone

            (2) leads to venous congestion
            (3) leads to Edema
      ii. Vasoconstriction
         (1) maintains BP
         (2) increased cardiac work
      iii. Increased sympathetic tone
         (1) Catecholamines, Epinephrine
         (2) increased HR & cardiac work
      iv. Hypertrophy
         (1) unloads individual myo. fibers
         (2) may lead to myopathy
      v. Collagen deposition
         (1) stiff ventricle
         (2) impairs filling
2. Forms of CHF
   a. Forward Theory
      i. Low BP & CO
      ii. lead to Renin, angiotensin, aldosterone secretion
      iii. leads to Na & water retention
      iv. results in edema
   b. Backward Theory
      i. Damming effect
      ii. increased venous congestion/edema
   c. Cor Pulmonale
      i. COPD
   d. Left Heart Failure

        i.   backs up into lungs
        ii. increased PAW, PE, SOB
        iii. Orthopnea
   e. Right Heart Failure
        i.   backs up into peripheral veins
        ii. liver congestion
        iii. distended neck veins
        iv. tissue (pitting) edema
        v. ascites

3. Hemodynamics of CHF
   a. Swan-Ganz PAW pressure monitoring
        i.   elevated PAW >28 is severe
        ii. PAW = PCW = LA = LVedp
   b. CVP pressure monitoring
        i.   elevated CVP = RA
   c. Starling's hypothesis (water balance)
        i.   Oncotic pressure
        ii. hydrostatic pressure (PAW)
        iii. time to build up edema
        iv. lymphatic flow
   d. Reduced SV & EF
   e. increased EDV (dilatation)
        i.   Stretching mitral annulus
        ii. leads to Mitral Regurgitation

4. Signs & Symptoms of CHF
   a. Physical Exam
        i.   Lung Base Rales
        ii. tissue edema
        iii. ascites
        iv. cyanosis
        v. renal failure
        vi. New York Heart Classification
           (1) I, II, III, IV
   b. Symptoms
        i.   Orthopnea
        ii. SOB, Dyspnea
        iii. Frothy expectorations
   c. High output failure
        i.   pink, warm skin
        ii. high CO, SV & HR
        iii. good BP
        iv. AV fistula, thyrotoxicosis, beriberi, anemia and pregnancy

5. Management of CHF
   a. Increasing perfusion pressure
        i.   Inotropic medications
           (1) Dubutamine
           (2) Digitalis (Lanoxin)
   b. Reducing cardiac Work
        i.   vasodilators (Nitro.)
        ii. beta blockers
           (1) Inderol
   c. Control Na and water retention
        i.   Low salt diet
        ii. diuretics
           (1) reduce preload
        iii. ACE inhibltors
           (1) inhibit Angiotensin mechanism
   d. Mechanical Support
        i.   IABP
        ii. rotating tourniquets
   e. Starling curves in CHF
        i.   Inotropic state (different curve)

        ii. failure on "downslope" of curve
           (1) compensated CHF
           (2) decompensation CHF
        iii. preload level
        iv. Forrester subsets
        v. plotting patients curve
        vi. how various therapies effect patient's position on Starling curve

6. General Pathology of Shock
   a. Definitions
   b. Shock = insufficient blood flow to vital organs (brain, heart...)
           (1) Redirected flow to vital organs
           (2) Anaerobic Metabolism (Acidosis)
           (3) Shock Lung - ARDS
        ii. Vasogenic Shock
           (1) Distributive Low-Resistance
        iii. Septic Shock
           (1) Distributive High-Resistance
        iv. Obstructive Shock
           (1) E.g.,Pulmonary Embolism
           (2) DIC
        v. Cardiogenic Shock
           (1) Pump failure
           (2) Myocardial Infarction
           (3) Untreated mortality 100%
        vi. Hypovolemic Shock
           (1) E.g. hemorrhage
           (2) (Anaphylactic Shock)
        vii. Anaphylactic
           (1) hypersensitivity to any agent
              (a) respiratory distress
              (b) skin rash
              (c) vascular collapse
              (d) pooling of venous blood
        viii. irreversible stage of shock

7. Signs & symptoms of Shock
   a. Cold clammy skin
   b. collapsed neck veins
   c. decreased urine output
   d. hypotension
   e. increased HR
   f. stupor, coma
   g. reduced CO
   h. Usually elevated PAW pressure
   i. Pulmonary Edema

8. Management and therapy of Shock
   a. Increase O2 delivery to tissues
        i.   Administer Oxygen
        ii. Ventilation, Intubation
   b. Increase CO
        i.   IABP
        ii. Increase preload
           (1) elevate legs
           (2) administer IV fluid
        iii. Inotropic agents
           (1) Epinephrine
   c. Reduce LV Work
        i.   IABP
        ii. vasodilators (Nitro.)

Congenital Heart Disease

1. Review of Normal Congenital Anatomy

Pediatric Cath was removed in 2013 from RCIS. Expect basic shunt ID questions.

1050. In normal anatomy the right pulmonary artery is positioned _____ to the SVC and the left PA is positioned _____ to the descending AO.

   a.   Anterior,   Anterior
   b.   Anterior,   Posterior
   c.   Posterior,   Posterior
   d.   Posterior,   Anterior

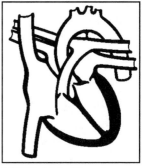

ANSWER d. Posterior, Anterior. The RPA and RPV normally lie behind the SVC, whereas the LPA lies in front of the descending AO. Note how the aortic arch curves up in front of the RPA and descends behind the LPA just to the left of the vertebra. This becomes important in distinguishing various types of transposition.
See: Braunwald, chapter on "Congenital Heart Disease." **Keywords:** RPA posterior to the SVC, LPA anterior to the AO

NORMAL Heart

1051. Normal anatomic positioning with the LA and LV apex on the patient's left side is termed:

   a.   Situs inversus, levocardia
   b.   Situs inversus, dextrocardia
   c.   Situs solitus, levocardia
   b.   Situs solitus, dextrocardia

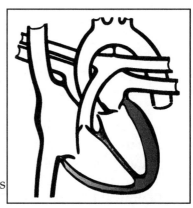

ANSWER c. Situs solitus is Latin for normal visceral position (E.g. Liver on the right side.) This means the venous blood enters the RA on the right side. When the viscera are mirror image reversed it is termed situs inversus. Here the RA and liver are on the left side.

    Levocardia refers to a left sided LV apex ("levo" means "left"). When the LV apex points to the patient's right side it is termed "dextrocardia."

Situs solitus & levocardia

See: Braunwald, chapter on "Congenital Heart Disease." **Keywords:** Normal = Situs Solitus, Levocardia

1052. **Inversion of the atria (RA on left side) is usually associated with _____ and a _____ sided IVC.**
  a.   Situs solitis,   Left
  b.   Situs solitis,   Right
  c.   Situs inversus,   Left
  d.   Situs inversus,   Right

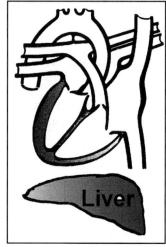

ANSWER c. Situs Inversus, Left. Situs refers to the Rt-Lt. sidedness of the viscera and atria. When "inverted" the situs inversus creates a left sided liver, IVC, SVC, and RA. This diagram shows complete inversion at all three levels of the heart: Atria, ventricles, and great vessels. Here everything is reversed: Situs inversus, ventricular inversion, and right sided descending AO. The ventricle is identified by the trabeculations. The most heavily trabeculated chamber is the RV. The LV has a smooth walled endocardium.
See: Braunwald, chapter on "Congenital Heart Disease."
Keywords: Atrial inversion = situs inversus

Total Inversion

1053. **In certain congenital anomalies it may be difficult to angioqraphically distinguish RV from LV. In normal anatomy the RV has __ and____.**
  a.   Coarse trabeculations, conus between tricuspid and pulmonic valve.
  b.   Course trabeculations, continuity of tricuspid and pulmonic valve
  c.   Smooth endocardial wall, conus between tricuspid and pulmonic valve
  d.   Smooth endocardial wall, continuity of tricuspid and pulmonic valve

ANSWER a. Coarse trabeculations, conus between tricuspid and pulmonic valve. The endocardial wall is different between the two ventricles. The RV has a rough trabeculated surface, while the LV is relatively smooth walled. This may be appreciated on the ventriculogram. and allows the physician to detect ventricular inversion (situs).

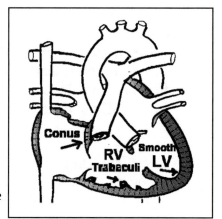

   The continuity between the AV and semilunar valves is also quite different between the two chambers. The two right sided valves are quite separate, being separated by the conus arteriosus. Whereas, the base of the mitral valve hinges off the aortic valve annulus. This is easily detected on echocardiography and angiography. In addition to the discontinuity the tricuspid valve is normally slightly caudad (lower) to the mitral valve.
See: Braunwald, chapter on "Congenital Heart Disease."

Trabeculations in RV, discontinuous TV-PV

1054. Congenital heart defects are usually caused by pathological:
- a. Atherosclerosis
- b. Rheumatic fever
- c. Bacterial infections
- d. Embryological development

ANSWER d. Embryological development. Congenital heart defects develop because the embryological development goes wrong. For example transposition of the great vessels develops when the normal truncus arteriosus fails to spiral normally.

Most causes of these defects are unknown. However, some of these defects are associated with environmental and genetic factors. Mothers who develop certain diseases or use certain drugs have a higher incidence of defective babies. These include rubella (German measles), thalidomide and alcohol abuse.

Some congenital diseases can be inherited from the parents. Children born of parents with congenital defects have a 2-10 times greater incidence of these defects. Genetically transmitted defects can include ASD, VSD, pulmonary hypertension, situs inversus and others.

See: Braunwald, chapter on "Congenital Heart Disease." **Keywords:** Causes congenital heart disease.

BOTH QUESTIONS BELOW REFER TO THIS DIAGRAM.

1055. This is a diagram of the normal prenatal circulation. Identify the structure seen at # 2.
- a. Portal vein
- b. Hepatic vein
- c. Umbilical vein
- d. Ductus venosus

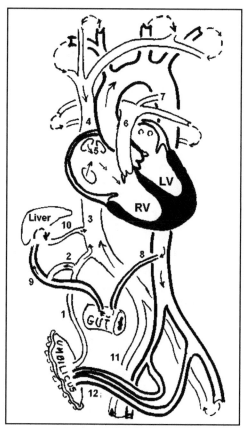

Prenatal Circulation

1056. Which prenatal structure in this diagram has the highest O2 saturation?
- a. Aorta
- b. Pulmonary vein
- c. Umbilical artery
- d. Umbilical vein

BOTH ANSWERS LISTED TOGETHER BELOW.

1078. ANSWER d. Ductus venosus
**BE ABLE TO CORRECTLY MATCH ALL
ANSWERS BELOW.**
  1. Umbilical Vein
  2. Ductus Venosus
  3. IVC
  4. SVC
  5. Patent Foramen Ovale
  6. PA
  7. PDA
  8. Mesenteric Artery
  9. Portal Vein
  10. Hepatic Vein
  11. AO & Iliac Artery
  12. Umbilical Artery

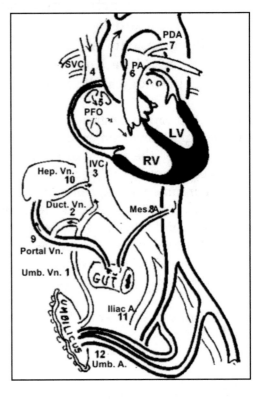

The chief structures of interest are:
  #2 the Ductus Venosus, an extension of the
umbilical veins which supplies the liver and IVC
with the only source of oxygenated blood - the
placenta.
  #5 the Patent Foramen Ovale (Ostium Secundum) between the RA and LA. It is a normal
R-L shunt carrying the oxygenated blood (approx. 62% sat.) into the LV, ascending AO,
coronary arteries, and brain (which badly needs it).
  # 7. PDA which carries the PA blood (52% O2 sat.) into the descending AO and lower
trunk and extremities. Note how all 3 of these normal shunts bridge other structures to get
the most O2 rich blood to the tissues that need it most - the liver, brain, and heart.
See: Braunwald, chapter on "Congenital Heart Disease." **Keywords:** ID structures in
prenatal circulation

1079 ANSWER d.   Umbilical Vein The placenta is the only source of O2 for fetal life.
Oxygen and CO2 are exchanged across the placenta. The umbilical arteries bring the dark
venous blood and the umbilical vein carries blood averaging only 80% O2 saturation.
That's as good as it gets for the fetus. It survives and grows with less oxygen than us "air
breathers" are used to.
  Some of this oxygenated blood passes through the liver. The brain gets the next highest
concentration of O2 and that only averages 62% O2 sat. The blackest blood comes back
from the SVC (approx. 25% sat.) because the brain extracts so much O2.
  The blood going into the lungs is only 52% O2 sat. and the pulmonary veins lower yet at
42%.
See: Braunwald, chapter on "Congenital Heart Disease." **Keywords:** Highest O2 in
umbilical vein

2. General Congenital Heart Disease

1080. **Identify the type of atrial septal defect (ASD) shown at #3 on the diagram.**
   a.   **Sinus venosus defect**
   b.   **Ductus venosus**
   c.   **Ostium secundum defect**
   d.   **Ostium primum defect**

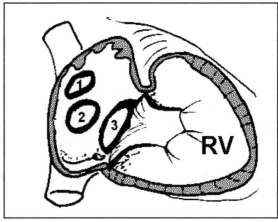

Locations of ASDs

ANSWER. d. Ostium primum defect
CORRECTLY MATCHED ANSWERS ARE:
1. SINUS VENOSUS DEFECT
   Remember that the sinus venosus forms the most inferior part of the cardiac tube. When the tube folds these lower veins form the vena cava and pulmonary veins. For this reason sinus venosus defects are near the SVC and are often associated with anomalous pulmonary veins.
2. OSTIUM SECUNDUM DEFECT:

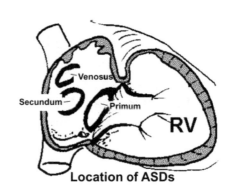

Location of ASDs

   These are located mid-atrial septum. They are often large and the most common. They are often called "Patent Foramen Ovale" because it is located where the normal fossa ovale occurs. But it is much larger. The foramen ovale normally closes at the first breath. When LA pressures exceed RA pressures a flap in the LA covers the foramen ovale. It normally seals itself to the atrial septum. But about 25% of normal adults have a "probe patent" foramen ovale which can be passed with a stiff catheter.
3. OSTIUM PRIMUM DEFECT:
   These are the lowest ASDs. They occur just above the tricuspid valve and are crescent shaped. They are also called "AV canal" or "atrioventriuclaris communis" ASDs. Since they are so low they are often associated with endocardial cushion defects where part of the mitral valve is absent.
4. DUCTUS VENOSUS: (Not shown on diagram)
   This is NOT an ASD. It is a normal shunt in the abdomen, that carries red blood from the umbilical vein through the liver and into the IVC.
See: Braunwald, chapter on "Congenital Heart Disease." **Keywords:** Types of ASDs

1081. **The most common ASD is termed the _____.**
   a. **Ostium primum**
   b. **Ostium secundum**
   c. **Sinus venosus**
   d. **Ductus venosus**

ANSWER b. Ostium secundum. These defects are often called "Patent Foramen Ovale." It is located mid-septum in the normal fossa ovale. An ostium secundum is abnormal and larger than a normal foramen ovale.

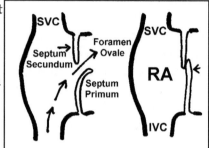

Remember, the foramen ovale normally closes at the first breath of life. When LA pressures exceed RA pressures a flap (septum primum) in the LA covers the foramen ovale. It normally grows into and seals to the atrial septum. But about 25% of normal adults have a "probe patent" foramen ovale which can often be passed with a stiff catheter.

Despite a large amount of L-R shunting, this defect is seldom recognized in infants until they become older and develop pulmonary hypertension.

Sealed Fossa Ovalis

See: Braunwald, chapter on "Congenital Heart Disease."
Keywords: Most common ASD = Ostium Secundum

1082. **A cyanotic cardiac shunt implies a:**
   a. **Low Systemic Vascular Resistance (SVR)**
   b. **High Systemic Vascular Resistance (SVR)**
   c. **Low Pulmonary Vascular Resistance (PVR)**
   d. **High Pulmonary Vascular Resistance (PVR)**

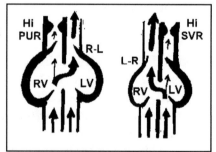

ANSWER d. High (PVR) Pulmonary Vascular Resistance. Shunts go from high pressure to low pressure areas. For a shunt to be cyanosis, it must shunt from the right side of the heart to the left side (diluting the red blood). Cyanosis lesions must have high pressures on the right side of the heart. The right sided pressures usually build up over the years to overcome high resistance in the pulmonary arterioles and capillaries.

High Pulm. resistance

Shunts are like a river which divides. If the right leg of the river is dammed up (high pulmonary resistance) the flow will be diverted into the left side of the river. This is how a R-L shunt develops. If the right sided resistance is low (low PVR) the river will take its normal route through the low resistance path and away from the peripheral circuit's high resistance.

See: Braunwald, chapter on "Congenital Heart Disease." **Keywords:** Cyanosis shunt = high PVR

1083. The degree of cyanosis in Tetralogy of Fallot is determined mainly by:
- a. Size of the ASD
- b. Size of the VSD
- c. Systemic vascular resistance
- d. Pulmonary vascular resistance

ANSWER: d. Pulmonary vascular resistance determines the amount of pulmonary blood flow and level of cyanosis. Braunwald says, " In the absence of alternative sources of pulmonary blood flow, the degree of cyanosis reflects the severity of right ventricular outflow track obstruction and the level of systemic vascular resistance. There is R-L shunt shunting across the VSD. " When the pulmonary resistance rises to equal systemic resistance, pressures equalize on both sides of the heart. Then flow across a shunt becomes bidirectional or reverses. Severe R-L shunts produce cyanosis with blue skin. L-R shunts are acyanotic with pink skin.
See: Braunwald, chapter on "Congenital Heart Disease" **Keywords:** cyanosis=high PVR

1084. Identify the location of the VSD labeled #3 on the diagram.
- a. Muscular - anterior VSD
- b. Muscular - posterior VSD
- c. Membranous - inferior VSD
- d. Membranous - infracristal VSD
- e. Membranous - subpulmonic VSD

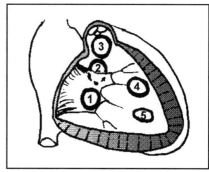
Location of VSDs - RAO view

ANSWER e. Membranous - subpulmonic VSD.
BE ABLE TO MATCH ALL ANSWERS BELOW.
1. MEMBRANOUS - inferior VSD: Beneath the septal tricuspid leaflet in the membranous IV septum.
2. MEMBRANOUS - infracristal VSD: Beneath the aortic valve at the right margin.
3. MEMBRANOUS - subpulmonic VSD: These are also called "subpulmonary" or "outlet" VSDs.
4. MUSCULAR - anterior VSD: Through the thick anterior aspect of the interventricular septum. There may be multiple small fenestrations which close with time.
5. MUSCULAR - posterior VSD: Through the thick inferior-posterior aspect of the interventricular septum. There may be multiple small fenestrations which close with time.
See: Braunwald, chapter on "Congenital Heart Disease." **Keywords:** VSD locations, membranous supracristal

1085. The most common type of VSD is located in the:
- a. Membranous septum
- b. Mid IV septum
- c. Apical IV septum
- d. Muscular septum, with multiple holes (fenestrated type)

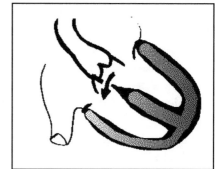

ANSWER a. Membranous septum. The membranous

Membranous IV septum

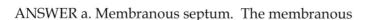

septum is the thin upper border of the IV septum. These VSDs can be even larger than the membranous septum itself. They are also called "peri" or "para" membranous VSDs. The amount of shunt through a VSD depends on its size and the amount of pulmonary vascular resistance present. A large shunt can begin as a large L-R shunt. Then pressures increase in the RV and PA, leading to elevated pulmonary vascular resistance. The shunt may then reverse - into a R-L shunt with cyanosis (Eisenminger's syndrome). Small VSD shunts may be innocent and close with time.
See: Braunwald, chapter on "Congenital Heart Disease." **Keywords:** Most common VSD = membranous septum

1086. **The most common defect causing CHF in the preterm infant "preemie" is:**
   a.   **ASD**
   b.   **VSD**
   c.   **PDA**
   d.   **Ductus Venosus**

ANSWER c. PDA . Virtually all "preemies" have a PDA which complicates their course. Preemies often have breathing problems and ARDS due to undeveloped hyaline membrane and surfactant production. The low oxygen levels may keep the PDA from constricting normally. So they may have two causes of cyanosis: a R-L shunt and ARDS. The LV volume overload may lead to CHF and pulmonary edema which again complicates the respiration problems.

   Normally the arterial PO2 and pH increase with the first breath. These cause secretion of the vasoconstrictor "prostoglandin" that begins shrinking the PDA into a vestigial "ligamentum arteriosum" and may take weeks or months to close. These vasoconstricting prostoglandins are not to be confused with the therapeutic drug "Prostaglandin E1" which has the opposite (vasodilatory) effect on the PDA.
See: Braunwald, chapter on "Congenital Heart Disease." **Keywords:** CHF in preemies usually PDA

1087. **The most common congenital heart defect found at a full term birth is:**
   a.   **ASD**
   b.   **VSD**
   c.   **PDA**
   d.   **Ductus Venosus**

ANSWER b. VSD. Approximately 0.8% of all live term births have some congenital defect. 30% of these are VSDs. The next most common are ASDs and PDAs which comprise another 10% each. So ½ of all congenital defects are simple ASD, VSD, or PDA defects.

   This 0.8% is low. The true percentage of congenital defects is underestimated because most of these children die stillborn. (Stillborn babies have a 10X higher incidence of congenital heart defects than term birth babies.) It also discounts the PDAs found in all preemies and the more common but less pathological bicuspid AO valve and mitral valve prolapse.
See: Braunwald, chapter on "Congenital Heart Disease." **Keywords:** VSD most common at term birth

1088. The most common valvular abnormality found in children is:
a. MR
b. TS with TR
c. PS
d. AS

ANSWER: c. PS. Pulmonary valve stenosis is a valvular heart disease in which outflow of blood from the right ventricle of the heart is obstructed at the level of the pulmonic valve. This results in the reduction of flow of blood to the lungs. Valvular pulmonic stenosis accounts for 80% of right ventricular outflow tract obstruction. While the most common cause of pulmonary valve stenosis is congenital heart disease, it may also be due to rheumatic heart disease or a malignant carcinoid tumor.
See: https://www.nlm.nih.gov/medlineplus/ency/article/001096.htm
Keywords: common valve = PS

1089. Which of the following is considered to be an "acyanotic" congenital heart lesion?
a. **Transposition (TGV)**
b. **Tetralogy of Fallot**
c. **Common ventricle**
d. **Tricuspid atresia**
e. **Total anomalous venous return (TAPVR)**
f. **Truncus arteriosus**

ANSWER c. Common ventricle. Note that the only answer that does NOT begin with a "T" is "Common Ventricle". The other five are the "**cyanotic - terrible T's**" all of which feature R-L shunts. Other cyanotic (blue babies) defects that do not happen to start with "T" are:
●Double outlet RV
●ASD with Pulmonary Stenosis
●Ebstein's anomaly
●Pulmonary AV fistula

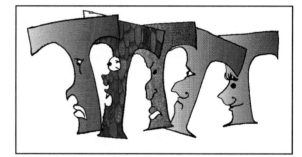
The 5 Terrible T's:

Common ventricle could be cyanotic if the pulmonary resistance was high enough to divert the RV blood into the LV.
See: Braunwald, chapter on "Congenital Heart Disease." **Keywords:** 5 cyanotic, terrible T's

1090. An elevated pulmonary resistance may become fixed by obstructive changes in the pulmonary vascular bed. This would be most likely found in a cyanotic child with chronic:
a. ASD
b. Tetralogy of Fallot
c. Transposition of great vessels
d. Transposition with pulmonary stenosis

ANSWER c. Transposition of great vessels. The congenital lesions most associated with pulmonary hypertension are: Complete Transposition of Great Vessels (TGV), single ventricle, large VSD, double outlet RV, and truncus arteriosus. Lesions that protect the lungs from high pressures like TET and TGV with PS, are less likely to develop pulmonary hypertension. These lesions provide a natural form of "pulmonary banding". Banding is a surgical band placed around the PA to constrict it. In severe L-R shunts it protects the lungs from this irreversible hypertensive condition. Atrial shunts normally cannot generate the pressures necessary for pulmonary hypertension.

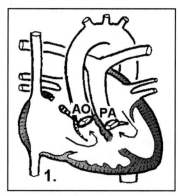

Transposition of Great Vessels (TGV)

See: Braunwald, chapter on "Congenital Heart Disease."
Keywords: Fixed high PVR in TGV

1091. A child has the hemodynamic findings shown in the box. Calculate the pulmonary vascular resistance (PVR).
  a.   1 Wood or Hybrid Resistance Unit
  b.   4.2 Wood or Hybrid Resistance Units
  c.   8.0 Wood or Hybrid Resistance Units
  d.   10.0 Wood or Hybrid Resistance Units

HEMODYNAMIC FINDINGS
CO = 2.2 L/min.
PA press. =   35 / 15 / 28 mmHg
RV press. =   36 / 0 / 5 mmHg
PA wedge =   7 / 10 / 6 mmHg

ANSWER d. 10.0 wood or Hybrid Resistance Units. Formula for Pulmonary Vascular Resistance is:

$$PVR = (PA\ mean\ pressure - Wedge\ Mean) / CO$$

PVR = (28-6)/2.2 = 22/2.2 = 10 mmHg/L/min, HRUs, or Wood units
This is an elevated PVR (0.6-1 is normal). She will be UNABLE to tolerate and benefit from corrective surgery unless the PVR can be reduced. If it drops to 1 HRU with vasodilators or O2 then corrective surgery may be considered and her prognosis improved.
See: Braunwald, chapter on "Congenital Heart Disease." **Keywords:** Calculate PVR

1092. The most common intracardiac shunts are the _____ defects that shunt blood from ___ to ___.
  a.   Cyanotic, R-L
  b.   Cyanotic, L-R
  c.   Acyanotic, R-L
  d.   Acyanotic, L-R

ANSWER d. Acyanotic, L-R. Normally pressures are higher on the left side of the heart. This directs most shunts from L-R. And since this dilutes the blue right heart blood with oxygenated red blood from the left heart, it does not effect the systemic circulation. Acyanotic babies are pink. In acyanotic congenital disease it is the heart's right side which becomes overloaded and may begin to fail. **See:** Braunwald, chapter on "Congenital Heart

Disease." **Keywords:** Most common shunts acyanotic from L → R

1093. **Cyanotic cardiac shunts show a _____ in O2 saturation on the ___ side of the heart.**
   a.   Step-up,   Left
   b.   Step-up,   Right
   c.   Step-down, Left
   d.   Step-down, Right

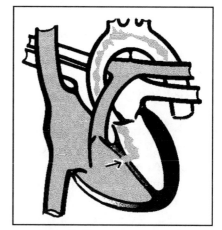

R to L Shunt = cyanosis

ANSWER c. Step-down, left. Cyanotic lesions shunt from Right to Left (R-L). The dark venous blood is shunted into the red arterial blood lowering its O2 saturation.

   Large shunts which have balanced pressures may show both R-L and L-R shunting. This is termed a "bidirectional shunt." These rare shunts show both saturation step-up on the right side and step-down on the left side.

See: Braunwald, chapter on "Congenital Heart Disease." **Keywords:** Cyanotic = sat. step-down on left side

1094. **This diagram shows an infant's blood oxygen saturation data taken at cath. From the data what type of shunt is shown? (Note that the shunt is NOT diagramed.)**
   a.   R-L ASD
   b.   L-R ASD
   c.   Bi-directional ASD
   d.   Endocardial cushion defect

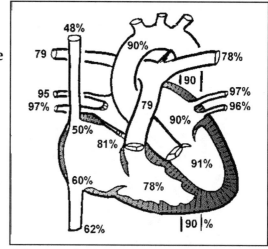

O2 sats. taken at Cath

ANSWER c. Bidirectional ASD shunts show both step-up in the right heart and step-down in the left heart. The RA shows a 30% step-up (Big L-R ASD). The LA shows a PV average of 96% which drops to 90% in the LA. This is a 6% step-down, indicating a small R-L ASD. Calculation of Qp/Qs is misleading and low. E.g. if the amount of R-L shunt = the amount of L-R shunt the Qp/Qs would be normal. A special long formula must be used for exact calculation.

See: Grossman, chapter on "Shunt Detection and Measurement." **Keywords:** Bi-directional ASD

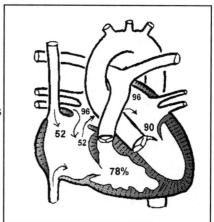

O2 sats. taken at Cath

1095. During a pediatric heart catheterization on a child with an ASD the physician is unable to enter the PA. In order to accurately evaluate pulmonary resistance, how can the PA mean pressure be estimated?
a. Transeptal puncture of AV septum
b. Pulmonary venous wedge through LA
c. Use RV systolic
d. Use LV diastolic

ANSWER b. Pulmonary venous wedge through LA. In pediatric cases it may be easy to enter the LA through an ASD or VSD. After entering the pulmonary veins a balloon tip catheter can be inflated to measure the PA wedge pressure directed into the catheter tip. Although not always reliable, PV wedge approximates the mean PA, just like a PA wedge approximates the LA. It is most useful to evaluate CHANGES in PA pressure with O2 or vasodilator testing for pulmonary reactivity.
See: Braunwald, chapter on "Congenital Heart Disease." art Disease." desaturation

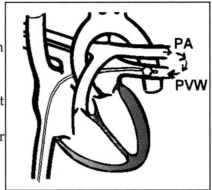

Pulm. Venous Wedge

3. Identification of Congenital Heart Disease

BOTH QUESTIONS BELOW REFER TO THIS DIAGRAM.

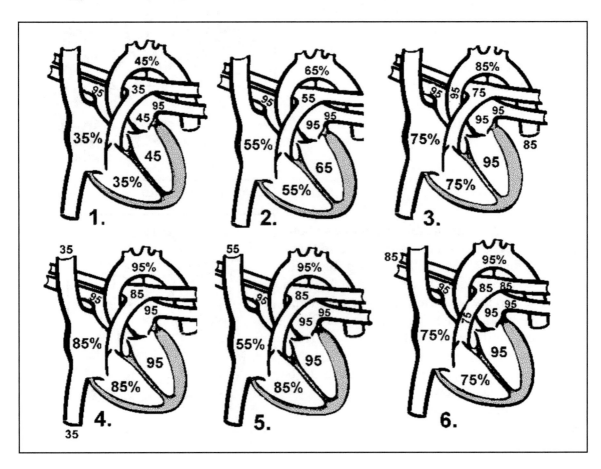

1096.   These diagrams represent the O2 saturation samples taken at heart cath. Identify the type of shunt labeled #4 on the diagram.

a.   **L-R, VSD**
b.   **L-R, PDA**
c.   **L-R, ASD**
d.   **R-L, VSD**
e.   **R-L, PDA**
f.   **R-L, ASD**

1097. Using the O2 saturation data in the diagram labeled #2, calculate the ratio of pulmonary blood flow to systemic blood flow (Qp/Qs).

a.   **1:2**
b.   **1:4**
c.   **1:6**
d.   **2:1**
e.   **4:1**
f.   **6:1**

BOTH ANSWERS LISTED TOGETHER BELOW. BE ABLE TO CORRECTLY MATCH ALL ANSWERS BELOW.

1096. ANSWER c. L-R, ASD.
CORRECTLY MATCHED ANSWERS ARE:
  1. R-L, ASD step-down in O2 from 95% to 45% in LA
  2. R-L, VSD step-down in O2 from 95% to 65% in LV
  3. R-L, PDA step-down in O2 from 95% to 85% in AO
  4. L-R, ASD step-up in O2 from 35% in vena cavae to 85% in RA
  5. L-R, VSD step-up in O2 from 55% to 85% in RV
  6. L-R, PDA step-up in O2 from 75% to 85% in PA
  Normally the RA should be an average between the IVC and SVC blood O2 sat.
  Identify the type of shunt from O2 sat. data. Note the jump in saturation from 35 to 85%. This is a HUGE jump in saturation. It must be a HUGE shunt. The step-up begins in the RA, so it must be an ASD coming into the RA from left to right.
See: Braunwald, chapter on "Congenital Heart Disease." **Keywords:** ID direction and location of shunts, L-R, VSD

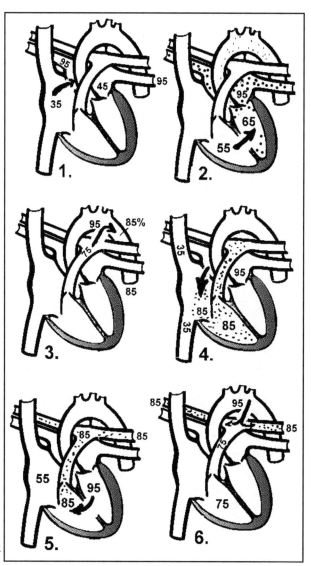

O2 Sats. taken at Cath.

1097. ANSWER b. 1:4. Diagram #2 is a 1:4 shunt from R-L into the LV. This means that the LV pumps four times as much as the RV. You can tell it is a large shunt because the LV drops in saturation from 95% to 65%.

BE ABLE TO CORRECTLY MATCH ALL ANSWERS BELOW:

1.= 1:6 = (45-35)/(95-35) = HUGE R-L shunt
2.= 1:4 = (65-55)/(95-55) = Large R-L
3.= 1:2 = (85-75)/(95-75) = Small R-L
4.= 6:1 = (95-35)/(95-85) = HUGE L-R shunt
5.= 4:1 = (95-55)/(95-85) = Large L-R
6.= 2:1 = (95-75)/(95-85) = Small L-R

Note how the side of the heart from which the shunt originates always has constant saturation. E.g. in all R-L shunts the right heart O2 sat is always the same in RA, RV, & PA, with only slight variation due to streaming and incomplete mixing. While in all L-R shunts the O2 sat. is the same in LA, LV, and AO. Also, note that pulmonary venous saturation is 95% regardless of the direction of shunt. This is true if the lungs are oxygenating well. (Grossman says you can usually estimate PV at 98% sat. even if you can't get in to sample it.) The ratio of pulmonary to systemic blood flows (Qp/Qs) formula is:

$$\frac{Qp}{Qs} = \frac{(SA - SV)}{(PV - PA)} = \frac{\text{Systemic A-V dif.}}{\text{Pulm. A-V dif.}} \approx \frac{AO - RA}{PV - PA}$$

SA = Systemic Arterial (usual distal AO)
SV = Systemic venous (usually IVC, SVC average or RA whichever is lower)
PV = Pulmonary venous (usually PV average or LA whichever is higher)
PA = Pulmonary arterial (usually PA or distal PA)

This formula, which is easily derived from the Fick formulae, is the ratio of the reciprocal A-V differences of the two systems. Note how Qp (pulmonary) is in the left numerator but, the systemic A-V difference is in the numerator - on the right side of equation. This is

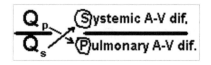

because of the inverse relation between A-V difference and CO. It looks weird, Qp looks opposite to pulmonary A-V difference. **But that is the way this formula is always set up.**

The only tricky part occurs in ASDs and PDAs. The mixing of shunt blood with non-contaminated blood, presents the question of which O2 saturation to put into the Qp/Qs equation. In response, always select the samples closest to the **capillary system** named.

#1. In diagram #1 which sample best represents the pulmonary venous O2 sat? 45% or 95%? Well 95% is closer to the lung capillary system, so 95% is the pulmonary venous O2 sat. before the shunt dumps in. Qp/Qs = (45-35)/(95-35) = 10/60 = 1:6 .

This means six times as much blood goes through the systemic capillary bed as through the pulmonary system.

#2. In the 2nd diagram: SA = AO = 65% sat.

SV = RA = 55%
PV = LA = 95%
PA = PA = 55%

- Substituting into the Qp/Qs formula we get:

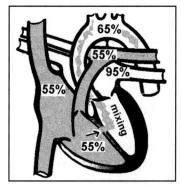

#2. R-L VSD shunt

$Qp/Qs = (65-55)/(95-55) = 10/40 = 1/4 = 1:4$ shunt

#3. Which sat. represents the best mixed systemic arterial sample 95% or 85%? Since we always select the sample closest to its capillary system, here the AO feeds the systemic capillaries, so the distal AO 85% best represents the systemic arterial O2 sat (although some 95% sat blood flows to the arch vessels).

#4. In #4 which sat. best represents the systemic venous sat? Since the IVC & SVC are closest to the systemic capillary bed they represent the O2 sat of the blood draining it. So SV = 35%. $Qp/Qs = (95-85)/(95-35) = 10/60 = 1:6$ ratio.

#5. This is a straightforward L-R VSD. RV blood increases from 55% to 85%. $Qp/Qs=(95-55)/(95-85) = 40/10 = 4:1$

#6. Which sat. best represent PA blood 95% or 85%? The 85% feeds the pulmonary capillary bed, so it best represent pulmonary arterial blood. $Qp/Qs= (95-85)/(95-75) = 10/20 = 1:2$ shunt.

Note the dotted blood in the diagram represents the mixed arterial and venous blood downstream from the shunt. These shunts are exaggerated and simplified for teaching purposes. **See:** Braunwald, chapter on "Congenital Heart Disease."

REFERENCES:

Baim, D. S and Grossman W.., Cardiac Catheterization, Angiography, and Intervention, 7th Ed., Lea and Febiger, 2006

Kern, M. J., Ed., The Cardiac Catheterization Handbook, 6th Ed., Mosby-Year Book, Inc., 2016

Braunwald, Eugene, Ed., HEART DISEASE A Textbook of Cardiovascular Medicine, 9th Ed., W. B. Saunders Co., 2012

Fink, B.W., *"Congenital Heart Disease, a deductive approach,"*3rd Ed., C.V. Mosby, 1991

OUTLINE: C5 - Congenital Heart Disease

1. REVIEW OF NORMAL CONGENITAL ANATOMY
   a. Prenatal structures/flow
      i. Umbilical Vein
      ii. Ductus Venosus
      iii. IVC
      iv. SVC
      v. Patent Foramen Ovale
      vi. PA
      vii. PDA
      viii. Mesenteric Artery
      ix. Portal Vein
      x. Hepatic Vein
      xi. Iliac Artery
      xii. Umbilical artery
   b. Normal Situs
      i. Levocardia
      ii. Right sided vena cava
      iii. Left sided AO
   c. Angiograpy
      i. RV trabeculations
      ii. LV smooth wall
      iii. Great vessels
   d. Fetal Shunts and flows
      i. Foramen Ovale
         (1) Oxygenated blood passes
         (2) assures brain & heart O2
      ii. Ductus Arteriosus
      iii. Ductus Venosus
2. GENERAL CONGENITAL HEART DISEASE
   a. Closure of fetal shunts
      i. Foramen Ovale - 1st breath
      ii. Ductus Venosus - cutting umbilicus
      iii. Ductus Arteriosus - 1-3 days past term
         (1) Preemies retain PDA
   b. Most common defects
      i. Preemies - PDA
      ii. full term - VSD
   c. Pulmonary Vascular Resistance
      i. Calculation of PVR
         (1) Pulm. Flow. or CO
         (2) PA mean pressure
         (3) Wedge LA mean pressure
      ii. Elevated PVR
         (1) pulmonary hypertension
         (2) Reversible - Oxygen reactivity
         (3) Irreversible - fixed PVR
            (a) Eisenmingers
         (4) Associated with R-L shunts (Cyanosis)
      iii. Acyanotic
         (1) L-R SHUNT
            (a) most common shunt direction
            (b) ASD

                    (i)   L-R ASD
                    (ii)   bi-directional ASD
                    (iii) endocardial cushion defect
              (c)   VSD
              (d)   PDA
         (2)   Obstructive lesions
         (3)   Other congenital lesions
    iv.   Cyanotic
         (1)   R-L SHUNT
              (a)   Transposition (TGV)
              (b)   Tetralogy of Fallot
              (c)   Tricuspid Atresia
              (d)   Total Anomalous Venous
                     Return (TAPVR)
              (e)   Truncus Arteriosus
              (f)   Persistent Fetal Pathway
         (2)   implies elevated PVR
  d.   Locations ASDs
    i.   Sinus Venosus defect
    ii.   Ostium Secundum defect
    iii. Ostium Primum defect
  e.   Locations VSDs
    i.   Muscular - anterior VSD
    ii.   Muscular - posterior VSD
    iii. Membranous - inferior VSD
    iv. Membranous - infracristal VSD
    v.   Membranous - supracristal VSD

3.   PHYSICAL EXAM IN CONGENITAL HEART
DISEASE
  a.   Cyanosis
    i.   central (low P_aO2)
         (1)   more than 3 gm% desaturated Hgb.
              (usually <80% sat)
         (2)   Pulmonary Hypoxemia

                    (3)   R-L shunt - cyanosis
        ii.   peripheral (vasoconstriction)
  b.   Clubbing of fingers
  c.   Murmurs
    i.   ASD
    ii.   VSD
    iii. PDA

4.   IDENTIFICATION OF CONGENITAL HEART
DISEASE
  a.   Hemodynamics
    i.   Catheter positions in heart
         (1)   Normal x-ray silhouette
         (2)   VSD
         (3)   Left SVC
         (4)   PDA
         (5)   Anomalous venous return
    ii.   O2 saturation data
         (1)   Diagnostic run during cath
              (a)   Step up in Rt. Ht. = L-R shunt
              (b)   Set down in Lt. Ht. = R-L Shunt
         (2)   Calculation Qp/Qs
              (a)   Qp/Qs normally = 1.0
              (b)   Qp/Qs <1 is R-L shunt
              (c)   Qp/Qs >1 is L-R shunt
         (3)   Cardiac Pressures
              (a)   Normal Elevated Right sided
                   pressures
              (b)   PA wedge
              (c)   PV wedge
    iii. O2 consumption/BSA elevated
         (1)   high metabolic rate
  b.   Angiography
  c.   Echocardiography

Vascular Disease

1. General Vascular

1098. The abbreviation used in vascular procedures labeled at #2 (Compression of subclavian artery or nerves) is:

a. TIA
b. CVA
c. TOS
d. EVAR
e. DVT
f. AVF (AVM)
g. AAA
h. FMD
I. RVH
j. Bruit

Vascular Abbreviations

1. Bulging aorta in abdomen
*2. Compression of subclavian artery or nerves
3. Hyperplastic web or fibrosing lesions in artery
4. Increased BP due to renal artery stenosis
5. Small stroke
6. Stroke
7. Clotting of leg veins
8. Aortic stentgrafts
9. Shunt between artery and vein (usually for dialysis)
10. Murmur of arterial stenosis

ANSWER #2. = c. = TOS = Thoracic Outlet Syndrome = COMPRESSION OF SUBCLAVIAN ARTERY OR NERVES as they exit the thorax, resulting in arm numbness and pain.

BE ABLE TO CORRECTLY MATCH ALL ANSWERS.

<u>**VASCULAR ABBREVIATIONS = DEFINITION**</u>
1. **AAA =** Abdominal Aortic Aneurysm = BULGING AORTA in the abdomen
2. **TOS =** Thoracic Outlet Syndrome = COMPRESSION OF SUBCLAVIAN ARTERY OR NERVES as they exit the thorax, resulting in arm numbness and pain
3. **FMD =** Fibro-Muscular Dysplasia = HYPERPLASTIC WEB OR FIBROSING LESIONS IN ARTERY. Usually increased medial fibrous tissue with mural aneurysms (Ectatic).
4. **RVH =** Reno-Vascular Hypertension = INCREASED Blood Pressure (Hypertension) DUE TO RENAL ARTERY STENOSIS or other obstruction to renal blood flow that activates the Renin-Angiotensin vasoconstrictor system
5. **TIA =** Transient Ischemic Attack = SMALL STROKE (Temporary interference with the brains blood supply) - resolves in 24 hours
6. **CVA =** Cerebral Vascular Accident = STROKE = Pathologic Ischemia or hemorrhage within the brain (Apoplexy) - Effects last over 24 hours
7. **DVT =** Deep Vein Thrombosis = CLOTTING of deep LEG VEINS (in 25% DVT leads to PE/Pulmonary Embolism.)
8. **EVAR =** Endovascular Aortic Repair usually of aortic aneurysms with stents or stentgrafts.
9. **AVF/AVM =** Arterio Venous Fistula or Malformation = SHUNT BETWEEN ARTERY AND VEIN (Usually for Renal DIALYSIS)
10. **BRUIT** (not an abbreviation) = Stenotic arterial (or venous) murmur = Sound of blood rushing through a constricted vessel
See: Kandarpa, appendix of "Abbreviations." **Keywords:** Vascular abbreviations

1099.   **In the USA what is the most frequent reason for a cardiovascular patient to visit a physician and the leading indication for a prescription?**
a. **Coronary artery disease**
b. **Peripheral atherosclerotic disease**
c. **Pulmonary hypertension**
d. **Systemic hypertension**

ANSWER d. Systemic hypertension is found in 60,000,000 US citizens. It is the most common CV risk factor in all developing countries. In recent years there has been an explosion of hypertensive patients. This is because of the aging population and lower criteria for diagnosing hypertension. In the 1970's a BP over 160/95 mmHg. defined hypertension. Then the limit was 140 mmHg. Recently it has been lowered even further to 130 mmHg systolic or 80 mmHg diastolic for stage 1 hypertension. Lowering the diagnostic criteria has doubled the population of hypertensive patients. Lowering the diagnostic criteria is justified because of the devastating effects of hypertension and the efficiency with which it can be controlled.
See: ACC, 2017 Guideline for High Blood Pressure in Adults

1100.   **Which arterial wall is primarily involved with arteriosclerotic changes?**
- a. **Intima**
- b. **Media**
- c. **Basement membrane**
- d. **Adventia**

ANSWER a. Intima. Although secondary changes may sometimes be found in the media, most atherosclerotic changes occur in the inner wall of the arteries (intima). Intimal changes associated with atherosclerosis are: intimal injury, denudation, platelet aggregation, deposition of fat, proliferation of smooth muscle from the media, and eventually thrombus formation from associated injury. The diagram shows a section of normal epithelium (#1) and an injured (denuded) arterial wall (#2). Platelets are attracted, aggregate and attach to the injured area. If the internal elastic wall is broken, medial cells may also migrate into the area of injury.

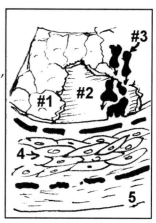

Intimal injury

    Any kind of damage to the intimal wall will eventually induce atherosclerotic-like lesions. Injury inducing stressors include: hypertension (shear stress), smoking (injurious hydrocarbons), diabetes, elevated cholesterol, and elevated catecholamine. Labeled are:
    1. Intimal wall (a single layer of endothelial cell)
    2. Denuded (injured) arterial wall
    3. Platelets
    4. Media - smooth muscle cells
    5. Adventia (tunica externa)
See: Underhill, chapter on "Pathogenesis of Atherosclerosis." **Keywords:** Arterial wall, atherosclerotic changes

1101.   **Which type of atherosclerotic lesion is most often associated with unstable angina, thrombus formation, and myocardial infarction?**
- a. **Fatty lesions**
- b. **Fibrous plaque**
- c. **Calcified plaque**
- d. **Smooth muscle proliferation**

ANSWER c. The "calcified plaque" or "complicated lesion" is an unstable ruptured plaque. They tend to ulcerate, bleed, and thrombose. The three phases of ASHD shown in arterial walls are:
    1. Fatty streaks develop from foam cells(cells with fat in them), which balloon out but usually don't obstruct blood flow.

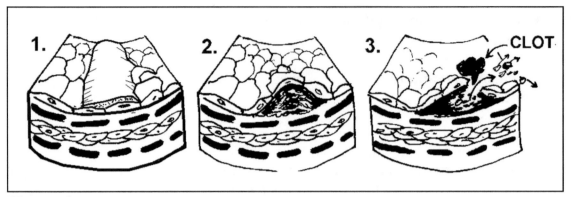

Fibrous plaques

2. Raised fibrous plaques are characteristic and stable protrusions in the lumen. These plaques include smooth muscle cells which migrate in to help cover the injury. These growths and inclusions of fat push up the intima. A fibrous plaque eventually covers the lesion. These plaques are believed to be irreversible.

3. Complicated lesions are calcified fibrous plaques which have plaque rupture, hemorrhage into the plaque, and/or thrombus formation. This unstable plaque may rupture, attracts clot and often results in complete occlusion and STEMI myocardial infarction. Many of these unstable plaques have remodeled the vessel so the enlargement does not narrow the vessel lumen, but makes the vessel bulge outward. That makes them invisible to angiography.

See: Underhill, chapter on "Pathogenesis of Atherosclerosis." **Keywords:** calcified plaque, complicated lesion

1102. **What are the 4 main modifiable risk factors associated with peripheral vascular disease? (Select 4 below.)**
a. **Diabetes mellitus**
b. **Hypercholesterolemia**
c. **Cigarette smoking**
d. **Hypertension**
e. **Family history of PAD**
f. **Black race**
g. **Male gender**

ANSWERS: a, b, c, & d. Diabetes mellitus, Hypercholesterolemia, Cigarette smoking, and Hypertension are the greatest risk factors that patients can modify. They have relative risks of PAD 2.0 to 5 times normal.

Braunwald says, "The well known modifiable risk factors associated with CAD also contribute to atherosclerosis of the peripheral circulation.... [nonmidifiable factors are] PAD prevalence is greater in men than in women in some studies, and greater in blacks than in non-hispanic whites." **See:** Braunwald, chapter on "Peripheral Artery Disease"

1103. Check the 3 general conditions that predispose to vascular thrombosis formation in the body, known as Virchow's Triad. (Select 3 below)
a. Arterial calcification
b. Blood turbulence
c. Stagnation of blood
d. Injury to the vessel wall
e. Sharp vessel angulation
f. Blood hypercoagulability
g. Endothelial nitric oxide
h. Elevated plasma cholesterol & triglyceride

ANSWERS: c, d, & f. Stagnation of blood, injury to the vessel wall, and blood hypercoagulability. In the diagram of Virchow's Triad note the various pathologies under each of 3 major coagulation factors.

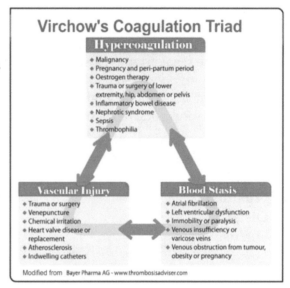

Braunwald says, "In 1856, Rudolf Virchow postulated a triad of factors that predispose to intravascular coagulation: local trauma to the vessel wall, hypercoagulability, and stasis." **See:** Braunwald, chapter of Pulmonary Embolism

Kyrle & Eichinger, say: "Venous thrombi are formed in the setting of low flow and low shear stress and mainly consist of fibrin strands, red blood cells, and a few platelets. In 1856, Rudolf Virchow postulated that abnormalities in blood flow, hypercoagulability of the blood, and injury to the vessel wall are causally related to thrombus formation. Reduced venous blood flow during, for instance, immobilization, prolonged bed rest, limb paresis, long-distance travel, or in obese or pregnant individuals, has been convincingly shown to increase the risk of deep vein thrombosis (DVT). In keeping with Virchow's concept, alterations of the coagulation system that induce a hypercoagulable state also confer an increased risk of DVT. For example, patients with high clotting factor levels have an increased risk of both a first and a recurrent DVT. Alterations of the vessel wall that lead to plaque formation and plaque rupture play a key role in the development and progression of arterial occlusive disease." **See:** Kyrle & Eichinger, "Is Virchow's triad complete?" Blood Journal, 2009

Virchow's Triad enumerates the general prothrombotic factors but fails to take into account the antithrombotic factors like natural anticoagulants and endothelial nitric oxide. The coagulable state is a balance between these prothrombotic and antithromboti factors.

1104. In what part of the body does the most peripheral artery disease occur?
a. Legs
b. Arms
c. Renal arteries
d. Carotid arteries

ANSWER: a. Legs. Braunwald says, "Lower limb peripheral artery disease (PAD) is the third leading cause of atherosclerotic vascular morbidity after coronary heart disease and stroke." **See:** Braunwald chapter on Peripheral Artery Disease

1105.   **Renal fibromuscular dysplasia (FMD) usually occurs in the _____ and is treated with _____.**
   a. **Distal renal artery, POBA**
   b. **Distal renal artery, Stenting**
   c. **Proximal renal artery, POBA**
   d. **Proximal renal artery, Stenting**

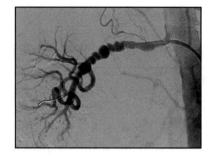

ANSWER: a. Distal renal artery, POBA. FMD has a distinctive angiographic appearance with a beaded, aneurysmal pattern and web stenosis in the distal 2/3 and branches of the renal arteries closest to the kidney. On the other hand atherosclerotic renal artery stenosis involves a smooth narrowing of the proximal main renal arteries and is frequently bilateral. Balloon angioplasty is all that is usually needed for FMD, but stenting is best for atherosclerotic renal artery stenosis.

1106.   **Where is atherosclerotic renal artery stenosis usually located?**
   a. **Ostial**
   b. **Proximal**
   c. **Distal**
   d. **Diffuse**

ANSWER: a. Ostial. "Most atheromatous renal artery stenosis is due to aortic plaques encroaching on the ostium of the renal artery." See: http://www.ncbi.nlm.nih.gov/pmc/articles/PMC1127255/

1107.   **To evaluate renal artery stenosis with a pressure wire what vasodilator is optimal?**
   a. **Adenosine**
   b. **Papaverine**
   c. **Isuprel**
   d. **Diltiazem or Verapamil**

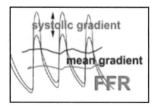

ANSWER: b. Papaverine. To evaluate the significance of RAS, evaluate the FFR using papaverine instead of adenosine as the hyperemic agent.

   Kern says, "Similar to the practice in CAD, there has been a recent movement to define significant RAS, not by anatomic severity, but rather by physiologic impact using pressure wire evaluation with induction of hyperemia. Of note, adenosine should not be used in the renal vasculature for the induction of vasodilation because it can paradoxically provoke renal artery vasoconstriction. The optimal vasodilator for the renal vasculature is papaverine, which must be used with heparin-free saline, because the combination of these two drugs leads to formation of a precipitate that may provoke microvascular injury. Some studies have evaluated the use of other vasodilators, including dopamine. A hemodynamically significant RAS is characterized by one of the following conditions: (1) resting pressure distal to stenosis/pressure in the aorta (Pd/Pa) <0.90, (2) hyperemic Pd/Pa called fractional flow reserve (FFR) for the coronary circulation <0.80, (3) hyperemic mean gradient >20 mm Hg, (4) hyperemic systolic gradient >20 mm Hg, and (5) minimal luminal area (MLA) by intravascular ultrasound (IVUS) imaging of 8.6 mm2 or less. Given the limitations of angiography, any intermediate stenosis should likely be assessed using one of these techniques." **See:** Kern, chapter on "Peripheral Artery Disease and Angiography"

2A. Hypertension - General & Types

1108. **Right ventricular dilatation and hypertrophy secondary to pulmonary hypertension is termed:**
   a. **Cor pulmonale**
   b. **Hyaline membrane disease**
   c. **Asymmetric septal hypertrophy**
   d. **Hypertrophic cardiomyopathy**

ANSWER a. Cor pulmonale. "Cor" = heart; "Pulm" = lungs. Pulmonary hypertension and hypertrophy. This is a backing up of blood in the PA due to increased pulmonary vascular resistance usually due to chronic lung disease.
See: Medial dictionary. **Keywords:** Cor pulmonale

1109. **Secondary hypertension may be due to:**
   a. **Renal artery stenosis**
   b. **Hepatic artery stenosis**
   c. **Vena cava obstruction**
   d. **Valvular heart disease**

ANSWER a. Reno-vascular obstructive disease involves older men. The stenosis occurs is the proximal third of the main renal artery. These are usually amenable to angioplasty if they are not in the renal artery orifice itself.

The remainder of reno-vascular disease occurs in younger women, and occurs in the distal 2/3 and branches of the renal arteries. This latter is termed fibro-muscular disease (FMD). These are small aneurysms appearing in the distal renal artery as a "string of pearls." (See: left renal FMD in the diagram.) A rare type of FMD is intimal fibroplasia. This type of renal stenosis manifests as a web of fibers in the distal artery. FMD is usually easy to angioplasty.

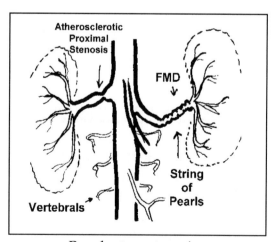

Renal artery stenosis

Only 5% of hypertensives have renal stenosis. But it is the most common secondary form of hypertension that is correctable. It is standard practice to shoot a renal arteriogram after every heart cath on patients with hypertension.
See: Braunwald, chapter on "Systemic Hypertension."

1110. The most common cause of renal artery stenosis is:
a. FMD
b. Hypertension
c. Arteriosclerosis
d. intimal hyperplasia

ANSWER: c. Areriosclerosis. Grossman says, "It is important to distinguish between the two major causes of renal artery stenosis: fibromuscular dysplasia (FMD and the more common atherosclerotic disease." **See:** Grossman, chapter on "Peripheral Interventions"

1111. Mainstem renal artery stenosis is best imaged with small amounts of contrast using:
a. DSA
b. IVUS
c. MRA
d. CTA

ANSWER: a. DSA. King say, "...angiography remains the gold standard for the detection of RAS...." Digital subtraction angiography improves contrast resolution and may decrease the volume of contrast needed to as little as 15 mL.

Khan, 2013 article in Medscape says, "Conventional angiography remains the criterion standard for the detection of RAS, although CTA and MRA are increasingly being used.... Lesions occluding more than 50% of the diameter of the artery are considered significant. ...Generally, flush aortography suffices for mainstem RAS, but if branch stenosis is suspected, selective renal angiography may better define the lesion.... CTA or MRA may cause the clinician to overlook mild cases of fibromuscular dysplasia (FMD) that are detectable with digital subtraction angiography (DSA)...." Khan, "Imaging in Renal Artery Stenosis/Renovascular Hypertension " Medscape, April 2013

2B. Hypertension - Pathology

1112. The vast majority of high blood pressure is caused by:
a. Stress and drug side effects
b. High salt and cholesterol diet
c. Renal or endocrine disease
d. Primary and unknown factors

ANSWER d. Primary and unknown factors. 90% - 95% of all hypertensive patients have no evident medical cause for it. This is termed "primary," "essential," or "idiopathic" hypertension; as opposed to the 5-10% of secondary hypertensions which have a distinct cause.

The most common "secondary" cause of hypertension is "chronic renal" disease such as: glomerulonephritis, renal failure, polycystic renal disease, chronic pyelonephritis, and nephropathy. These chronic renal diseases account for the largest category of secondary hypertension. These comprise approximately 5% of all hypertensives. Discrete renovascular stenosis accounts for only 1% of all hypertension.

We do know that primary hypertension often runs in families, and has some hereditary component. There are also, many associated risk factors, such as salt intake which in themselves are not the "cause" of hypertension. They are only "associated with it."
See: Underhill, chapter on "High Blood Pressure." **Keywords:** majority of hypertension = primary, essential

1113. The chief sequelae (consequence) associated with uncontrolled hypertension is:
a. Sudden death
b. Dilated heart (dilated cardio-myopathy)
c. Acceleration of atherosclerosis
d. Dilation and rupture of aortic aneurysms

ANSWER c. Acceleration of atherosclerosis. Hypertension accelerates the atherosclerotic process. If left untreated, most hypertensive patients eventually die of some form of atherosclerotic cardio-vascular disease. 50% die of coronary artery disease or CHF, 33% die of stroke, and 10-15% die of renal disease secondary to the hypertension.
See: Braunwald, chapter on "Systemic Hypertension."

1114. Increased blood levels of _____ can control and reduce a patient's tendency toward high BP.
a. Catecholamines & angiotensin
b. Prostocyclins and nitric oxide
c. Thromboxane A2 and endothelin
d. Na+ and aldosterone

ANSWER b. Prostocyclins and nitric oxide are naturally occurring potent vasodilators released by the endothelium (termed EDRF). They act by increasing Na+ and water excretion.
a. NO, CATECHOLAMINES & ANGIOTENSIN: are both potent vasoconstrictor humors.
b. YES, PROSTOCYCLINS AND NITRIC OXIDE: are potent vasodilator humors also termed "Endothelial Derived Relaxation Factors (EDRF)". Remember, that prostoglandin E2 is a potent vasodilator used to keep PDAs open and also cause erections in impotency. They are stimulated by bradykinin's. These also act to increase Na+ and water excretion. Note the naturally occuring hormones dilate the peripheral resistance vessels and are shown in the diagram below.
c. NO, INCREASED NA+ AND ALDOSTERONE: both act to retain water and increase the circulating volume and hence the cardiac output through increased preload. The renin - angiotensin - aldosterone system is a major contributor to hypertension.

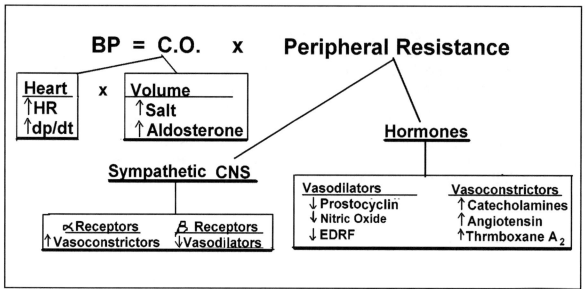

Factors increasing the blood pressure, BP = CO x SVR
CO is increased by heart and volume factors.
SVR (Systemic or Peripheral Resistance) is increased by hormones-
vasoconstrictor drugs and sympathetic CNS, alpha receptor stimulation.

d. NO, THROMBOXANE A2 AND ENDOTHELIN are endothelial derived constrictor
factors (EDCFs).

See: Braunwald, chapter on "Systemic Hypertension." **Keywords:** Regulate high BP =
prostocyclin, nitric oxide, EDRF

1115. **An example of an acute hypertensive emergency "crisis," where an extremely
elevated BP needs to be rapidly reduced (in 1 hr), is in hypertensive patients
with:**
a. **Widow-maker coronary lesion**
b. **Accelerating angina**
c. **Acute aortic dissection**
d. **Post op. CABG patient**

ANSWER c. Acute aortic dissection is a life threatening emergency, especially in the
ascending AO, where cerebral and coronary arteries may be blocked by a flap of intima.
High blood pressure must be rapidly reduced since it accelerates the tearing process. Type
A dissections are a surgical emergency. The other pathologies listed are "urgent" but not
quite as "emergent" as the dissecting aneurysm. Other hypertensive emergencies are:
  • Acute pulmonary edema
  • Pheochromocytoma crisis (tumors in adrenal cortex)
  • Intracranial hemorrhage
  • Eclampsia (convulsions and coma complication of pregnancy)
See: Underhill, chapter on "High Blood Pressure." **Keywords:** Hypertensive emergency =
AO Dissection

1116. Isolated systolic hypertension (E.g., BP of 160/80mmHg) is associated with:
a. Oral contraceptive use
b. Renal parenchymal disease (E.g., Nephritis)
c. Coarctation of the aorta (Post-ductal type)
d. Elderly rigid atherosclerotic aorta.

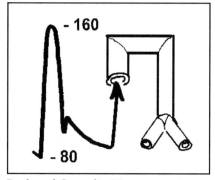

Isolated Systolic Hypertension

ANSWER d. Elderly rigid atherosclerotic aorta. Isolated systolic hypertension (ISH) occurs when systole alone is elevated and diastole is not. As atherosclerosis progresses in elderly individuals, the large arteries become calcified, non-compliant, and rigid. They become like old metal pipes that "hammer" when the water is turned off and on.

But, when the systolic BP exceeds 160 mmHg increased cardiovascular risk still exists. Longstanding hypertension like this should be reduced slowly. The other answers are possible causes of regular systolic and diastolic hypertension.

See: Underhill, chapter on "High Blood Pressure." **Keywords:** Isolated systolic hypertension = elderly rigid atherosclerosis

1117. An accelerated extreme form of hypertension has a diastolic BP over 130 or 140 mmHg with associated retinal hemorrhages and impaired vision. This is termed _____ hypertension.
a. Metastatic
b. Malignant
c. Ocular
d. Labile

ANSWER b. Malignant hypertension is a severe hypertensive state with a poor prognosis. It is characterized by edema of the ocular fundus with vascular exudates and hemorrhage. The media of small arterioles is thickened, as is the LV wall. This dangerous form of hypertension must be treated quickly and aggressively to avoid stroke and blindness.
See: Underhill, chapter on "High Blood Pressure." **Keywords:** Malignant hypertension

2C. Hypertension - Diagnosis

1118. The "cut point" above which "mild or borderline" hypertension begins is a BP greater than:
a. > 160/105 mmHg.
b. > 160/90 mmHg.
c. > 140/90 mmHg.
d. > 130/80 mmHg.

ANSWER d. >130/80 mmHg is the new threshold above which the patient has "hypertension." Using this threshold, a patient with a BP of 135/85 would get anti-hypertensive treatment.

People in the mild and borderline hypertensive range are followed with repeated BP readings over the next year. It has been shown that many in this "borderline" range will have lower subsequent BP readings - perhaps in the normal range. This artifact is termed "White Coat Hypertension" and is apparently due to the temporary stress of the medical exam. General health measures should be followed such as: weight reduction, exercise, and Na and cholesterol restricted diet. If "general health" regimens are not successful in maintaining normal BP, then antihypertensive agents are considered. Research continues on this borderline group to determine how aggressive anti-hypertensive therapy should become.

AHA ACC guidelines 2017 are:
- Normal: Less than 120/80 mm Hg;
- Elevated: Systolic between 120-129 and diastolic less than 80
- Stage 1: Systolic between 130-139 or diastolic between 80-89
- Stage 2: Systolic at least 140 or diastolic at least 90 mm Hg
- Hypertensive crisis: Systolic over 180 and/or diastolic over 120, with patients needing prompt changes in medication if there are no other indications of problems, or immediate hospitalization if there are signs of organ damage.

See: Braunwald, chapter on "Systemic Hypertension."

1119. At the time of heart catheterization an "accelerating angina" patient is found to have diffuse severe multi-vessel coronary disease. CABG surgery is openly discussed with the patient. He has diabetes and elevated blood creatinine and BUN levels. His BP has recently elevated from 150/90 to 190/110 mmHg. Besides LV and coronary angiography, what additional angiography should be done at this time?
a. Ilio-femoral arteriogram (for IABP insertion pre-surgery)
b. Carotid arteriography (for stroke prevention)
c. Renal arteriography (possible reno-vascular stenosis)
d. IMA arteriography (evaluate IMA for CABG)

ANSWER c. Renal arteriography (possible reno-vascular stenosis). Several factors should make you suspect secondary reno-vascular hypertension.
1. Clinical signs including recent onset and rapid progression of hypertension.
2. Extensive coronary or peripheral vascular disease suggests extensive atherosclerosis in peripheral vessels as well.
3. History or signs of renal failure, in this case suggested by the elevated creatinine and BUN levels.

Most hypertensive patients with these findings have obstructive renal artery stenosis. Renal artery stenosis causes renal ischemia which triggers the renin, angiotensin and aldosterone reflex.

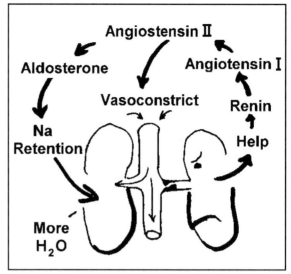
Renovascular Hypertension

As the kidney becomes more deprived of blood it sends out a hormone (renin - angiotensin) call for help (I NEED MORE BLOOD!). The angiotensin vasoconstricts the periphery and raises the BP. It also triggers production of aldosterone that increases sodium retention and contributes to the hypertension. The first hormone produced is renin. It is easily measured in the renal venous blood. Renin triggers angiotensin I & II release (vasoconstrictor) and aldosterone (a water retainer). All of this may lead to a hypertension which can be cured by renal artery angioplasty or surgery.

Braunwald says "Clearly the renal arteries should be examined in every hypertensive patient undergoing angiography if possible. If renal artery stenoses are seen, additional evidence must then be obtained to prove the functional significance of the lesions before correction is attempted.", p. 835. Most authors, however, do not consider renal arteriography a general "screening tool."
See: Braunwald, chapter on "Systemic Hypertension." **Keywords:** Patient with CAD, and hypertension ➜ check renal arteries at cath.

3. Aortic Aneurysms

1120. **AAAs enlarge over time. When should EVAR be recommended?**
  a. **When aneurysm diameter exceeds 3-4.5 cm**
  b. **When aneurysm diameter exceeds 5-5.5 cm**
  c. **When aneurysm walls begins to thrombose**
  d. **Never (Surgery is recommended only when symptoms develop)**

ANSWER: b. When aneurysm diameter exceeds 5-5.5 cm.
Aortic aneurysms usually expand even while the patient is asymptomatic. The risk of rupture increases with increasing wall tension and diameter. For an average sized man Endovascular Aortic Repair (EVAR) with a stent graft is recommended at a diameter of 5.5 cm. - women lower at 5.0 cm.

Topal say, "However, in general, the clinical recommendation remains to offer treatment for aneurysms between 5 and 5.5 cm,... An exception to this guideline is that intervention should be offered despite the size of the aneurysm if symptoms develop or if the aneurysm increases in size by 1 cm per year. In addition, if the patient is a woman with smaller native vessels, the relative size that represents aneurysmal disease may be less than the conventional 5- to 5.5-cm range." **See:** Topal, chapter on "Lower Extremity Interventions"

1121. Most aortic aneurysms are _____ in shape and arise in the _____.
  a. Fusiform, Thoracic AO
  b. Saccular, Thoracic AO
  c. Fusiform, Abdominal AO (below renals)
  d. Saccular, Abdominal AO (above renals)

ANSWER c. Fusiform, Abdominal AO (below renals). 3/4 of all aneurysms arise in the abdominal AO between the renal and iliac arteries. Most of these are circumferential or fusiform in shape around the entire circumference of the aortic wall.
See: Braunwald, chapter on "Diseases of the Aorta." **Keywords:** Majority aneurysms = fusiform, Abdominal below renals

1122. What is the most common type of aortic aneurysm?
  a. Ascending type A asymmetrical
  b. Ascending type B symmetrical
  c. Descending type A asymmetrical
  d. Descending type B symmetrical

ANSWER: d. Descending type B symmetrical. Also termed infrarenal type B fusiform dissection.
   Braunwald says, "Aortic aneurysms are either fusiform or saccular. Fusiform aneurysms are most common and are characterized by a general symmetric dilation with a fairly uniform shape involving the entire aortic wall circumference.... AAAs occur in 3% to 9% of men older than 50 years and are the most common form of aortic aneurysms. Most AAAs arise in the infrarenal aorta, but up to 10% may involve the pararenal or visceral aorta, and some extend into the thoracoabdominal segment." **See:** Braunwald, chapter on "Aortic Aneurysms"

1123. What is a characteristic of the descending thoracic aneurysm shown at #2 on the diagram?
  a. Associated with severe atherosclerotic heart disease in other areas
  b. Associated with syphilis or Marfan's syndrome
  c. Most common location for an aortic aneurysm

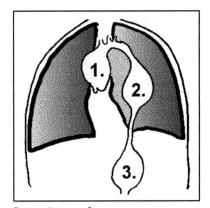
Locations of aneurysms

ANSWER a. Associated with severe atherosclerotic heart disease in other areas.
BE ABLE TO CORRECTLY MATCH ALL ANSWERS.
1. ASCENDING AO ANEURYSM: Associated with syphilis or Marfan's syndrome
2. THORACIC AO ANEURYSM: Associated with severe atherosclerotic heart disease in other areas
3. ABDOMINAL AO ANEURYSM: Most common location for aneurysms
See: Braunwald, chapter on "Diseases of the Aorta." **Keywords:** location & associations with aneurysms: thoracic, ascending AO

1124. When aortic aneurysms reach a certain point they continue to weaken and expand ever more rapidly. Whose law predicts this?
a. Poiseuille's law
b. Starling's law
c. Bernoulli's law
d. Laplace's law

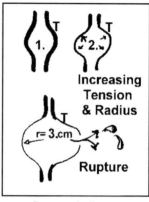

Lapace's Law

ANSWER d. Laplace's law states that $T = p \times r$.
Wall Tension = lumen pressure x vessel radius.
E.g., since 100 mmHg = 2 psi and a 3-cm radius is about 1 inch (2.54 cm/in).

$T = 2 \text{ lb/in}^2 \times 1 \text{ in.} = 2 \text{ lb/in}$

As vessel radius increases the wall tension increases. This increased tension causes it to stretch and thin. The more it thins the more tension in the wall. It continues to stretch, until it ruptures. This is the vicious circle of an enlarging aneurysm. They continue to grow, like a bulge in a car tire, until they pop, and in the aorta that's a catastrophe! Because of this risk, aortic aneurysms are carefully followed and given early surgery.

This indicates the danger point where aneurysms rapidly enlarge is a tension of about 2 lb/in. So if you had a 1 inch wide strip of aorta, and hung a 2 lb. weight on it, it would continue to stretch and thin over time until it eventually ruptured. (Probably a gross over-simplification but the concept is there.)
See: Braunwald, chapter on "Diseases of the Aorta."

1125. Aortography in patients with aortic aneurysms generally:
a. Is contraindicated if symptoms are present, because when symptoms develop they are likely to rupture
b. Is contraindicated unless alternate routes of entry allow entry above the aneurysm
c. Underestimates the diameter of an aneurysm, because laminated clot is usually present
d. Overestimates the diameter of aneurysms, because pressure injection enlarges it.

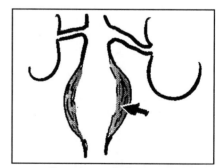

Laminated clot

ANSWER c. Underestimates the diameter of an aneurysm. Laminated clots are frequently present in longstanding large aneurysms. Since the clot may not be opacified by angiographic dye, it is difficult to distinguish the true inner lumen.

In experienced hands, aortography is safe. The angiographic complication rate is only 2%. Although ultrasound, CT scans, and MRI usually make the definitive diagnosis. Angiography is currently recommended if the diagnosis is questionable or if other cardiovascular disease is suspected (E.g., coronary disease). Braunwald's text recommends it routinely for patients being considered for surgery "to facilitate perioperative management." **See:** Braunwald, chapter on "Diseases of the Aorta."

1126. **Which type of aneurysm is labeled at #3 on the diagram?**
a. **Normal**
b. **True Aneurysm - fusiform**
c. **True Aneurysm - saccular**
d. **False Aneurysm - loculated**
e. **False Aneurysm - herniated**
f. **Dissected Aneurysm**

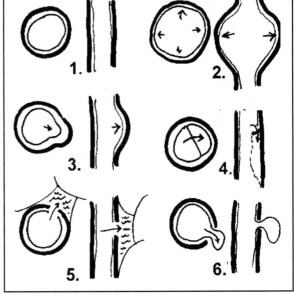

Types of aortic aneurysms

ANSWER c. True Aneurysm - Saccular.

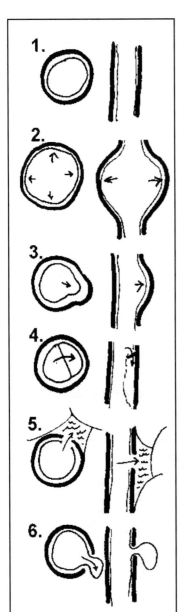

Types of Aneurysms

1. NORMAL: The ascending AO is normally 3 cm in diameter. The abdominal AO is 2 cm in diameter. When it has expanded to 4 cm and above it is a clinically significant aortic aneurysm.

2. TRUE ANEURYSM - FUSIFORM: True aneurysms involve all 3 layers of the aortic wall. "Fusiform" aneurysms are also termed "circumferential" because the entire wall of the aorta is dilated.

3. TRUE ANEURYSM - SACCULAR: True aneurysms involve all 3 layers of the aortic wall. The saccular shape is like a "sack" and bulges out one side of the aortic wall.

4. DISSECTED ANEURYSM: The layers of the aorta are torn apart. Usually blood enters at the tear and fills the sack between intima and media - creating a false lumen. The blood may continue to split the wall apart and the intima may overlap and obstruct branch vessels.

5. FALSE ANEURYSM- LOCULATED: False aneurysms do not involve all 3 walls of the AO. Several wall layers are ruptured. The blood communicates with the aneurysm through a narrow neck. Loculated means the blood is localized in a cavity and surrounded by other tissue, which encloses and contains the hematoma.

6. FALSE ANEURYSM- HERNIATED: False aneurysms do not involve all 3 walls of the AO. Here only one or two layers are ruptured and the remaining layer herniates through the separation. These are also termed "pulsating" aneurysms,

because they are contained by a thin wall of the aorta. A narrow neck allows blood to pass back and forth, making these aneurysms pulsatile.
See: Braunwald, chapter on "Diseases of the Aorta." **Keywords:** Types of aneurysms

1127. **The ACC/AHA guidelines recommend that elective repair of AAAs be done when:**
a. The aneurysm reaches a 3.5 cm diameter
b. The aneurysm reaches a 5.5 cm diameter
c. Thrombus begins to line the walls of the AAA
d. Embolism occurs to the lower extremities

ANSWER b. The aneurysm reaches a 5.5 cm diameter. Lanzer says, "According to recently published ACC/AHA guidelines, patients with infrarenal or juxtarenal AAAs ≥5.5 cm in diameter should undergo repair and those with AAAs measuring 4.0 to 5.4 cm in diameter should be monitored by ultrasound or CT every 6 to 12 months." However, many physicians prefer to place a stent-graft sooner. As the aneurysm expands and approaches the rupture point surgery or stent-graft are lifesaving.
See: Braunwald, chapter on "Diseases of the Aorta."

1128. **What abnormality is shown on this aortogram?**
a. Mycotic AAA
b. Fusiform AAA
c. False thoracic aortic aneurysm
d. Wide neck, true renal aneurysm

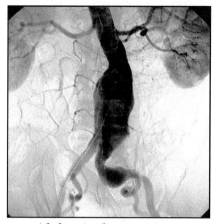
Abdominal aortogram

ANSWER b. Fusiform AAA. Abdominal aortic aneurysms (AAAs) are aortic wall dilations that bulge evenly on all sides of the aorta. AAAs are the most common type of aortic aneurysm. Most are true aneurysms that involve all three layers (tunica intima, tunica media and tunica adventitia), and are generally asymptomatic before rupture. Approximately 95 percent of aortic aneurysms are caused by atherosclerosis. High blood pressure (hypertension) intensifies the force of blood on the walls of the arteries and contributes to the ballooning of aneurysms. Abdominal aortic aneurysms maybe either fusiform, if circumferential, or saccular, if more localized. **See:** Braunwald, chapter on "Acute MI." **Keywords:** fusiform LV aneurysm

1129. **What type of surgery is usually performed to repair fusiform abdominal aortic aneurysms?**
a. Resect and replace it with a Dacron graft
b. Resect and replace it with Teflon pledgets
c. Wrap and constrict it within a Dacron tube
d. Bypass it with a large vein graft

ANSWER a. Resect and replace it with a Dacron graft. The diseased section is usually resected and replaced with a Dacron graft. These grafts can be used to replace most of the aorta if necessary. Some saccular aneurysms may be resected and the healthy walls merely sutured back together. Some ascending aortic aneurysms develop aortic regurgitation and the valve needs to be replaced. Here the diseased valve and ascending aorta are replaced with a Dacron tube with a valve implanted in the proximal end.

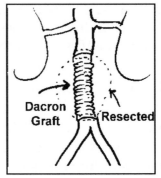

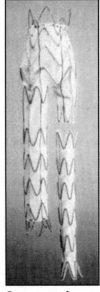

AO An. Surgery

An invasive catheter based therapy is being developed using cloth covered stents or stent-grafts. These are self expanding nitinol stents coated with graft material as shown.
See: Braunwald, chapter on "Diseases of the Aorta." **Keywords:** Surgery of AO aneurysms = resect, Dacron graft

Stent-graft

4. Aortic Dissections

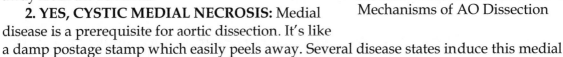

1130.   **Three mechanisms involved in the etiology (origin) of aortic dissections are:**
1. Torn intima at entry point
2. Cystic medial necrosis
3. Medial hemorrhage
4. Extravasation hematoma
    a. 1, 2, 3
    b. 1, 2, 4
    c. 1, 3, 4
    d. 2, 3, 4

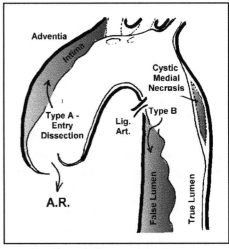

ANSWER a. **1, 2, 3**
    1. YES, TORN INTIMA AT ENTRY POINT: Most dissections have an entry point where the blood enters the false lumen. This column of blood driven by the blood pressure then strips the intimal wall away from the adventia.
    2. YES, CYSTIC MEDIAL NECROSIS: Medial disease is a prerequisite for aortic dissection. It's like

Mechanisms of AO Dissection

a damp postage stamp which easily peels away. Several disease states induce this medial disease: Marfan syndrome, Ehlers-Danlos syndrome, and atherosclerosis.
    3. YES, MEDIAL HEMORRHAGE: Some dissections begin as a hemorrhage within the media. This splits the walls apart from within. The pressure buildup may cause rupture into the aorta. Then the aortic pressure continues to erode the media and peel off intima.
    4. NO, EXTRAVASATION HEMATOMA: This is a false aneurysm or aortic rupture which bleeds into the mediastinum. **See:** Braunwald, chapter on "Diseases of the Aorta."
Keywords: Mechanisms AO dissection = torn intima, medial necrosis, medial hemorrhage

1131. These drawings depict the Debakey classification of aortic dissections. What type of AO dissection is shown at #3 (in the descending AO)?
a. Type I
b. Type II
c. Type IIIa
d. Type IIIb

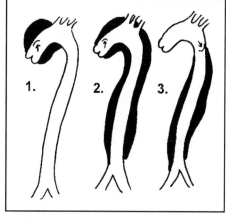

Debakey classes of AO dissection

ANSWER c. Type IIIa - Debakey class. **BE ABLE TO CORRECTLY MATCH ALL ANSWERS.**
1. TYPE II - Originates in the ascending AO and is confined to it.
2. TYPE I - Originates in the ascending AO and extends into the descending AO.
3. TYPE IIIa - Originates in the descending thoracic AO and propagates distally into the thorax.
4. TYPE IIIb - Originates in the descending thoracic. AO and propagates down the thoracic and past the diaphragm into the abdominal aorta.
See: Braunwald, chapter on "Diseases of the Aorta."

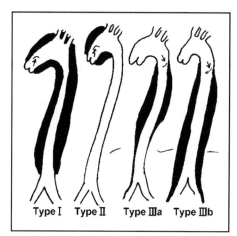

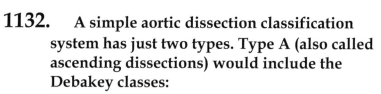

Type I   Type II   Type IIIa   Type IIIb

Debakey classes of AO dissection

1132. A simple aortic dissection classification system has just two types. Type A (also called ascending dissections) would include the Debakey classes:
a. I
b. II
c. I & II
d. I & III

ANSWER c. Debakey type I and II (Both originate in the ascending aorta and would be called type A.) Type A dissections originate in the proximal or ascending AO - Type B in the descending or distal AO. This classification system does not care where they propagate to. They may or may not extend into the thoracic AO or abdominal AO. Most type B dissections originate from the area below the left subclavian artery, near the ligamentum arteriosus. **See:** Braunwald, chapter on "Diseases of the Aorta." **Keywords:** A & B - classification AO dissections

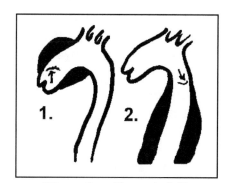

Dissection: Type A & B

1133. Identify 5 common classic causes of aortic dissections. (Select 5 below.)
a. Abdominal soft tissue trauma
b. Marfan or Ehlers-Danlos syndromes
c. Bicuspid AO valve or coarctation of AO
d. Atherosclerotic plaques
e. Hypertension
f. Pregnancy
g. Low cardiac output

ANSWERS: b, c, d, e, & f.
a. **CAR ACCIDENT OR OTHER ABDOMINAL SOFT TISSUE TRAUMA: NO.** Braunwald states that "Trauma almost never causes a classic aortic dissection, although a localized tear in the region of the aortic isthmus is common following massive chest trauma." The isthmus is where the ligamentum arteriosus is located - just below the left subclavian artery. This is where most type B dissections originate.
b. **MARFAN OR EHLERS-DANLOS SYNDROMES: YES.** These are both connective tissue disorders which involve degeneration of the media. Dissection is common in advanced cases.
c. **BICUSPID AO VALVE OR COARCTATION OF AO: YES.** These congenital defects somehow weaken the aortic wall predisposing it to dissection.
d. **ELDERLY MEN WITH ATHEROSCLEROTIC PLAQUES: YES.** Elderly men are more prone to ASHD. Their atherosclerotic plaques may rupture within the aortic wall. The resulting bleeding tears the intima and may split the wall leading to dissection.
e. **HYPERTENSION: YES.** A common denominator found in ½ of all dissections is high blood pressure. Hypertension creates stress within the aortic wall and causes degenerative changes within the media. There are no ECG changes as there are in ischemic heart disease.
f. **PREGNANCY: YES.** The hypertension often seen in pregnant women may predispose them to dissection.
G. **Low CO: NO.** It is high CO and high velocity jets that are more likely to cause dissection.
See: Braunwald, chapter on "Diseases of the Aorta."

1134. Aortography in patients with aortic dissection generally:
a. Is contraindicated because the catheter may extend the intimal tear
b. Is contraindicated unless alternate routes of entry allow entry above the dissection (E.g., Brachial approach)
c. Should be done by venous injection only using digital subtraction angiography
d. Is safe if contrast is not injected into the false channel

ANSWER d. Is safe if contrast is not injected into the false channel. Usually ultrasound or chest films are the initial lab tests to discover aortic dissections. The post-op follow up study is also usually noninvasive (CT or MRI). However, Braunwald states that "Aortic angiography is the single most important study in the diagnosis of aortic dissection. ..The retrograde approach is now the method of choice. The hazards of the approach have proved

minimal, provided the catheter is carefully inserted and contrast material is not injected into the false channel. Aortic angiography has three objectives: (1) to establish a definite diagnosis, (2) to identify the site of origin of the dissection, and (3) to delineate the extent of the dissection and the distal circulation to vital organs. One additional feature to be assessed by angiography is the degree to which the false channel is opacified..., and the procedure is well tolerated by even critically ill patients."
See: Braunwald, chapter on "Diseases of the Aorta." **Keywords:** Pain of AO dissection

1135. **The pain associated with aortic dissection:**
   a. **Is described as "ripping, tearing, or stabbing"**
   b. **Continues to accelerate and crescendo**
   c. **Often migrates down the left arm**
   d. **Is remittent or transient**

ANSWER a. Is described as "ripping, tearing, or stabbing." This pain is often "cataclysmic" in onset. It may be all but unbearable, and patients may writhe in agony. It is unlike angina pain in that it is usually as severe as it is going to get during the initial dissection, whereas angina usually increases as time goes on. Neither does this pain migrate down the arm as angina does. The location of the pain is usually in the anterior chest for proximal dissections, in the neck or jaw for arch dissections, or in the back for distal dissections.
See: Braunwald, chapter on "Diseases of the Aorta."

1136. **Braunwald's suggested therapy for most "uncomplicated" acute distal (descending) aortic dissections is:**
   a. **Medication only**
   b. **Surgical repair**
   c. **Angioplasty**
   d. **Stent placement**

ANSWER a. Medication only. Although somewhat controversial, Braunwald currently recommends medical therapy for simple descending AO dissections. Medications are directed at reducing the BP and aortic flow rate (dV/dT).

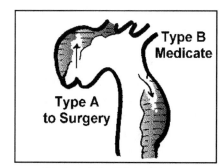

Rx for AO. Dissections

An emergency surgical replacement is recommended only for dissections of the ascending (proximal) aorta. This is because the proximal dissections are so much more critical. Proximal dissections often progress, involve the aortic valve and compromise cerebral flow. Surgery is also recommended for those with progression of the dissection, vital organ compromise, aortic rupture, AI, or Marfan syndrome.
See: Braunwald, chapter on "Diseases of the Aorta."

1137. Recommended treatment of type A aortic dissections is _____ .
a. EVAR
b. Surgery
c. Endarterectomy
d. Medical therapy

ANSWER: b. Surgery. Type A dissections are in the ascending AO and are a surgical emergency because of the risk of MI, aortic valve tear, and pericardial tamponade. Type B dissections are in the descending AO. All are initially treated by lowering the BP, HR, and force of contraction, because if these are elevated the dissection is likely to tear the intima even further.

Braunwald says, "Aortic dissection is a highly lethal condition. ... Emergency surgery improves survival in acute type A dissections, whereas initial medical therapy is recommended for acute type B dissections.... Surgical therapy for type A aortic dissection has dramatically improved survival for this lethal condition. The goals of surgical therapy arc to treat or prevent the common complications of dissection, such as cardiac tamponade, aortic regurgitation, aortic rupture, stroke, and visceral ischemia." **See:** Braunwald, chapter on "Aortic Dissection"

1138. Your young patient arrives in the ER with stabbing back pain. Ultrasound shows type A aortic dissection with pericardial tamponade and sinus tachycardia. BP is 110/80 and falling. The patient is on IV beta blocker and nitroprusside medications. The physician calls for a pericariocentesis tray. Your suggestion is:
a. Recommend a stent-graft first
b. Recommend coronary angiography first
c. Caution about risky pericardiocentesis
d. Proceed with emergency pericardiocentesis

ANSWER: c. Caution about risky pericardiocentesis. If it is a large tear into the pericardium, it will continue to bleed, and you will never drain the pericardium. Even coronary arteriography should be postponed until after surgery.

Braunwald says, "Routine coronary angiography is not recommended before surgery for acute type A aortic dissection because of concern about delay in emergency surgery.... In addition to the time delay incurred, coronary angiography may be technically difficult

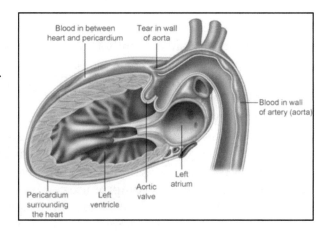

in the setting of dissection. Arterial access may fail to gain entry into the true lumen.... Cardiac tamponade, occurring in 19% of acute type A dissections, is one of the most common mechanisms for death in this disorder.... Because hemodynamic instability with hypotension often complicates hemopericardium in acute dissection, pericardiocentesis is commonly considered as initial therapy in this condition, to attempt to stabilize these patients before surgery. But sudden death from pulseless electrical activity has been reported minutes after pericardiocentesis in this setting. The relative increase in intra-aortic pressure that occurs after pericardiocentesis may lead to a reopening or resurgence of blood under pressure from the false channel into the pericardial space, resulting in acute hemorrhage and fatal cardiac tamponade. Therefore, in the relatively stable patient with acute type A dissection and cardiac tamponade, the risks of pericardiocentesis likely outweigh its benefits. The initial strategy should be to proceed emergently to the operating room for open surgical repair of the aorta and drainage of the pericardium under direct visualization, but when managing such a patient, with pulseless electrical activity or refractory hypotension, an attempt at resuscitation with pericardiocentesis may be lifesaving. In this case, one should attempt to aspirate only enough pericardial fluid to stabilize the patient, and then proceed to emergency surgery.... " **See:** Braunwald, chapter on "Aortic Dissection"

Topol says, "In type A dissections, interventional endo vascular strategies have no clinical application except to relieve critical malperfusion before surgery of the ascending aorta." **See:** Topol, chapter on "Peripheral Vascular Interventions"

1139. **While awaiting diagnosis or surgery, patients with suspected aortic dissection should receive early "EMERGENCY MEDICAL THERAPY" which includes IV administration of: (Select 2 answers)**
1. Epinephrine
2. Atropine
3. Nitroprusside
4. Dopamine
5. Beta-adrenergic blockers
   a. 1, 3
   b. 1, 4
   c. 2, 5
   d. 3, 5

ANSWER d. 3 & 5 (Nitroprusside & Beta-adrenergic blockers.) Initial therapy is to admit the patient to the ICU where both the blood pressure and the dV/dT should be lowered. The vasodilator nitroprusside lowers the BP but not necessarily the dV/dT. The dV/dT is the rate of change of aortic blood flow velocity. This is reduced with beta blockers like Inderol. Lowering these parameters reduces the shearing forces which extend the intimal tear.

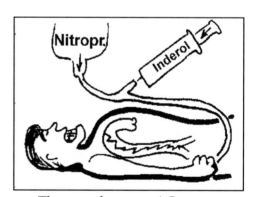

Therapy for acute AO dissection

The incorrect responses (dopamine, epi, and atropine) are contraindicated because they increase CO and BP, and thus increase the shearing stress on the aorta. **See:** Braunwald, chapter on "Diseases of the Aorta." **Keywords:** Medication for AO dissection = nitroprusside & beta blockers

5. Pulmonary Embolism

1140. Which of the following hyper-coagulable clinical conditions are associated with a pulmonary embolism?

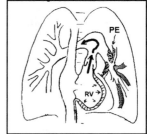

Pulmonary Embolism

1. Oral contraceptive use or post pregnancy bed rest
2. Bed rest or venous trauma
3. Central venous alimentation or Swan-Ganz catheters
4. Anemia or thrombocytopenia
5. Tumors or malignancy
    a. 1, 2, 3, 4
    b. 1, 3, 4, 5
    c. 1, 2, 4, 5
    d. 1, 2, 3, 5

ANSWER d. 1, 2, 3, 5 are risk factors for developing PE.
1. **YES**, ORAL CONTRACEPTIVE USE OR POST PREGNANCY BED REST: Oral contraceptives have shown to be thrombus inducing in the heart, brain, and lungs. Pregnancy is also associated with PE.
2. **YES**, BED REST OR VENOUS TRAUMA: Damaged veins containing stagnant blood tend to clot.
3. **YES**, CENTRAL VENOUS ALIMENTATION (Hickman) OR SWAN-GANZ CATHETERS: Long term venous catheters can clot and lead to a pulmonary embolism.
4. NO, ANEMIA OR THROMBOCYTOPENIA: Deficiency of red blood cells or thrombocytes (platelets) makes the blood LESS prone to clotting.
5. **YES**, TUMORS OR MALIGNANCY: Neoplastic disease is associated with an increased incidence of PE. PE may be predictive of a malignant tumor as yet undiscovered.
These are the "secondary" hyper-coagulable states that are more common than the inherited "primary" hyper-coagulable states such as antithrombin deficiency. In these secondary states the molecular mechanism causing thrombosis is not known - only the associated clinical conditions. **See:** Braunwald, chapter on "Pulmonary Embolism." **Keywords:** Associated conditions

1141. What pathology is termed the "Great Masquerader" because it may present such varied symptoms such as: chest pain, dyspnea, fever, cough, or hemoptysis?
a. RV infarction
b. Pulmonary hypertension
c. CHF
d. PE

ANSWER d. Pulmonary embolism diagnosis is often missed because it "masquerades" as other diseases such as: pneumonia, CHF, MI, or primary pulmonary hypertension. Braunwald's text recommends that when one of these diseases is unresponsive to therapy a diagnosis of coexisting PE should be considered.

PE is the third most common cardiovascular disease, after MI and stroke. Yet its diagnosis is commonly missed and recognized only at autopsy. PE is intimately associated with deep vein thrombosis which embolizes into the lungs.

See: Braunwald, chapter on "Pulmonary Embolism." **Keywords:** "Great masquerader" = PE

1142. **Most pulmonary emboli originate in the:**
   a. **Pulmonary artery (lungs)**
   b. **Vena cava**
   c. **Deep thigh veins**
   d. **Superficial calf veins**

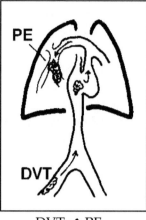

DVT ➜ PE

ANSWER c. Deep thigh veins. Most PE arises from the clots in the deep veins of the leg, usually the thigh (50%). About 30% arise from the deep veins of the calf. An embolism rarely occurs from the upper extremity or superficial veins.

Most of these thrombo-embolisms occur because of extended bed rest, immobility, clotting defects, and trauma to the vein. Therefore, you should ambulate post-op. patients early to prevent this "thrombo-phlebitis."

The thrombus usually fills and obstructs the vein. These clot "casts" of the thrombosed veins may break loose from the vein and float (embolize) into the lung. The larger the clot and the more it obstructs blood flow the more severe the PE. PE is the leading nonsurgical cause of death to hospitalized patients. **See:** Braunwald, chapter on "Pulmonary Embolism." **Keywords:** PE results from emboli from deep thigh veins

1143. **The "Gold Standard" now used to diagnose deep vein thrombosis (DVT) is:**
   a. **Clinical evaluation (leg tenderness, discoloration...)**
   b. **Venography and pulmonary angiography (filling defects in veins)**
   c. **B-mode ultrasound (compressing veins while imaging them)**
   d. **Impedance plethysmography (changes in electrical "impedance" of the legs)**

ANSWER c. B-mode ultrasound venous scan. B-mode is "brightness" mode. It is a 2-D fan shaped ultrasound scan with the most reflective tissues showing brightest. Braunwald says "The introduction of B-mode ultrasonography has revolutionized the diagnosis of DVT... The inability to compress these veins is highly accurate indication of DVT proximal to the calf... B-mode ultrasound ...is so reliable, inexpensive, safe, and nontraumautic that it is rapidly supplanting leg phlebography as the Gold Standard."

   a. CLINICAL EVALUATION (leg tenderness, discoloration...): helpful but too variable.
   b. VENOGRAPHY AND PULMONARY ANGIOGRAPHY (filling defects in veins): many deep veins are missed because the entry site bypasses them.

c. B-MODE ULTRASOUND (compressing veins while imaging them): The femoral and popliteal veins are imaged with a 2-D transducer in cross section. Slight pressure is applied to the transducer and a normal vein should compress easily. Clotted veins remain distended. Color flow Doppler imaging can also visualize blood flow and its absence. Now used extensively and very sensitive.

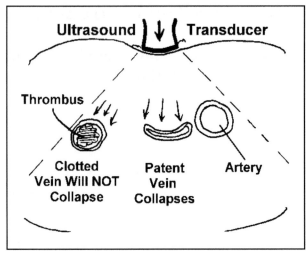

Dx of DVT with B-mode Ultrasound

d. IMPEDANCE PLETHYSMOGRAPHY (changes in leg electrical resistance). The patient's legs and abdomen are encircled with metal tapes that conduct low voltage high frequency electricity. The electrical resistance changes in edematous thrombo-phlebitic legs. This test has been superseded by the more sensitive and specific B-mode ultrasound venous scan.

See: Braunwald, chapter on "Pulmonary Embolism." Keywords: DVT ➜ B mode ultrasound diagnoses

1144. **A 70 year old woman is in the hospital recovering from hip replacement surgery. She develops chest pain and SOB. A lung V/Q scan diagnoses an acute pulmonary embolism. What therapy is indicated?**
a. **Streptokinase IV**
b. **IV heparin**
c. **IVC filter implant**
d. **Knee high compression stockings**

ANSWER b. IV heparin will prevent the formation of further clots. Thrombotic therapy in PE is still controversial, but would be avoided post surgery. The compression stockings "Sup-hose" should be "thigh-high" not just over the foot and calf, since most throbo-emboli originate from above the knee.
See: Braunwald, chapter on "Pulmonary Embolism."

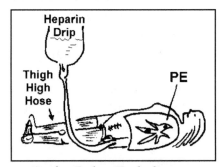

Rx for Pulm. Embolism

1145. **Hemodynamics associated with a massive pulmonary embolism include:**
a. **Low PA blood pressure**
b. **Dilatation and pressure overload of left ventricle**
c. **IV septum bulges into LV reducing LV-EDV**
d. **Pulmonic valve regurgitation**

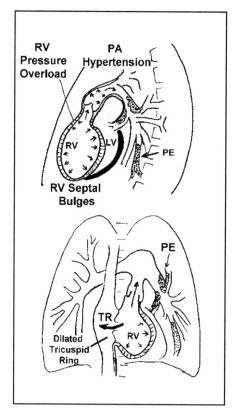

ANSWER c. IV septum bulges into LV reducing LV-EDV. In severe cases with increased pulmonary pressure and reduced blood pressure thrombolytics may be used to dissolve the clot.
a. NO, PULMONARY ARTERY HYPOTENSION: The obstruction of the PA causes the RV to increase its pressure resulting in pulmonary HYPERTENSION.
b. NO, LV DILATATION AND PRESSURE OVERLOAD: It is the RV which is dilated and pressure overloaded.
c. YES, IV SEPTUM BULGES INTO LV REDUCING LV-EDV: The obstructed PA causes RV pressure overload. The RV distends maximally but is limited by the pericardium. This causes the RV septum to bulge into the LV, reducing LV preload and CO. This RV pressure overload effect is also seen in cardiac tamponade. Reflexive tachycardia compensates for the decreased LV stroke volume.
d. NO, PULMONIC VALVE REGURGITATION: As the RV dilates the tricuspid ring dilates causing tricuspid regurgitation.

See: Braunwald, chapter on "Pulmonary Embolism." **Keywords:** Hemodynamics of PA = IV septal bulging into LV reducing LV-EDV.

1146. **Identify the IVC filter labeled on the diagram at #3.**
a. **Simon nitinol filter**
b. **Bard Denali or G2 filter**
c. **Greenfield filter (Medi-Tech.)**
d. **Giantuarco-Roehm "bird's nest" filter (Cook)**
e. **TrapEase filter (Cook)**

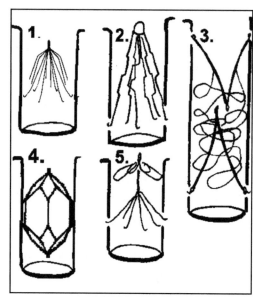

ANSWER d. Giantuarco-Roehm "bird's nest" filter (Cook Co.) All these filters can be implanted percutaneously. **BE ABLE TO CORRECTLY MATCH ALL ANSWERS.**

Vena caval filters

1. BARD DENALI or G2 FILTER: Can be removed by hooking and collapsing in IVC.
2. GREENFIELD FILTER (MEDI-TECH): Has a cone to collect thrombus and six stainless steel legs with hooks on their ends that spring open and catch in the IVC. These legs filter the IVC blood and funnel it into a cone at the tip - pointed up. Has a large 24 French size.
3. GIANTUARCO-ROEHM "BIRD'S NEST" FILTER (COOK): Has been on the market since 1989. Two springs open at each end of the system locking it into the IVC. The fine coils of steel between the springs form a tangle resembling a "nest" which trap and dice emboli. Braunwald's text recommends it as the filter of choice.
4. TRAPEASE FILTER (COOK): Laser cut from hypo tube. Six struts are joined at each end, so that the device has no head or tail. Self expanding.
5. SIMON NITINOL FILTER: Made of a nickel-titanium alloy with a heat dependent memory. It is cooled in ice water which makes it pliable before insertion. Body heat allows it to open up and take the shape instilled in it's memory with time and heat. Similar to the Greenfield filter with six hooked legs it has a metal cap to align itself with the IVC.

See: Braunwald, chapter on "Pulmonary Embolism."or **See:** Wojtowycz, chapter on "Vena Cava Filters." **Keywords:** types of vena caval filters

1147. **Where should vena caval filters normally be placed in the IVC?**
a. **Above the renal veins**
b. **Below the renal veins**
c. **Superior to the femoral bifurcation**
d. **Inferior to the femoral bifurcation**

ANSWER b. Below the renal veins. An inferior vena cavogram is done first to ascertain the diameter of the IVC and that it is clot free. The renal veins usually enter the IVC at L1-L2. Kandarpa says, "The apex of the filter should be below the lowest renal vein. Here the blood flow is laminar and allows entrapment of thrombi (larger than 3 mm) within the apex, allowing the intrinsic lytic system to dissolve them." He also states that it may be placed above the renal veins via the internal jugular vein if a clot is present below the renal veins.
See: Underhill, chapter on "Vascular Diseases."
Keywords: Thromboangiitis Obliterans, Buerger's Disease

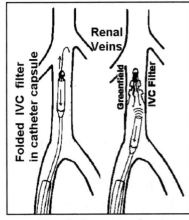

IVC filter below renal veins

1148. **Thrombolysis of massive pulmonary embolism may use the an ultrasound-assisted Catheter-directed thrombolysis catheter. In the EKOS system what is the ultrasound used for?**
a. **Vibrate and break up the clot for aspiration**
b. **Visualize the clot with forward looking transducers**
c. **Visualize the clot with IVUS side looking transducers**
d. **Accelerate penetration of tPA into the clot**

ANSWER: d. Accelerate penetration of tPA into the clot. Note the 2 EKOS catheters in image.

Safadi says, "EkoSonicEndovascular System for the ultrasound facilitated, controlled and selective infusion of physician-specified fluids, including thrombolytics, into the vasculature for the treatment of pulmonary embolism (PE). The EKOS® ultrasonic devices are designed to gently accelerate the penetration of thrombolytic agents into thrombus, providing high levels of lysis." See: Safadi, Ultrasound-Assisted, Catheter-Directed, Low-Dose Thrombolysis: A Safer Alternative to Systemic Thrombolytics for Pulmonary Embolism, Cath Lab Digest, 2014

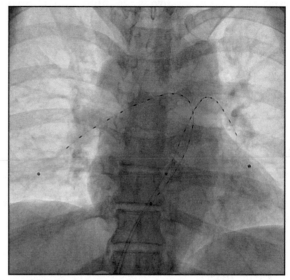

EKOS ultrasound catheters in PA

Weinber says, "The mainstay of treatment for pulmonary embolism is anticoagulation. Thrombolysis for pulmonary embolism should be reserved for sicker patients.....One type of catheter directed thrombolysis for pulmonary embolism is with the EKOS catheter. The EKOS catheter delivers thrombolytic agents into the clot in a unique fashion. The catheter has ultrasound ports near its tip. Ultrasound energy is used to spray the thrombolytic agent into the clot. The EKOS catheter is inserted into the pulmonary embolism. It is left there for several hours while thrombolysis is taking place. Typically tPA is used. It is dripped at a pace of 1 mg/hour for several hours and then the rate is reduced to 0.5 mg/hour for several hours more. Heparin is given in tandem, mainly to prevent catheter thrombosis." See: http://www.angiologist.com/thrombosis-section/thrombolysis-for-pulmonary-embolism/ 2017

1149. A patient who has smoked for years presents with syncope, painless dyspnea, tachycardia and tachypnea. Right heart cath shows severely increased PA and RA pressures and decreased wedge pressure. This suggests a diagnosis of:
a. Aortic stenosis
b. Pulmonary embolism
c. Pericardial tamponade
d. Pulmonary hypertension

ANSWER: b. Pulmonary embolism when massive and acute clots may occlude the lungs so much that the pressure backs up into the right heart. Decreased pulmonary flow may reduce the left heart preload and wedge pressure. Grossman says, "The most common symptoms include dyspnea, chest pain, cough, and hemoptysis....The presence of syncope and severe painless dyspnea usually indicate a hemodynamically significant PE, particularly when accompanied by tachycardia and tachypnea. Many PE patients without cardiopulmonary disease have normal hemodynamics....acute increase in RV afterload with a systolic pressure above 50 or 60 mm Hg will result in acute right ventricular dilation and systolic failure....As a result of RV diastolic dysfunction, the RV diastolic pressure approximates pulmonary artery diastolic pressure and typically shows a prominent dip and

rapid rise. RA pressure is elevated, with a prominent A wave and steep x descent. RV dilation and dysfunction evolve, reduced right ventricular output impairs LV filling....Left ventricular cardiac output is decreased, ..."
See: Grossman, chapter on "Pulmonary Angiography"
Keywords: PE symptoms

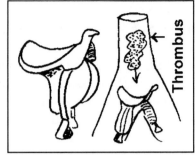

Saddle Thrombus

6. Arterial Embolism

1150. **A blood clot that has broken from its place of formation and is circulating in the blood is called a/an:**
   a. **Embolus**
   b. **Hemorrhage**
   c. **Phlebitis**
   d. **Thrombus**

ANSWER a. An embolus is a clot or other plug (could be air or fat) brought by the blood from another vessel and forced into a smaller one. This obstructs the circulation, resulting in probable necrosis of the tissue fed by the artery.
See: Medial dictionary **Keywords:** embolus

1151. **A large thrombus lodged at the bifurcation of the main PA or iliac artery is termed a/an:**
   a. **Anastomosis**
   b. **Subtotal obstruction**
   c. **Massive embolism**
   d. **Saddle embolism**

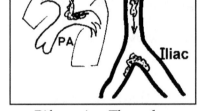

Bifurcation Thrombus

ANSWER d. Saddle embolism. Large clots can float into the bifurcation and straddle the arterial bifurcation with one leg down each branch of the artery.
See: Braunwald, chapter on "Diseases of the Aorta."
Keywords: Saddle embolism

1152. **Most large acute arterial embolisms of the leg originate from:**
   a. **The right side of the heart**
   b. **The left side of the heart**
   c. **Aortic aneurysms**
   d. **Deep veins of the leg**

ANSWER b. 90% of these clots form in the LEFT SIDE OF THE HEART.
   a. NO, RIGHT SIDE OF THE HEART: Right heart

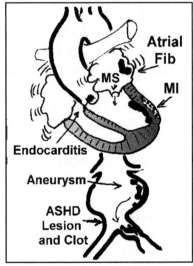

Sources of arterial emboli

thrombi usually lodge in the lungs (PA) but may pass through a PDA or ASD if R-L shunts are present.

b. YES, LEFT SIDE OF HEART: Specific left heart sites for origin of pulmonary emboli include:
1. LA (Atrial fib induced)
2. LV mural thrombus (MI)
3. Mitral stenosis prone to turbulence, atrial fibrillation and associated thrombi
4. Endocarditis lesions can clot but usually send out showers of micro-vegetations.

c. NO, AORTIC ANEURYSMS: Are prone to developing layered thrombi, but the heart is the chief source of aortic emboli due to the motion and turbulence in the heart.

d. NO, DEEP LEG VEINS: Are a major source of emboli for the VENOUS system, but they are filtered out by the lungs and never get into the arterial system. **See:** Braunwald, chapter on "Diseases of the Aorta." **Keywords:** Arterial thrombi originate in Lt. Ht.

1153. **Identify the 5 clinical signs and symptoms of acute femoral arterial occlusion. (Check all 5 that apply.)**
a. **Leg pain**
b. **Leg paralysis**
c. **Warm, sweaty leg**
d. **Pulseless leg**
e. **Leg numbness**
f. **Pale or mottled leg color**

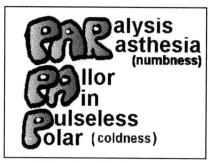

6 P's - Art. Occlusion

ANSWERS: a, b, d, e, & f
A "warm, sweaty leg" is NOT a sign or symptom of acute femoral arterial occlusion. Below the occlusion the leg is cool to the touch due to poor capillary flow. This is sometimes termed "polar" coldness - like the "North Pole." Note they all have words starting with P.

The 6 P's of acute arterial occlusion are:
1. PAIN
2. PARALYSIS
3. PARAESTHESIA (Numbness)
4. PALLOR
5. POLAR (coldness - NOT a warm, sweaty leg)
6. PULSELESS

See: Underhill, chapter on "Abnormalities of Coagulation, Bleeding and Clotting." P's

1154. **Identify the approved therapies for acute leg arterial thrombosis and occlusion (Select 4.)**
a. **Arterial stent**
b. **AngioJet**
c. **Bypass graft**
d. **Endarterectomy**
e. **Thrombolytic medication**
f. **Impella or LVAD**

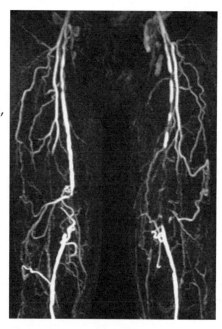

ANSWERS: b, c, d, & e.
The therapy for arterial occlusion centers around removing or bypassing the obstruction. Thrombi may be removed by thrombolytic drugs or AngioJet catheter thrombectomy. Surgical therapy involves either arterial bypass surgery or endarterectomy. Stents are only good for keeping a vessel open. They will not prevent a clot from lodging in the patent vessel. LV assist is not needed at this time.

   Other emergency therapy includes:
Pain control with narcotics. Keeping the patient very warm to relieve arterial spasm. A warm room 80-85 degrees helps. Wrap the involved extremity loosely in cotton to preserve body heat and protect it from trauma. Icing the limb is contraindicated as long as there is hope for survival of the limb. But once gangrene has set-in and amputation is inevitable, packing the limb in ice may reduce pain and delay emergency surgery. Elevation and application of heat are contraindicated as they may hasten gangrene. **See:** Hurst and Logue, chapter on "Vascular Disease." and Braunwald, chapter on "Diseases of the Aorta."

1155.   **Following LV angiography, a patient's leg becomes cool, pale, and painful from acute femoral artery occlusion. Initial therapy should include:**
a. **Heparin infusion**
b. **Vasodilator infusion**
c. **Cooling or icing the extremity**
d. **Elevating the extremity**

ANSWER a. Heparin infusion. Initial therapy is to anticoagulate the patient to prevent further embolization and clot extension. Definitive treatment is surgical removal of the clot, usually with Fogarty catheters.

   Other emergency therapy includes: Pain control with narcotics. Keeping the patient very warm to relieve arterial spasm. A warm room 80-85 degrees helps. Wrap the involved extremity loosely in cotton to preserve body heat and protect it from trauma. Icing the limb is contraindicated as long as there is hope for survival of the limb. But once gangrene has set in and amputation is inevitable, packing the limb in ice may reduce pain and delay emergency surgery. Elevation and application of heat are contraindicated as they may hasten gangrene. **See:** Hurst and Logue, chapter on "Vascular Disease." Also, **See:** Underhill, chapter on "Vascular Diseases." **Keywords:** Rx for arterial occlusion = heparin

1156.   **Which form of arterial occlusive peripheral vascular disease is most common?**
a. **Upper extremity**
b. **Lower extremity**
c. **Carotid arteries**
d. **Renal arteries**

ANSWER: b. Lower extremity. Rooke says, "Lower extremity PAD affects 10%-15% of community-dwelling older men and women. PAD affects 25% to 30% of men and women aged 50 years and older.... Intermittent claudication is the most classic manifestation of PAD." Braunwald says, "Peripheral arterial disease (PAD) generally refers to a disorder that obstructs the blood supply to the lower or upper extremities. It is most commonly caused by atherosclerosis..." **See:** Rooke, chapter on "Lower Extremity Occlusive Arterial Disease" and

Braunwald, chapter on "Peripheral Arterial Disease". **Keywords:** Leg PAD most common

7A. Other Vascular: Atherosclerosis

1157. Surgical repair of extensive and long atherosclerotic lesions in the iliac and superficial femoral arteries usually involves:
a. Replacement of these vessels with Dacron grafts
b. Replacement of these vessels with saphenous vein grafts
c. AO-iliac-femoral Dacron bypass grafts
d. AO-iliac-femoral saphenous vein bypass grafts

ANSWER c. AO-iliac-femoral Dacron bypass grafts. In the leg bypass grafts are usually preferred to total replacement because of the many takeoff vessels and the many layers of muscle which must be removed to reach the deep leg arteries. **See:** Braunwald, chapter on "Diseases of the Aorta." **Keywords:** AO-iliac-femoral graft

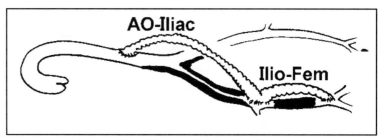
Aorto-iliac-Femoral skip Graft

1158. What is the recommended treatment for a patient with acute ischemic TIA or CVA, two hours after symptoms develop?
a. Thrombolysis
b. Thrombectomy
c. Heparin anticoagulation
d. Angioplasty and carotid artery stent

ANSWER: a. Thrombolysis must be administered within 3 hours of initial symptoms.
Topol say, "The only approved treatment for acute ischemic stroke is intravenous thrombolysis for patients presenting within 3 hours of the onset and without contraindications." **See:** Topol, chapter on "Carotid and Cerbrovascular Intervention"
Braunwald says, "As with acute coronary syndromes, time is of the essence in the treatment of patients with acute ischemic stroke. ... In the period immediately following the onset of ischemic symptoms, however, evaluation should center on determining whether the patient would benefit from reperfusion therapy.... The indications for acute anticoagulation of patients with ischemic stroke are extremely limited. The most recent American Heart Association/American Academy of Neurology guidelines specifically discourage emergent anticoagulation with the goal of improving neurologic outcomes or preventing early recurrent stroke in patients with acute ischemic stroke because of a high risk of intracranial bleeding complications, and do not recommend the initiation of anticoagulant therapy within 24 hours of treatment with intravenously administered rt-PA"
See: Braunwald, chapter on "Stroke"

1159. The time window to effectively administer tPA thrombolysis to treat patients with a stroke is ____, while the effective thrombolysis time window for massive PE is____.
a. 3 hrs, 6 hrs
b. 3 hrs, 14 days
c. 6 hrs, 3 hrs
d. 6 hrs, 14 days

ANSWER: b. 3 hrs, 14 days. PE window for effective thrombolysis is MUCH wider.
    Braunwald says,"Intravenous recombinant tissue plasminogen activator (rt-PA) is currently the only specific treatment for acute ischemic stroke that has received approval from the FDA. The treatment aims to lyse a clot occluding a cerebral artery.... The drug must be given <u>within 3 hours</u> of the onset of symptoms, which means that the patient must generally arrive at a properly equipped and organized hospital within 2 hours of symptom onset to have the necessary evaluations (including a brain computed tomography [CT] scan to exclude hemorrhage or other conditions) completed. Within the 3-hour window, the sooner treatment can be given, the greater the likelihood of a favorable response" **See:** Braunwald, chapter on "Stroke"
    "The FDA has approved alteplase [tPA] for massive PE, in a dose of 100 mg as a continuous infusion during 2 hours, without concomitant heparin. Unlike patients receiving myocardial infarction thrombolysis [or stroke], patients with PE have a wide 'window' for effective use of thrombolysis. Those who receive thrombolysis up to 14 days after new symptoms or signs maintain an effective response, probably because of the bronchial collateral circulation." **See:** Braunwald, chapter on "Pulmonary Embolism"

BOTH QUESTIONS BELOW REFER TO THESE ANGIOGRAMS.

1160. This is a right carotid arteriogram and DSA. Identify the artery labeled #2?
a. Right common carotid
b. Right internal carotid
c. Right external carotid
d. Right vertebral

1161. What atherosclerotic lesion is seen?
a. Right external carotid eccentric plaque
b. Right internal carotid eccentric plaque
c. Right common carotid Bifurcation lesion
d. Right internal carotid string of pearls lesion

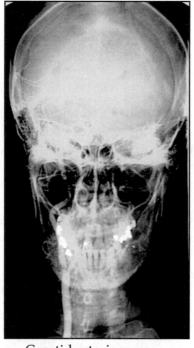
Carotid arteriogram

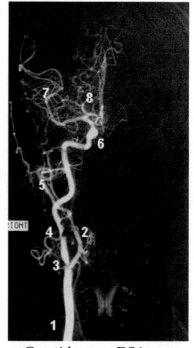
Carotid artery DSA

BOTH ANSWERS LISTED BELOW.
1160. ANSWER c. Right external carotid. The smaller branch off the common carotid crosses in front of the internal carotid to supply the temple and face.
ARTERIES SHOWN ARE:
    1. Right common carotid artery
    2.& 5. Right external carotid artery
    3. Carotid bifurcation or carotid sinus
    4 & 6. Right internal carotid artery
    7. Middle cerebral artery and branches
    8. Anterior cerebral artery and branches
See: Johnsrude, chapter on "Aortic Arch and Brachiocephalic Angiography." **Keywords:** Identify carotid artery anatomy

1161. ANSWER c. Right common carotid bifurcation lesion. Note the pinching at the division of the common carotid artery. Most strokes and carotid bruit murmurs are thought to originate from this site. The carotid sinus is the most common location of carotid artery stenosis. Johnsrude says, "Although stenosis is usually localized to the origin of the brachiocephalic vessels and their major bifurcations, significant lesions can occur high in the cervical course... " The two "bites" out of the internal carotid artery, labeled #4, are due to metallic dental fillings that were inadequately subtracted from the DSA image. These are clearly seen on the initial angiographic image to overlie the internal carotid artery.
See: Johnsrude, chapter on "Aortic Arch and Brachiocephalic Angiography." **Keywords:** Carotid bifurcation lesion

1162. **Surgical repair of obstructive atherosclerotic lesions in the carotid arteries usually involves:**
a. **Carotid artery balloon angioplasty**
b. **Carotid endarterectomy**
c. **Carotid artery bypass surgery with saphenous veins**
d. **Carotid artery bypass surgery with Dacron grafts**

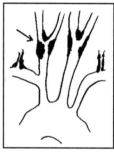
Carotid Stenosis

ANSWER b. Carotid endarterectomy. Most atherosclerotic lesions in the carotid arteries are localized within the carotid sinus - where the internal and external carotids divide. The carotid endarterectomy surgeon opens the carotid sinus. He then peels off the atheroma and plaque from the vessel wall and sews it back together.

When the size of the carotid sinus is too small or constricted due to scarring from previous surgery, a patch graft is performed. Here a patch of Dacron cloth is sewed over the arteriotomy to increase the size of the carotid sinus. This allows more blood flow through the area.
See: Braunwald, chapter on "Diseases of the Aorta."

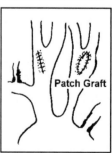
Carotid Endarterectomy

1163. In treating carotid artery bifurcation stenosis, placing a balloon expandable stent:
a. Is not recommended, because carotid endarterectomy is the gold standard
b. Is not recommended, because they may cause distal kinking and poor apposition
c. Is recommended, because they can more fully dilate a calcified artery than self expanding stents
d. Is recommended, because they result in less restenosis than self expanding stents

ANSWER b. Is not recommended. Self expanding stents are preferred in carotids (NOT BALLOON EXPANDABLE) because they are so flexible. Self expanding stents maintain a constant pressure on the vessel wall, can bend with neck motion, and don't stretch the vessel, which may result in distal kinking, as shown. Yadav says, "conventional balloon-expandable stents were too rigid and resulted in kinking of the internal carotid artery in the length between the stent and the petrous portion of the artery.., and balloon-expandable stents were associated with a high incidence of loss of apposition between the stent and vessel wall. These considerations led to the development of

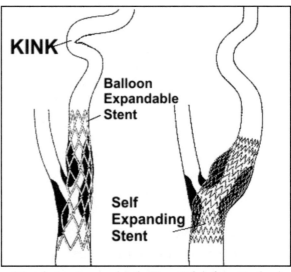

Rigid stent may kink Carotid (after Yadov)

nitinol self-expanding stents that have performed well..." See: Yadav, Casserly & Sachar, "Manual of Peripheral Vascular Intervention", Lippincott Williams & Wilkins, 2005

1164. Cerebral Vascular Accidents (CVAs) and Transient Ischemic Attacks (TIAs) in hypertensive patients occur at a rate four times those of normal individuals. Most of these "strokes" are due to:
a. Subarachnoid hemorrhage
b. Hyalinotic obstructive lesions (lacunar infarcts)
c. Cerebral micro-aneurysms (hyalinosis)
d. Cerebral embolism and infarct

ANSWER d. Cerebral embolism and infarct. Cerebral infarcts cause 80% of the CVAs and TIAs in hypertensive persons. Carotid arterial atherosclerosis is just like coronary atherosclerosis. It leads to thrombi in the carotid vessels which embolize to the cerebral vessels and the brain. That is why carotid endarterectomy is so common because it prevents stokes. CE surgery removes the atherosclerotic plaques in the carotid sinus which is the usual site of clot formation. **See:** Underhill, chapter on "High Blood Pressure." **Keywords:** Chief cause CVA = embolism

1165. A patient is brought to the cath lab to get an Amplatzer PFO occluder. He is most likely getting this because of a history of:
a. L-R shunt
b. DVT with PE
c. Diabetic PAD
d. Cryptogenic stroke

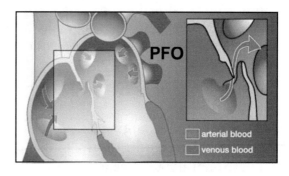

ANSWER: d. Cryptogenic stroke is a stroke within an unknown cause. If a patient has a patent foramen ovale (PFO) this is the most likely site for R-L shunting, especially if the person has DVT and elevated right heart pressures. This is not considered an ASD because there is no fixed hole in the atrial septum. PFO is a trap door type of defect with R-L shunting only when the septum secundum/primum flap is pushed open. This can occur with a valsalva maneuver or transient high RA pressure. Only then can R-L shunting occur with possible passage of thrombi into the systemic circulation & brain.

Topol says, "in 35% to 40% of patients who suffer CVAs, the etiologies remain unknown even after a thorough evaluation, and the CVAs are classified as cryptogenic.... In situ thrombosis, paradoxical embolization, and predisposition to atrial arrhythmias have been proposed as mechanisms for PFO-associated cryptogenic strokes. Paradoxical embolization—the passage of a venous thrombus into the systemic circulation through a PFO—has been the predominant theory. Evidence that supports the role of PFOs in cryptogenic strokes includes case reports of the transit of thrombi across PFOs; cerebral distribution of cryptogenic CVAs, which suggests an embolic nature; and the increased frequency of deep venous thrombosis (DVT) in patients who had cryptogenic CVAs.... The Amplatzer PFO occluder is a self-expanding, double-disk device made from 0.005-inch nitinol wire, with a polyester fabric sewn into both disks" **See:** Topol, chapter on "Percutaneous Closure of Foramen Ovale"

1166. Progressive obstruction of the femoral artery with intermittent claudication describes:
a. Expanding aortic aneurysm
b. Acute femoral thromboembolism
c. Thromboangiitis obliterans
d. Atherosclerosis obliterans

ANSWER d. Atherosclerosis obliterans is common below the descending aorta where the main vessels divide. This develops slowly over the years and may eventually completely "obliterate" the leg arteries. Claudication describes the hallmark pain of "atherosclerosis obliterans." Claudication describes a leg pain that comes on with ischemic exercise and exertion. Since blood flow is inadequate to meet the metabolic demands of walking, the characteristic ischemic claudication pain sets in. However, it goes away shortly after resting.

Because of the stenosis, during exercise the leg pulses and

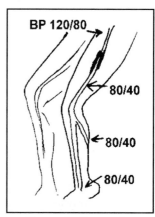

Fem. A. Stenosis

blood pressure diminish. Blood pressures taken at different points on the leg immediately after exercise, localize the obstruction. Popliteal stenosis will show a sudden drop in BP from thigh to calf. Femoral angiography confirms the % obstruction before corrective surgical bypass of the stenosis. **See:** Underhill, chapter on "Vascular Diseases."

1167.   **A cramping leg pain brought on by walking or running and that goes away with rest describes:**
   a. **Intermittent leg angina**
   b. **Intermittent claudication**
   c. **Exertional paraesthesia**
   d. **Exertional amaurosis fugax**

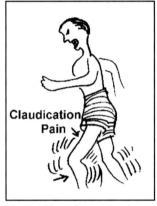

ANSWER b. Intermittent claudication. This pain is typical of atherosclerotic disease of the legs. It occurs during walking or exercise and goes away with rest. The ischemic pain results not so much from O2 deficits, but more from the accumulation of metabolic waste (lactic acid buildup) in the muscles due to inadequate blood flow.

   The location of the pain is below the obstruction usually in the calf. **See:** Underhill, chapter on "Vascular Diseases."

Claudication

1168.   **What is the usual pattern of peripheral artery disease (PAD) found in patients with severe diabetes and critical limb ischemia (CLI)?**
   a. **Diffuse arterial stenoses below the knee**
   b. **Diffuse arterial stenoses above the knee**
   c. **Discrete superficial femoral artery occlusion**
   d. **Discrete popliteal artery occlusion**

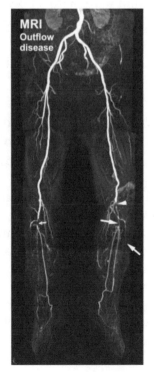

ANSWER: a. Diffuse arterial stenoses below the knee.
   Topol says, "Diabetes-associated vascular disease of the lower extremities is characterized by extensive vascular calcification and a more frequent infrapopliteal involvement. The lower limb amputation rate among diabetic patients is up to 13-fold compared with that among nondiabetic individuals.... Up to a quarter of patients with CLI [critical limb ischemia] have lesions isolated to arteries below the knee, and they occur mostly in those with diabetes...." **See:** Topol, chapter on "Peripheral Vascular Interventions"
   The American Diabetes Association says, "In contrast to the focal and proximal atherosclerotic lesions of PAD found typically in other high-risk patients, in diabetic patients the lesions are more likely to be more diffuse and distal.... Also, diabetic patients who have been identified with PAD are more prone to the sudden ischemia of arterial thrombosis or may have a pivotal event leading to neuroischemic ulceration or infection that rapidly results in an acute presentation with critical limb ischemia and risk of

amputation." **See:** "Peripheral Arterial Disease in People With Diabetes" online at
http://care.diabetesjournals.org/content/26/12/3333

1169. **PAD patients with the highest risk of gangrene, leg amputation and death are those with:**
a. **Chronic Staphylococcus infections unresponsive to antibiotics**
b. **Class 4 claudication pain at rest**
c. **Type 2 Diabetes and are cigarette smokers**
d. **Critical Limb Ischemia**

ANSWER: d. Critical Limb Ischemia.

Schanzer, says, "Critical limb ischemia (CLI), defined as chronic ischemic rest pain, ulcers, or gangrene attributable to objectively proven arterial occlusive disease, is the most advanced form of peripheral arterial disease. Traditionally, open surgical bypass was the only effective treatment strategy for limb revascularization in this patient population. However, during the past decade, the introduction and evolution of endovascular procedures have significantly increased treatment options. In a certain subset of patients for whom either surgical or endovascular revascularization may not be appropriate, primary amputation remains a third treatment option." See: Schanzer, Critical Limb Ischemia, Curr Treat Options Cardiovasc. Med., 2010

Dr. Davies says, "Critical limb ischemia [CLI] is found in 12% of the U.S. adult population. Its clinical presentation varies from no symptoms to intermittent claudication, atypical leg pain, rest pain, ischemic ulcers, or gangrene. Those with critical limb ischemia have a high incidence of cardiovascular comorbidities that reflect a significant systemic atherosclerotic burden; they have increased functional impairment and increased rates of functional decline compared with persons without critical limb ischemia.... At 1 year, 25% of patients will be dead, 30% will have undergone amputation, and only 45% will remain alive with both limbs. At 5 years, more than 60% of patients with critical limb ischemia will be dead.

The ABI is a simple test that can be conducted in the office and typically confirm the presence of disease. It is calculated by dividing the ankle pressure by the highest brachial pressure. An ABI <0.9 is abnormal and indicates critical limb ischemia." See, Criticial Limb Ischemia: Epidemiology, by Mark G. Davies, https://www.ncbi.nlm.nih.gov/pmc/journals , 2012

1170. **Identify the type of arterial graft labeled #3 on the diagram.**
a. **AO end-to-end; Iliac end-to-side graft**
b. **AO - femoral - pop skip graft**
c. **Aorto - femoral; End-to-side**
d. **Femoral - pop; End-to-side graft**
d. **In situ; Femoral vein graft**

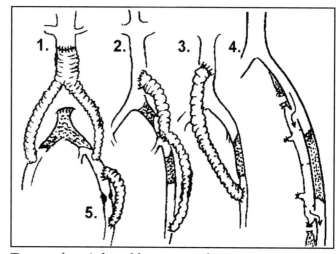

Types of peripheral bypass grafts

ANSWER c. Aorto -femoral; end-to-side anastomosis. These are Dacron cloth knit grafts which are sewn proximal and distal to the stenosis. Although endovascular therapy has almost replaced this surgery, there are still lots of patients with these grafts.

1. AO END-TO-END; ILIAC END-TO-SIDE GRAFT: The iliac bifurcation is clotted. A Dacron "Y" graft is attached end-to-end with the descending AO, and anastomosed end-to-side with the iliac artery.

2. AO - FEMORAL - POP SKIP GRAFT: Skips over clotted left iliac and femoral segments.

3. AORTO - FEMORAL END-TO-SIDE ANASTOMOSIS: A Dacron graft is attached to the descending AO end-to-side and then to the femoral artery, bypassing the blocked left iliac segment.

4. IN SITU FEMORAL VEIN GRAFT. The femoral vein is ligated at 2 ends and attached side-to-side with the femoral artery. This way the vein does not have to be removed from along-side the native artery. Arterial blood shunts into the femoral vein and runs retrograde through the vein. Venous valves must be cut to allow retrograde blood flow.

5. FEMORAL - POP END-TO-SIDE GRAFT: The ends of a simple Dacron graft are attached to the side of the femoral artery, bypassing the stenosis. **See:** Underhill, chapter on "Vascular Diseases."

1171. Hemodialysis access requires high blood flows into the dialysis machine from the patient's arm circulation. These patients may have had a surgical procedure where an arm artery was anastomosed to an adjacent superficial arm vein. This artery to vein communication is termed a/an:
a. Collateral shunt
b. PEG tube
c. AV fistula
d. AV graft

ANSWER c. AV fistula. This is a direct communication between an arm artery and vein. These fistulas are cannulated to draw large amounts of blood into the dialysis machine, cleanse it and return the purified blood into the vein. The fistula, artery, and vein may increase dramatically in flow causing a loud bruit because there is no interposed resistant capillary bed. If a conduit is used it is termed an AV graft. **See:** Sales, chapter on "Hemodialysis Access"

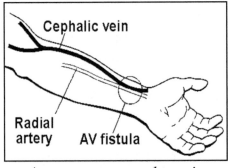
Artery anastomosed to vein

7B. Other Vascular: Varicose Veins

1172. Patients with secondary varicose veins of the lower extremity have:
a. Increased venous pressure
b. Decreased venous pressure
c. Incompetent venous valves
d. Stenotic venous valves

ANSWER c. Incompetent venous valves. Varicose veins are dilated and distended and associated with leaky venous valves. The distension of the veins causes the venous valves to leak and become incompetent. This results in back flow and pooling of blood in these veins. It is a vicious cycle. The more the valves leak, the more they are distended, the more they leak, etc.

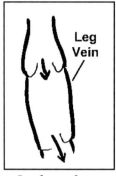
Leaky valves

Secondary varicose veins are caused by deep vein insufficiency or obstruction. Primary varicose veins may be hereditary and not associated with deep venous pathology. Varicose veins may be found in tissues other than the legs such as: scrotum (varicocele), esophagus (esophageal varices), and anus (hemorrhoids).

They leak not because of high venous pressures (although that may make it worse) but because the distended valves fail to coapt properly. Varicose veins are associated with obesity, chronic standing, and pregnancy: all things which impede venous return. **See:** Sales, chapter on "Venous Disease"

1173. **Two catheter therapies to heat and fibrose symptomatic saphenous varicose veins include: (Select 2 below.)**
a. **Vein stripping**
b. **Foam sclerotherapy**
c. **Laser ablation**
d. **Radio frequency ablation**
e. **Infrathermal ablation**
f. **Ambulatory phlebectomy**

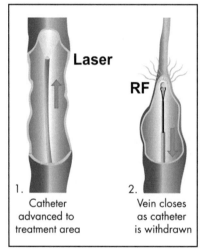
Vein ablation

ANSWERS: c. Laser ablation & d. Radio frequency ablation. Varicose vein treatment, also known as endovenous ablation, uses radiofrequency or laser energy to heat, cauterize and close varicose veins. Sclerotharapy injects caustic solutions to shrink the veins & sclerose them. Ambulatory phlebectomy uses slits in the skin to engage varicosities near the surface. Vein stripping actually surgically removes the varicosed veins.

7C. Other Vascular: Vasospastic, Raynaud's, Buerger's, etc.

1174. **A young woman has attacks of intermittent vasospasm in both of her hands when exposed to cold or if she becomes emotional. Her fingers become white, numb, and painful. These signs and symptoms are most likely due to:**
a. **Thromboangiitis Obliterans**
b. **Atherosclerosis Obliterans**
c. **Raynaud's Disease**
d. **Takayasu's Arteritis**

ANSWER c. Raynaud's disease is the cold finger disease of young women (feet may also become involved). The cooled fingers become pale then cyanotic, but immediately following the attack they turn red (rubor). This vasospastic action is probably due to a defect in the sympathetic nervous system supplying the extremities. Sympathetic ganglion-ectomy usually cures the symptoms, especially if the feet are involved. Vasodilator drugs such as nitroglycerine paste may improve the vasoconstriction. **See:** Underhill, chapter on "Vascular Diseases."

1175. **A child has coarctation of the aorta. When taking the child's vital signs you would expect to observe:**
a. **Higher BP in upper extremities**
b. **Weak, thready radial pulses**
c. **Irregular heart rhythm**
d. **Bradycardia**

ANSWER a. Higher BP in upper extremities than in lower extremities. This is because of the pressure gradient in the aorta. Arteries branching from below the coarctation will have a lower pressure than those above the stenosis. **See:** Braunwald, ch. on "Diseases of the AO."

1176. **A 30-year-old woman has low BP in both arms but normal BP in the legs (reverse coarctation sign). An arterial biopsy shows intimal proliferation and fibrosis within the subclavian arteries and descending aorta. This pathology describes:**
a. **Pseudo-coarctation**
b. **Syphilitic aortic disease**
c. **Giant cell arteritis**
d. **Takayasu's arteritis**

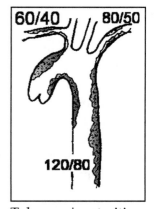

ANSWER d. Takayasu's arteritis is mostly found in young Asian or African women. This inflammation of the major arteries leads to arterial obstruction (easily seen on angiogram) and isolated aneurysms. The intima and adventia become markedly thickened and the vasa vasorum is destroyed (the inside of the aorta looks like tree bark.) The cause of Takayasu's disease is unknown.

Takayasu's arteritis

The reduced arm BP is termed "reverse coarctation" because in post ductal coarctation the distal AO and leg pressures are reduced, opposite from Takayasu's arteritis. **See:** Braunwald, chapter on "Diseases of the Aorta." **Keywords:** Takayasu's arteritis

1177. **A male smoker has painful cold hands and fingers. An occlusive inflammatory disease of the small peripheral arteries and veins that might cause this is:**
a. **Thromboangiitis Obliterans**
b. **Atherosclerosis Obliterans**
c. **Raynaud's Disease**
d. **Takayasu's Arteritis**

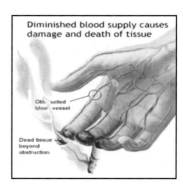

ANSWER a. Thromboangiitis Obliterans (Buerger's disease) is the cold finger disease of young smoking men. Although the specific cause is unknown, it is always associated with cigarette smoking. Small thrombi form in the finger and toe arteries leading to inflammation and obstruction of the small arteries and veins. Continued obstruction often leads to painful ischemia, non-healing skin ulcers, or gangrene of the upper extremity. **See:** Underhill, chapter on "Vascular Diseases." **Keywords:** Thromboangiitis Obliterans, Buerger's Disease

1178. **In explaining Raynaud's disease to your patient, you should explain that it is important for her to avoid:**
a. **Fatty food diet**
b. **Smoking cigarettes**
c. **Drinking alcoholic beverages**
d. **Excessive hand exercises**

ANSWER b. Smoking cigarettes. Raynaud's disease typically attacks fingers and toes. The affected areas feel cold, numb, and prickly due to poor circulation, due to vasospasm. Because nicotine in cigarettes causes vasoconstriction, cigarette smoking should be avoided by the person with Raynaud's disease. **See:** Underhill, chapter on "Vascular Diseases" **Keywords:** Raynaud's, no cigarettes

1179. **As Raynaud's or Buerger's disease progresses, the patient's fingers and toes are likely to develop:**
a. **Contractures**
b. **Chronic swelling**
c. **Thickened fingernails**
d. **Ulcers with superficial gangrene**

ANSWER d. Ulcers with superficial gangrene are typical as Raynaud's or Buerger's disease progresses. The lesions are easily infected and healing is slow due to poor circulation to the extremities. Thickening of fingernails, chronic swelling of the fingers, and contractures of the fingers are not associated with these diseases. Leg ulcers often heal slowly due to insufficient blood supplies to the tissue. **See:** Underhill, chapter on "Vascular Diseases" **See:** Lewis, chapter on "Cardiovascular"

REFERENCES

Baim, D. S and Grossman W.., Cardiac Catheterization, Angiography, and Intervention, 7th Ed., Lea and Febiger, 2006
Braunwald, Eugene, Ed., HEART DISEASE A Textbook of Cardiovascular Medicine, 9th Ed., W. B. Saunders Co., 2012
Hurst, J. W., and Logue, R. B., et. al., *THE HEART*, 3rd Ed., McGraw-Hill Book Co., 1974
Kandarpa, K., *Handbook of Cardiovascular and Interventional Radiologic Procedures*, 1st Ed., Little Brown and Co., 1989
Kern, M. J., Ed., The Cardiac Catheterization Handbook, 6th Ed., Mosby-Year Book, 2016
Lewis, LuVerne Wolff, RN, Lippincott State Board Review for NCLEX-PN, J.B. Lippincott, 1990
Rooke, et, al., Vascular Medicine and Endovascular Interventions, Blackwell Futura, 2010
Sales, C.M., Goldsmith, R., Veith, F.J., Ed., *Handbook of Vascular Surgery*, Quality Medical, Publishing, 1994
Taylor, E. J. Ed., *Dorland's Medical Dictionary*, 27th ed., W. B. Saunders Co.,1988 Underhill, S. L., Ed., *CARDIAC*

NURSING, 2nd Ed., J. B. Lippincott Co., 1989

OUTLINE: C6 - Vascular Disease

1. GENERAL VASCULAR
   a. Abbreviations
      i. TIA, CVA, ICA, PAD, DVT, AVF (AVM), AAA, . FMD, NO, BRUIT, EVAR, rt-PA, & ABI
   b. Frequency
      i. Hypertension most common Dr. Apt.
      ii. PE = Great masquerader
      iii. Stroke = Most disability & institutionalization
      iv. PAD - most common arterial occlusive peripheral pathology
      v. Atherosclerosis = global high risk of: PAD, CAD, MI, stroke, diabetes
2. ARTERIAL ANATOMY REVIEW
      i. Largest @ AO valve - tapers down
      ii. Intima - endothelium
      iii. media - muscle
      iv. adventitia - strongest
3. AORTIC ANEURYSMS
   a. Types
      i. True Aneurysm- Fusiform
      ii. True Aneurysm- Saccular
      iii. False Aneurysm- loculated
      iv. False Aneurysm- herniated
      v. Dissected Aneurysm
   b. Pathology
      i. 50% larger diameter than normal AO
      ii. Inflamation & degeneration of elastic media & adventia
      iii. Abdominal Ao. Aneu. (AAA) most common
         (1) mostly older men (x5)
      iv. Risk Factors:
         (1) Smoking (x5) COPD
         (2) hypertension
         (3) hyperlipidemia
      v. Ruptured AA
         (1) exsanguination :(
      vi. Laplace's Law
         (1) T = P x r
         (2) Fix at 5 -5.5 cm
   c. Diagnosis
      i. Angiography
      ii. CT, MRI scan, Ultrasound
   d. Interventions for AA
      i. Surgical Repair
         (1) Dacron graft
      ii. Endograft (EVAR)
         (1) Thoracic stent-grafts
            (a) AAA many side branches
            (b) May use periscopes, fenestrated, or branched grafts
         (2) Abdominal AO stent-grafts
            (a) Y shaped stent-grafts
            (b) Requires 2nd leg addition
         (3) Dacron covered metal stent
            (a) False lumen clots off
         (4) Proximal & distal fixation
            (a) Hooks at top & bottom
            (b) Endo leaks (most common problem)
4. AORTIC DISSECTIONS
   a. Intima tears from wall in media (flap)
      i. Like loose wallpaper
   b. Entry point
      i. May be due to intimal injury or hematoma (vaso

vasorum)
      ii. True lumen
         (1) main blood flow (cath OK here)
      iii. False lumen
         (1) stay out - cath may increase tear
         (2) may clot
         (3) may reenter (exit point)
      iv. May extend & cut of side branches
         (1) may extent prox. or distal
   c. Classification
      i. Stanford A
         (1) Ascending (most die)
         (2) Requires stat surgery
         (3) Risk to coronary artery & MI
         (4) May tamponade
      ii. Stanford B descending AO
         (1) Not usually lethal
         (2) Not surgery
      iii. Connective tissue disorders
         (1) Marfan syndrome
         (2) Other genetic syndromes
         (3) AO wall may be feel like wet toilet paper
   d. Diagnosis
      i. Sharp stabbing chest/back pain
      ii. CT, Ultrasound, MRI scan
      iii. Angiography (avoid false lumen)
   e. Surgery
      i. Beta blockers, Nitroprusside
      ii. Open heart lung bypass
      iii. May glue flap down
      iv. Replace dissected area Dacron graft
5. CAROTID ARTERY PATHOLOGY
   a. Cerebral Artery Anatomy review
   b. R & L Common Carotids
      i. R & L Int & Ext. Carotids
   c. R & L Vertebrals
      i. Basilar
   d. Circle Willis
      i. Communicating arteries
      ii. Built in collateral for stroke protection
   e. Cerebral pathology
   f. TIA (symptoms <24 hrs)
   g. Stroke (>24 hrs)
      i. Ischemic stroke (85%)
         (1) Emboli (clot or plaque) from
            (a) ICA (most common)
            (b) LA appendage (AF)
            (c) LV clot post MI
      ii. Intracerebral hemorrhage (15%)
         (1) Localized bleeding injury
         (2) + CT scan means no lysis, no tPA
      iii. Cryptogenic stroke
         (1) Patent Foramen Ovale (PFO)
         (2) R-L ASD through PFO
         (3) Embolism through PFO
         (4) PFO closure device
   h. Surgery
      i. Carotid Endarterectomy
         (1) Removal of plaque
         (2) Patch graft
   i. Thrombolysis
      i. rt-PA
      ii. 3 hour window

        iii.   IV or intra-arterial
    j.   Stent (long term results = CE)
        i.   ICA Distal protection required
            (1)   Until placed, never pass ICA stenosis
        ii.   Tapered self expanding stent
        iii.   Complications
            (1)   Hemodynamic depression
                (a)   Temporary hypotension & bradycardia
                (b)   Due to stent pressure on baroreceptors
            (2)   Hyperperfusion syndrome
                (a)   Sudden temp. increase brain flow
                (b)   Headache
                (c)   feared risk of intracranial bleed

6.   PULMONARY EMBOLISM
    a.   Pathophysiology
        i.   Thrombotic emboli to lung
        ii.   Emboli lodge in small branches of PA
            (1)   Saddle embolus
        iii.   Virchow's clotting triad
            (1)   Absence of flow (stagnation)
            (2)   Hypercoagulability (easy clotting)
            (3)   Abnormal vessel wall (endothelium)
        iv.   Deep Leg Vein thrombosis (90%)
            (1)   diagnosed with B mode ultrasound
    b.   Associated findings
        i.   Immobility (Post pregnancy or surgery)
            (1)   Bed or chair immobility
            (2)   Loss of muscle venous pump
            (3)   Insufficient venous valves
        ii.   Venous trauma
        iii.   Catheters
            (1)   Hickman Alimentation cath
            (2)   Swan-Ganz catheters
    c.   Diagnosis
        i.   CT Pulmonary angiogram
        ii.   Angiography (Gold standard)
            (1)   abrupt vessel cut off
            (2)   intralumen filling defects
        iii.   PA & RV pressures increase
            (1)   from mean >20 mild
            (2)   to >40 severe
        iv.   RV dilates with IV sepal bulge
        v.   Right heart failure (Cor Pulmonale)
        vi.   Eventually decreases CO & BP
        vii.   Obstructive shock may develop
        viii.   V/Q mismatch , <O2 sat, > PCO2
        ix.   D-Dimer assay
    d.   Therapy
        i.   O2
        ii.   Anticoagulation (3 months)
            (1)   Heparin 1st (bridge then DC)
            (2)   Coumadin, Vit. K antagonist
        iii.   Thrombolytic agents
            (1)   fibrinolysis, rt-PA
            (2)   EKOS cath, ultrasound
        iv.   Surgery   v.   IVC filters
            (1)   Metal traps for emboli - prevent PE
            (2)   Placed in IVC below renal veins
            (3)   Removable by hooking & retracting
            (4)   Used only if poor anticoagulation or large emboli

7.   ARTERIAL EMBOLISM
    a.   Atherosclerosis chief cause
    b.   Emboli
        i.   Float downstream
            (1)   to any arterial bed
            (2)   Most dreaded = stroke
            (3)   Leg, post cath
        ii.   Saddle (AO bifurcation)

    c.   Signs and symptoms (6 P's)
        i.   Pain
        ii.   Paralysis
        iii.   Paraesthesia (Numbness)
        iv.   Pallor
        v.   Polar (Coldness)
        vi.   Pulseless
    d.   Therapy
        i.   Heparin
        ii.   Thrombolytic agents
        iii.   Fogarty embolectomy
            (1)   pass through clot
            (2)   inflate balloon
            (3)   pull clot out
        iv.   Surgical bypass

8.   PERIPHERAL ARTERY DISEASE (PAD)
    a.   Atherosclerosis usual cause
    b.   Usually indicates global atherosclerosis
            (a)   CAD, Stroke risk...
    c.   PAD Indicator of global CV risk
        i.   Smoking, hypertension, age, cholesterol
        ii.   Diabetes (risk of foot lesions or amputation)
            (1)   Ulcers, infection, gangrene
            (2)   Diffuse 3-vessel calf disease
            (3)   Not amenable to revascularization
    d.   Critical Limb Ischemia
        i.   High-risk for amputation
    e.   Subclavian stenosis
        i.   Subclavian steal - shunt down vertebral
        ii.   Coronary Subclavian steal - shunt up IMA
    f.   ilio-femoral
        i.   symptom - Claudication
            (1)   Leg pain when walking fixed distance
        ii.   Ankle Brachial Index (ABI)
            (1)   Highest systolic arm BP / ankle syst. BP
            (2)   <0.9 = PAD
            (3)   ABI drops further with treadmill exercise
            (4)   ABI indicates severity of stenosis (<0.4 severe)
            (5)   Segmental pressures moving down leg
                (a)   Localize level of stenosis
    g.   Imaging
        i.   Color Duplex Doppler
        ii.   MRI or CT angiogram
        iii.   Invasive Angiography
            (1)   DSA
            (2)   Runoff X-ray films
    h.   Medical Therapy
        i.   Exercise program
        ii.   Cilostazol (Pletaal) drug - vasodilator
        iii.   Antiplatelet drugs
        iv.   Statins
    i.   Endovascular Therapy
        i.   Retrograde crossover sheath Ilio-femoral
            (1)   contralateral over AO-iliac bifurcation
        ii.   Angioplasty
            (1)   Coated balloon angioplasty
        iii.   Stent
            (1)   BMS vs DES ?
            (2)   Self expanding stent at flexion points
        iv.   Thrombolysis
            (1)   Infusion wire/catheter
            (2)   Pulsed spray
            (3)   Trellis infusion catheter
        v.   Mechanical thrombecomy
            (1)   Angiojet
    l.   Surgery - Arterial Bypass Veins/Grafts
        i.   AO. end-to-end
        ii.   Iliac end-to-side graft
        iii.   AO. - Fem. - pop; skip graft
        iv.   Aorto - Femoral; end-to-side

v.   Fem. - Pop; end-to-side graft
vi.   In situ; Femoral vein graft
9.   RENAL ARTERY STENOSIS
  a.   Risk factors same as CAD & PAD
  b.   90% lesions atherosclerotic
    i.   Discrete usually ostial
  c.   Fibromuscular dysplasia (FMD)
    i.   String of pearls angio
    ii.   Common cause RAS in young females
  d.   Renovascular hypertension
    i.   Decreased renal flow > Rennin hormone
    ii.   Angiotensin I & II (vasoconstrictor)
    iii.   Stimulates Aldosterone & Na reabsorption
    iv.   Volume overload
  e.   Diagnoses
    i.   Elevated BNP
    ii.   Duplex color US
    iii.   Angiography
      (1)   LAO views best
      (2)   AO gram
    iv.   Translesion Pressure gradient
      (1)   Significant if >10 mmHg pressure gradient
      (2)   Significant if >20 mmHg gradient with vasodilator
        (a)   Dopamine/papaverine (not adenosine) induction
  f.   Endovascular Therapy
    i.   Stenting technuque
      (1)   Use short sheath 35 cm
      (2)   No touch technique
        (a)   Avoids deep throating into lesion
      (3)   Telescoping exchange technique
        (a)   Wire Renal artery through 4-Fr soft cath
        (b)   Exchange for 6 Fr sheath
      (4)   Balloon inflation
        (a)   pain suggests risk of rupture
          (i)   Deflate & withdraw
        (b)   Embolic Protection Device (EPD)
          (i)   Appropriate if high-risk patient
          (ii)   If long landing zone in Renal Art.
          (iii)   May reduce atheroma embolization
      (5)   Balloon expandable stent
        (a)   Should protrude 1-2 mm from ostium
        (b)   May use Pro stent positioning foot cath
        (c)   Flare proximal stent end in os
          (i)   Post stent deployment
          (ii)   As deflating, advance tapered   tip cath
          (iii)   Cath tip dilates, flares ostial portion
            1)   while balloon holds stent position
    ii.   Percutaneous Sympathetic Denervation
      (1)   Renal artery nerves contribute hypertension
      (2)   RF burn of nerves in renal artery adventia
      (3)   < Rennin, <Na reabsorption, & >renal flow
      (4)   experimental in resistant hypertension
10.   HYPERTENSION
  a.   General and types
    (1)   Primary = Essential = unknown cause
      (a)   most common type   (2)
    (3)   Reno Vascular Hypertension
      (a)   Secondary to renal artery stenosis
      (b)   Rennin-Angiotensin-Aldosterone system
      (c)   Diagnose with Renal arteriogram

    (4)   Systolic Hypertension
      (a)   >140 mild
      (b)   >160 moderate
      (c)   >180 severe
    (5)   Diastolic Hypertension
    (6)   Increases all atherosclerosis
      (a)   PAD, CAD, stroke...
    (7) Risk: Stroke, PAD, blindness, MI, CHF, Kidneys
        Acceleration of atherosclerosis
  b.   Diagnosis Hypertension
    i.   Noninvasive BP measurement
    ii.   Arterial Line
    iii.   BP Calculation
      (1)   BP = SVR x CO
    iv.   Prostoglandins/Kinin's
      (1)   Vasodilators
  c.   Risk factors
    i.   High salt diet
    ii.   Cigarette smoking
    iii.   Diabetes Mellitus
    iv.   High Cholesterol
  d.   Associated Hormones
    i.   Aldosterone
    ii.   Angiotensin
    iii.   Catecholamines
    iv.   Loss autoregulation (NO)
  e.   Associated sympathetic neural
    i.   Alpha (vasoconstriction)
    ii.   Beta (HR, contractility)
11.   OTHER VASCULAR
  a.   Varicose veins -
    i.   Leaky venous valves
    ii.   Dilated ectatic veins Rx
      (1)   Compression stockings
      (2)   Catheter ablation by RF or laser energy
      (3)   Vein stripping & other surgery
  b.   Vasospastic Disease
    i.   Thromboangiitis Obliterans
      (1)   Smokers
    ii. Raynaud's disease
      (1) Cold white fingers
      (2) Young women
      (3) May lead to superficial finger ulcers
      (4) Avoid nicotine
    iii. Takayasu's arteritis
      (1) Young Asian and African women
      (2) Intima - like tree bark
      (3) Arterial obstructions & aneurysms
      (4) BP may be higher in legs than arms
      (5) Reverse ABI / reverse coarctation
  c.   AV fistula stenosis
    i.   Arterial-venous shunt
    ii.   AV graft
    iii.   Usually for dialysis access
      (1)   2 needle sites: Artery & vein
    iv.   Stenosis &/or thrombosis
      (1)   PTA or surgery
  d. Cirrhosis of Liver
      Increased resistance to renal blood flow
      Portal hypertension
      Dilates portal veins

BASIC CV - FORMULAS

MEASUREMENTS/ CONVERSION
*Linear (length) : **1 in = 2.54 cm**
*Mass (Weight) : **1 Kg = 2.2 lb**
Volume : 1 L = 1000 ml = 1.05 qt.
*Pressure : **1 atmosphere = 760 mmHg or Torr = 15 psi**

PHYSICS FORMULAS *(Vol. 1, Chapter A3)*
*Velocity : **$V = d / t$** =distance / time
Force : $F = m \times a$ = Mass x Acceleration
Work : $W = F \times d$ = Force x distance
Power : $P_w = F \times d / t$ = Force x distance / time
*Pressure : **$P = F / A$** = **Force / Area**
*Density : **$D = wt/vol.$**
Acceleration : $a = V / t$ = Velocity / time
Area (square) : **b x w = base x width**
Area (triangle) : ½ b x h = ½ base x height
Volume (rectangular): b x w x h = base x width x height
*Temperature : **$F = [(9/5)\ C] + 32$**
F = degrees Fahrenheit, C = degrees Celsius

PHYSICAL PRINCIPLES *(Vol. 1, Chapter A3)*
*Distance : **$D = V \times t$**
Distance = Velocity x time
Acceleration : $A = V / t$ = Velocity / time = D / t^2

Graham's Law Diffusion: $$D = \frac{\Delta P \times A \times S}{d \times \sqrt{MW}}$$

D = rate of diffusion, ΔP = Pressure gradient
A = Area, S = Solubility, d = density, MW = Molecular Weight
Henry's Law Gases : $S = C \times P / t$ =Sol. coef. x Partial Pr. / temp.
Dalton's Law Gases: $P_t = P_1 + P_2 + ... P_n$ = Sum of partial pressures

ULTRASOUND : *(Vol. 1 Chapter A3)*
*Period = 1/ frequency
*Wavelength = propagation speed / frequency
Wavelength = propagation speed x Period
*(note: in soft tissue propogation speed = 1540 M/sec)

PHYSIOLOGY   *(Vol. 1, Chapter A3)*

Ohm's Law (fluid)   :   R = (Pi - Po) / Q   = Pressure drop/blood flow
Continuity Eqn.   :   Q = V x A   = Velocity x Area
Poisieulle's Law   :

$$Q = \frac{\pi(P_i - P_o)\,r^4}{8\eta l}$$

Q = flow, P_i= Pressure in, r= radius, η=viscosity, l = length
or since R = (P_i - P_o) / Q

Poiseuille's Resistance: R= 8(Viscosity)(Length) / (π)(radius)^4
                                      =(revised   Ohm's law)

Laplace Law   :   T = P x R   Tension = Pressure x radius
Kinetic Energy   :   ½mv^2 = 1/2   mass x velocity ^{2}
Potential Energy :   mgh   =   mass x gravity x height
Bernoulli Eqn.   :   K = 1/2mv^2 + mgh
Starling's Eqn. :   Fluid Movement = k(P_c+π_i) - (P_i+π_p).
                              where k = constant
                              π_p = plasma protein oncotic pressure
                              P_c = hydrostatic capillary pressure

HEMODYNAMICS   *(See: Review Book Vol. III)*

*Heart Rate   :   HR = 60/RR interval = 60 x paper speed/mm. RR int.
*Stroke Volume   :   SV = EDV - ESV
*Ejection Fraction :   EF = SV/EDV x 100%
                              SV=End Systolic LV vol - End Diast. LV Vol.
*Regurgitant Fraction   Regurg./min/   LVMF   x 100%
*Cardiac Output   :   CO = SV x HR
                              This CO also termed LVMF (LV minute Flow)
*Cardiac Index   :   CI = CO/BSA
                              CO = Cardiac Output;   BSA = Body Surface   Area
*Arterial Pulse Pressure: pp = s - d   = systolic - diastolic
*Mean Blood Pressure   :mean BP = (s + 2 d)/3 = (systolic + 2 x diastolic) / 3
*Systemic Vasc. Resistance: SVR   = (mean BP - mean CVP) / CO
                              usually SVR   = (mean AO- mean RA) / CO
 mean BP   :   mean BP = CO x SVR
*Compliance   :   ΔV / Δ P   = change in Volume / change in Press.

PHARMACOLOGY *(Vol. IV, F6 & F7)*
*Concentration   :   C = wt/vol.   = solute/solvent
*Amount   :   Amount = C x V   = Conc. x Volume
*Administration rate: Amount/min = C x V/t   = Conc. x Vol./time

RCIS exam will require you to learn additional formulas.
        See, Vol 3 Hemodynamics

ACID BASE & O2   *(Review Book, Vol. I, ch. B2)*

pH   :   pH = log [1/H$^+$]   where H$^+$ = Hydrogen ion conc.

*Hgb. O2 Content :   CaO2 =1.39 x Hgb x O2 Sat/100

Plasma O2 Content: Physically dissolved O2 = .004 X PO$_2$ =   CpO2 in vol%.
Total O2 Cont   C$_t$O2   = Hgb O2 + Plasma O2 content in vol. %
                                        = 1.39 x O2 Sat x Hgb +   .004 X PO$_2$
Hgb. O2 Capacity :   O2 Cap. =1.39 x 100% Sat x Hgb

*% O2 Saturation   :   CaO2 / O2 Capacity

ELECTRICITY   *(Vol. 1, Chapter A3)*
Series Resistance   :   R$_{eff}$ = R$_1$ + R$_2$ ...+ R$_n$
                                        Effective total Resistance = Sum Res.

Parallel Resistance :

$$\frac{1}{R_{eff}} = \frac{1}{R_1} + \frac{1}{R_2} + ... \frac{1}{R_n}$$

Ohm's Law   :   V = I x R
Voltage = Current x Resistance
Power   :   Watts = V x I   = Voltage x Current
 Energy   :   Energy = Power x time = V x I x t   = Watt Sec or Joules

*Indicates an **important formula** worth **memorizing**. Understand the relationships
described by each equation, and how to solve for each variable.

Cardiovascular Review Books & Interactive media

These PERFECT TO:

Self Study for at home
Help staff pass the Cath Lab Registry Exams.
Resource for new employee in-service
Assess your cath lab knowledge and skills.
Text to accompany CV Review CD & USB

ORDER TODD's CV REVIEW BOOKS

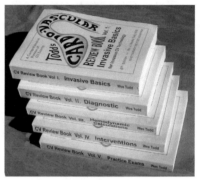

- Vol. I: Invasive Basics
            Includes Pt. Care, A&P, Pathology
- Vol. II: Cath Lab **Diagnostic Techniques**
- Vol. III: Cath Lab **Hemodynamics**
- Vol. IV: Cath Lab **Interventions**
- Vol. V: Practice Exams, Includes **8 Invasive Mock Exams**

5 Vol. Book Set

ORDER TODD's CV REVIEW CD or USB

- CV Review **CD or USB**, includes all above chapters and questions, Plus:

New interactive lectures & games
Mock RCIS exams
Main resource for RCIS online class
Site License and new serial numbers available
Evaluate your strengths & weaknesses
Fast & enjoyable way to scan RCIS material
Recommended for all cath lab staff, Invasive students, Cath lab nurses & Technicians.

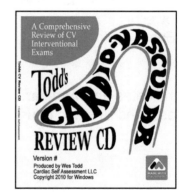

Todd's CV Review CD

We recommend that your prepare for your exam using all 5 books in the set *and* the CD or USB. *They complement each other.*

Order from amazon.com
Or www.westodd.com

More information at http://www.westodd.com
Or Email info@westodd.com

Made in the USA
Thornton, CO
04/14/24 11:08:47

8a73bd9d-a199-4350-9891-181d265c062cR01